THE AHA CLINICAL CARDIAC CONSULT

SECOND EDITION

Associate Editors

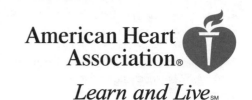

American Heart
Association®

*Learn and Live*sm

SECOND EDITION

THE AHA CLINICAL CARDIAC CONSULT

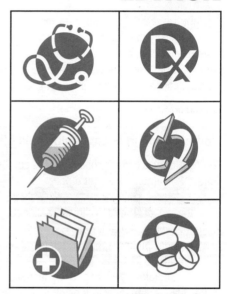

EDITOR

J. V. (Ian) Nixon, M.D.

Professor of Medicine
Department of Internal Medicine and Cardiology
Virginia Commonwealth University School of Medicine
VCU Health System
Richmond, Virginia

Lippincott Williams & Wilkins
a Wolters Kluwer business
Philadelphia · Baltimore · New York · London
Buenos Aires · Hong Kong · Sydney · Tokyo

Acquisitions Editor: Fran DeStefano
Managing Editor: Joanne Bersin
Production Manager: David Murphy
Senior Manufacturing Manager: Benjamin Rivera
Marketing Manager: Angela Panetta
Design Coordinator: Doug Smock
Production Services: Techbooks
Printer: Courier Westford

© 2007 by LIPPINCOTT WILLIAMS & WILKINS- a Wolters Kluwer business

530 Walnut Street
Philadelphia, PA 19106 USA
LWW.com

Printed in the USA

Library of Congress Cataloging-in-Publication Data

The AHA clinical cardiac consult.—2nd ed. / [edited by] Joseph Alpert, Ian Nixon ; associate editors, Gerard P. Aurigemma . . . [et al.].
      p. ; cm.
   Rev. ed. of: The AHA clinical cardiac consult / editor, Joseph S. Alpert ; associate editors, Gerard P. Aurigemma . . . [et al.]. c2001.
   Includes bibliographical references.
   ISBN 0-7817-6490-4 (case)
   1. Cardiology—Handbooks, manuals, etc. 2. Heart—Diseases—Handbooks, manuals, etc. 3. Cardiological manifestations of general diseases—Handbooks, manuals, etc. I. Alpert, Joseph S. II. Nixon, Ian. III. American Heart Association. IV. Title: Clinical cardiac consult.
   [DNLM: 1. Cardiovascular Diseases—diagnosis—Handbooks. 2. Cardiovascular Diseases—therapy—Handbooks.   WG 39 A285 2007]
RC669.15.A36 2007
616.1′2—dc22   2006028394

PREFACE

The second edition of *The American Heart Association Clinical Cardiac Consult* is the result of the success of the first edition. A property owned by the Council on Clinical Cardiology of the American Heart Association, the first edition's success was due to the extraordinary efforts of the editor and associate editors.

In accepting the invitation to edit the second edition of the book, my primary goal was to capitalize on the success of the first edition and where possible to improve, to update, and to expand its comprehensive coverage. To this end, the format of the book is unchanged, as are the majority of the topics covered by the book. To ensure that the book remains a contemporary reference text of clinical cardiology, some topics have been omitted or consolidated into other topics, the remaining topics have been updated, and new topics have been included to cover primary and secondary cardiovascular preventive care, metabolic syndrome, and acute coronary syndromes. Furthermore, multiple selected topics such as cardiac surgery and cardiomyopathies have been grouped together, and the appendix tables have been revised and updated.

It is impossible to single-handedly complete a project of this magnitude in a timely fashion without significant assistance and cooperation. My overwhelming gratitude is extended to many individuals for their assistance, especially including the following:

- The Long Range Planning Committee of the Council on Clinical Cardiology of the American Heart Association for the invitation to be the editor and to carry out this important task.

- My co-editor, Joseph S. Alpert, MD, who has been for many years a colleague and very good friend. Joe was the editor of the first edition of the book, and his availability, assistance and advice have been invaluable.

- My associate editors for their incredible industry and promptness. A book of this type is not possible without the collaboration of a willing group of associate editors, and this group more than fulfils the necessary criteria. Because several associate editors of the first edition were unable to assist in the second edition, three colleagues were added to the group: Ann Bolger, MD, Jere Fletcher, MD, and Peter Ott, MD. Seven of the original associate editors continued their collaboration. As stated, all of the associate editors were uniformly helpful and complied with some rigid deadlines. Without their prompt assistance and cooperation, none of this would have been possible.

- The staff of the publishers, Lippincott Williams & Wilkins for their assistance. Fran DeStefano, Joanne Bersin, and Mary Choi provided expert direction to someone performing this task for the first time. My gratitude is also extended to Renée Redding of Techbooks, Inc. for her expertise and her persistence.

It is hoped by all involved in the publication of this book that its readers will find the topics easy to find, precisely and contemporarily discussed, and will find the book a useful and frequently used addition to their professional reference library.

J. V. (IAN) NIXON

CONTRIBUTING AUTHORS

*An asterisk by an author's name in the chapters designates a first edition author whose original work was utilized but did not contribute to the second edition.

Christopher Abadi, M.D.
Cardiologist
Cardiovascular Associates of Rhode Island, Inc.
Providence, Rhode Island

Linda J. Addonizio, M.D.
Professor of Pediatrics
Department of Pediatrics
Columbia University
Medical Director, Pediatric Heart Transplant
   Program
Department of Pediatrics
Children's Hospital of New York-Presbyterian
New York, New York

Carlos A. Aguilar-Salinas, M.D.
Medical Researcher
Department of Endocrinology and Metabolism
Instituto Nacional de Ciencias Médicas y
   Nutrición
Vice-head of the Department of Endocrinology
   and Metabolism
Department of Endocrinology and Metabolism
Instituto Nacional de Ciencias Médicas y
   Nutrición
México City, Mexico

Jorge R. Alegria, M.D.
Fellow in Cadiovascular Diseases
Mayo Graduate School of Medicine
Mayo Clinic
Rochester, Minnesota

Joseph S. Alpert, M.D.
Robert S. and Irene P. Flinn Professor of
   Medicine
Head, Department of Medicine
University of Arizona College of Medicine and
   Health Sciences Center
Tucson, Arizona

Karen Altmann, M.D.
Assistant Professor of Clinical Pediatrics
Columbia University
College of Physicians and Surgeons
New York Presbyterian Hospital
New York, New York

Nezar L. Amir, M.D.
Cardiology Fellow
Department of Medicine
UCSF Medical Center
San Francisco, California

Paul Anaya, M.D.
DeKalb Medical Center
Decatur, Georgia

Howard D. Apfel, M.D.
Assistant Professor of Clinical Pediatrics
Department of Pediatric Cardiology
Columbia University
Attending Cardiologist
Department of Pediatric Cardiology
The Presbyterian Hospital
New York, New York

Gerard P. Aurigemma, M.D.
Division of Cardiovascular Medicine
Department of Medicine
University of Massachusetts Medical School
Worcester, Massachusetts

David S. Bader, M.D.
Department of Cardiology
Boston University Medical Center
Boston, Massachusetts

Maria Cecilia Bahit, M.D.
Duke Clinical Research Institute
Durham, North Carolina

Robyn J. Barst, M.D.
Professor of Pediatrics
Columbia University College of Physicians
   and Surgeons
Attending Physician
Director, Pulmonary Hypertension Center
New York Presbyterian Hospital
New York, New York

Deepak L. Bhatt, M.D.
Associate Professor of Medicine
Department of Cardiology
Cleveland Clinic Lerner College of Medicine
Case Western Reserve University
Interventional Cardiology
Department of Cardiology
Cleveland Clinic
Cleveland, Ohio

Ann F. Bolger, M.D.
William Watt Kerr Professor of Clinical Medicine
Department of Medicine
University of California, San Francisco
Director, Echocardiography
Division of Cardiology
San Francisco General Hospital
San Francisco, California

Joseph L. Bouchard, M.D.
Division of Dermatology
University of Massachusetts Medical
   School
Worcester, Massachusetts

David Brick, M.D.
Instructor in Clinical Pediatrics
Columbia University
College of Physicians and Surgeons
New York Presbyterian Hospital
New York, New York

Craig M. Brodsky, M.D.
Instructor of Clinical Medicine
Atlanta Veterans Affairs Medical Center
Decatur, Georgia

Bernard R. Chaitman, M.D.
Professor of Medicine
Director of Cardiovascular Research
Division of Cardiology, Department
   of Medicine
St. Louis University School of Medicine
St. Louis, Missouri

Dinesh Chandok, M.D.
Division of Cardiovascular Medicine
Department of Medicine
University of Massachusetts Medical School
Worchester, Massachusetts

Gerald A. Charlton, M.D.
Director, Cardiology Fellowship Program
Department of Medicine
University of New Mexico School of Medicine
Director, Cardiology Clinical Service
Cardiology Section
New Mexico VA Health Care System
Albuquerque, New Mexico

Richard Chen, M.D.
Cardiology Fellow
Department of Medicine
Division of Cardiology
Emory University School of Medicine
Atlanta, Georgia

Jeffrey P. Ciaramita, M.D.
Cardiology Fellow
Department of Internal Medicine
Division of Cardiology
St. Louis University Hospital
St. Louis, Missouri

Contributing Authors

Gerald Cioce, M.D.
Department of Internal Medicine
University of Massachusetts Memorial Medical
  Center
Worcester, Massachusetts

Rubin S. Cooper, M.D.
Professor of Clinical Pediatrics
Department of Pediatrics
Weill Cornell Medical College
Chief/Director
Department of Pediatrics
New York Presbyterian
New York, New York

Michael H. Crawford, M.D.
Professor and Lucie Stern Chair
  in Cardiology
Department of Medicine
University of California, San Francisco
Chief of Clinical Cardiology
Department of Medicine
UCSF Medical Center
San Francisco, California

L. Van-Thomas Crisco, M.D.
Interventional Cardiology Fellow
Department of Medicine
Division of Cardiology
Emory University School of Medicine
Northside Cardiology, PC
Atlanta, Georgia

David A. Crowe, M.D.
Assistant Professor of Pediatrics
Department of Cardiology
Columbia University
Attending Physician
Department of Pediatrics
Children's Hospital of New York
New York, New York

Rajesh Dash, M.D., Ph.D
Chief Fellow
Division of Cardiology
University of California, San Francisco
UCSF Medical Center
San Francisco, California

Harold L. Dauerman, M.D.
Department of Medicine
Division of Cardiovascular Medicine
University of Massachusetts Memorial Medical
  Center
University Campus
Worcester, Massachusetts

Rajat Deo, M.D.
Cardiology Fellow
University of California
San Francisco, California

Chandan Devireddy, M.D.
Assistant Professor
Division of Cardiology
Emory University School of Medicine
Atlanta, Georgia

Christopher K. Dyke, M.D.
Assistant Professor of Medicine
Department of Cardiology
Duke University Medical Center
Durham, North Carolina

Deborah L. Ekery, M.D.
Department of Cardiology
Austin Heart Hospital
Austin, Texas

Luis Eng-Ceceña, M.D.
Medical Director
Hospital Fátima
Los Mochis, Sin. México

Andrew E. Epstein, M.D.
Professor of Medicine
Division of Cardiovascular Disease
Department of Medicine
University of Alabama
Professor of Medicine
University of Alabama Hospital
Birmingham, Alabama

Gordon A. Ewy, M.D.
Professor of Medicine
Director, Sarver Heart Center
University of Arizona College of Medicine
Director
Department of Diagnostic Cardiology
University Medical Center
Tucson, Arizona

Husam H. Farah, M.D.
San Francisco General Hospital
San Francisco, California

Kevin P. Fitzgerald, M.D.
Cardiology Fellow
Department of Cardiology
St. Louis University
St. Louis, Missouri

Gerald F. Fletcher, M.D.
Preventive Cardiology
Department of Cardiovascular Disease
Mayo Clinic College of Medicine
Jacksonville, Florida

Michael J. Forsberg, M.D.
Interventional Fellow
Division of Cardiology
St. Louis University
St. Louis, Missouri

Gary S. Francis, M.D.
Professor of Medicine
Department of Cardiology
Cleveland Clinic Lerner College
  of Medicine
Case Western Reserve University
Section Head
Department of Clinical Cardiology
Cleveland Clinic
Cleveland, Ohio

Mary Frisella, M.D.
Internal Medicine
UMass Memorial Medical Center
Worcester, Massachusetts

Samer Garas, M.D.
Chief Cardiology
Department of Interventional Cardiology
St. Vincent's Hospital
Jacksonville, Florida

Efrain Gaxiola, M.D.
Chief
Interventional Cardiology Department
Instituo Cardiovascular de Guadalajara
Guadalajara, Mexico

Deborah R. Gersony, M.D.
Assistant Professor of Clinical Medicine and
  Pediatrics
Department of Cardiology
Columbia University Medical Center
New York, New York

Welton M. Gersony, M.D.
Alexander S. Nadas Professor
  of Pediatrics
Division of Pediatric Cardiology
Columbia University
College of Physicians and Surgeons
Morgan Stanley Children's Hospital of
  New York Presbyterian
New York, New York

Helene Glassberg, M.D.
Director, Preventive Cardiology
  and Lipid Center
Temple University School of Medicine
Philadelphia, Pennsylvania

Peter C. Grow, M.D.
Fellow
Department of Cardiology
Emory University School of Medicine
Atlanta, Georgia

Robert A. Harrington, M.D.
Professor of Medicine
Department of Medicine
Duke Clinical Research Institute
Interventional Cardiologist
Division of Cardiology
Duke University Medical Center
Durham, North Carolina

Ian S. Harris, M.D.
Cardiology Research Fellowship
Barnes-Jewish Hospital
Washington University
St. Louis, Missouri

Constance J. Hayes, M.D.
Professor of Clinical Pediatrics
Department of Pediatrics
Columbia University
Pediatric Cardiologist
Department of Pediatrics
New York Presbyterian Hospital
New York, New York

William E. Hellenbrand, M.D.
Professor of Clinical Pediatrics
Department of Pediatric Cardiology
Children's Hospital of New York
Director
Department of Pediatric Cardiac Catheterization
  Lab
Children's Hospital of New York
New York, New York

Steven C. Hermann, M.D., Ph.D.
Adjunctive Assistant Professor
Department of Physiology and Pharmacology
St. Louis University School of Medicine
Director
Cardiovascular Services
Bradford Regional Medical Center
Bradford, Pennsylvania

Robert Hogan, M.D.
Interventional Cardiology Fellow
Division of Cardiology
University of Massachusetts Medical School
Worcester, Massachusetts

Allan J. Hordof, M.D.
Professor
Department of Pediatrics
Columbia University
Interim Director
Department of Pediatric Cardiology
Morgan Stanley Children's Hospital
New York, New York

Brenda J. Hott, M.D.
Fellow
Department of Medicine
Division of Cardiology
Emory University School of Medicine
Atlanta, Georgia

Daphne T. Hsu, M.D.
Professor of Clinical Pediatrics
Department of Pediatrics
College of Physicians and Surgeons, Columbia
  University
Attending Physician
Department of Pediatrics
Morgan Stanley Children's Hospital of
  New York-Presbyterian
New York, New York

Patrick Hu, M.D., Ph.D.
Cardiology Fellow
Department of Medicine
Division of Cardiology
University of California, San Francisco
San Francisco, California

Michael P. Hudson, M.D.
Cardiology, Internal Medicine
Henry Ford Health System
Detroit, Michigan

Brian C. Jensen, M.D.
Cardiology Fellow
Department of Medicine
Division of Cardiology
University of California, San Francisco
San Francisco, California

Jesse P. Jorgensen, M.D.
Fellow
Department of Internal Medicine
Division of Cardiology
Emory University School of Medicine
Atlanta, Georgia

Apur R. Kamdar, M.D.
Cardiology Fellow
Department of Cardiology
Cleveland Clinic
Cleveland, Ohio

Vineet Kaushik, M.D.
Clinical Cardiology Fellow
Division of Cardiology
Department of Medicine
Emory University
Atlanta, Georgia

Jeffrey H. Kern, M.D.
Clinical Associate Professor
Department of Pediatrics
Weill Medical College of Cornell University
Attending Physician
Department of Pediatrics
New York Presbyterian Hospital
New York, New York

James A. Kong, M.D.
The Ohio Heart and Vascular Center
Cincinnati, Ohio

Peter A. Kringstein, M.D.
Clinical Instructor in Medicine
Department of Cardiology
University of Rochester, SMH
Clinical Instructor in Medicine
Department of Cardiology
Strong Memorial Hospital
Rochester, New York

Stephen C. Kuehn, M.D.
Fellow and Assistant Clinical Professor
Departments of Cardiology and Internal
  Medicine
St. Louis University School of Medicine
Fellow
Department of Cardiology
St. Louis University Hospital
St. Louis, Missouri

Jarvis W. Lambert, M.D.
Internal Medicine and Cardiology Associate
Healthfirst Family Care Center, Inc.
Falls River, Massachusetts

Jacqueline M. Lamour, M.D.
Assistant Professor
Department of Pediatrics
Columbia University
Assistant Attending Physician
Department of Pediatrics
Children's Hospital of New York
New York, New York

Jonathan Langberg, M.D.
Professor of Medicine
Cardiology Division
Emory University School of Medicine
Director
Cardiac Electrophysiology Laboratory
Emory University Hospital
Atlanta, Georgia

Joshua M. Larned, M.D.
Cardiology Fellow
Division of Cardiology
Emory University
Atlanta, Georgia

Jennifer Lash, M.D.
Fellow
Division of Cardiology
St. Louis University
St. Louis University Hospital
St. Louis, Missouri

Donald A. Leichter, M.D.
New York Presbyterian Hospital
Columbia University Medical Center
Morgan Stanley Children's Hospital
New York, New York

Contributing Authors

Stéphanie Levasseur, M.D.
Assistant Professor
Department of Pediatrics
Columbia University
Assistant Attending Physician
Department of Pediatric Cardiology
Morgan Stanley Children's Hospital of
    New York-Presbyterian
New York, New York

Leonardo Liberman, M.D.
Assistant Professor of Clinical Pediatrics
Department of Pediatric Cardiology
Columbia University
Physician
Department of Pediatric Cardiology
New York Presbyterian Hospital
New York, New York

Francisco Lopez-Jimenez, M.D., M.Sc.
Assistant Professor of Medicine
Department of Cardiovascular Diseases
Mayo Clinic College of Medicine
Consultant
Department of Cardiovascular Diseases
Mayo Clinic
Rochester, Minnesota

Jerre Lutz, M.D.
Associate Professor of Medicine
Department of Medicine
Division of Cardiology
Emory University School of Medicine
Atlanta, Georgia

Zvi S. Marans, M.D.
Associate Clinical Professor of Pediatrics
Department of Pediatrics
Columbia University
Associate Attending Physician
Department of Pediatrics
Columbia-Presbyterian Medical Center
New York, New York

Deryk McDowell, M.D.
Cardiology Fellow
Division of Cardiology
St. Louis University
St. Louis, Missouri

Rosemary Mehl, M.D.
Staff Physician
Brockton/West Roxbury Veterans Affairs
    Medical Center
Instructor in Medicine
Harvard Medical School
Brockton, Massachusetts

Roopa Mehta, M.D.
Department of Endocrinology and Metabolism
Instituto Nacional de Ciencias Médicas y
    Nutricion
Mexico City, Mexico

Theofanie Mela, M.D.
Department of Cardiology
Massachusetts General Hospital
Harvard Medical School
Boston, Massachsetts

Seema Mital, M.D.
Assistant Professor
Department of Pediatrics
Columbia University
Assistant Clinical Attending Physician
Department of Pediatrics
Morgan Stanley Children's Hospital of New York
    Presbyterian
New York, New York

Duy T. Nguyen, M.A., M.D.
Cardiology Fellow
Department of Medicine
UCSF
Cardiology Fellow
Department of Medicine
UCSF Medical Center
San Francisco, California

J. V. (Ian) Nixon, M.D.
Professor of Medicine
Department of Internal Medicine and
    Cardiology
Virginia Commonwealth University School of
    Medicine
VCU Health System
Richmond, Virginia

Peter Ott, M.D.
Assistant Professor of Clinical Medicine
Director of Electrophysiology Laboratory and
    Arrhythmia Service
University of Arizona Health Sciences Center
Department of Internal Medicine, Section of
    Cardiology
Sarver Heart Center
Tucson, Arizona

Robert H. Pass, M.D.
Assistant Professor of Pediatrics
Department of Pediatrics
Columbia University
Director of Pediatric Electrophysiology
    Services
Department of Pediatrics
New York Presbyterian-Children's Hospital of
    New York
New York, New York

Amar D. Patel, M.D.
Cardiology Fellow
Department of Medicine
Division of Cardiology
Emory University School of Medicine
Atlanta, Georgia

Timothy E. Paterick, M.D.
Cardiologist
Division of Cardiovascular
Mayo Clinic
Jacksonville, Florida

Timothy James (T. J.) Paterick, M.D.
Research Assistant
Department of Cardiology
Mayo Clinic
Jacksonville, Florida

Stefano Perlini, M.D.
Associate Professor
Director, Echocardiography Lab
Clinica Medica II, Internal Medicine
IRCCS San Matteo, University of Pavia
Pavia, Italy

Priya Pillutla, M.D.
Resident
Department of Internal Medicine
University of California, San Francisco
San Francisco, California

Ferdos Khan Pohlel, M.D.
Cardiology Fellow
Department of Medicine
Division of Cardiology
Emory University School of Medicine
Emory University Hospital
Atlanta, Georgia

Joseph L. Polizzi, M.D.
Fellow
Division of Cardiology
St. Louis University
St. Louis University Hospital
St. Louis, Missouri

Ashwin Prakash, M.D.
Assistant Professor of Pediatrics
Division of Pediatric Cardiology
Columbia University College of Physicians and
    Surgeons
Attending Pediatric Cardiologist
Division of Pediatric Cardiology
Morgan Stanley Children's Hospital of New York
    Presbyterian
New York, New York

Benjamin Prentiss, M.D.

Daniel T. Price, M.D.
Assistant Professor of Medicine
Section of Cardiology
Boston University School of Medicine
Boston Medical Center
Boston, Massachusetts

Beth Feller Printz, M.D., Ph.D.
Assistant Professor of Pediatrics (in Radiology)
Department of Pediatrics
Columbia University
Assistant Attending Physician in Pediatrics
Department of Pediatrics
Morgan Stanley Children's Hospital of
    New York-Presbyterian
New York, New York

Julie J. Ramos, M.D.
Cardiology Fellow
Division of Cardiology
Emory University
Cardiology Fellow
Department of Cardiology
Emory University Hospital
Atlanta, Georgia

Rajni K. Rao, M.D.
Clinical Instructor
Cardiology Division
Department of Medicine
University of California, San Francisco
Moffitt-Long Hospital
San Francisco, California

Jason S. Reingold, M.D.
Senior Medicine Resident
Department of Medicine
University of California, San Francisco
Moffitt-Long Hospital
San Francisco, California

John Respass, M.D.
Department of Internal Medicine
University of Massachusetts Medical Center
Worcester, Massachusetts

John A. Riddick, M.D.
Cardiology Fellow
Division of Cardiology
Emory University School of Medicine
Atlanta, Georgia

Bryan Ristow, M.D.
Cardiology Fellow
Department of Cardiology
California Pacific Medical Center
San Francisco, California

Carlos A. Roldan, M.D.
Associate Professor of Medicine
University of New Mexico School
    of Medicine
Staff Cardiologist
Director
Echocardiography Laboratory
Department of Medicine
Veterans Affairs Medical Center
University of New Mexico
Albuquerque, New Mexico

Erica Berman Rosenzweig, M.D.
Assistant Professor of Pediatrics (in Medicine)
Department of Pediatrics, Division of Pediatric
    Cardiology
Columbia University College of Physicians and
    Surgeons
Assistant Attending Pediatrician
Department of Pediatrics, Pediatric Cardiology
New York Presbyterian Hospital
New York, New York

Adhar Seth, M.D.
UMass Memorial Medical Center
Worcester, Massachusetts
Beth Israel Deaconess Medical Center
Boston, Massachusetts

Sanjiv J. Shah, M.D.
Fellow in Cardiovascular Medicine
Department of Medicine
University of California
Fellow in Cardiovascular Medicine
Department of Medicine
University of California, San Francisco Medical
    Center
San Francisco, California

Abdul M. Sheikh, M.D.
Cardiology Fellow
Department of Medicine
Emory University School of Medicine
Atlanta, Georgia

Helge U. Simon, M.D.
Department of Cardiovascular Medicine
University of Massachusetts Medical Center
Memorial Campus
Worcester, Massachusetts

David Singh, M.D.
Department of Medicine
University of California, San Francisco
San Francisco, California

Harsimran S. Singh, M.D., M.Sc.
Internal Medicine Resident
Department of Internal Medicine
University of California, San Francisco
Internal Medicine Resident—PGY II
Department of Internal Medicine
University of California, San Francisco
San Francisco General Hospital
San Francisco, California

David E. Solowiejczyk, M.D.
Associate Professor
Department of Pediatrics
Columbia University
Attending Physician
Department of Pediatrics
Morgan Stanley Children's Hospital of
    New York-Presbyterian
New York, New York

Virend K. Somers, M.D., Ph.D.
Department of Medicine
Division of Cardiovascular Medicine
Mayo Clinic College of Medicine
Rochester, Minnesota

Thomas J. Starc, M.D.
Professor of Clinical Pediatrics
Columbia University College of Physicians and
    Surgeons
Attending Physician
New York Presbyterian Hospital
Columbia University Medical Center
New York, New York

Mark Steiner, M.D.
Fellow
Department of Medicine
Division of Cardiology
Emory University School of Medicine
Atlanta, Georgia

Kimara L. Targoff, M.D.
Instructor in Pediatrics
Department of Pediatrics, Division
    of Cardiology
Columbia University
Attending Physician
Department of Pediatrics, Division of
    Cardiology
Children's Hospital of New York, Columbia
    Presbyterian Medical Center
New York, New York

John A. Ternay, M.D.
Department of Cardiology
East Tennessee Heart Consultants
Knoxville, Tennessee

Randal J. Thomas, M.D., M.S.
Assistant Professor
Department of Internal Medicine
Mayo Medical School
Director
Department of Cardiovascular Health
    Clinic
Mayo Clinic
Rochester, Minnesota

Donna M. Timchak, M.D.
Assistant Clinical Professor
Department of Pediatrics
Columbia University
New York, New York
Associate Attending
Department of Pediatrics
Morristown Memorial Hospital
Morristown, New Jersey

Contributing Authors

Jorge F. Trejo, M.D., M.H.S.
Assistant Professor of Medicine
Consultant
Department of Cardiovascular Diseases and
    Internal Medicine
Mayo Clinic College of Medicine
Rochester Minnesota
Mayo Clinic
Jacksonville, Florida

Quynh A. Truong, M.D.
Clinical Research Fellow
Department of Radiology
Massachusetts General Hospital
Clinical Research Fellow
Department of Radiology
Massachusetts General Hospital
Boston, Massachusetts

Pradyumna E. Tummala, M.D.
Assistant Professor of Medicine
Division of Cardiology
Gainesville Radiology Group, PC
Gainesville, Georgia

Christopher S. Vaccari, M.D.
Fellow in Cardiovascular Medicine
Division of Cardiology
Emory University School of Medicine
Emory University Hospital
Atlanta, Georgia

Vasanth Vedantham, M.D.
Division of Medical Sciences
Harvard Medical School
Boston, Massachusetts
MA General Hospital—Nuclear Magnetic
    Resonance Center
Charlestown, Massachusetts

Michele P. Voeltz, M.D.
Cardiology Fellow
Department of Internal Medicine
Division of Cardiology
Emory University School of Medicine
Atlanta, Georgia

Rishi R. Vohora, D.O.
Resident
UMass Memorial Medical Center
Worchester, Massachusetts

Nanette K. Wenger, M.D.
Professor of Medicine (Cardiology)
Department of Medicine (Cardiology)
Emory University School of Medicine
Chief of Cardiology
Department of Medicine (Cardiology)
Grady Memorial Hospital
Atlanta, Georgia

S. Patrick Whalen, M.D.
Fellow, Cardiac Electrophysiology
Department of Medicine
Emory University
Emory University Hospital
Atlanta, Georgia

Matthew E. Wiisanen, M.D.
Resident
Internal Medicine
Mayo Clinic
Mayo School of Graduate Medical Education
Rochester, Minnesota

B. Robinson Williams III, M.D.
Cardiology Fellow
Department of Medicine
Emory University School of Medicine
Atlanta, Georgia

Ismee A. Williams, M.D., M.S.
Fellow, Pediatric Cardiology
Department of Pediatrics
Columbia University College of Physicians and
    Surgery
Fellow, Pediatric Cardiology
Department of Pediatrics
Morgan Stanley Children's Hospital of New York
New York, New York

Marcus Williams, M.D.
Professor
Department of Surgery
James H. Quillen College of Medicine
Staff Surgeon
Veterans Affairs Medical Center
Cardiac Surgeon
Johnson City Medical Center
North Side Hospital
Johnson City, Tennessee

Benoy J. Zachariah, M.D.
Clinical Assistant Professor of Medicine
Department of Medicine
Boston University School of Medicine
Staff Cardiologist
Department of Medicine
Boston Medical Center
Boston, Massachusetts

CONTENTS

Contents

SECOND
EDITION

THE AHA
CLINICAL
CARDIAC
CONSULT

ACROMEGALY AND THE HEART

Apur R. Kamdar
Deepak L. Bhatt
Gary S. Francis

 ## BASICS

DESCRIPTION
Excess production of growth hormone, usually from a pituitary adenoma or rarely an ectopic site, results in biventricular hypertrophy and possible diastolic and, eventually, systolic heart failure.
- Due in part to associated hypertension, diabetes, and coronary artery disease
- There may be a causal relationship with high levels of growth hormone.

EPIDEMIOLOGY
Up to one third of patients with acromegaly have ventricular hypertrophy and congestive heart failure.

Incidence
Approximately 900 new cases are diagnosed yearly in United States

RISK FACTORS
- Hypertension is a risk factor for development of heart failure in the acromegalic patient.
- Genetics

Pregnancy Considerations
Not advisable in someone with symptomatic congestive heart failure

ETIOLOGY
Excess growth hormone can have a direct effect on cardiac hypertrophy.
- Concomitant hypertension, present in about one third of patients, leads to ventricular enlargement and failure.
- Difficult to distinguish the mechanism of heart failure in patients with acromegaly, because severe hypertension and obesity frequently coexist.

ASSOCIATED CONDITIONS
- Hypertension
- Diabetes mellitus
- Coronary artery disease
- Hyperthyroidism, especially if arrhythmias are present
- Obesity
- Obstructive sleep apnea
- Gastrointestinal (GI) malignancy, colonic polyps

 ## DIAGNOSIS

SIGNS AND SYMPTOMS
- Dyspnea on exertion and at rest
- Orthopnea
- Paroxysmal nocturnal dyspnea
- Decreased exercise tolerance
- Arrhythmia
- Cardiomegaly
- Left ventricular hypertrophy (LVH)
- Left ventricular lift
- S_3 (third heart sound)
- S4 (fourth heart sound)
- Hypertension
- Large hands
- Prominent forehead
- Obesity

TESTS
- Cardiac catheterization often shows premature coronary artery disease. Small-vessel disease also may be present.
- Myocardial biopsy can show massive myocardial hypertrophy. Lymphocyte infiltration and interstitial fibrosis also may be seen, although these findings are not specific.

Lab
- Elevated serum growth hormone levels at baseline and nonsuppressibility after glucose loading
- Measurement of insulinlike growth factor 1 levels
- Electrocardiogram (ECG) commonly shows LVH, ST-wave depression, septal Q-waves, T-wave inversion, bundle branch block, and atrial or ventricular ectopy.

Imaging
- Chest X-ray
  - Shows cardiomegaly by the fifth decade of life
- Echocardiography
  - Shows LVH, right ventricular hypertrophy (RVH), and asymmetric hypertrophy of the septum
  - Diminished ejection fraction and left ventricular dilation also may be seen.
  - Tissue Doppler shows diastolic dysfunction.

Pathologic Findings
- Interstitial fibrosis may precede hypertrophy
- Disordered and hypertrophied left ventricular architecture
- Thickened arterial intimal layers

DIFFERENTIAL DIAGNOSIS
- Other causes of cardiomegaly
- Other possible coexisting causes of hypertension are pheochromocytoma and aldosteronoma.
- Hyperthyroidism should be sought if atrial fibrillation is present.

 ## TREATMENT

GENERAL MEASURES
Low-sodium diet is particularly effective in treating heart failure in these patients.

MEDICATION (DRUGS)

- Management of the underlying condition, previously with bromocriptine but now with somatostatin analogs (octreotide), can lead to rapid reversal of even severe ventricular dysfunction. May actually reverse interstitial fibrosis.
- Growth hormone receptor antagonist, pegvisomant, may be used in somatostatin-resistant patients.
- Standard therapy for congestive heart failure (CHF)
- Diuretics are particularly effective.
- Antihypertensive therapy

SURGERY
- Surgery and irradiation of the pituitary gland are the principal types of management for acromegaly and may result in a dramatic improvement in cardiac function.
- Treatment of hypertension is important.
- Heart transplantation has been performed for acromegalic cardiomyopathy.

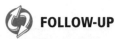 **FOLLOW-UP**

Admission Criteria
Standard for heart failure of any etiology

PROGNOSIS
- Risk of sudden death and ventricular arrhythmias.
- Risk of premature coronary artery disease
- Two- to threefold higher overall mortality
- Younger patients may have better prognosis than elderly.

PATIENT MONITORING
- These patients are usually obese.
- At risk for development of diabetes

REFERENCES
1. Trainer PJ, Drake WM, Katznelson L, et al. Treatment of acromegaly with the growth hormone-receptor antagonist pegvisomant. *N Engl J Med*. 2000;342:1171.
2. Topol EJ, ed. *Textbook of Cardiovascular Medicine*. Philadelphia: Lippincott Williams & Wilkins, 2002.
3. Zipes DP. Braunwald's Heart Disease: A Textbook of Cardiovascular Medicine, 7th ed., 2005.
4. Martins JB, Kerber RE, Sherman BM, et al. Cardiac size and function in acromegaly. *Circulation*. 1977;56:863–869.
5. McGuffin WL, Sherman BM, Roth J, et al. Acromegaly and cardiovascular disorders—a prospective study. *Ann Intern Med*. 1974;81:11–18.
6. Chanson P, Timsit J, Masquet C, et al. Cardiovascular effects of the somatostatin analog octreotide in acromegaly. *Ann Intern Med*. 1990;113:921–925.
7. Albat B, Leclercq F, Serre I, et al. Heart transplantation for terminal congestive heart failure in an acromegalic patient. *Eur Heart J*. 1993;14:1572–1575.

CODES
ICD9-CM
- 428.0 Failure, heart, congestive
- 425.4 Cardiomyopathy

PATIENT TEACHING
- Standard for heart failure of any etiology
- Risks of hypertension, diabetes, coronary artery disease, colon cancer

ACUTE CORONARY SYNDROME(S)

F. Khan Pohlel
Nanette K. Wenger

BASICS

DESCRIPTION
- Acute coronary syndrome (ACS) is described as a clinical spectrum of ischemic discomfort resulting from atheromatous plaque rupture leading to thrombus formation. Its spectrum ranges from unstable angina (UA) to non–ST elevation myocardial infarction (NSTEMI) to ST elevation myocardial infarction (STEMI). The diagnosis depends on the characteristics of the chest pain, level of serum cardiac biomarkers, and electrocardiographic (ECG) abnormalities.
- In its most severe form, an occlusive thrombus results in STEMI.
- NSTEMI is differentiated from UA by the presence of abnormal cardiac biomarkers.

GENERAL PREVENTION
Reduction and modification of coronary risk profile

EPIDEMIOLOGY
Leading cause of death in the United States with nearly 1.2 million people sustaining a myocardial infarction yearly and a mortality rate of 40%

RISK FACTORS
- Hypertension
- Hyperlipidemia
- Diabetes mellitus and glucose intolerance
- Family history of premature coronary heart disease (age before 55 in father, or age before 65 in mother)
- Cigarette smoking
- Metabolic syndrome and obesity
- Chronic kidney disease
- Sedentary lifestyle
- Cocaine use

PATHOPHYSIOLOGY
- Atheromatous plaque rupture resulting in platelet activation, aggregation, and deposition at the injury site. This forms a thrombus after the coagulation cascade is activated.
- Inflammation including lymphocyte and macrophage activation contributes to plaque instability.

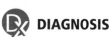

DIAGNOSIS

SIGNS AND SYMPTOMS
- Symptoms: severe, crushing substernal chest pain with a tightness or pressure quality radiating to the neck or arms. Associated symptoms of diaphoresis, dyspnea, fatigue, lightheadedness, nausea, or vomiting are common.
- Signs: Physical exam may be nonspecific, but may reveal a third heart sound (S3), distended neck veins, pulmonary edema, new or worsening mitral regurgitation murmur, or, in late presenting cases, a murmur of ventricularseptal defect (VSD).

TESTS
- ECG changes of ST depression or T-wave inversion can be consistent with UA/NSTEMI
- ECG changes of ST-segment elevation greater than 1 mm in two contiguous leads or new left bundle branch block (LBBB) is consistent with STEMI.
  - Inferior: II, III, aVF
  - Anterior: V1-V6
  - Anteroseptal: V1-V3
  - Lateral: I, aVL, V4-V6
- ECG changes of ST-segment depression greater than 1 mm in V1-V3 consistent with a posterior STEMI
- Cardiac biomarkers: creatine kinase (CK)-MB, troponin I (TnI) or T (TnT), and myoglobin.
  - TnI or TnT is specific for cardiac injury and rise in 4–6 hours with a gradual fall in up to 10 days. Good specificity with prognostic implications
  - CK-MB has a rapid rise in 4–6 hours with a rapid fall over 36–48 hours.
  - Serial evaluation should be performed every 6–8 hours for 24 hours.
- Echocardiogram: can visualize regional wall-motion abnormalities and determine left ventricular (LV) function. Poor LV function portends a worse prognosis.
- If diagnosis of ACS is unclear, echocardiography, chest computed tomographic (CT) scan, or magnetic resonance imaging (MRI) may help differentiate from acute aortic dissection or pulmonary embolus.
- High-sensitivity C reactive protein (Hs-CRP) may be useful in predicting higher risk individuals with more complex lesions.
- Brain natriuretic peptide (BNP) is an independent predictor of mortality in NSTEMI.

Imaging
Myocardial perfusion imaging using thallium scans with exercise testing or pharmacologic stress or dobutamine echocardiography may evaluate low risk patients with UA for inducible ischemia.

Diagnostic Procedures/Surgery
- Cardiac catheterization should be considered in patients with congestive heart failure (CHF), depressed LV function, malignant ventricular arrhythmias, persistent or recurrent ischemia, large perfusion defect on noninvasive functional test, or prior revascularization procedures.
- Pulmonary artery catheter monitoring may be considered for progressive hypotension, cardiogenic shock, or with suspected mechanical complications of myocardial infarction (MI) such as muscle rupture.
- Intra-aortic balloon counterpulsation is recommended for cardiogenic shock to stabilize for revascularization.

DIFFERENTIAL DIAGNOSIS
- Cardiac: Pericarditis, myocarditis
- Aorta: Acute aortic dissection
- Lung: Pulmonary embolism
- Gastrointestinal
  - Esophageal disorders
  - Acute cholecystitis

TREATMENT

GENERAL MEASURES
- Treatment of STEMI requires immediate reperfusion of blocked vessel.
- Treatment of UA/NSTEMI involves stabilization of unstable plaques and activated platelets.
- Risk scores such as thrombolysis in myocardial infarction (TIMI), global utilization of strategies to open occluded coronary arteries (GUSTO), and Braunwald classifications help stratify patients with UA/NSTEMI according to risk level, and correlate to risk of recurrent ischemia and death. These risk scores identify higher risk individuals needing more aggressive interventions.
- In general, an early invasive strategy in ACS provides better mortality and morbidity benefit compared to a conservative approach.

MEDICATION (DRUGS)

- Aspirin (ASA) should be administered as soon as possible and continued indefinitely. Initial dose should be 162–325 mg. (Class I)
- Clopidogrel should be administered at 75 mg daily for those unable to tolerate ASA or when an early noninterventional approach is planned for at least one month and up to 9 months. (Class I)
  - Should be held for 5–7 days prior to elective CABG to reduce risk of bleeding. (Class I)
  - Should be continued for 1 month with bare metal stent implantation and 3–6 or more months with drug eluting stent implantation.
- Antianginal therapy with nitrates and β-blockers should be started if hemodynamics permit.
  - Nitrates should be avoided in patients with hypotension (systolic blood pressure, SBP <90 mmHg), suspected right ventricular (RV) infarction, or with recent use of phosphodiesterase type 5 inhibitors such as sildenafil.
  - β-Blockers relieve myocardial ischemia by lowering myocardial oxygen demand. Goals of therapy are a resting heart rate of 50–60 beats/minute. Cardioselective β-blockers have fewer noncardiac side effects.
  - Morphine sulfate intravenous (IV) is analgesic of choice if required at 2–4 mg doses over 5–15 minutes interval.
  - Calcium channel blockers are second line therapy in patients with a contraindication to β-blockers or when β-blockers and nitrates fail to relieve symptoms of ischemia. They are preferred in variant angina or cocaine-induced vasospasm. They are to be avoided if LV dysfunction, atrioventricular block, or signs or symptoms of congestive heart failure are present.
  - Oxygen supplementation as needed
- Unfractionated heparin (UFH) or subcutaneous low-molecular-weight heparin (LMWH) should be added to aspirin or clopidogrel therapy. (Class I)
  - Enoxaparin is preferable to UFH in the absence of renal failure or planned coronary artery bypass grafting (CABG) within 24 hours in UA/NSTEMI. (Class IIa)

- Direct thrombin inhibitors such as bivalirudin is acceptable alternative to UFH, especially in setting of heparin-induced thrombocytopenia.
- Platelet glycoprotein (GP) IIb/IIIa antagonist should be administered in addition to ASA and heparin if early catheterization and intervention are planned. (Class I)
  - Eptifibatide or tirofiban should be given for patients with ongoing ischemia, elevated troponin, or other high-risk features despite conservative management. (Class IIa)
  - Abciximab is reserved for patients undergoing primary percutaneous coronary intervention (PCI)
- Angiotensin-converting-enzyme (ACE) inhibitors are indicated with LV dysfunction (ejection fraction, EF <.40), anterior infarction, or pulmonary congestion and improve survival and ventricular remodeling. An angiotensin receptor blocker (ARB) is an acceptable alternative for ACE intolerant individuals.
- Lipid-lowering therapy with hydroxymethylglutaryl coenzyme A (HMG-CoA) reductase inhibitors (statins) should be started before lipid levels measured with a goal low density lipoprotein (LDL) <100 mg/dL or optional <70 mg/dL in very high risk patients.
- Aldosterone blockade such as spironolactone or eplerenone should be considered post-MI in patients with CHF in the absence of renal dysfunction or hyperkalemia.
- Hemodynamically significant ventricular arrhythmias should be treated with amiodarone or lidocaine.
  - Prophylactic use of antiarrhythmic agents such as flecainide (Class Ic antiarrhythmic agents) for ventricular ectopy is associated with increased mortality.
- Fibrinolytic agents such as alteplase (tPA), reteplase, or tenecteplase (TNK) for STEMI decrease mortality and improve LV function.
  - Should be administered within 12 hours of symptom onset in the presence of ST elevation greater than 1 mm in 2 contiguous leads or a new LBBB in absence of contraindications.
  - If presentation is within 3 hours of symptom onset, no preference between fibrinolytic therapy versus invasive strategy.
  - Individuals with high risk features of STEMI such as cardiogenic shock, increased risk of bleeding, or late presentation should be managed with an invasive strategy.
  - No benefit for fibrinolytic therapy in UA/NSTEMI.
- Diuretics such as furosemide for signs and symptoms of congestive heart failure
- Dobutamine 2–20 mcg/kg/minute IV with SBP between 70 and 100 mmHg if signs of acute pulmonary edema or low output cardiogenic shock
- Dopamine 5–15 μcg/kg/minute IV if signs and symptoms of shock present.
- IV fluids should be administered for RV infarction.
- Insulin infusion may be necessary to normalize blood glucose levels.

First Line
- Reperfusion therapy is the primary goal in management of STEMI or new LBBB MI.
- Survival benefit of reperfusion is greatest in those treated the earliest.
- Risk of death, nonfatal MI, and recurrent ischemia is significantly reduced with early invasive strategy with percutaneous coronary interventions (PCIs)

- If facilities are available, treatment with immediate coronary angiography and PCI is preferred method with a goal door-to-balloon time of 90 minutes.
- An early invasive strategy is beneficial in UA/NSTEMI, especially with high-risk features such as recurrent angina/ischemia at low levels of activity with or without CHF symptoms despite anti-ischemic therapy, elevated TnT or TnI, new ST depression, high-risk findings on noninvasive stress testing, depressed LV function (EF <.40), hemodynamic instability, sustained ventricular tachycardia, PCI within 6 months, or prior CABG.

SURGERY
CABG may be indicated in patients with left main occlusion or equivalent lesions, three-vessel disease or two-vessel including proximal left anterior descending disease, patients with diabetes mellitus and significant coronary disease, and depressed LV function.

 FOLLOW-UP

Patients should be seen 2–4 weeks after discharge to evaluate functional status and the presence of cardiopulmonary symptoms and for medication changes

DISPOSITION
Exercise testing following an MI may be considered to guide postdischarge exercise prescription.

PROGNOSIS
Patients with reduced LV function (EF <.30) at least 1 month following MI, or who have hemodynamically significant ventricular arrhythmias more than 2 days after MI, have indications for implantable cardioverter-defibrillator (ICD) due to high risk of sudden cardiac death from malignant ventricular arrhythmias.

COMPLICATIONS
- Ventricular septal rupture occurred in 1–2% in prethrombolytic era, usually 2–5 days after MI.
  - Occur in older, female, hypertensive, anterior infarction, worse Killip class on admission
- Mitral regurgitation
- Cardiac rupture occurs in 3% following MI (90% in first 2 weeks).
- Pseudoaneurysm
- Cardiogenic shock
- RV failure following inferior wall MI
- Ventricular aneurysm
- Arrhythmias can affect up to 90% of patients with MI.
- Pericarditis affecting 10% early after MI. Late pericarditis or Dressler syndrome occurs up to 8 weeks after MI.

PATIENT MONITORING
- Telemetry monitoring for low-risk UA
- Cardiac care unit (CCU) monitoring for moderate to high-risk UA, NSTEMI, or STEMI

REFERENCES
1. 2006 Heart and Stroke Statistical Update. Dallas, Texas. American Heart Association 2006.
2. Braunwald E, Antman EM, Beasley JW, et al. ACC/AHA 2002 guideline update for the management of patients with unstable angina and non–ST-segment elevation myocardial infarction—summary article: a report of the American College of Cardiology/American Heart Association task force on practice guidelines. *J Am Coll Cardiol*. 2002;40:1366–1374.
3. Antman EM, Anbe DT, Armstrong PW, et al. ACC/AHA guidelines for the management of patients with ST-elevation myocardial infarction—executive summary: A report of the American College of Cardiology/American Heart Association Task Force on practice guidelines. *J Am Coll Cardiol*. 2004;44:671–719.
4. Grundy SM, Cleeman JL, Bairey Merz CN, et al. for the Coordinating Committee of the National Cholesterol Education Program: Implications of recent clinical trials for the National Cholesterol Education Program Adult Treatment Panel III Guidelines. *Circulation*. 2004;110:227–239.
5. Sabatine MS, Antman EM. The thrombolysis in myocardial infarction risk score in unstable angina/non-ST-segment elevation myocardial infarction. *J Am Coll Cardiol*. 2003;41:89S–95S.
6. Cannon CP, Braunwald E, McCabe CH, et al. for the Pravastatin or Atorvastatin Evaluation and Infection Therapy—Thrombolysis in Myocardial Infarction 22 Investigators (PROVE-IT-TIMI 22). Intensive versus moderate lipid lowering with statins after acute coronary syndromes. *N Engl J Med*. 2004;350:1495–1504.

CODES
ICD9-CM
- 410 STEMI
- 410.7 NSTEMI
- 411.1 Unstable Angina

PATIENT TEACHING
Diet
Low-fat, low-cholesterol diet consistent with an AHA Step II diet. Low sodium with hypertension (HTN) and CHF

Activity
- Driving can be resumed within 1 week.
- Sexual activity can be resumed within 1 week. Sildenafil is contraindicated with nitrate use.
- Can return to most work within 2 weeks in absence of symptoms
- Performance on an exercise test can be used to determine activity levels. Performance of at least 5 metabolic equivalent (MET) on a submaximal exercise test has good long-term prognosis in absence of angina or ischemia.

Prevention
- Exercise regimen at least 3–4 days per week for a minimum of 30 minutes.
- Cardiac rehabilitation recommended
- Weight control
- Smoking cessation
- Risk factor modification

ADENOSINE

Stefano Perlini
Gerald P. Aurigemma

 BASICS

DESCRIPTION

- Adenosine is an endogenous purine derived from high-energy adenosine phosphates (ATP, ADP, and AMP).
  - Intracellular adenosine can cross the cell membrane and diffuse to the extracellular space, where it may act as an autocoid (i.e., it can exert its effects on adjacent cells).
  - Adenosine also can be generated in the extracellular space by the ectonucleotidase metabolism of plasma ATP that is released from vascular cells, thrombocytes, and sympathetic nerves during ischemia.
  - In the interstitial space, adenosine has a very short half-life. The cell actively reuptakes adenosine, by either simple or facilitated diffusion via a nucleoside transport system that can be pharmacologically inhibited (e.g., by dipyridamole).
- Adenosine receptors
  - The physiologic effects of adenosine are mediated by specific G protein—coupled receptors (also known as purinergic P1 receptors) that belong to the family of the seven transmembrane domain receptors.
  - At present, four adenosine receptors have been characterized: A1, A2a, A2b, and A3.
    - The Al and the A3 receptors both couple to inhibitory Gi/o G proteins (hence causing an inhibition of adenyl cyclase), can activate phospholipase C via G-protein subunits, and can activate protein kinase C.
    - The high-affinity A2a and the low-affinity A2b receptors both couple to Gs, but the A2b receptor also can couple to Gq/11 to mobilize calcium.

- Adenosine cardiovascular effects
  - Vascular tone
    - Coronary vasodilation (the A2a receptor mainly at the level of resistance vessels and the A2b receptor at the level of conductance vessels), via both potassium ATP (KKATP) channel and nitrous oxide (NO)-mediated mechanisms
    - Renal vasoconstriction (A1)
    - Peripheral vasodilation (A2)
  - Electrophysiology
    - Negative chronotropic effect (sinoatrial node, A1)
    - Negative dromotropic effect [atrioventricular (AV) node, A1]
    - Depression of automaticity (A1)
  - Mechanical performance
    - Negative inotropic effect (atrial myocardium, A1)
    - Direct positive inotropic effect [A2a receptor, via cyclic AMP (cAMP)-dependent and -independent effects].
    - Indirect negative inotropic effect, by attenuating the cardiac responsiveness to beta-adrenergic stimulation
    - A2-mediated modulation of A1 receptor activity
  - Adrenergic responsivity: A1 receptor stimulation attenuates the responsiveness by reducing the β-adrenergic-mediated increase in cAMP (A1)
    - Presynaptic nerve endings: Adenosine attenuates the release of norepinephrine caused by adrenergic nerve stimulation (A1).
    - Myocardial metabolism: attenuation of the metabolic effects of beta-adrenergic stimulation
    - Endothelial cells: proliferation (and angiogenesis)
- Adenosine as a retaliatory metabolite
  - Adenosine acts as a negative feedback modulator of β-adrenoceptor-mediated responses in the heart and as a negative feedback regulator that inhibits norepinephrine release from the sympathetic nerve endings. These effects are already present at physiologic adenosine interstitial concentrations.

- In several pathophysiologic conditions, adenosine concentrations in the intracellular space may increase significantly (e.g., during β-adrenergic catecholamine stimulation, cardiac ischemia, cardiac hypoxia, and increased cardiac workload caused by volume or pressure overload). In these situations, characterized by an unfavorable oxygen supply-demand ratio, adenosine can induce coronary vasodilation, attenuate the metabolic and inotropic response to β-adrenergic stimulation, and modulate the release of norepinephrine from the sympathetic nerve endings.
- Cardioprotection against the ischemic–reperfusion injury
  - During ischemia, the antiadrenergic effect of adenosine reduces the norepinephrine available for stimulating the flow-deprived heart and reduces the metabolic and inotropic effects of β-adrenergic receptor stimulation. At the same time, adenosine is a potent coronary vasodilator.
  - Adenosine can therefore protect against ischemia-induced cell death and against reperfusion injury. Moreover, adenosine attenuates ischemia-induced myocardial stunning and decreases the incidence of arrhythmias.
- Ischemic preconditioning
  - Adenosine plays an important role in triggering and mediating the cardioprotective effect of ischemic preconditioning, via the activation of A1 and A3 adenosine receptors. By mechanisms yet to be completely elucidated, adenosine release during an ischemic episode interacts with KATP channels to induce a protective effect against subsequent periods of acute ischemia. Adenosine-induced protein kinase C activation may be involved as well.

- Cardiovascular diagnosis
  Arrhythmias
  - The cardiac electrophysiologic actions of adenosine are mediated by the A1 receptor and are either cAMP independent (at the level of nodal or atrial tissue) or cAMP dependent, that is, mediated by the inhibition of the stimulatory effects of adenylyl cyclase (at the level of atrial and ventricular myocytes).
  - Due to these electrophysiologic effects, adenosine can be used in the electrophysiology laboratory as a diagnostic tool:
    - Adenosine may transiently suppress (but not terminate) automatic atrial tachycardia.
    - Because adenosine may transiently block AV nodal conduction, it plays an important role in the diagnosis of reentrant arrhythmias in which the AV node is a critical component of the tachycardia circuit.
    - Adenosine causes transient suppression of adrenergically mediated automatic arrhythmias.
    - Adenosine is useful to identify ventricular arrhythmias due to triggered activity.
    - Adenosine may be used to diagnose latent preexcitation, to localize the region of the accessory pathway, and to assess the immediate efficacy of accessory pathway ablation.

- Ischemic heart disease
  - In the setting of coronary atherosclerosis artery disease, adenosine-induced coronary vasodilation may induce acute regional ischemia due to flow maldistribution (coronary steal in the myocardial area perfused by a stenotic artery). This paradoxical effect of coronary vasodilation can be exploited as a diagnostic tool by allowing the evaluation of the consequences of acute inducible ischemia. To this end, endogenous adenosine accumulation induced by dipyridamole infusion is used as a pharmacologic stress test in combination with two-dimensional echocardiography or radionuclide perfusion scans. The former will allow the identification of wall-motion abnormalities induced by regional ischemia, whereas the latter will assess the relative flow heterogeneity caused by dipyridamole in the presence of coronary artery disease.
  - The short-lasting effect of dipyridamole, which acts by blocking the reuptake of adenosine by the cells, and the availability of the antidote theophylline, which blocks adenosine receptors, make dipyridamole stress testing a safe and effective choice for cardiac imaging in ischemic heart disease.

- Possible role in cardiovascular therapy arrhythmias
  - Adenosine can terminate sinus node reentry, paroxysmal reciprocating atrial tachycardia, nodal reciprocating tachycardia, and effort-related ventricular tachycardia due to triggered activity. Dipyridamole-induced increase in endogenous adenosine may slow or terminate AV nodal reentrant tachycardia and AV reciprocating tachycardia.
  - Adenosine receptor blockade by theophylline may be effective in treating bradycardia in patients with sick sinus syndrome, in increasing the ventricular response rate in patients with atrial fibrillation, and in reversing complete heart block in the setting of acute myocardial infarction.
  - Adenosine administration may cause atrial flutter and/or fibrillation, AV block, sinus bradycardia, and sinus pauses.
- Myocardial cardioprotection
  - Adenosine is a potentially beneficial additive to cardioplegic solutions during open heart surgery, and it is used to control blood pressure in the setting of postoperative systemic and pulmonary hypertension. Its possible role in protecting the ischemic myocardium during coronary angioplasty and in acute myocardial infarction is under extensive clinical evaluation.

AGING HEART

Amar D. Patel
Nanette K. Wenger

BASICS

DESCRIPTION

- Current estimates suggest more than 35 million people 65 years of age or older in the United States; it is expected this number will double by the year 2030.
- Advanced age has strong associations with diseases such as hypertension, coronary atherosclerotic heart disease, congestive heart failure, valvular disease, and conduction system abnormalities.
- Age-related changes in cardiac structure and function play an important role in several of these conditions.

GENERAL PREVENTION

Primary and secondary prevention measures should be aggressively used in the elderly in an attempt to reduce the risk of future adverse cardiac events.

PATHOPHYSIOLOGY

- Remodeling cardiac structures
  - Increased left ventricular (LV) wall thickness
    - Delayed diastolic filling
    - Increased likelihood for diastolic heart failure
    - Increased intracardiac filling pressures
    - Left ventricular hypertrophy
  - Increased left atrial size
    - Increased likelihood for atrial fibrillation
  - Valve structural changes
    - Aortic sclerosis
    - Mitral annulus thickening and calcification
    - Mild mitral regurgitation
  - Conduction system degeneration
    - Sinus bradycardia, sinoatrial nodal block, sinoatrial arrest, sick sinus syndrome, PR prolongation, atrioventricular (AV) block
  - Coronary atherosclerotic heart disease
    - Stable angina, unstable angina, myocardial infarction
    - Development of ischemic cardiomyopathy
- Alteration in cardiac function
  - Decrease cardiac reserve
    - Lowers threshold and increases severity for heart failure development
    - Leads to inability to tolerate changes in systemic processes that have secondary effects on the cardiovascular system (i.e., sepsis, hypovolemia, hypervolemia)
  - Diminished threshold for cellular calcium overload
    - Increased susceptibility for atrial and ventricular arrhythmias
    - Increased myocardial fibrosis and necrosis
    - Diminished systolic and diastolic function

ETIOLOGY

- Remodeling of cardiac structures
  - Increased LV wall thickness
    - Possible mechanisms include increase in LV myocyte size, decrease in myocyte number via necrosis and apoptosis, altered regulation of growth factors, and focal collagen deposition
  - Increased left atrial size
    - Possible mechanisms include increased left atrial pressure and volume
  - Valvular structural changes
    - Thickening and calcification of valve leaflets
  - Conduction system degeneration
    - Decrease in the number of sinus node cells by 50–75% in the aged heart. The number of atrioventricular node cells remains fairly well preserved
    - Fibrosis of the conduction system
  - Coronary atherosclerotic heart disease
    - Development of both stable and unstable atherosclerotic plaques, with the latter more prone to cause an acute coronary syndrome due to its large thrombogenic lipid core
    - Injury to the endothelium by chemical, mechanical, or inflammatory events incites the process of atherosclerosis. Oxidation of low-density lipoprotein cholesterol propagates an inflammatory state in the endothelial lining of the vessel after deposition, causing development of atherosclerotic plaques.
    - Commonly, in the aging heart, there is a greater degree of subcritical stenoses spanning the length of the vessel. This diffuse disease limits blood flow to the distal vascular bed.
- Alteration in cardiac function
  - Decreased cardiac reserve
    - Possible mechanisms include decreased intrinsic myocardial contractility, increased vascular load, increased plasma catecholamine levels, and altered β-adrenergic modulation of heart rate and myocardial contractility
  - Diminished threshold for cellular calcium overload
    - Possible mechanisms include altered gene expression that regulates calcium handling, increased polyunsaturated fatty acid ratios in cardiac membranes

ASSOCIATED CONDITIONS

- Aortic sclerosis is associated with atherosclerotic disease, especially coronary atherosclerotic heart disease.
- Peripheral vascular disease and cerebrovascular disease are associated with coronary atherosclerotic heart disease

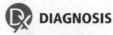

DIAGNOSIS

SIGNS AND SYMPTOMS

- Symptoms: Fatigue, confusion, lethargy, weight gain, reduced exertional tolerance, presyncope, syncope, visual disturbances, headaches, cough, shortness of breath, orthopnea, chest discomfort, and palpitations
- Signs/physical examination findings: Hypertension, tachycardia, bradycardia, irregular rhythm, elevated jugular venous pressure, displaced and/or sustained apical impulse, third heart sound (S_3), fourth heart sound (S_4), regurgitant or stenotic valvular murmurs, pulmonary rales or wheezing, lower extremity edema, cool extremities, poor capillary refill

Diagnostic Procedures/Surgery

- Diagnostic procedures may lend information regarding cardiac structural remodeling
  - Electrocardiogram (ECG): Rhythm abnormalities, LV hypertrophy, and left atrial abnormality, old Q-waves, ST-segment abnormalities
  - Chest x-ray: Cardiomegaly, LV chamber enlargement, left atrial enlargement, enlarged central pulmonary arteries, pulmonary edema
  - Echocardiography with Doppler: Enlarged left atrium/LV, LV hypertrophy, abnormal mitral valve inflow velocities, impaired relaxation, diastolic dysfunction, systolic dysfunction, wall motion abnormalities, valvular regurgitation, stenosis, or calcification
  - Stress testing: All testing gives risk assessment.
    - Exercise ECG stress testing: Exercise tolerance, ST-segment depression suggestive of myocardial ischemia
    - Stress echocardiography: Stress-induced wall motion abnormalities, change in LV ejection fraction
    - Nuclear Stress: perfusion defects, transient ischemic dilation
    - Cardiac magnetic resonance perfusion imaging: Perfusion defects, subendocardial perfusion defect localization, transmyocardial perfusion gradients, stress-induced wall motion abnormalities, change in LV ejection fraction
  - Cardiac catheterization: Identification of angiographically significant coronary disease

MEDICATION (DRUGS)

Depending on the disease, medications prescribed for younger patients should be also offered to elderly patients. Initiation of medications should be closely monitored and started at lower doses, as the elderly are more prone to side effects such as bradycardia, hypotension, conduction system disturbances, and hepatic or renal toxicity.

SURGERY

Although increased periprocedural complications are directly associated with age, surgical intervention should not be withheld from the elderly. Careful consideration of the overall clinical status of the patient must be taken into consideration prior to intervention.

REFERENCES

1. Cheitlin MD, Zipes DP. Cardiovascular disease in the elderly. In Braunwald E, Zipes DP, Libby P, eds. *Heart Disease*, 6th ed. Philadelphia: WB Saunders, 2001.
2. Lakatta EG, Levy D. Arterial and cardiac aging: Major Shareholders in Cardiovascular Disease Enterprises. Part II: The Aging Heart in Health: Links to Heart Disease. *Circulation*. 2003;107:346–354.
3. Lakatta EG. Cardiovascular regulatory mechanisms in advanced age. *Physiol Rev*. 1993;73:413–467.
4. Varagic J, Susic D, Frohlich ED. Heart, aging, and hypertension. *Curr Opin Cardiol*. 2001;16: 336–341.
5. Wei JY. Advanced aging and the cardiovascular system. In Wenger NK (ed): *Cardiovascular Disease in the Octogenarian and Beyond*. London, Martin Dunitz, 1999.

ADDITIONAL READING

1. Otto CM, Lind BK, Kitzman DW, et al. Association of aortic-valve sclerosis with cardiovascular mortality and morbidity in the elderly. *N Engl J Med*. 1999;341:142–147.
2. Stratton JR, Levy WC, Cerqueira MD, et al. Cardiovascular Responses to Exercise. Effects of Aging and Exercise Training in Healthy Men. *Circulation*. 1994;89:1648–1655.

 MISCELLANEOUS

PATIENT TEACHING

All patients must be educated regarding their disease and how concurrent comorbid illness affects the overall clinical condition.

Diet

Dietary modifications must be made depending on concurrent comorbidities (i.e. diabetes mellitus, dyslipidemia, heart failure).

Activity

• Regular physical activity should be encouraged
  – Reduces blood pressure
  – Reduces insulin resistance
  – Increases high-density lipoprotein cholesterol
    Goal should be walking 30 minutes per day for at least 4 days a week

Prevention

• Tobacco use cessation using a structured approach
• Weight control

AICDs

Peter Ott

 BASICS

DESCRIPTION

- Sudden cardiac death (SCD) is a major public health problem and responsible for approximately 350,000 deaths in the U.S. alone.
- Ventricular tachycardia (VT) and ventricular fibrillation (VF) are the main mechanisms for SCD.
- Implantable cardioverter defibrillators (ICDs) are highly effective in treating VT and VF.
- Patients with significant structural heart disease are at increased risk for SCD and may be candidates for ICD therapy.

RISK FACTORS

- Ischemic cardiomyopathy, reduced systolic function (left ventricle ejection fraction [LVEF] <35%), and nonsustained VT on Holter, with inducible sustained VT on electrophysiologic (EP) study (refractory to intravenous Procainamide) (MADIT 1 study)
- Ischemic cardiomyopathy, reduced systolic function (LVEF <30%) (MADIT 2 study)
- Ischemic or nonischemic cardiomyopathy with reduced systolic function (LVEF <30%) and class II/III heart failure (SCDHeFt study)
- Survivors of cardiac arrest not due to clearly reversible causes or patients with documented sustained VT, especially if heart disease is present (AVID, CIDS studies)
- Patients with primary electrical disorders, such as long QT syndrome or Brugada syndrome, may require an ICD.

Genetics

Certain primary electrical disorders, such as long QT syndrome or Brugada syndrome, are genetically determined and thus inherited.

PATHOPHYSIOLOGY

- VT termination often is accomplished with overdrive pacing through the ICD-antitachycardia pacing.
- Both VT and VF can be cardioverted/defibrillated successfully.

 DIAGNOSIS

SIGNS AND SYMPTOMS

- Symptoms related to VT (palpitations, syncope) and VF (sudden collapse, sudden death)
- Antitachycardia pacing is painless.
- Cardioversion and defibrillation shocks can be quite painful.

History

- Palpitations, syncope, collapse, resuscitated sudden death
- History of prior heart disease, heart failure, or myocardial infarction (MI)

Physical Exam

Possible signs of heart disease or heart failure

TESTS

Imaging

- Echocardiogram for LV systolic function, coronary angiography
- CXR for device follow-up to assess stable lead position

Diagnostic Procedures/Surgery

Some patients may require an EP study to clarify the role of ICD therapy.

DIFFERENTIAL DIAGNOSIS

- VT need to be differentiated from supra ventricular tachycardia (SVT) with wide QRS complex. SVT can be cured with catheter ablation.
- In patients with Wolff-Parkinson-White (WPW) syndrome VF is caused by atrial fibrillation and can be cured by catheter ablation.

 TREATMENT

GENERAL MEASURES

ICD is implanted by a cardiac electrophysiologist with special training. Typically performed under conscious sedation in a cath-lab/EP lab setting. The implant procedure is similar to that of a pacemaker. Device testing (VF induction and defibrillation) performed after device implanted.

 MEDICATION (DRUGS)

- Optimal therapy of the underlying cardiac condition is mandatory.
- Up to 30% of ICD patients may require therapy with an antiarrhythmic drug, either to reduce the number of VT/VF episodes or to treat other arrhythmias primarily atrial fibrillation.

First Line

Often-used antiarrhythmic drugs: Amiodarone or sotalol

SURGERY

- Surgical ICD implant is rare.
- Patients undergoing open heart surgery who have an ICD indication should have the device implanted transvenously after the surgery procedure.

⚡ FOLLOW-UP

- Routine follow-up (in device clinic), typically every 3 months, is required to evaluate device function and battery status.
- After ICD shock or symptoms suggesting significant arrhythmias, ICD evaluation should be performed. The device data storage can be extremely helpful in evaluating symptoms.

DISPOSITION

Often joined patient follow-up between cardiologist/primary care physician and cardiac electrophysiologist

Admission Criteria

Admission for ICD implant: Typically 1 night stay, same-day discharge may be feasible in selected patients.

Discharge Criteria

- Chest radiograph and ICD interrogation performed just prior to discharge to assess stable lead position and verify proper device function and programming
- Underlying heart disease should be stable.

COMPLICATIONS

- Device implant-related complications are rare but include infection, bleeding, vein thrombosis, pneumothorax, pericardial tamponade, stroke, myocardial infraction, lead dislodgement.
- Inappropriate device therapy (anti-tachycardia pacing or shock therapy) occurs in 15 –25% of patients. It is mostly due to sinus tachycardia or atrial arrhythmias with fast ventricular rates. Proper device programming can largely avoid such events.

PATIENT MONITORING

Routine (typically every 3 months) device interrogation, sooner if symptoms.

REFERENCES

1. AVID investigators. A comparison or antiarrhythmic drug therapy with implantable defibrillators in patients resuscitated from near fatal ventricular arrhythmias. *N Engl J Med* 1997;337:1576–1583.
2. Bardy GH, Lee KL, Mark DB, et al. Amiodarone or an implantable defibrillator for congestive heart failure. *N Engl J Med* 2005;352:225–237.
3. Moss AJ, Hall WJ, Cannom DS, et al. Improved survival with an implantable defibrillator in patients with coronary artery disease at high risk for ventricular arrhythmias. *N Engl J Med* 1996;335:1933–1940.
4. Moss AJ, Zareba W, Hall WJ, et al. Prophylactic implantation of a defibrillator in patients with myocardial infarction and reduced ejection fraction. *N Engl J Med* 2002;346:877–883.

AIDS AND THE HEART

Chandan Devireddy

BASICS

DESCRIPTION
Clinical syndrome caused by infection with human immunodeficiency virus (HIV)
- An enormous spectrum of clinical presentations secondary to primary effects of HIV, opportunistic infection, neoplastic transformation, and of therapeutic agents themselves
- Cardiac involvement also has been demonstrated with similar diversity in presentation.

EPIDEMIOLOGY
In the United States:
- 2 million estimated have been diagnosed with AIDS
- 1 million estimated HIV positive
- Globally:
  - Estimated 60–70 million adults infected with HIV
  - 13.9 million deaths since 1981

Incidence
Estimated incidence of dilated cardiomyopathy in HIV-positive patients: 1.59%/year

Prevalence
Prevalence of cardiac involvement uncertain: 5–70%

RISK FACTORS
- Homosexual sex
- Intravenous drug abuse
- High-risk sexual practice (unprotected sex, money for sex)
- Use of blood products (hemophiliacs), immigration from area of high prevalence (sub-Saharan Africa, South Asia)

ETIOLOGY
- HIV retrovirus possessing reverse transcriptase infecting CD4 T-helper lymphocytes; profound immunodeficiency resulting primarily from a progressive quantitative and qualitative deficiency of the subset of T lymphocytes referred to as helper or inducer T cells
- Etiology of cardiac disease is as broad as range of opportunistic infections in AIDS.
- HIV cardiomyopathy has been identified with causation secondary to HIV myocyte infection or autoimmune process.
- Multiple opportunistic agents also can involve the myocardium, pericardium, or endocardium. Heart failure can result secondary to other co-morbidities caused by AIDS.

DIAGNOSIS

SIGNS AND SYMPTOMS
- Congestive heart failure
  - Dyspnea, orthopnea, paroxysmal nocturnal dyspnea, lower extremity edema, tachycardia, pulmonary rales on auscultation, third heart sound (S_3), jugulovenous distention, ascites
- Pericardial involvement
  - Inspiratory chest pain, pain relieved by sitting up/leaning forward, pericardial friction rub on auscultation, distant heart sounds and absent PMI (point of maximal impulse) if prominent effusion, tamponade (elevated neck veins, pulsus paradoxus, shock)
- Myocarditis
  - Chest pain/pressure, shortness of breath, fever, may be asymptomatic

TESTS
- ECG (electrocardiogram): Nonspecific, but acute myocarditis may mimic ischemia/infarction
- Myocardial biopsy: Current evidence does not support utility.

Lab
- CD4+ T-cell count: Useful for prognosis (< increased opportunistic events)
- HIV-positive plasma viral RNA level: Useful for determining timing of and response to treatment
- Complete blood count (CBC)

Imaging
- Chest X-ray: Nonspecific, but look for cardiomegaly, pulmonary edema, or other source of pulmonary pathology.
- Echocardiography: Evaluate for impaired left ventricular shortening, left ventricular dilation, pericardial effusion, vegetation/thrombus, overall right and left ventricular function

DIFFERENTIAL DIAGNOSIS
Myocardial Involvement
- HIV-related infections
- Bacterial
  - Mycobacterium tuberculosis
  - Mycobacterium avium-intracellulare
- Fungal
  - *Cryptococcus neoformans*
  - *Aspergillus fumigatus*
  - *Candida albicans*
  - *Histoplasma capsulatum*
  - *Coccidioides immitis*
- Protozoan
  - *Toxoplasma gondii*
- Viral
  - Cytomegalovirus
  - HIV
  - Herpes simplex
  - Coxsackievirus

Noninflammatory Myocardial Disease
- Microvascular spasm
- Catecholamine excess
- Coronary artery disease
- Infection
- Toxic drug reaction (antiretroviral therapy)
- Malnutrition (particularly selenium deficiency)

Inflammatory Myocardial Disease
- Autoimmune process induced by HIV or other viruses, systemic lupus erythematosus
- Right Ventricular Hypertrophy or Dilation
- Pulmonary infections, pulmonary emboli
- Neoplastic
- Kaposi's sarcoma, lymphoma
- Pericardial Involvement
- Infectious
  - Bacterial: M. tuberculosis, M. avium-intracellulare, Nocardia
  - Viral: Herpes simplex
  - Fungal: Histoplasma capsulatum, Cryptococcus neoformans
  - Neoplastic: Kaposi's sarcoma, lymphoma

Endocardial Involvement
- Marantic endocarditis (nonbacterial thrombotic endocarditis)
- Infective endocarditis (bacterial, fungal)

TREATMENT

GENERAL MEASURES
Currently, a cure for HIV is nonexistent.
- Aggressive antiretroviral therapy to limit the onset of opportunistic pathogens and neoplasms
- Only supportive treatment exists for HIV-specific cardiomyopathy, similar to that of typical congestive heart failure.
- Maintain wide differential, including cardiac etiologies, for any presenting symptoms given the broad spectrum of offending pathology in HIV/AIDS.
- If other causative etiology is found, tailor therapy accordingly (e.g., removal of cardiotoxic agent, antiinfective therapy, dialysis, etc.)

MEDICATION (DRUGS)

First Line
- Antiretroviral therapy (typically two nucleoside analogs and protease inhibitor, although multiple alternative regimens exist and are in development)
- Antiinfectives should be targeted to etiologic agent if treatment is possible.
- Supportive therapy for congestive heart failure

SURGERY
- None. Significant concern exists regarding transmission to health care workers.
- Risk of transmission after documented parenteral exposure in health care setting is 0.29% per exposure.
- Physician may not ethically refuse to treat patient solely because he or she is HIV positive.

FOLLOW-UP

DISPOSITION
Admission Criteria
Specific to individual patient presentation

Discharge Criteria
Specific to individual patient presentation

PROGNOSIS
- Median time from primary HIV infection to the development of AIDS is approximately 10 years.
- Onset of congestive heart failure commonly marks onset of terminal stages of disease.
- Dilated cardiomyopathy on echocardiography is an independent adverse prognostic factor, with 50% mortality within 6 months.
- Patients with congestive heart failure may demonstrate initial symptomatic response to standard agents.

PATIENT MONITORING
- Plasma CD4+ and HIV-positive plasma RNA every 3–6 months
- Close monitoring for development of clinical manifestations of opportunistic processes

REFERENCES
1. Alexander RW, et al., eds. *Hurst's the Heart*, 9th ed. New York: McGraw-Hill, 1998.
2. Fauci AS, et al., eds. *Harrison's Principles of Internal Medicine*, 14th ed. New York: McGraw-Hill, 1998.
3. Kaul S, et al. Cardiac manifestations of acquired immune deficiency syndrome: A 1991 update. *Am Heart J*. 1991;122:535–544.
4. Lipshultz SE. Dilated cardiomyopathy in HIV-infected patients. *N Engl J Med*. 1998;339:1153–1155.

CODES
ICD9-CM
- 421.9 Acute endocarditis, unspecified
- 422.90 Acute myocarditis, unspecified
- 422.91 Idiopathic myocarditis
- 425.4 Idiopathic cardiomyopathy
- 423.9 Pericardial disease, unspecified

PATIENT TEACHING
Centers for Disease Control and Prevention website:http://www.cdc.gov/nchstp/hiv_aids/dhap.htm

ALCOHOL AND THE HEART

Deepak L. Bhatt
Gary S. Francis
Apur R. Kamdar

 BASICS

DESCRIPTION

Excess consumption of alcohol leads to a dilated cardiomyopathy.

- The definition of excess, however, is not clear.
- Varying levels of alcohol intake can lead to cardiomyopathy in a particular individual, including amounts considered "social drinking."
- Binge drinking also can lead to cardiomyopathy.
- Individuals with left ventricular dysfunction of any etiology should likely avoid consumption of even small quantities of alcohol, especially to avoid reverting to alcoholism.
- Complete abstinence and decreasing to moderate amounts of alcohol may achieve similar cardiac outcomes.
- Alcohol can even depress cardiac function in people with normal hearts.
- Although alcohol in small quantities may have a beneficial effect on the lipid profile and possibly even a protective effect against ischemic cardiomyopathy, the clinical significance of this is controversial.

EPIDEMIOLOGY

- Potentially one-third of cases of nonischemic cardiomyopathy are caused by alcohol.
- Found most often in men 30–55 years of age with a long history of heavy alcohol consumption, usually for at least a decade
- However, the prevalence of cardiomyopathy is similar among male and female alcoholics.
- Women may be more sensitive to toxic effects of alcohol on the heart.

RISK FACTORS

- Heavy alcohol use
- Malnutrition

Pregnancy Considerations

Contraindicated in someone who drinks heavily

Genetics

Definite genetic variability in individual susceptibility and in alcohol metabolizing enzymes

ETIOLOGY

- Alcohol can damage the heart due to a direct toxic effect on the myocardium.
- Acetaldehyde and acetate, metabolites of ethanol, are known to inhibit myocardial protein synthesis and disrupt the myofibrillary structure.
- In certain circumstances, iron or cobalt added to alcohol may predispose to cardiomyopathy.
- Certain individuals may have a genetic predisposition to develop alcoholic cardiomyopathy.
- Women may develop this disorder with a lower cumulative intake of alcohol compared with men.
- Nutritional deficiencies also may play a role.
- Thiamine deficiency, known to occur in alcoholics, can cause beriberi.

ASSOCIATED CONDITIONS

- Atrial fibrillation, either due to the cardiomyopathy or to alcohol ingestion, is a common initial presentation.
- Supraventricular arrhythmia
- Cirrhosis of the liver
- Pancreatitis
- Gastritis
- Myopathy
- Hypertension
- Subarachnoid hemorrhage
- Thiamine and folate deficiency

 DIAGNOSIS

SIGNS AND SYMPTOMS

- Fatigue
- Weakness, especially muscle weakness
- Exertional dyspnea
- Orthopnea
- Paroxysmal nocturnal dyspnea
- JVD (jugulovenous distension)
- Edema
- Hypertension
- Narrow pulse pressure
- S3 (third heart sound)
- S4 (fourth heart sound)
- MR (mitral regurgitation), TR murmurs (tricuspid regurgitation)
- Hepatomegaly (either from right-sided failure or alcoholism)
- Telangiectasia
- Spider angiomata

TESTS

Myopathy is often present on skeletal muscle biopsy.

Lab

ECG (electrocardiogram) may show atrial arrhythmia, ectopy, or bundle branch block.

- QT interval may be prolonged.
- Poor R-wave progression and hypertrophy also may be seen.

Imaging

- Chest x-ray may show cardiomegaly and pulmonary congestion.
- Echocardiography shows biatrial and biventricular dilatation.
- Both systolic and diastolic dysfunction are present.
- Mitral and tricuspid regurgitation may be present.

Pathologic Findings

Nonspecific interstitial fibrosis, myocyte hypertrophy

DIFFERENTIAL DIAGNOSIS

Other causes of dilated cardiomyopathy

TREATMENT

GENERAL MEASURES
- Alcohol cessation or significant reduction of intake is recommended.
- Concomitant tobacco abuse, often present, also should be discouraged.
  - Hypophosphatemia, hypokalemia, and hypomagnesemia also may be present and should be corrected.

 MEDICATION (DRUGS)

Intravenous thiamine administration is standard.

SURGERY
Heart transplantation would not be considered unless a period of abstinence could be shown.

 FOLLOW-UP

DISPOSITION
Admission Criteria
- As for heart failure of any etiology
- Hospitalization (and observed alcohol cessation) is particularly useful.

PROGNOSIS
- With complete abstinence or reduction to moderate levels of alcohol use, the cardiomyopathy may partially, or even completely, resolve.
- The majority of improvement occurs in the first several months of abstinence.
- Continued, sometimes covert, drinking makes it difficult to gauge the true effect of abstinence.
- Continued heavy alcohol abuse may lead to myocardial failure and death.
- An increased risk of sudden death, even in the absence of overt cardiac dysfunction

PATIENT MONITORING
- Standard for heart failure of any cause
- Observe for any clues that the patient has started drinking again.

REFERENCES
1. Lee WK, Regan TJ. Alcoholic cardiomyopathy: is it dose-dependent? *Congest Heart Fail*. 2002;8: 303–306.
2. Piano MR. Alcohol and heart failure. *J Card Fail*. 2002;8:239–246.
3. Zipes DP. *Braunwald's Heart Disease: A Textbook of Cardiovascular Medicine*, 7th ed., 2005.

CODES
ICD9-CM
- 428.0 Failure, heart, congestive
- 425.5 Alcoholic cardiomyopathy

SELECTED REFERENCES
1. Walsh CR, Larson MG, Evans JC, et al: Alcohol consumption and risk for congestive heart failure in the Framingham Heart Study. *Ann Intern Med*. 2002;136:181.
2. Topol EJ, ed. *Textbook of Cardiovascular Medicine*. Philadelphia: Lippincott Williams & Wilkins, 2002.
3. Rodkey SM, Ratliff NB, Young JB. Cardiomyopathy and myocardial failure. In: Topol EJ, ed. *Comprehensive Ccardiovascular Medicine*. Philadelphia: Lippincott Williams & Wilkins, 1998:2610–2611.
4. Fernandez-Sola J, Estruch R, Nicolas JM, et al. Comparison of alcoholic cardiomyopathy in women versus men. *Am J Cardiol*. 1997;80:481–485.
5. McKenna CJ, Codd MB, McCann HA, et al. Alcohol consumption and idiopathic dilated cardiomyopathy: A case control study. *Am Heart J*. 1998;135:833–837.
6. Jacob AJ, McLaren KM, Boon NA. Effects of abstinence on alcoholic heart muscle disease. *Am J Cardiol*. 1991;68:805–807.
7. Regan TJ. Alcohol and the cardiovascular system. *JAMA* 1990;264:377–381.
8. Reeves WC, Nanda NC, Gramiak R. Echocardiography in chronic alcoholics following prolonged periods of abstinence. *Am Heart J*. 1978;95:578–583.

PATIENT TEACHING
The need for abstinence or significant reduction in alcohol use must be stressed.

AMYLOID HEART DISEASE

Apur R. Kamdar
Deepak L. Bhatt
Gary S. Francis

 ## BASICS

DESCRIPTION
Deposition of amyloid proteins into the myocardium leads to a restrictive cardiomyopathy.

EPIDEMIOLOGY
- Familial amyloidosis is transmitted via an autosomal-dominant mode of inheritance and can lead to cardiomyopathy in 25% of patients.
- A certain type of amyloidosis, called trans-thyretin (isoleucine 122), is more prevalent among African Americans.

RISK FACTORS
Multiple myeloma

Pregnancy Considerations
Poorly tolerated, as with other restrictive cardiomyopathies

PATHOPHYSIOLOGY
Restrictive cardiomyopathy develops as normal myocardium and is replaced by amyloid tissue. Over time, the myocardium becomes rubbery and nonpliant.

ETIOLOGY
- Primary amyloidosis is caused by excess production of immunoglobulin light chain (called AL), whereas secondary amyloidosis is caused by production of a protein (called AA).
- Cardiac involvement is much more common in the primary form than in the secondary form.
- Familial and senile types of amyloidosis are both due to deposition of a protein called transthyretin (also called prealbumin) and also frequently involve the heart.

ASSOCIATED CONDITIONS
- Primary amyloidosis is often associated with multiple myeloma. Renal involvement is common.
- Peripheral and autonomic neuropathy
- Systemic and pulmonary emboli
- Malabsorption

DIAGNOSIS

SIGNS AND SYMPTOMS
- Orthostatic hypotension
- Right-sided heart failure
- Jugulovenous distension
- Hepatomegaly
- Splenomegaly
- Edema
- S3 (third heart sound)
- Mitral and tricuspid valve regurgitation
- Narrow pulse pressure
- Macroglossia
- Angina
- Neuropathy

TESTS
- Chest X-ray
  - May show cardiomegaly, pleural effusions, and pulmonary congestion
- Echocardiography with Doppler imaging
  - Massive hypertrophy, with small left and right ventricular cavities
  - The hypertrophied walls have a sparkling pattern due to increased echogenicity.
  - Both atria are usually dilated, with thickening of the atrioventricular valves.
  - Valvular regurgitation, and less commonly, stenosis, can occur.
  - A small pericardial effusion is often present.
  - Abnormal diastolic function, with variable degrees of systolic dysfunction, is present.
  - Thrombus may be seen in either the atria or ventricles.
- Doppler measurements are able to predict cardiac death more reliably than is two-dimensional echocardiography.

Lab
- The electrocardiogram (ECG) classically shows low voltage, despite echocardiographic hypertrophy; this is an important differentiating feature from other causes of left ventricular hypertrophy and is present in about half of cases of cardiac-amyloid.
- Q waves may be present.
- Atrial fibrillation is common.
- PVCs (premature ventricular contractions) and ventricular arrhythmias may be seen.
- Sick sinus syndrome and conduction block may be observed.
- Serum and urine protein electrophoresis often can be used to detect a monoclonal protein in primary amyloidosis.
- Endomyocardial biopsy remains the gold standard for diagnosis; however, extracardiac biopsy may be sufficient for diagnosis with the right clinical picture.

Imaging
- Chest X-ray
  - May show cardiomegaly, pleural effusions, and pulmonary congestion
- Echocardiography with Doppler imaging
  - Massive hypertrophy, with small left and right ventricular cavities
  - The hypertrophied walls have a sparkling pattern due to increased echogenicity.
  - Both atria are usually dilated, with thickening of the atrioventricular valves.
  - Valvular regurgitation, and less commonly, stenosis, can occur.
  - A small pericardial effusion is often present.
  - Abnormal diastolic function, with variable degrees of systolic dysfunction, is present.
  - Thrombus may be seen in either the atria or ventricles.
- Doppler measurements are able to predict cardiac death more reliably than two-dimensional echocardiography.

Pathologic Findings
- Congo red staining produces apple-green birefringence under polarized light.
- The characteristic fibrillar pattern of the amyloid deposits can be seen by electron microscopy.

DIFFERENTIAL DIAGNOSIS
Other causes of restrictive cardiomyopathy

TREATMENT

GENERAL MEASURES
- Treatment of any underlying disease process, such as multiple myeloma, may help the heart.
- Salt restriction

MEDICATION (DRUGS)

- Digitalis toxicity can occur at much lower doses than one would expect because it is bound extracellularly by amyloid fibrils; if used, caution must be exercised.
- Diuretics can be useful for symptom control, but can precipitate hypotension.
- Calcium channel blockers, by binding to amyloid fibrils, can lead to impaired cardiac contractility and hypotension.
- Angiotensin-converting enzyme (ACE) can be useful, but would not be prudent if there is preexisting orthostatic hypotension.
- Coumadin is used for treatment of thrombi; bleeding due to vessel fragility can be problematic.
- Intravenous melphalan has been used to treat primary amyloidosis as well as the associated cardiomyopathy.

SURGERY
- Amyloid is generally considered a contraindication to heart transplantation.
- Cardiac transplantation has been used, but results have not been good due to recurrence of amyloid.
- In the familial form, combined heart and liver transplantation has been performed because liver transplantation cures the disorder.
- Pacemakers are indicated for advanced heart block.

FOLLOW-UP

DISPOSITION
Admission Criteria
As for other etiologies of heart failure

Discharge Criteria
As for other etiologies of heart failure

PROGNOSIS
- Progressive heart failure occurs.
- Heart failure, especially in primary amyloidosis, is associated with a poor short-term prognosis. In AL amyloidosis, the median survival with symptoms of congestive heart failure (CHF) is only 6 months.
- Sudden death can occur as a result of arrhythmias or from infiltration of the conduction system.

PATIENT MONITORING
As for other etiologies of heart failure

REFERENCES
1. Falk RH. Diagnosis and management of cardiac amyloidoses. *Circulation*. 2005;112:2047–2060.
2. Topol EJ, ed. *Textbook of Cardiovascular Medicine*. Philadelphia: Lippincott Williams & Wilkins, 2002.
3. Zipes DP. *Braunwald's Heart Disease: A Textbook of Cardiovascular Medicine*, 7th ed., 2005.
4. Reisinger J, Dubrey SW, Lavalley M, et al. Electrophysiologic abnormalities in AL (primary) amyloidosis with cardiac involvement. *J Am Coll Cardiol*. 1997;30:1046–1051.
5. Kashyap K, Hosenpud J. Cardiac amyloidosis. *Curr Treatment Options Cardiovasc Med*. 1999;1:209–217.
6. McCarthy RE, Kasper EK. A review of the amyloidoses that infiltrate the heart. *Clin Cardiol*. 1998;21:547–552.
7. Klein AL, Hatle LK, Taliercio CP, et al. Prognostic significance of Doppler measures of diastolic function in cardiac amyloidosis: A Doppler echocardiography study. *Circulation*. 1991;83:808–816.

CODES
ICD9-CM
- 428.0 Failure, heart, congestive
- 277.3 [425.7] Amyloidosis, heart

PATIENT TEACHING
As for other etiologies of heart failure

ANEMIA AND THE HEART

Deepak L. Bhatt
Gary S. Francis
Apur R. Kamdar

 BASICS

DESCRIPTION
- Chronically low hemoglobin (<3–4 g/dL) can lead to high-output heart failure.
- A postulated mechanism is that hemoglobin normally degrades nitric oxide.
- Anemia leads to elevated levels of nitric oxide with resultant vasodilation.
- Lower viscosity is another potential mechanism leading to elevated cardiac output.
- Neurohormonal activation can be triggered by the low blood pressure and lead to sodium and water retention.
- Acute blood loss does not lead to heart failure.

EPIDEMIOLOGY
- Anemia is common among hospitalized patients.
- Anemia as an isolated cause of heart failure is rare in the United States.
- In the developing world, anemia is more common due to conditions such as hookworm infection.

RISK FACTORS
Poor nutrition (iron, folate, or vitamin B_{12} deficiency)

Pregnancy Considerations
Severe degrees of anemia would need to be corrected before pregnancy to reduce risks to both mother and fetus.

ETIOLOGY
- Any cause of profound, chronic anemia
- Hookworm infection (and subsequent chronic blood loss)
- Sickle cell disorder
- Thalassemia

ASSOCIATED CONDITIONS
- Pericarditis is common in thalassemia.
- Pulmonary infarction, stroke in sickle cell anemia

 DIAGNOSIS

SIGNS AND SYMPTOMS
- Pale conjunctivae
- Fatigue
- Exertional chest pain, dyspnea
- S3 (third heart sound)
- S4 (fourth heart sound)
- Systolic and diastolic flow murmurs
- Duroziez sign
- Quincke pulse
- Edema

TESTS
Right-heart catheterization reveals increased cardiac output and low systemic vascular resistance.

Lab
- Iron, folate, or vitamin B12 levels may be low.
- The electrocardiogram (ECG) may show ischemic changes with profound anemia.
- Left ventricular hypertrophy also may be present. In sickle cell anemia right ventricular hypertrophy may occur.

Imaging
- Chest X-ray shows cardiomegaly.
- Echocardiography shows a dilated ventricle with thickened walls.

DIFFERENTIAL DIAGNOSIS
Other causes of high-output heart failure

 TREATMENT

GENERAL MEASURES
- Transfusion may be necessary.
  - If performed, red blood cells should be transfused slowly and given with diuretic agents.
- Chelation therapy in cases of iron overload

MEDICATION (DRUGS)

Iron, folate, or vitamin B_{12}, as appropriate

SURGERY

Splenectomy is useful in patients with thalassemia.

FOLLOW-UP

DISPOSITION

Admission Criteria
As for heart failure of any etiology

Discharge Criteria
As for heart failure of any etiology

PATIENT MONITORING
Follow blood counts.

REFERENCES

1. Amsterdam PB. Hematologic and oncologic disorders and the heart. In: Topol EJ, ed. *Comprehensive Cardiovascular Medicine,* Philadelphia: Lippincott Williams & Wilkins, 1998:970–974.
2. Anand IS, Chandrashekhar Y, Ferrari R, et al. Pathogenesis of edema in chronic severe anemia: studies of body water and sodium, renal function, hemodynamic variables, and plasma hormones. *Br Heart J.* 1993;70:357–362.
3. Shulman LN, Braunwald E, Rosenthal DS. Hematological–oncological disorders and heart disease. In: Braunwald E, ed. *Heart Disease: A Textbook of Cardiovascular Medicine,* 5th ed. Philadelphia: WB Saunders, 1997:1786–1792.
4. Topol EJ, ed. *Textbook of Cardiovascular Medicine.* Philadelphia: Lippincott Williams & Wilkins, 2002.
5. Zipes DP. *Braunwald's Heart Disease: A Textbook of Cardiovascular Medicine,* 7th ed., 2005.

CODES

ICD9-CM
428.0 Failure, heart, congestive

PATIENT TEACHING
Watch for signs of blood loss.

AORTIC ANEURYSM

Duy Nguyen
Helene Glassberg

 BASICS

DESCRIPTION

Localized dilation of the aorta with a diameter at least 1.5 times normal
- Morphologically, fusiform (symmetrical dilation) or saccular (localized outpouching)
- The majority of aortic aneurysms are located in the abdominal aorta (abdominal aortic aneurysms [AAAs]).
- Thoracic aortic aneurysms (TAAs) are classified according to location:
  - Aortic root/ascending aorta (most frequent)
  - Transverse aortic arch
  - Traumatic, usually distal to left subclavian artery
  - Descending thoracic aorta
  - Thoracoabdominal aorta

EPIDEMIOLOGY

Incidence
- Increases rapidly after 55 years of age in men and 70 years in women
- The incidence of aortic aneurysms has increased two- to threefold over the last few decades.

Prevalence
- Present in 4–9% of persons older than 60, although most are not clinically significant and have a diameter <3.5 cm.
- Sex
  - Male–female ratio 4–5:1

RISK FACTORS
- Increased age
- Atherosclerotic disease
- Hypertension
- Hypercholesterolemia
- Smoking
- Aortic dissection
- Connective tissue disorders

ALERT

Pregnancy Considerations
When aneurysms present during pregnancy, they typically do so with rupture and shock; the mortality rate is 65%.

PATHOPHYSIOLOGY
- Unclear in most patients.
- Uncertain whether atherosclerosis is a primary cause or a secondary consequence.
- Defects in and destruction of structural proteins in the aortic wall are implicated.
- Inflammation may play a role as well.

ETIOLOGY
- AAAs
  - Atherosclerosis
  - Genetic predisposition: those with a family history of AAA have a 30% increased risk of developing an AAA.
- TAAs
  - Atherosclerosis (arch, descending aorta)
  - Connective tissue disorder or cystic medial necrosis: Most commonly Marfan syndrome (ascending aorta), also Ehlers-Danlos syndrome
  - Inflammatory disease: Granulomatous, giant cell arteritis, Takayasu arteritis
  - Syphilis (now rare)
  - Aortic dissection
  - Aortic trauma
  - Infectious: often secondary to direct spread from aortic valve bacterial endocarditis

ASSOCIATED CONDITIONS
- Aortic dissection
- Aortic rupture
- Annuloaortic ectasia
  - A subset of patients with TAA have idiopathic dilatation of the proximal aorta and aortic annulus leading to pure aortic regurgitation

 DIAGNOSIS

SIGNS AND SYMPTOMS

Abdominal Aortic Aneurysms
- Majority are asymptomatic, often discovered incidentally.
- Most common symptoms:
  - Hypogastric pain
  - Lower back pain
- Most common signs:
  - Palpable, pulsatile abdominal mass (occasionally tender)
  - Abdominal bruit
  - Diminished femoral/distal pulses

Thoracic Aortic Aneurysms
- 40% are asymptomatic (including traumatic thoracic aneurysms, in which patients often remain asymptomatic for 10–20 years)
- Most common symptoms:
  - Chest pain/back pain due to compression of intrathoracic structures or bony erosion
  - Wheezing, cough, dyspnea (may be positional) due to tracheal compression
  - Hemoptysis, recurrent pneumonitis
  - Hoarseness due to compression of the recurrent laryngeal nerve
  - Dyspnea, orthopnea, paroxysmal nocturnal dyspnea, edema due to congestive heart failure from aortic regurgitation and left ventricular failure
  - Angina/myocardial infarction due to local compression of coronary arteries
  - Thromboembolism causing stroke, lower extremity ischemia, renal infarction, mesenteric ischemia
  - Local mass effect precipitating superior vena cava syndrome
  - Dysphagia due to esophageal compression

- Signs
  - Tracheal deviation, aortic regurgitation murmur with or without peripheral manifestations, wide pulse pressure.
  - Rarely, a left paravertebral bruit will be heard with a descending aortic aneurysm

Physical Exam
Assess for asymmetric pulses or blood pressures in all extremities.

TESTS

Imaging
- Chest x-ray
  - Frequently a TAA is initially identified as an incidental finding on chest x-ray; it appears as widening of the mediastinal silhouette, dilatation of the ascending aorta, enlargement of the aortic knob, or tracheal deviation.
- Abdominal ultrasonography
  - Most practical screening method
  - Nearly 100% sensitive for AAA
  - Can accurately define size to within ±0.3 cm
  - Unable to define associated mesenteric and renal arterial anatomy or cephalad or pelvic extent of disease
- Computed tomography (CT)
  - Extremely accurate for diagnosis and sizing to within ±0.2 cm
  - Better defines aneurysm and local anatomy than ultrasonography
  - More expensive, less available than ultrasonography, requires intravenous contrast
  - Can differentiate TAA from other lung parenchymal/mediastinal masses
- Aortography
  - Has long been the standard preoperative imaging technique; however, its routine use in evaluation of AAA is under debate
  - Excellent definition of extent of the aneurysm and evaluation of aortic root involvement
  - May underestimate the size of the aneurysm due to the presence of mural thrombus
- Magnetic resonance angiography (MRA)
  - Alternative to aortography for preoperative evaluation
  - Useful in defining aortic branch vessel anatomy and extent of disease; better than CT to evaluate aortic root.
  - Transthoracic echocardiography
  - Can image aortic root but limited examination of other thoracic aortic segments.
- Transesophageal echocardiography
  - Much more accurate than transthoracic echocardiography in assessing thoracic aorta; commonly used for detection of aortic dissection.

DIFFERENTIAL DIAGNOSIS
- In AAAs, renal colic, musculoskeletal pain, GI disorders
- In TAAs, congestive heart failure from other causes, acute coronary syndromes, musculoskeletal back pain, primary lung process, bronchogenic carcinoma, mediastinal tumor

TREATMENT

GENERAL MEASURES

- Risk factor modification, including cholesterol lowering, smoking cessation, and treatment of hypertension
- Routine ultrasonography or CT scan yearly to detect either rapid expansion (more than 0.5 cm expansion within 6-month interval) or increase in diameter to 5.0 cm or larger, either of which is an indication for surgery; consider follow-up scan every 3–6 months for higher risk patients (e.g., those with saccular aneurysms, Marfan syndrome)
- Traumatic aneurysms that have been present and are asymptomatic >10 years after injury may be periodically observed versus elective excision.

MEDICATION (DRUGS)

- β-Blockers reduce the risk of aneurysm expansion and rupture. Once β blockers are maximized, persistent hypertension should be controlled with other medications to bring systolic blood pressure to a range of 105–120 mm Hg.
- The long-term outcome of medical management of TAAs has not been examined, however, β-blocker treatment in patients with Marfan syndrome significantly slows the rate of aortic dilation, reduces clinical end points (death, aortic dissection, aortic regurgitation, aortic root >6 cm), and decreases mortality.

SURGERY

Size of AAA is the primary indicator for repair of asymptomatic aneurysms; rapid AAA expansion is another indication.

- Surgery is indicated for symptoms, AAA diameter size >5.5 cm, or if AAA increases >0.5 cm in 6-month interval.
- For asymptomatic AAA with diameter 4–5.5 cm, options include careful surveillance with abdominal ultrasound or surgery, particularly if female gender (who rupture at smaller sizes), strong family history, or high risk features.
- Approximately half of all perioperative deaths from aneurysm repair are due to myocardial infarction; therefore, preoperative cardiac risk assessment is recommended and risk reduction strategies should be considered.

- In general, unless the aneurysm is quite small, prompt excision should be considered for TAAs; most recommend elective surgery for ascending TAAs 5.5–6 cm, descending TAAs 6–7 cm, and 7.0 cm or larger in patients at high operative risk. Surgical indications for smaller TAAs include rapid rate of expansion, associated significant aortic regurgitation, or the presence of aneurysm-related symptoms.
- In patients with Marfan syndrome, bicuspid aortic valve, or familial syndromes, surgery should be considered at 4.5–5.0 cm given the higher risk of dissection and rupture.
- Surgical repair of AAAs consists of resection of the aneurysm and insertion of a synthetic prosthetic graft.
- Endovascular repair of AAA is a possible alternative to surgical repair; however, its precise role, in terms of cost effectiveness and morbidity/mortality benefits compared to surgery, remains to be defined; the use of a transluminally placed endovascular stent graft may be an alternative approach to the surgical management of descending TAAs.
- TAAs are generally resected and replaced with an appropriately sized prosthetic sleeve; when significant aortic regurgitation is present in ascending TAAs, either a separate valve or composite graft with a prosthetic valve sewn into one end is used.

FOLLOW-UP

PROGNOSIS

- Abdominal aortic aneurysms 4–4.9 cm have a 0–5% annual risk of rupture; 5–5.9 cm have a 3–15% annual risk, 6–6.9 cm have a 10–20% annual risk, and >7 cm AAAs have a 20–50% annual risk. AAA rupture carries >80% mortality. Mean rate of AAA expansion is approximately 0.4 cm/year but is variable and unpredictable across population.
- Survival following AAA repair has been reported as 1-, 5-, and 10-year survival rates of 93%, 63%, and 40%, respectively. Operative mortality is 4–6% overall and is as low as 2% in low risk patients.
- Those with concomitant coronary artery disease have a 10% lower rate of survival than those without coronary artery disease.

- Mean rate of rupture or dissection is <2% for TAAs <5 cm diameter, 3% for TAAs 5–5.9 cm, but increases sharply to 7% for TAAs >6 cm. Mean rate of growth for all TAAs is 0.1 cm/year.
- Rupture occurs in 32–68% of patients with TAAs not treated with surgery; mortality rate is 76% at 24 hours after rupture.
- Elective surgical repair of ascending and descending TAAs has an 86–97% early survival rate.

COMPLICATIONS

- The incidence of neurologic injury after aortic arch repair is 0–15%; incidence of paraplegia with descending TAA repair ranges from 0–17%, and is 5–6% in most up-to-date series.
- Most common causes of early postoperative death are myocardial infarction, congestive heart failure, stroke, renal failure, hemorrhage, respiratory failure, and sepsis.

REFERENCES

1. Isselbacher EM. Diseases of the aorta. In: Braunwald E, ed. *Heart Disease*, 7th ed. Philadelphia: WB Saunders, 2005:1403–1435.
2. Safi HC, Miller CC. Thoracic vasculature. In: Brunicardi FC, et al. *Schwartz's Principles of Surgery*, 8th ed. New York: McGraw-Hill, 2004:1313–1338.
3. Zarins CK, Hill BB, Wolf YG. Aneurysmal vascular disease. In: Brunicardi FC, et al. *Schwartz's Principles of Surgery*, 8th ed. New York: McGraw-Hill, 2004:1357–1372.

CODES

ICD9-CM

- 441.9 Aortic aneurysm (unspecified)
- 441.4 Abdominal aortic aneurysm (unspecified)
- 441.2 Thoracic aortic aneurysm (unspecified)

PATIENT TEACHING

- Screening with ultrasonography is indicated for relatives of patients with AAAs, because the estimated relative risk for first degree relatives of affected individuals is 11.6 times greater than for non–first-degree relatives.
- Compliance with antihypertensive management and smoking cessation are critical.

ANGINA WITH NORMAL CORONARY ARTERIES

Michele D. Voeltz
Nanette K. Wenger

 BASICS

DESCRIPTION

Syndrome X is a heterogeneous syndrome, characterized by both typical and atypical anginal chest pain with exertion, ST-segment depression on exercise testing, and normal coronary arteries at angiography, most often due to dysfunction of the coronary microvasculature, caused by endothelial dysfunction and abnormal pain perception with enhanced sensitivity to intracardiac pain.

EPIDEMIOLOGY

- May occur in up to 30% of patients undergoing coronary angiography for anginal chest pain
- Predominant sex: Females > Males
- Predominant age: Mean age at onset 49

Incidence

Increasing since discovered in 1973

RISK FACTORS

- Female sex
- Postmenopausal status
- Hypertension
- Hyperlipidemia
- Diabetes mellitus
- Smoking

PATHOPHYSIOLOGY

Coronary microvascular dysfunction leading to myocardial ischemia and angina

ETIOLOGY

- Imbalance in vasodilator and vasoconstrictor forces produced by the endothelium:
  - Abnormal coronary flow reserve elevated endothelin-1 (ET-1) levels and reduced nitric oxide (NO) levels
  - Abnormal autonomic control with increased sympathetic activation
  - Increased levels of serum C-reactive protein (CRP), a marker of inflammation
- Estrogen deficiency in postmenopausal female patients
- Increased platelet aggregability
- Decreased threshold for pain perception, also known as the "sensitive heart syndrome"

ASSOCIATED CONDITIONS

30% of patients with Syndrome X have a treatable psychiatric disorder

 DIAGNOSIS

SIGNS AND SYMPTOMS

- Symptoms: Typical or atypical anginal chest pain with normal epicardial coronary arteries; can occur with exercise or at rest
- Signs: Exercise electrocardiogram (ECG) with ST-segment depression typical of myocardial ischemia; rare ST-segment elevation; may have abnormal myocardial perfusion imaging; left ventricular (LV) function usually normal at rest and with stress

TESTS

Must rule out coronary atherosclerotic heart disease with cardiac catheterization prior to diagnosis

Diagnostic Procedures/Surgery

- Exercise ECG testing: May reveal ST-segment depression with exercise and at rest
- Myocardial perfusion imaging: Often abnormal
- Cardiac magnetic resonance imaging (MRI): May demonstrate subendocardial hypoperfusion during intravenous (IV) adenosine administration suggestive of ischemia
- Coronary angiography with intravenous or intracoronary ergonovine challenge to evaluate for epicardial vasospasm
- Repeat exercise testing after nitrate administration (administration of short-acting nitrate may worsen Syndrome X, in contrast to Prinzmetal and coronary atherosclerotic heart disease (CASHD), which often improve)
- Other testing (gastrointestinal [GI], musculoskeletal, psychiatric) as appropriate to evaluate noncardiac causes of chest pain

DIFFERENTIAL DIAGNOSIS

- Coronary atherosclerotic heart disease
- Prinzmetal angina due to epicardial coronary vasospasm
- Noncardiac chest pain
  - GI: Esophageal dysmotility, gastroesophageal reflux disease, esophageal mass, gastric mass
  - Pulmonary: Bronchitis, pulmonary embolism
  - Musculoskeletal: Costochondritis, muscular chest pain, fibromyalgia

 TREATMENT

GENERAL MEASURES

- AHA/ACC guidelines for management
  - Class I: Reassurance, medical therapy, risk factor reduction
  - Class IIb: Intravascular ultrasound to evaluate for missed coronary stenosis, coronary angiography with provocative testing
  - Class III: Medical therapy for patients with noncardiac causes of chest pain
- Exercise training may decrease symptoms, increase exercise capacity, and improve endothelial function
- Medical therapy, psychiatric treatment, and physical training should be used together to reduce symptoms and improve quality of life

 MEDICATION (DRUGS)

- Goal of pharmacologic therapy is to decrease symptoms
- Hormone replacement therapy, although used in the past because of favorable effect on endothelial function, not currently recommended due to increased cardiovascular and other risks

First Line

- Calcium channel blocking agents
  - Effective in reducing frequency and severity of angina and improving exercise tolerance
- β-Blocking agents
  - May be most effective in patients with increased sympathetic activation
- Angiotensin converting enzyme (ACE) inhibitors
  - Have favorable effects on endothelial function, vascular remodeling, and sympathetic activity
- Hydroxymethylglutaryl coenzyme A (HMG-CoA) reductase inhibitors
  - Improves endothelial function and exercise stress test responses
- Nitrates and nicorandil
  - No large randomized studies of these agents in patients with angina and normal coronary arteries
  - Effective in up to 50% of patients with Syndrome X
- Trimetazidine
  - Vasodilator, which acts at cellular level
  - Improved time to ST-segment depression in patients with Syndrome X

Second Line
- Imipramine
  - May improve the decreased pain perception threshold
- Aminophylline
  - May favorably effect exercise-induced angina and increase exercise tolerance through adenosine antagonism

INTERVENTION
- Transcutaneous electrical nerve stimulation (TENS)
  - Stimulation of A-B fibers via the skin, indirectly delivering low-voltage electrical impulses to the spinal cord
  - May reduce myocardial oxygen demand
- Spinal cord stimulation
  - Direct stimulation of the spinal cord via an electrode percutaneously placed into the epidural space
  - May improve exercise tolerance and ECG findings

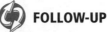 **FOLLOW-UP**

PROGNOSIS
- Excellent prognosis, mortality similar to age- and sex-matched healthy controls
- Markedly better survival than seen in patients with coronary atherosclerotic heart disease
- In patients with ejection fraction of $\geq 50\%$, 7-year survival rate 96% with normal coronary angiogram

REFERENCES
1. Kaski JC, Aldama G, Cosin-Sales J. Cardiac syndrome X. *Am J Cardiovasc Drugs.* 2004;4:179–194.
2. Kemp HG, Kronmal RA, Vlietstra RE, et al. 7-year survival of patients with normal or near-normal coronary arteriograms: A CASS registry study. *J Am Coll Cardiol.* 1986;7:479–483.
3. Morrow DA, Gersh BJ, Braunwald EJ. Chest pain with normal coronary arteriogram. In: Zipes DP, Libby P, Bonow RO, Braunwald E, eds. *Braunwald's Heart Disease,* 7th ed. St. Louis: WB Saunders, 2005:1328–1329.
4. Mirza MA. Angina like pain and normal coronary arteries. *Postgrad Med online.* 2005;117:41–46.
5. Crea F, Lanza GA. Angina pectoris and normal coronary arteries: cardiac syndrome X. *Heart.* 2004;90:457–463.
6. Panting JR, Gatehouse PD, Yang GZ, et al. Abnormal subendocardial perfusion in cardiac syndrome X detected by cardiovascular magnetic resonance imaging. *N Engl J Med.* 2002;346:1948–1953.

CODES
ICD9-CM
413.9 Cardiac Syndrome X

PATIENT TEACHING
- Internet resources
  - NHLBI http://www.NHLBI.nih.gov
  - AHA http://www.americanheart.org

ANGINA, PRINZMETAL'S VARIANT ANGINA

John A. Ternay
Brenda J. Hott*
Nanette K. Wenger

 ## BASICS

DESCRIPTION
Variant angina, described in the 1930s, is characterized by angina at rest associated with spontaneous transient ST-segment elevation on electrocardiogram (ECG).
- Exercise tolerance is preserved.
- ST segments rapidly return to baseline with relief of chest discomfort.
- Circadian variation of symptoms
- Symptoms often occur in the early morning hours.
- Most commonly occurs in the right coronary artery, but can occur in the left, and, less commonly, in coronary artery bypass grafts.
- Synonym(s): Prinzmetals angina
- System(s) Affected: Cardiovascular

EPIDEMIOLOGY
- More often occurs in younger patients than does exertional angina
- Average age 48
- Affects women more than men

Incidence
- Exact incidence unknown
- Overall less common than exertional angina

Prevalence
Exact prevalence unknown

RISK FACTORS
- Smoking most important risk factor
- Cocaine may precipitate vasospasm.
- Patients with pure vasospasm younger than patients with exertional angina (average age 48), more likely to be female
- Traditional coronary disease risk factors may be lacking.

Genetics
- Increased prevalence in certain geographic locations, including Canada, Italy, and Japan.
- Recent evidence suggests that specific mutations in the eNOS gene are found with significantly greater incidence in patients with variant angina versus controls.

PATHOPHYSIOLOGY
- Several mechanisms implicated
  - Abnormalities in cardiac sympathetic tone
  - Endothelial dysfunction

ETIOLOGY
- Transient coronary artery spasm, usually focal, with normal coronary anatomy or at site of atherosclerotic plaque coronary spasm may be contributing factor in development, progression of atherosclerosis.
- Vasospasm superimposed on a fixed obstructive coronary heart disease (CHD) lesion has worse prognosis
- IVUS (intravascular ultrasound) often demonstrates atherosclerotic plaque at site of spasm even in angiographically normal coronary arteries
- Thrombus may form at the site of vasospasm.

ASSOCIATED CONDITIONS
- Migraine headaches
- Raynaud phenomenon
- Ocular spasm
- Aspirin-induced asthma
- Hypomagnesemia
- Hyperinsulinemia
- Hyperthyroidism
- Churg-Strauss syndrome

 ## DIAGNOSIS

SIGNS AND SYMPTOMS
- Retrosternal discomfort that may radiate to arms, neck, or jaw usually occurs at rest, often in early morning hours.
- Exercise capacity preserved
- Physical examination usually normal
- Arrhythmia
  - Typically atrioventricular (AV) block is seen with right coronary involvement and ventricular arrhythmias with left coronary involvement.

History
- Seek provocative factor
  - Tobacco use
  - Cocaine use
  - Relationship to exercise
  - Hyperventilation

Physical Exam
- Often unremarkable
- A fourth heart sound can be present indicating ischemia.
- Congestive heart failure can be seen in cases of significant ischemia with resultant left ventricular dysfunction or ischemic mitral regurgitation.

TESTS
- ECG during pain and after relief of pain
- Ambulatory ECG monitoring helpful in establishing diagnosis
- Exercise testing may provoke angina, ST elevation.
- Patients with positive hyperventilation test more likely to have frequency of attacks, multivessel spasm, AV block, ventricular tachycardia

Imaging
- Coronary angiography recommended
- Consider provocative testing with ergonovine, which produces focal spasm in approximately 90% of patients with variant angina.

ALERT
Refractory vasospasm leading to malignant arrhythmia, myocardial infarction, and death can occur with ergonovine challenge. Such testing is recommended only in those with recurrent ischemic-type chest pain, no obstructive disease on coronary angiography, and a suspicion of vasospasm. If the diagnosis is confirmed clinically, provocative testing need not be performed.

Negative ergonovine test result makes diagnosis unlikely.

Pathologic Findings
Histologic examination of coronary artery plaques revealed neointimal hyperplasia significantly more often in variant angina than in chronic stable exertional angina (68% vs. 8%).

DIFFERENTIAL DIAGNOSIS
- Angina pectoris
- Pericarditis
- Aortic dissection
- Gastrointestinal disorders
- Neurologic disorders
- Pulmonary processes
- Musculoskeletal disorders
- Psychiatric disorders

 ## TREATMENT

GENERAL MEASURES
Symptoms should be treated immediately.
- Chest pain and electrocardiographic changes usually resolve with nitroglycerin.
- Patient is at highest risk for sudden death or myocardial infarction during acute, active phase of disease.
- Treatment goal is prevention of coronary spasm.
- Smoking cessation of utmost importance.
- Control risk factors for atherosclerosis.
- Avoid cocaine use.

 ## MEDICATION (DRUGS)

First Line
- Calcium channel blockers
  - Greater than 50% of patients become asymptomatic with calcium channel blocker therapy.
  - Dihydropyridine and nondihydropyridine agents have been shown effective.
  - High doses may be required.
  - If symptoms not completely relieved with one drug, may be beneficial to add second calcium channel blocker.
  - Calcium channel blocker may decrease risk of myocardial infarction.
- Long-acting nitrates effective, but patients may develop tolerance.
- Sublingual nitrates indicated for acute attacks
- Low-dose aspirin
- Consider imipramine, aminophylline
- Contraindications
  - β-Blockers, non-selective agents in particular, may exacerbate vasospasm.
  - Attacks may be provoked by 5-Fluorouracil, cyclophosphamide.
  - High-dose aspirin may exacerbate attacks by inhibiting coronary vasodilator prostacyclin.
- Precautions
  - Calcium channel blocker withdrawal may cause rebound.

Second Line
May be effective in refractory cases, but not approved for this use in the United States.
- Amiodarone

- Guanethidine
- Clonidine
- Prazosin
- Corticosteroids

SURGERY

- Consider percutaneous transluminal coronary angioplasty (PTCA)/stenting for patients with significant fixed coronary lesions.
- PTCA with stenting also used successfully in patients whose conditions are refractory to medical treatment without a fixed stenosis.
- Recurrence rate of symptoms and angiographic disease after PTCA/stenting higher in patients with variant angina than stable angina
- Reports of spasm recurring proximal to the stent
- Reports of continued symptoms in occasional patients without demonstrable spasm.
- Surgical Options
  – Consider coronary artery bypass graft surgery in patients with significant multivessel disease.
  – Surgical denervation and plexectomy have been used in refractory cases.

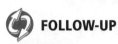 **FOLLOW-UP**

DISPOSITION

Admission Criteria

- Unstable symptoms
- Syncope
- Arrhythmia
- Myocardial infarction

PROGNOSIS

- Possible complications include sudden death, myocardial infarction, ventricular arrhythmias, AV block, syncope
- Greatest risk of adverse outcome during acute, active phase of disease
- Sudden death and myocardial infarction occur most often during acute active phase.
- Acute active phase usually lasts 3–6 months; then symptoms often remit.
- Arrhythmias or syncope during attacks increase risk of sudden death.
- ST elevations in both inferior and anterior leads on ECG mark increased risk of sudden death.
- Predictors of poor outcome include extensive and severe coronary artery disease, abnormal left ventricular function, absence of treatment with calcium channel blockers, continued tobacco abuse, and ventricular arrhythmias during attacks.
- In absence of underlying coronary atherosclerosis, once patient is past acute active phase, chance of long-term survival is excellent (89–97%).

PATIENT MONITORING

- Monitor for relief of symptoms.
- Telemetry
- Ambulatory ECG monitoring helpful as some patients have silent attacks

REFERENCES

1. Beller GA. Calcium antagonists in the treatment of Prinzmetal's angina and unstable angina pectoris. *Circulation*. 1989;80[Suppl IV]:IV-78–IV-87).
2. Gersh BJ, Cannon CP, Braunwald E, et al. Chronic coronary artery disease. Unstable angina and non-ST elevation myocardial infarction. In: Braunwald E, ed. *Heart Disease: A Textbook of Cardiovascular Medicine,* 5th, 7th ed. Philadelphia: WB Saunders,1997, 2005:1340–1343, 1264–1267.
3. Delehanty JM: Variant angina. In: Rose BD, ed. *UpToDate* Waltham, MA, 2005.
4. Hong MK, Park SW, Lee CW et al. l. Intravascular ultrasound findings of negative arterial remodeling at sites of focal coronary spasm in patients with vasospastic angina. *Am Heart J.* 2000;140:395–401.
5. Nakayama M, et al. T786 → C mutation in the 5;dp;-flanking region of the endothelial nitric oxide synthase gene is associated with coronary spasm. *Circulation*. 1999;99:2864–2870.
6. Theroux P, Waters D, O'Rourke RA. Diagnosis and management of patients with unstable angina. Unstable angina and non-ST elevation myocardial infarction: Clinical presentation, diagnostic evaluation, and medical management. In: Fuster V, Alexander RW, Schlant RC, et al., eds. *Hurst's The Heart,* 9th, 11th ed. McGraw Hill, 1998, 2004: 1332–1336, 1269–1276.
7. Suzuki H, et al. Histological evaluation of coronary plaque in patients with variant angina: Relationship between vasospasm and neointimal hyperplasia in primary coronary lesions. *J Am Coll Cardiol.* 1999;33:198–205.
8. Van Spall HG, Overgaard CB, Abramson BL. Coronary vasospasm: A case report and review of the literature. *Can J Card.* 2005;21:953–957.

CODES

ICD9-CM

- 413.1

PATIENT TEACHING

- Prevention/avoidance
- Smoking cessation of utmost importance
- Compliance with medications

Organizations
American Heart Association, National Center, 7272 Greenville Avenue, Dallas, Texas 75231-4596, phone 1-800-242-8721. American Heart Association website: www.americanheart.org

Diet

Low-fat, low-cholesterol diet because approximately two thirds of coronary spasm occurs at site of angiographic atherosclerotic coronary lesion.

Activity

As tolerated after consulting physician

ANGINA, STABLE

Abdul M. Sheikh
L. Van-Thomas Crisco*
Nanette K. Wenger

BASICS

DESCRIPTION
Stable angina is a symptom complex resulting from mismatched myocardial oxygen demand and myocardial oxygen supply, with no change in pattern in the previous 60 days.
- Typical angina
  - Brief (seconds to minutes) chest, jaw, neck, shoulder, back, epigastric, or arm discomfort, aggravated by physical exertion or emotional stress and relieved by rest or nitroglycerin
  - Other precipitants include smoking, meals, cold air, hyperthyroidism, anemia, infection, tachyarrhythmia, and uncontrolled hypertension.
- Atypical angina
  - Dyspnea, fatigue, or generalized weakness aggravated by exertion or emotional stress and relieved by rest or nitroglycerin
- Noncardiac chest pain
  - Chest discomfort syndromes without the preceding characteristics
- Unstable angina
  - See chapter Angina, Unstable.
- Angina, Prinzmetal, Variant
  - See chapter Angina, Prinzmetal, Variant.

EPIDEMIOLOGY
- The initial manifestation of coronary heart disease (CHD) in approximately one half of patients; affects 7 million Americans; costs over $150 billion per year.
- Predominant age
  - Middle-aged and older men and postmenopausal women
- Predominant sex
  - More male than female

RISK FACTORS
- Family history of premature CHD (first-degree relative, male <55 years, female <65 years of age)
- Primary or secondary dyslipidemia: hypercholesterolemia, elevated low-density lipoprotein (LDL) level, isolated low high-density lipoprotein (HDL), ↑ triglycerides
- Hypertension
- Metabolic syndrome
- Tobacco abuse
- Diabetes mellitus
- Male gender
- Advanced age
- Sedentary life-style
- Obesity

Genetics
Genetic susceptibility for CHD; family history very important

ETIOLOGY
- CHD with fixed atherosclerotic plaque; thrombus or plaque with associated thrombus
- Coronary spasm; endothelial dysfunction
- Severe valvular aortic stenosis; insufficiency
- Hypertrophic cardiomyopathy
- Primary pulmonary hypertension
- Severe hypertension or systemic hypotension
- Severe anemia
- Nonatherosclerotic coronary artery disease
  - Coronary artery anomalies
  - Primary coronary artery dissection
  - Coronary embolism
  - Radiation vasculopathy
  - Carbon monoxide poisoning
- Arteritis
  - Kawasaki's disease
  - Takayasu disease
  - Polyarteritis nodosa
  - Systemic lupus erythematosus
  - Giant cell arteritis
  - Buerger disease
  - Syphilis

ASSOCIATED CONDITIONS
- See Risk Factors (above)
- Cerebrovascular or peripheral vascular disease
- Chronic kidney disease

DIAGNOSIS

SIGNS AND SYMPTOMS
See preceding text for types of angina.
- Discomfort often radiates to the neck, shoulders, arms, or back.
- Often described as "pressure-like"
- Dyspnea on exertion; fatigue
- Discomfort often described as clenched fist over the sternum (Levine sign)

Physical Exam
- Often unrevealing
- Careful exam may reveal the presence of risk factors of coronary atherosclerosis or other etiologies, such as aortic valve disease or anemia.
- Tests
- Electrocardiogram (ECG)
  - Normal in ≤50% of patients with chronic stable angina, does not exclude severe CHD
- Prior Q-wave myocardial infarction (MI) on ECG, ST–T wave changes consistent with myocardial ischemia, or ECG changes of left ventricular hypertrophy favor diagnosis of angina pectoris
- Chest X-ray with signs or symptoms of heart failure (HF), valvular disease, pericardial disease, or aortic dissection/aneurysm
- Exercise ECG
  - Primary utility diagnostic; risk stratification

- Appropriate if diagnosis remains uncertain after history, physical examination, ECG, and chest X-ray
- Greatest utility with intermediate pretest probability of CHD (50%) based on age, gender, and symptoms
- Add imaging modality if baseline ECG abnormal (see Imaging, below)
- Echocardiography
  - Systolic murmur suggestive of aortic stenosis or hypertrophic cardiomyopathy
  - Evaluate ischemia severity during pain

Lab
- Hemoglobin (Hgb)
- Fasting glucose, Hgb A1C (glycosylated hemoglobin)
- Fasting lipid panel, including total cholesterol, HDL cholesterol, triglycerides, and LDL cholesterol
- If concern for unstable angina pectoris
  - ECG
  - Cardiac enzymes (creatine kinase-(CK)-MB, troponin I

Imaging
- Use when baseline ECG abnormal
- Nuclear perfusion imaging or stress echocardiography
- Increases sensitivity/specificity
- Pharmacologic stress for patients unable to exercise.

DIAGNOSTIC PROCEDURES/SURGERY
See Imaging

DIFFERENTIAL DIAGNOSIS
- Acute MI
- Anemia
- Aortic dissection
- Symptomatic cholelithiasis
- Chest wall pain, costochondritis (Tietze syndrome)
- Esophageal spasm, esophagitis
- Fibromyalgia
- Gastritis, peptic ulcer disease
- Gastroesophageal reflux disease
- Pancreatitis
- Panic disorder
- Pericarditis, myocarditis
- Pneumothorax
- Pulmonary embolism or hypertension
- Radiculopathy, shoulder arthropathy

Pregnancy Considerations
- Differential diagnosis of anginal symptoms must be considered (coronary artery dissection, pulmonary embolism, etc.).
- Co-management cardiologist, obstetrician
- Symptoms may increase with hemodynamic changes.
- Treatment options may be limited by pregnancy concerns.

Pediatric Considerations
Pediatric patients: suspect familial dyslipidemia or arteritis (Kawasaki disease)

TREATMENT

GENERAL MEASURES
- Control precipitating; exacerbating conditions
- Risk stratification by history, physical examination, ECG, chest X-ray, exercise ECG, or diagnostic imaging
- Patients with high likelihood (>1 chance in 2) of severe disease: consider angiography
- Treatment of stable angina to:
  – Prevent MI, death, need for revascularization
- Reduce symptoms of angina, occurrence of ischemia
- A handy mnemonic for appropriate initial health care is A, B, C, D, E:
  – A. Aspirin and antianginal therapy
  – B. β-Blocker and blood pressure
  – C. Cigarette smoking and cholesterol
  – D. Diet and diabetes
  – E. Education and exercise
- Risk factor modification
  – Blood pressure control The seventh Report of the Joint National Commitee on Prevention, Detection, Evaluation, and Treatment of High Blood Pressure (JNC VII) guidelines
  – Cholesterol lowering to National Cholesterol Education Program (NCEP) guidelines
  – Smoking cessation
  – Glycemic control
  – Weight control
  – Regular aerobic exercise
  – Dietary modification: low fat, low cholesterol, caloric restriction as needed, low-sodium diet for salt-sensitive hypertensive patients
- Stress reduction

MEDICATION (DRUGS)

First Line
Pharmacotherapy shown to prevent MI and death and reduce symptoms:
- Aspirin 81 mg daily, unless contraindications
- Clopidogrel 75 mg daily, when aspirin contraindicated
- Statin-based lipid-lowering therapy target LDL of <100 mg/dL
  – Statins significantly reduce risk of death, MI, stroke, and the need for revascularization in randomized trials
    - Pravastatin 10–80 mg daily
    - Simvastatin 10–80 mg daily
    - Lovastatin 10–80 mg daily
    - Atorvastatin 10–80 mg daily
  – Statins likely providing equal benefit (death, MI, stroke, revascularization)
    - Fluvastatin 10–80 mg daily
Pharmacotherapy shown to reduce ischemia and relieve symptoms:
- β-Blockers to target heart rate of 50–60 beats/minute, improve survival, reduce reinfarction
  – Atenolol 25–100 mg daily
  – Metoprolol 25–100 mg twice daily
  – Propranolol 30–100 mg two to three times daily

- Long-acting calcium antagonists
  – Verapamil 160–480 mg daily
  – Diltiazem 90–360 mg daily
- Avoid verapamil, diltiazem with decreased left ventricular function, atrioventricular block
  – Amlodipine 5–20 mg daily
  – Nifedipine 30–120 mg daily
- Short-acting dihydropyridine calcium antagonists should be avoided.
- Long-acting nitrates, sublingual nitroglycerin, or nitroglycerin spray for immediate relief of angina
  – All patients should receive a sublingual nitroglycerin prescription and usage education.
- Nitrate-free interval of 10–14 hours required with long-acting nitrates
- Should be prescribed with β-blocker or calcium antagonist

Second Line
Possible benefits:

Low-intensity anticoagulation with warfarin in addition to aspirin

Geriatric Considerations
- Elderly: Special attention to medication side effects, drug interactions
- Exacerbating conditions (anemia, hyperthyroidism) may elicit symptoms more than in younger patients.

SURGERY
- Medical therapy as effective as percutaneous transluminal angioplasty (PTCA) for death, MI outcome.
- PTCA does not improve survival.
- Neither PTCA nor coronary artery bypass grafting (CABG) decreases reinfarction.
- Quality of life is better with CABG or PTCA than with medical therapy.
- Stable angina refractory to medical therapy may benefit from revascularization.
  – Revascularization by PTCA or CABG offered for left main coronary artery stenosis, three-vessel coronary artery disease (CAD), or two vessel CAD with proximal left anterior descending coronary artery stenosis
  – Choice of therapy should include patient preference, tolerability of medical therapy

FOLLOW-UP

DISPOSITION
Admission Criteria
- Unstable symptoms require hospitalization and telemetry monitoring.
- Lack of response to medical therapy or significant; specific angiographic stenosis may indicate need revascularization by PTCA or CABG.

PROGNOSIS
- Overall annual mortality rate 3–4%
- Prognosis related to age of onset; disease etiology; disease severity; co-morbid conditions; left ventricular function; response to therapy

COMPLICATIONS
Ischemia, MI, arrhythmia, congestive heart failure (CHF), sudden death, mitral regurgitation, depression

PATIENT MONITORING
- Every 4–12 months with ECG
- Testing with changes in clinical status:
  – Chest X-ray and echocardiogram for CHF or MI by history or ECG
  – Echocardiogram for new or worsening valvular heart disease
  – Treadmill exercise ECG if no prior revascularization
  – Pharmacologic stress imaging if no prior revascularization and unable to exercise or with significant ECG abnormalities
  – Stress imaging with prior revascularization
  – Angina within 8 months of PTCA suggests restenosis
- Coronary angiography if marked limitation of ordinary activity (CCS class III) despite maximal medical therapy

REFERENCES
1. ACC/AHA/ 2002 Guideline update for the management of patients with chronic stable angina. *J Am Coll Cardiol*. 2003;41:159–168.
2. Heidenreich PA, et al. Meta-analysis of trials comparing beta-blockers, calcium antagonists, and nitrates for stable angina. *JAMA*. 1999;281:1927–1936.
3. Morrow DA, Gersh BJ, Braunwald E. Chronic coronary artery disease. In: *Braunwald's Heart Disease*, 7th ed. Philadelphia: Saunders, 2005: 1281–1308.

CODES
ICD9-CM
- 411.1 Angina, stable
- 413 Angina Pectoris
- 413.1 Prinzmetal angina
- 413.9 Angina, Unspecified

PATIENT TEACHING
Diet
Patient specific
- Low-cholesterol, low-fat diet (general population)
- Diabetic diet (diabetics)
- 2-g sodium diet (hypertensives)

Activity
- Symptom limited, after physician counseling
- Cardiac rehabilitation improves quality of life, functional status, symptom severity.

ANGIOGENESIS

Harold L. Dauerman
Dinesh Chandok

 BASICS

DESCRIPTION

Angiogenesis is the growth and development of supplemental collateral coronary vessels that will result in endogenous bypass arteries surrounding occluded coronary arteries.

- Mechanism
  - A complex process involving endothelial cell proliferation and migration, formation of new capillaries, attraction of macrophages, stimulation of smooth muscle cell proliferation and migration, formation of new vascular structures, and deposition of new matrix
- Target population

Patients with chronic ischemia and anginal symptoms due to advanced coronary artery disease, that is:
  - Refractory to antianginal medical therapy
  - Not amenable to percutaneous interventions
  - Not amenable to conventional coronary artery bypass grafting due to small, diffusely diseased distal target vessels
  - Found to have significant areas of viable, but underperfused myocardium
  - Not a candidate for cardiac transplantation
- Typical candidate patient profile
  - Elderly patient with class III or IV angina, mild to moderate reduction in ejection fraction, and multiple prior revascularization procedures
  - Most patients have had prior coronary bypass surgery within last 5–10 years and have occluded most bypass grafts.
  - Patients frequently have small, diffusely diseased coronary arteries in association with longstanding diabetes mellitus.
  - The estimated annual myocardial infarction and mortality rate for these patients is 26% and 15% per year, respectively.
- Goals of therapeutic myocardial angiogenesis
  - Increase growth of new blood vessels
  - Increase oxygen delivery
  - Decrease angina
  - Increase exercise capacity
  - Improve quality of life
- Rationale
  Natural History of Collateral Vessels
  Collateral vessels form from preexisting vascular structures in response to acute myocardial infarction or chronic ischemia in order to bypass occluded coronary artery territories. This can improve oxygen supply to ischemic muscle.

  - Patients with acute myocardial ischemia (AMI) have less myocardial damage if collaterals are more abundant.
  - There are intra- and interspecies differences in the collateral response to ischemia; collateral development response in humans is intermediate compared with species such as cats and rabbits.
  - These differences in collateral development may relate to different levels of endogenous angiogenic factors that would promote this process.
  - The signaling for collateral development is upregulated in situations of ischemia and infarction. For example, fibroblast growth factor receptors will be increased in numbers in ischemic myocardium.
  - Endogenous angiogenic stimulants include fibroblast growth factors (FGFs), vascular endothelial growth factors, platelet-derived growth factors, angiopoietin-1, hepatocyte growth factor, hypoxia inducible factor 1, interleukin 8, tumor necrosis factor alpha, and extracellular matrix protein.
- Animal studies
  - Canine and porcine models of acute coronary occlusion or chronic ischemia have been developed in order to assess the response of the coronary arteries to supplemental exogenous angiogenic factors to stimulate coronary collateral growth.
  - The following factors stimulate growth of coronary collateral vessels in these animal models:
    - Basic and acidic FGF
    - Vascular endothelial growth factor (VEGF)
    - Transmyocardial laser channels inducing inflammation and angiogenesis
- Methods
  Increased myocardial levels of angiogenic factors have been demonstrated by a variety of methods for the introduction of growth factors in animal models.
  - Intracoronary infusions
  - Heparin alginate slow-release intramyocardial pellets
  - Local perivascular delivery
  - Intrapericardial infusion
  - Direct myocardial injection
  - Direct or transthoracic laser channels
  - Treatment with genes, plasmids, or virus expressing the angiogenic protein factors rather than with the protein itself

---

 FOLLOW-UP

PROGNOSIS

Treatment Results
- VIVA Trial
  - A randomized, placebo-controlled trial of combined intravenous and intracoronary infusions of VEGF in 180 patients with unstable angina
  - No adverse effects reported
  - Although exercise tolerance and anginal symptoms improved in the VEGF arm, they also improved in the placebo arm, thus making definite conclusions about the efficacy of VEGF coronary infusions difficult.
  - By day 120, placebo-treated patients showed reduced benefit in all the measures but no significant difference from low-dose VEGF group
- FIRST Trial
  - A randomized, placebo controlled trial of a 20-minute intracoronary infusion of basic FGF in 337 patients with symptomatic, severe coronary artery disease
    - Trial is based on earlier phase I open label trial of basic FGF in 66 patients with severe symptomatic coronary artery disease demonstrating safety, maximum tolerated dose, and improvement in symptoms and exercise tolerance
    - No adverse outcome except for hypotension, which occurs with high doses
    - Trial did not improve exercise tolerance or myocardial perfusion but does show trend toward symptom improvement at day 90 (but not 180) days.
- AGENT Trial
  - A randomized, placebo controlled trial of single intracoronary infusion of replication defective adenovirus containing a human fibroblast growth factor in 79 patients
    - No serious adverse outcome reported
    - Results show evidence of favorable antiischemic effect compared to placebo with improvement in exercise tolerance
    - The subsequent AGENT 2 trial showed trend towards improved myocardial perfusion with single protein emission computed tomography (SPECT).
    - Transmyocardial laser trials

- Two randomized, nonblinded trials of transmyocardial laser revascularization in patients with refractory angina have reported improvement in symptoms and possible improvements in exercise tolerance.
- The mechanism of benefit is unclear and may include formation of new myocardial blood channels, promotion of angiogenesis, and cardiac sympathetic denervation.
- Results are controversial due to the possibility that a significant placebo effect may be present in patients undergoing surgical procedures.
- Direct trial is the only major blinded study on laser myocardial revascularization involving more than 300 patients. These results have been presented but not published; they failed to show any benefit over continued medical therapy.

Future Issues for Therapeutic Angiogenesis
- Proving efficacy versus the placebo effect
- Optimal route of delivery
- Duration of benefit
- Optimal method of angiogenesis: Laser, protein or gene therapy
- Long-term safety concerns
  - Neovascularization of nontargeted tissues
  - Tumorigenesis
  - Potential acceleration of atherosclerosis

REFERENCES

1. Charney R, Cohen M. The role of coronary collateral circulation in limiting myocardial ischemia and infarct size. *Am Heart J*. 1993;126:937–945.
2. Engler DA. Use of vascular endothelial growth factor for therapeutic angiogenesis. *Circulation*. 1996;94:1496–1498.
3. Grines CL, Watkins MW, Helmer G, et al. Angiogenic Gene Therapy (AGENT) trial in patients with stable angina pectoris. *Circulation*. 2002;105(11):1291–1297.
4. Grines CL, Watkins MW, Mahmarian JJ, et al. A randomized, double-bind, placebo-controlled trial of Ad5FGF-4 gene therapy and its effect on myocardial perfusion in patients with stable agina. *J Am Coll Cardiol*. 2003;42(8):1339–1347.
5. Henry TD, Rocha-Singh K, Isner JM, et al. Results of intracoronary recombinant human vascular endothelial growth factor (rhVEGF) administration trial. *J Am Coll Cardial*. 1998;31:65A.
6. Horrigan MC, MacIsaac AI, Nicolini FA, et al. Reduction in myocardial infarct size by basic fibroblast growth factor after temporary coronary occlusion in a canine model. *Circulation*. 1996;94:1927–1933.
7. Kornowski R, Hong MK, Leon MB. Current perspectives on direct myocardial revascularization. *Am J Cardiol*. 1998;81:44E–48E.
8. Laham RJ, Hung D, Simons M. Therapeutic myocardial angiogenesis using percutaneous intrapericardial delivery. *Clin Cardiol*. 1999;22:6–9.
9. Laham RJ, Simons M, Pearlman JD, et al. Biosense catheter direct laser myocardial revascularization improves 30 day angina class, regional wall motion, and perfusion of the treated zone using MRI. *J Am Coll Cardiol*. 1998;31:333A.
10. Losordo DW, Vale PR, Symes JF, et al. Gene therapy for myocardial angiogenesis. *Circulation*. 1998;98:2800–2804.
11. Losordo DW, Dimmerler Stefanie, et al. Therapeutic angiogenesis and vasculogenesis for ischemic disease. *Circulation*. 2004;109:2487–2491.
12. Schofield PM, Sharples LD, Caine N, et al. Transmyocardial laser revascularization in patients with refractory angina: A randomised controlled trial. *Lancet*. 1999;353:519–524.
13. Sellke FW, Laham RJ, Edelman ER, et al. Therapeutic angiogenesis with basic fibroblast growth factor: Technique and early results. *Ann Thorac Surg*. 1998;65:1540–1544.
14. Simons M, Annex BH, Laham RJ, et al. *Circulation*. 2002;105:788–793.
15. TI – A randomized, double-blind, placebo-controlled trial of Ad5FGF-4 gene therapy and its effect on myocardial perfusion in patients with stable angina.
16. Ware JA, Simons M. Angiogenesis in ischemic heart disease. *Nature Med*. 1997;3:158–164.

ANKYLOSING SPONDYLITIS AND THE HEART

Kevin P. Fitzgerald
Steven Hermann
Bernard R. Chaitman

 BASICS

DESCRIPTION
- Ankylosing spondylitis (AS) is a chronic inflammatory disorder predominantly affecting the axial skeleton.
- AS is classified as a seronegative spondyloarthropathy (category also includes reactive arthritis, inflammatory bowel disease–associated arthritis, psoriatic arthritis and a form of juvenile arthritis).
- Strong association exists between HLA-B27 gene and spondyloarthropathies.
- About 50% of patients with AS will have asymmetric involvement of peripheral large joints.
- AS may cause aortic root dilatation and aortic regurgitation (AR), and cardiac conduction defects, predominantly of the atrioventricular node (AVN).

EPIDEMIOLOGY
- Only 20% of HLA-B27-positive patients develop AS; 90% of patients who develop AS have the HLA-B27 gene.
- 1/3 of AS patients have cardiac conduction abnormalities.
- About 3/4 of patients with high-grade AVN conduction disease and AS have the HLA-B27 gene.

Prevalence
- In USA, approximately 206,000 whites and 5,000 blacks with AS
- Male to female prevalence is 3:1
- HLA-B27 prevalence:
  - North America: 0.2% in whites; much less in blacks and Asian Americans
  - Eskimo population: 25% to 40%
  - Japan: < 1%

RISK FACTORS
- A first-degree relative with AS increases a patient's risk by 5- to 16-fold.
- HLA-B27-positive children who have siblings with AS have a 10–20% risk of getting AS.
- Males have higher risk of AS.

Genetics
HLA-B27 is a strong genetic risk factor for cardiac conduction disease in males.

PATHOPHYSIOLOGY
- AS may cause AR through fibrotic thickening, retraction and rolling of the AV cusps, and aortic root dilatation.
- The AV lesions can extend down to the anterior mitral valve (MV) leaflet causing a "subaortic hump" and MV insufficiency.

ETIOLOGY
- Exact etiology of AS is not completely understood.
- No good evidence suggests that AS is a sequela of an infectious trigger, as with Reiter disease.
- All spondyloarthropathies appear to result from T cell–mediated autoimmune response.
- Autoantigen in AS may involve cartilage proteoglycans.

ASSOCIATED CONDITIONS
- AR associated with AS can present in children and can even precede joint manifestations.
- Extraskeletal involvement:
  - Cardiovascular: Aortic root disease, AR, conduction disturbances
  - Pulmonary: Apical lung fibrosis or restrictive lung disease secondary to spinal changes
  - Ophthalmologic: Anterior uveitis and cataracts
  - Renal: IgA nephropathy, renal amyloidosis, nonsteroidal anti-inflammatory drug (NSAID) nephropathy
  - Neurologic: Spinal cord compression
  - Gastrointestinal: Bowel ulcers and Crohn disease
  - Genitourinary: Varicocele

 DIAGNOSIS

SIGNS AND SYMPTOMS
- Back pain is most frequent symptom in AS.
- Patients with early AS may have nonspecific symptoms of fever, malaise, loss of appetite.
- Cardiac conduction disturbances may be intermittent and widely spaced in time.
- HLA-B27-associated heart block usually involves the AV node and not the His bundle.

History
- Chronic back pain
- Insidious onset of symptoms prior to age 45
- Pain worsens with inactivity and improves with exercise.
- Cardiac syndrome of AR and heart block may precede symptoms of AS.
- Alternating buttock pain
- Frequently a family history of a spondyloarthropathy in a first- or second-degree relative

Physical Exam
- Impaired spinal mobility
- Impaired chest expansion
- Asymmetric inflammatory arthritis or arthritis predominantly of the lower extremities
- May have sacroiliitis
- May have enthesitis; pain and inflammation at tendon insertion sites, especially Achilles tendon and plantar tendon
- Chronic AR may present as a high-pitched holodiastolic decrescendo murmur.

Lab
- HLA-B27 phenotype is found in 95% of patients with AS but is not a diagnostic test for AS.
- No serologic marker for disease diagnosis and activity
- Erythrocyte sedimentation rate (ESR) may be elevated, but normal ESR does not exclude active AS.
- Rheumatoid factor and antinuclear antibodies are negative.

Imaging
- Sacroiliitis on anteroposterior pelvis radiograph
- Classic "bamboo spine" on radiograph is diagnostic of AS.
- Impaired chest expansion on chest radiograph
- In early disease, MRI may show evidence of sacroiliitis and enthesitis prior to x-ray films.
- Spinal osteoporosis may be present with longstanding AS.
- Aortic root disease can be diagnosed by echocardiography, CT, or MRI.

Pathological Findings
- Aorta shows adventitial and medial scarring, intimal proliferation, and infiltration of the vaso vasorum with plasma cells and lymphocytes.
- Fibrous commissural bump is often prominent at the aortic valve cusp.
- AV cusps are short and thick.
- Fibrosis is common in the cardiac conduction system
- Coronary arteritis is not a feature of AS.
- Vascular changes seen with AS in the aorta and joints may also occur in the:
  - Sinus node artery: Sinus node dysfunction
  - AVN artery: AVN conduction block
  - Aortic root vasa vasorum: Aortic root dilatation
- Autopsy studies of AS patients have shown 100% involvement of aortic root and valve.
- Transesophageal echocardiogram studies of AS patients have shown 82% involvement of aortic root and valve.

DIFFERENTIAL DIAGNOSIS
- Rheumatoid arthritis
- Reiter syndrome
- Systemic lupus erythematosus
- Other causes of aortic insufficiency

 TREATMENT

GENERAL MEASURES
- All patients with AS should be encouraged to stop smoking.
- The skeletal involvement of AS is treated with regular exercise and NSAIDs.
- General osteoporosis prophylaxis and treatment should be considered.
- All patients with cardiac valve involvement should receive antibiotic prophylaxis for infective endocarditis.

MEDICATION (DRUGS)

First Line
- NSAIDs and possibly corticosteroid injections may be used for the musculoskeletal symptoms.
- TNF-α antagonists (infliximab, etanercept, adalimumab) have shown improvement of the musculoskeletal symptoms of AS but it is not known if these medications will curtail cardiovascular complications.
- Patients with chronic severe AR who are not surgical candidates or who do not yet meet the criteria for aortic valve replacement may be treated with medical therapy.
- Primary medical treatment of chronic severe AR is vasodilator therapy using angiotensin-converting enzyme (ACE) inhibitors, nifedipine, felodipine, or hydralazine.

Second Line
- Pamidronate and thalidomide may be of some benefit against the musculoskeletal symptoms.
- Limited data supports effectiveness of methotrexate.
- β-Blockers increase diastolic time and are a relative contraindication in AR.

SURGERY
- Total hip replacement and spinal surgery may be beneficial in some patients.
- Acute severe AR requires urgent surgery.
- Aortic valve surgery is indicated for AR in patients with symptoms or with abnormal left ventricular (LV) size or function (LV ejection fraction <50% or LV end diastolic dimension >75 mm or LV end systolic dimension >55 mm)
- High-degree heart block requires implantation of a permanent pacemaker.

 FOLLOW-UP

Issues for Referral
- Patients with chronic AR should be monitored by a cardiologist and referred to CTS when surgery is indicated.
- Consider referral to a rheumatologist for treatment of musculoskeletal manifestations of AS.

PROGNOSIS
- AS alone does not affect overall long-term mortality.
- Secondary amyloidosis and cardiovascular complications are the major causes of death due to AS.

COMPLICATIONS
- Aortic valve endocarditis has been described as a consequence of AS.
- AS patients may be at risk for spinal fractures and neurologic compromise.
- Atrial fibrillation may occur more commonly than expected in patients with AS.

PATIENT MONITORING
Monitoring for aortic regurgitation:
- Patients with mild to moderate AR and normal LV size and function must be followed by exam and echocardiography every 1–2 years.
- Asymptomatic patients with chronic severe AR and normal LV size and function need exams and echocardiograms every 6 months.
- Aortic valve surgery is indicated as soon as the patient develops symptoms or abnormal LV size or function (LV ejection fraction <50% or LV end diastolic dimension >75 mm or LV end systolic dimension >55 mm).

ALERT
Geriatric Considerations
- Limited data on surgical outcomes for AR in elderly patients
- Symptoms are generally the primary indication for aortic valve surgery in elderly patients >80 years old.

Pregnancy Considerations
- No contraindications exist for pregnancy with AS alone, but patients with AR need special consideration.
- Aortic regurgitation in pregnancy:
  - Patients with normal LV function and AR usually tolerate pregnancy well; cardiac output may improve due to pregnancy-related fall in systemic vascular resistance.
  - Patients with severe AR and abnormal left ventricular function (LVSF) are at risk for developing congestive heart failure and should have surgery prior to pregnancy.
  - May treat AR with nifedipine (pregnancy class C), hydralazine (C), furosemide (C), digoxin (C)
  - To avoid fetal renal agenesis, avoid ACEI and angiotensin II receptor blockers.
  - Controlled induced vaginal delivery preferred over cesarean delivery for patients with AR.
  - If patient has an aortic root diameter (ARD) >40 mm, pregnancy should be discouraged. If ARD is <40mm, treat with β-blockers and monitor via exams and echocardiograms during gestation.

REFERENCES
1. Peters MJ, van der Horst-Bruinsma IE, Dijkmans BA, Nurmohamed MT. Cardiovascular risk profile of patients with spondyloarthropathies, particularly ankylosing spondylitis and psoriatic arthritis. *Semin Arthritis Rheumat.* 2004;34:585–592.
2. Reveille JD, Arnett FC. Spondyloarthritis: update on pathogenesis and management. *Am J Med.* 2005;118:592–603.
3. Sims AM, Wordsworth BP, Brown MA. Genetic susceptibility to ankylosing spondylitis. *Curr Molec Med.* 2004;4:13–20.
4. Topol EJ, et al., eds. *Textbook of cardiovascular medicine,* 2nd ed. Philadelphia: Lippincott Williams & Wilkins, 2002.
5. Zipes DP, et al. *Braunwald's heart disease: A textbook of cardiovascular medicine,* 7th ed. Philadelphia: Elsevier Saunders, 2005.
6. Zochling J, Braun J. Management and treatment of ankylosing spondylitis. *Curr Opin Rheumatol.* 2005;17:418–425.

 MISCELLANEOUS

See also: Aortic Insufficiency; Rheumatoid Arthritis; Heart Block

CODES
ICD9-CM
720.0

PATIENT TEACHING
Diet
Low sodium diet if symptoms of heart failure develop

Activity
Activity limited by back and spine discomfort, and by heart failure symptoms if they develop.

Prevention
- Infective endocarditis prophylaxis is recommended with aortic or mitral valve involvement.
- Patient counseling for symptoms of HF or heart block

ANOMALOUS CORONARY ARTERIES

Seema Mital
Welton M. Gersony

 BASICS

DESCRIPTION
Anomalous coronary arteries include abnormal anatomy, origin, course, and/or termination of coronary arteries.

Normal Coronary Anatomy
- Left and right main coronary arteries arise from corresponding aortic sinuses.
  - Left main coronary artery (LMCA) divides into left anterior descending and left circumflex, which supply the left ventricular free wall.
  - Right coronary artery (RCA) is dominant in 90% of humans. It gives rise to the posterior descending coronary artery, which supplies the posterior interventricular septum, inferior left ventricle, and atrioventricular (AV) node.

EPIDEMIOLOGY
Prevalence
Overall prevalence ranges from 0.17–1% in the general population.

ETIOLOGY
Predominantly congenital in origin, they can occur in isolation or in association with other intracardiac malformations.

TYPES
Anomalies of Coronary Arterial Origin
- Pulmonary arterial origin
  - Anomalous LMCA from pulmonary artery (ALCAPA): 1 in 300,000 live births and 0.5% of all congenital heart disease
  - Origin of RCA or left anterior descending or left circumflex arteries from pulmonary artery is less common.
- Origin from inappropriate sinus
  - LMCA from right sinus of Valsalva: 1–3% of all major coronary anomalies
  - RCA from left sinus of Valsalva: 30% of all major coronary anomalies
  - Left circumflex coronary from RCA: 30% of all major coronary anomalies
  - Single coronary artery arising from a single ostium: 5–20% of all coronary anomalies

Anomalies of Coronary Artery Termination
- 0.2–0.4% of all congenital cardiac anomalies and 50% of congenital coronary anomalies
- These include coronary–cameral fistulas (connection between a coronary artery and a cardiac chamber) and coronary arteriovenous fistulas (between coronary artery and coronary sinus, superior vena cava or pulmonary artery).

Anomalies Intrinsic to the Coronary Artery
- Coronary artery aneurysm: Congenital or acquired (atherosclerosis, associated with coronary–cameral fistulas, Kawasaki disease, infectious, or traumatic)
- Congenital LCA stenosis or atresia
- Congenital coronary artery hypoplasia
- Myocardial bridges (muscle bridge overlying an epicardial artery) and coronary arterial loops (extreme coiling of the coronary arteries)

ASSOCIATED CONDITIONS
Coronary Artery Anomalies: Often associated with other congenital heart defects in particular with tetralogy of Fallot, d and l-transposition of great arteries, truncus arteriosus, pulmonary atresia, and univentricular hearts.

DIAGNOSIS

SIGNS AND SYMPTOMS
Many coronary anomalies are not clinically significant. Serious abnormalities may present with varying profiles and at different ages.

Anomalous left coronary artery from pulmonary artery of: As pulmonary resistance decreases in postnatal life, perfusion pressure decreases, collaterals develop between RCA and LCA, and there may be a pulmonary–coronary steal.
- Almost 90% of patients with this anomaly present in infancy with episodes of myocardial ischemia, mitral insufficiency with symptoms of congestive heart failure (CHF) (irritability, feeding difficulties, poor weight gain, diaphoresis, respiratory distress). Untreated, 65–85% die of intractable CHF in the first year of life (infantile type).
- Some present in later childhood or as young adults with angina of effort or CHF due to mitral incompetence (adult type).
- 15% remain asymptomatic, possibly because of extensive collaterals and a restrictive opening at the origin of the LCA.

Anomalous origins of the LCA or RCA: Are infrequently diagnosed in children and adolescents.
1. Many are discovered as incidental findings during echocardiography for innocent heart murmurs or screening for exercise participation.
2. Sudden death, especially in young asymptomatic athletic individuals, may frequently be the initial manifestation. Anomalous coronaries represent the second most frequent cause of athletic field deaths.

   Patients in whom the anomalous artery courses between the aorta and pulmonary artery (53%) are at greatest risk for exercise-induced sudden death or arrhythmias due to myocardial ischemia secondary to the slitlike ostium or compression of the coronary artery between the aortic and pulmonary roots as they distend during exercise. This is especially true if there are separate ostia from the right sinus of Valsalva. An interarterial course of an RCA is also associated with this risk, especially if there is a separate ostial origin from the left sinus. However the incidence of sudden death is much lower than that of anomalous LCA. A single ostium is less likely to be associated with sudden death, although it is not completely "protective." An intraseptal course for the anomalous LCA is "protective" against a sudden cardiac event, especially when associated with a single RCA ostium.
3. Premonitory symptoms such as chest pain and/or syncope or presyncope are reported in less than 30% patients. Symptoms are more likely to be reported by subjects with anomalous origin of the LMCA, and they usually occur in association with exercise.
- **Single coronary artery:** Mostly asymptomatic, except with atherosclerotic occlusion of the artery

- Congenital coronary artery aneurysm, congenital LCA stenosis, or atresia: Usually present with symptoms of myocardial ischemia with exercise
- **Coronary arteriovenous fistulas:** Physiology and presentation depend on the size and location of the shunt. Most patients younger than 20 years of age are asymptomatic; the majority older than 20 years become symptomatic with dyspnea on exertion, fatigue, angina, and palpitations. Most have only small left-to-right shunts.
  - Fistulas most often occur (in order of frequency) in the right ventricle, right atrium, and pulmonary artery. They also may drain into the left ventricle, left atrium, coronary sinus, or superior vena cava.
  - Complications: CHF, fistula rupture, infective endocarditis, myocardial ischemia/infarction, aneurysm formation

History
- In infants: Inquire about symptoms of CHF including irritability, feeding difficulties, failure to thrive, diaphoresis, and respiratory difficulties
- In children and older children: Inquire about symptoms of chest pain, exercise intolerance, syncope or near-syncope, and palpitations

Physical Exam
Physical findings are not pathognomonic but may aid in diagnosis. These include the following:
- Signs of CHF including hepatomegaly, rales, respiratory distress, left ventricular gallop, and holosystolic murmur of mitral insufficiency.
- Continuous murmur in patients with coronary arteriovenous fistula or adult type ALCAPA with collaterals
- Mitral regurgitation secondary to papillary muscle infarction in ALCAPA
- Findings of associated congenital heart defects

TESTS
Lab
There are no pathognomonic blood tests for diagnosis but peripheral markers of myocardial ischemia may aid in diagnosis.
- Cardiac troponin, creatine phosphokinase creatine kinase MB fraction levels may be elevated during episodes of ischemia
- Electrocardiogram (ECG)
- Resting ECG may be abnormal in symptomatic patients with evidence of myocardial ischemia (ST–T changes), ventricular hypertrophy, and arrhythmias depending on type and location of coronary artery abnormalities.
- Anterolateral infarct in an infant (i.e., abnormal Q waves in leads I, aVL, and precordial leads V4–V6 and abnormal R waves or R-wave progression in the left precordial leads) is highly suggestive of ALCAPA in an infant.
- Exercise Stress Test
  - May uncover ischemia due to underlying coronary anomaly, but is not always conclusive

Imaging
- Chest X-ray
  - May show cardiomegaly, pulmonary edema in patients with CHF, and abnormal cardiac silhouette in cases of large aneurysm.

- Transthoracic Echocardiography
  - Echocardiogram can diagnose most cases. Coronary anatomy is best visualized in the parasternal long, short, and high short-axis views. Echocardiographic features include the following:
  - Abnormal attachment of the origin of the coronary artery (in more than one view to avoid problems due to lateral dropout)
  - Doppler color-flow mapping showing flow away from the coronary artery into the pulmonary artery indicates ALCAPA.
  - A dilated coronary artery on two-dimensional echo should prompt a search for anomalous coronaries, e.g., ALCAPA (dilated RCA) or coronary arteriovenous fistula (dilated proximal portion of the coronary artery that feeds the fistula).
  - Intrinsic coronary artery abnormalities like aneurysm, stenosis, atresia, hypoplasia, fistulas
  - Chamber dilation secondary to shunting across large coronary fistula
  - Abnormalities of left ventricular size and function (i.e., enlarged left atrium and ventricle, diminished left ventricular function, global or regional wall motion abnormalities, endocardial fibroelastosis, and mitral regurgitation), especially in patients with ALCAPA
  - Associated congenital intracardiac anomalies and other causes of heart failure (e.g., cardiomyopathy)
- Ultrafast computed tomography (CT) with three-dimensional (3D) reconstruction may be useful in defining coronary anatomy
- Cardiac magnetic resonance imaging (MRI)
  - May occasionally be useful in defining coronary anatomy
- Stress Imaging
  - These include stress thallium imaging and dobutamine stress echocardiography. These studies have not been widely used in children. They may uncover ischemia due to underlying coronary anomaly but are not always conclusive due to false negative results.

DIAGNOSTIC PROCEDURES

Cardiac Catheterization and Angiocardiography remain a gold standard for diagnosis of most coronary anomalies. Injection of contrast into the aortic root and, in cases of anomalous origin, into the pulmonary artery can identify coronary abnormalities.

Screening Procedures

In general, standard testing with ECG is unlikely to provide clinical evidence of myocardial ischemia and is not reliable as a screening test in large athletic populations. A history of exertional syncope or chest pain requires exclusion of a coronary anomaly in athletes. Echocardiography and stress imaging are indicated in suspected cases.

DIFFERENTIAL DIAGNOSIS

ALCAPA is most often misdiagnosed as cardiomyopathy or myocarditis because of failure to identify the anomalous coronary artery. Every attempt must be made to define coronary artery anatomy in any young patient presenting with apparent cardiomyopathy or unexplained heart failure.

 TREATMENT

GENERAL MEASURES

- Medical treatment is usually supportive.
  - Treatment of CHF and arrhythmias to stabilize the patient with left ventricular dysfunction prior to surgery
  - Oral anticoagulation (aspirin, warfarin) in patients with aneurysms
  - Infective endocarditis prophylaxis

SURGERY

Corrective surgery is the treatment of choice for most coronary anomalies. However not all coronary artery anomalies require surgery.

Indications for Surgery

1. ALCAPA should be repaired urgently once diagnosis is made.
2. Anomalies that are associated with significant morbidity and mortality should be repaired once diagnosis is made regardless of symptoms (e.g., anomalous LCA from right coronary sinus, large coronary aneurysms, coronary arteriovenous fistulas). In general, a young patient (<35 years) with unequivocal diagnosis of anomalous coronary origin presenting with symptoms and/or signs of myocardial ischemia should undergo corrective surgery. A young asymptomatic patient with a coronary anomaly should also be considered for repair if engaged in heavy physical activity.
3. Patients with ARCAPA may require surgery in adult age.
4. As part of surgical repair of associated congenital heart defects. Failure to recognize an anomalous coronary artery may result in the artery being injured at surgery or inadequate myocardial protection when cardioplegia is given directly into the major coronary arteries.

Surgical Options

- Anomalous LCA or RCA
  - Unroofing procedure to move the coronary artery orifice to the appropriate sinus is the procedure of choice especially in the presence of a slitlike ostium.
  - Direct aortic reimplantation of the anomalous coronary artery (with a button of pulmonary artery around origin) provides the most physiologic repair in the absence of ostial abnormalities. The surgical mortality is less than 15%. Short-term use of left ventricular assistive device in the immediate postoperative period may assist recovery. Most often there is excellent recovery of normal or near-normal left ventricular function and regression of mitral insufficiency, usually within 6–24 months of corrective surgery.
  - Historical alternatives include creation of an intrapulmonary baffle or tunnel (Takeuchi procedure), primary angioplasty, and coronary artery bypass grafting.
  - **Aneurysm:** Ligation of aneurysm, aneurysmorrhaphy, aneurysmectomy with interposition of graft
  - **Fistulas:** Surgical ligation or transcatheter closure of coronary AV fistulas.
  - **Myocardial bridging:** Unroofing of myocardial bridge in symptomatic patients.

 FOLLOW-UP

PROGNOSIS

- Infants improve markedly after timely repair of ALCAPA, ventricular function normalizes, and over time mitral insufficiency lessens.
- In patients with anomalous origin of coronary arteries from the contralateral sinus and coronary AV fistulas, surgical repair is usually curative.

PATIENT MONITORING

Asymptomatic patients with mild abnormalities should be followed for development of symptoms or electrocardiographic or echocardiographic evidence of progression of lesion (e.g., enlarging aneurysm, chamber enlargement secondary to fistula, thromboembolism). According to AHA guidelines, patients with large coronary aneurysms secondary to Kawasaki disease should be followed with serial echocardiograms and exercise stress testing every 6 months to a year. Angiography may be required.

REFERENCES

1. Allen HD, Gutgesell HP, Clark EB, et al. *Moss and Adams' Heart Disease in Infants, Children and Adolescent.* 6th ed. Lippincott Williams & Wilkins, 2000.
2. Garson A, Bricker JT, Fisher DJ, et al. *The Science and Practice of Pediatric Cardiology,* 2nd ed. Baltimore: Williams & Wilkins, 1998.
3. Gowda RM, Chamakura SR, Dogan OM, et al. Origin of left main and right coronary arteries from right aortic sinus of Valsalva. *Int J Cardiol.* 2003;92:305–306.
4. Mirchandani S, Phoon C. Management of anomalous coronary arteries from the contralateral sinus. *Int J Cardiol.* 2005;102:383–389.
5. Pelliccia A. Congenital coronary artery anomalies in young patients. *J Am Coll Cardiol.* 2001;37:598–600.
6. Shirani J, Roberts WC. Solitary coronary ostium in the aorta in the absence of other major congenital cardiovascular anomalies. *J Am Coll Cardiol.* 1993;21:137–143.
7. Snider RA, Serwer GA, Ritter SB. *Echocardiography in Pediatric Heart Disease,* 2nd ed. St. Louis: CV Mosby, 1997.
8. Varghese A, Keegan J, Pennell DJ. Cardiovascular magnetic resonance of anomalous coronary arteries. *Coron Artery Dis.* 2005;16:35–64.

 MISCELLANEOUS

- Abbreviations
  - LMCA
  - RCA
  - ALCAPA
  - CHF

CODES
ICD9-CM

- 746.85
- 441.00
- 746.85

PATIENT TEACHING

Infective endocarditis prophylaxis for dental and invasive procedures

Activity

Avoid competitive sports for patients with residual coronary artery abnormalities.

ANOMALOUS PULMONARY VENOUS CONNECTIONS

Rubin S. Cooper
Welton M. Gersony

 BASICS

DESCRIPTION

- Total anomalous pulmonary venous connection (TAPVC) is a condition in which the pulmonary veins drain to a common pulmonary vein (CPV) that does not connect to the left atrium.
- TAPVCs are classified as:
  - Supracardiac (55%): Retrograde blood flow from CPV to left superior vena cava (vertical vein) to innominate vein to the superior vena cava (SVC) to the right atrium; or less commonly, CPV direct to right SVC
  - Intracardiac (30%): CPV to left SVC to coronary sinus
  - Infradiaphragmatic (13%): CPV to inferior cardinal vein to portal system to liver to inferior vena cava (IVC) to right atrium
  - Mixed (connections at two or more levels) (2%)

EPIDEMIOLOGY
Incidence
In autopsy series the incidence of TAPVCs varies from 1–5% of congenital heart disease.

RISK FACTORS
Pregnancy Considerations
Pregnancy should be well tolerated, following successful repair in childhood.

Genetics
There are limited data.
- The possibility of small chromosome translocations or a single autosomal gene mutation has been raised.
- There may be a multifactorial inheritance pattern.

PATHOPHYSIOLOGY
- The CPV drains into one or more alternate channels (embryonic cardinal veins), which eventually reach the right atrium.
- Systemic blood flow is maintained by right-to-left blood flow across a foramen ovale or atrial septal defect to the left atrium.
- If the channels returning blood from the CPV to the systemic venous system are obstructed, a neonate presents with the picture of severe left heart obstruction (e.g., mitral stenosis).
- If obstruction is mild, the infant will present later with high pulmonary blood flow, pulmonary hypertension, and congestive heart failure.
- With no obstruction, a patient may present later in childhood with the clinical profile of a large atrial septal defect.

ASSOCIATED CONDITIONS
- 2/3 of TAPVCs exist as isolated lesions with an atrial communication.
- 1/3 are associated with other congenital heart lesions
  - Single ventricle
  - Patent ductus arteriosus
  - Truncus arteriosus
  - Atrioventricular canal
  - Hypoplastic left heart syndrome (HLHS)
  - Transposition of the great vessels

- Pulmonary stenosis and/or atresia
- Heterotaxy syndrome with anomalies of the atriovisceral situs: Asplenia, right isomerism
- Absent morphologic left atrium and thus virtually always associated with TAPVCs via confluence to the right atrium, or right or left superior vena cava
- Associated noncardiac malformations include: Abdominal visceral heterotaxy, malrotation of the gastrointestinal tract, and bilateral right lungs

 DIAGNOSIS

SIGNS AND SYMPTOMS
Infants with severe obstruction of TAPVC
- Present with cyanosis and/or respiratory distress shortly after birth or within the first few days of life.
- Obstruction usually occurs at the connection of the pulmonary venous channel to the systemic venous system (e.g., portal vein, innominate vein, SVC, etc.), rarely at the atrial septum.
- In the infradiaphragmatic type, severe obstruction is usual when the chamber connects to the portal vein and the ductus venosus closes. It also may occur with supracardiac connections, especially when the common pulmonary vein connects directly to the right superior vena cava. With mild to moderate obstruction, the patient presents later in the first month or two of life with symptoms of heart failure:
- Dyspnea
- Difficulty feeding
- Failure to thrive
- Cyanosis with saturation of 80–85%
Patients with nonobstructed TAPVC may escape detection in infancy and present later in childhood, similar to atrial septal defect. Such patients may be asymptomatic.

History
See Signs and Symptoms.

Physical Exam
- Loud murmurs are infrequent.
- Grade 1 or 2 short systolic pulmonic flow murmurs can occur.
- S2 (second heart sound) may be loud.
- Pulses are normal.
- Blood pressure generally is normal. In the presence of severe pulmonary venous obstruction or a restrictive atrial communication in a neonate, there is decreased systemic output and low blood pressure.
- Hepatomegaly

TESTS
- Electrocardiogram (ECG)
  - Right ventricular hypertrophy: QR in V_3R or V_1 or pure R waves in V_3R are often present. Upright T waves in V1 and V_3R are consistent with systemic pressure in the right ventricle.
  - Left ventricular forces may be decreased.

Lab
Oximetry: Arterial oxygen saturation is often reduced to 85–90%; lower with obstruction. The umbilical venous saturation may be as high (90–100%), with infradiaphragmatic TAPVC to the portal system.

Imaging
Radiography
- Chest X-ray with pulmonary venous obstruction
  - Evidence of a ground-glass appearance with a diffuse linear reticular pattern or pulmonary edema associated with Kerley B lines.
  - Heart size is normal or small.
- Chest X-ray without severe pulmonary venous obstruction
  - Heart is enlarged.
  - Pulmonary vascular markings are increased.
  - Supracardiac type may have a "snowman" appearance with TAPVCs to the SVC via a vertical vein to the left innominate vein. This configuration may be obscured by thymus.
Echocardiography
- Should be diagnostic for all types of TAPVCs with demonstration of the pulmonary venous confluence draining to the:
  - Vertical vein (left SVC) to the left innominate vein, which drains to the right SVC and RA.
  - Right SVC
  - Coronary sinus or RA
  - Portal system or to hepatic sinusoids below the diaphragm may be recognized by fetal echocardiography.
MRI
- Multiplane gated magnetic resonance imaging (MRI)in older patients can be useful if transthoracic or transesophageal echocardiography is not diagnostic.
Cardiac Catheterization
- Generally not needed in the newborn period. Two-dimensional (2D) echocardiogram, Doppler, and Doppler color studies are most often definitive.
- In the presence of pulmonary venous obstruction below the diaphragm, cardiac catheterization may delay surgical treatment and increase morbidity.
- May be necessary to evaluate associated cardiac or pulmonary disease
- Urgent balloon septostomy may be useful in rare cases when the atrial communication is restrictive and surgery must be delayed.

DIFFERENTIAL DIAGNOSIS
Newborn
- Hypoplastic left heart syndrome
- Interrupted aortic arch or severe coarctation of the aorta
- Hypoplastic right heart syndromes (tricuspid and pulmonary atresia)
- Transposition of the great arteries
- Pulmonary vein stenosis or pulmonary vein atresia
- Cor triatriatum
- Persistent pulmonary hypertension of the newborn (PPHN)
- Respiratory distress syndrome or hyaline membrane disease
In older infants and children
- Large atrial septal defect
- Common atrium
- Partial anomalous pulmonary venous return

TREATMENT

GENERAL MEASURES

- Infants with cyanosis or respiratory distress may require ventilator support.
  - Prostaglandin E_1 0.03–0.1 μg/kg/minute IV may be required to maintain patency of the ductus arteriosus and thus maintain cardiac output.
  - All types of TAPVCs are generally surgically corrected in the newborn period soon after diagnosis.

MEDICATION (DRUGS)

- Prostaglandin E_1 to maintain patency of ductus arteriosus
- Diuretics and inotropics in the presence of pulmonary venous congestion and obstruction
- Possible use of nitric oxide in the presence of severe pulmonary artery hypertension

First Line

- Prostaglandin E_1 at .03–0.1 μg/kg/minute
- Preoperative and postoperative extracorporeal membrane oxygenation (ECMO) may be useful with severe pulmonary venous obstruction and pulmonary artery hypertension

Second Line

- ECMO
- Postoperative use of nitric oxide may be helpful in treating severe pulmonary artery hypertension.

SURGERY

- Establish connection of confluence of pulmonary veins (CPV) to the left atrium utilizing a generous left atrial anastomosis, usually with pericardial augmentation, as well as ligation of the common vertical vein.
- With prompt surgical intervention, mortality is low, especially with supracardiac and cardiac types.
- Surgical mortality is significantly higher when TAPVR is associated with complex lesions such as single ventricle, heterotaxy with atrial isomerism, and transposition of the great vessels.

FOLLOW-UP

DISPOSITION

Admission Criteria

Any patient diagnosed with a condition with or without obstruction should undergo surgical repair.

PROGNOSIS

- Long-term postoperative survival of isolated TAPVCs usually is excellent. Early or late postoperative problems could include the following:
  - Obstruction at the anastomotic site or proximal within the pulmonary veins.
  - Obstruction of intrapulmonary venules, causing pulmonary hypertension.
  - Pulmonary vein stenosis with medial hypertrophy may be present in utero and persist or progress postoperatively. These patients have increased morbidity and mortality.
  - Pulmonary vein stenting has had limited success.
- Clinically important atrial arrhythmias may develop in some patients, including sinus bradycardia, supraventricular tachycardia, atrial flutter, and sinus node dysfunction. Ventricular arrhythmias are rare.

COMPLICATIONS

- Pulmonary venous obstruction
- Pulmonary artery hypertension

PATIENT MONITORING

Postoperatively patients should be monitored for:
- Early and late signs of pulmonary venous congestion and/or obstruction
- Rhythm disturbances
- Pulmonary hypertension
- Pregnancy may be well tolerated in selected patients with excellent status.

REFERENCES

1. Freedom RM, Benson LN, Smallhorn JF. *Neonatal Heart Disease*. New York: Springer-Verlag, 1992.
2. Freedom RM, Mawson JB, Yoo S, et al. *Congenital Heart Disease—Textbook of Angiocardiology*. New York: Futura, 1997.
3. Garson A Jr, Bricker JT, Fisher DJ, et al. *The Science and Practice of Pediatric Cardiology*, 2nd ed. Baltimore: Lippincott Williams & Wilkins, 1998.
4. Moss AJ, Adams FH, Emmanouilides GC. *Heart Disease in Infants, Children and Adolescents*, 2nd ed. Baltimore: Williams & Wilkins, 1977.
5. Stark J, deLeval M. *Surgery for Congenital Heart Defects*. New York: Grune & Stratton, 1983.

CODES

ICD9-CM

747.41

PATIENT TEACHING

- Full activities and a regular diet appropriate for age
- Patients should be followed by clinicians in a pediatric cardiology or adult congenital heart program.

Activity

Full activity

ANOREXIA NERVOSA AND THE HEART

Maria Cecilia Bahit

 BASICS

DESCRIPTION
Refusal to maintain body weight (85% of expected weight), or significant weight loss; intense fear of gaining weight or becoming fat; disturbance in the way in which one's body shape is experienced; in postmenarcheal females, amenorrhea (not due to physical disease)
- Several systems affected
  - Endocrine, Gastrointestinal (GI), Metabolic, Hematologic, Immunologic, Dermatologic, Cardiovascular, and Psychiatric

EPIDEMIOLOGY
- Anorexia nervosa occurs in 0.2–1.3% of the general population, approximately 1% of women.
- Predominantly affects females during adolescence and young adulthood.

RISK FACTORS
Perfectionistic personality, compulsivity, low self-esteem, high self-expectations, ambivalence about dependence/independence, stress caused by multiple responsibilities, weight dissatisfaction. Starvation-induced hypophosphatemia, hypokalemia, and hypomagnesemia are risk factors for the refeeding syndrome.

Pregnancy Considerations
Rare due to amenorrhea

ETIOLOGY
Etiology of anorexia nervosa is unknown, but likely multifactorial (sociocultural, psychological, familial, and genetic factors).
- Some cardiac abnormalities are common adaptations to starvation (bradycardia, low blood pressure).

- Myofibrillar destruction is associated with protein caloric malnutrition.
- Refeeding syndrome is multifactorial in origin and may be the result of restoring of circulatory volume while left ventricular (LV) mass is still reduced.
- Leads to fluid retention; if this is severe, patient may develop congestive heart failure (CHF).

ASSOCIATED CONDITIONS
Major depression or dysthymia in 50–70% of patients; obsessive–compulsive disorder in 10% of patients

 DIAGNOSIS

SIGNS AND SYMPTOMS
- General
  - Patient is emaciated.
  - Skin is dry with excessive growth of downy hair.
  - Skin also may be yellowish due to carotenodermia.
  - Brittle nails
  - Thinning scalp hair
  - Hypothermia
- Cardiovascular
  - Bradycardia and hypotension are common.
  - Peripheral edema may be present.

TESTS
Electrocardiogram (ECG): Low voltage, T-wave inversions, nonspecific ST-segment depression, prolonged QT intervals (rare)

Lab
- No specific test for anorexia
- Findings related to starvation
  - Leukopenia, thrombocytopenia, anemia, reduced erythrocyte sedimentation rate, reduced complement levels, low CD4/CD8 counts
  - Metabolic alkalosis, hypocalcemia, hypokalemia, hypomagnesemia, hypophosphatemia, hypercholesterolemia
  - Endocrine abnormalities: Decreased follicle-stimulating hormone, luteinizing hormone, thyroxine (T4), triiodothyronine (T3), and estrogens; increased cortisol, growth hormone
  - Diminished blood urea nitrogen, creatinine clearance
  - Flat glucose tolerance curve

Imaging
Transthoracic echocardiogram: Mitral valve prolapse, reduced cardiac indices, reduced LV mass, impairment of LV filling

DIFFERENTIAL DIAGNOSIS
- Depression with loss of appetite
- Inanition due to physical disorder
- Schizophrenia
- Conversion disorder
- Endocrine disorder (hypo- or hyperthyroidism, Addison disease, diabetes mellitus, panhypopituitarism)
- GI disorders (celiac disease, Crohn disease, parasitosis)
- Infectious disease (AIDS, tuberculosis, chronic infection)
- Cardiovascular disease (other causes of cardiomyopathy, such as idiopathic, viral, hypertensive, Chagas disease, rheumatic fever)
- Malignancy

TREATMENT

GENERAL MEASURES

- A multidisciplinary approach (psychological, medical, and nutritional support) is needed.
- A goal weight should be set, and the patient should be initially monitored at least once a week.
- Weight gain should be gradual (1–3 lb/week) to avoid precipitating CHF.
- Strategies to avoid refeeding syndrome
  - Identify patients at risk (chronically malnourished or has not eaten for 7 days).
  - Measure serum electrolyte level and correct abnormalities before refeeding.
  - Obtain serum chemistry values every other day for the first 7–10 days, then weekly during remainder of refeeding.
  - Slowly increase daily caloric intake every 3–4 days.
  - Monitor patient carefully for development of tachycardia and edema.

MEDICATION (DRUGS)

First Line

- Pharmacologic treatment has no role in anorexia nervosa unless major depression or another psychiatric disorder is present.
- CHF due to volume overload is treated conventionally (diuretics and vasodilators).

FOLLOW-UP

DISPOSITION

Admission Criteria

- Hospitalization is recommended in the following situations:
  - Severe dehydration or electrolyte imbalance
  - ECG abnormalities (prolonged QT interval, arrhythmias)
  - Significant hemodynamic instability (hypotension, orthostatic changes)

PROGNOSIS

- Short-term prognosis is good if a strict program is followed but long-term prognosis is less favorable.
- Approximately 20% make a full recovery, 20% remain chronically ill, and 60% have recurrent episodes.
- Mortality rate 5%
  - Causes of death: Suicide, electrolyte abnormalities, sudden death, starvation

COMPLICATIONS

- Cardiac Complications
  - Arrhythmias, bradycardia, ECG abnormalities, hypotension, LV dysfunction, mitral valve motion irregularities, reduced work capacity, refeeding cardiomyopathy

PATIENT MONITORING

- Electrolyte levels, especially during refeeding
- Routine ECG monitoring, especially in patients with prolonged QT interval

REFERENCES

1. de Simone G, et al. Cardiac abnormalities in young women with anorexia nervosa. *Br Heart J.* 1994;7:287.
2. Goroll AH, May LA, Mulley AG, eds. *Primary Care Medicine,* 3rd ed. Philadelphia: Lippincott, 1995.
3. Mehler P. Eating disorders: Anorexia nervosa. *Hosp Pract.* 1996;31:109–113.
4. Schocken D, et al. Weight loss and the heart: Effects of anorexia nervosa and starvation. *Arch Intern Med.* 1989;149:877–881.

CODES

ICD9-CM

307.1 Anorexia nervosa

PATIENT TEACHING

For patient education materials, contact Anorexia Nervosa & Related Eating Disorders, P.O. Box 5102, Eugene, OR 97405, (503)344-1144; National Association of Anorexia Nervosa and Associated Disorders (ANAD), P.O. Box 7, Highland Park, IL 60035, (708)831-3438.

ANTIPHOSPHOLIPID ANTIBODY SYNDROME

Maria Cecilia Bahit

 BASICS

DESCRIPTION

Clinical constellation of venous and arterial thrombosis, recurrent fetal loss, or both, in association with persistent antiphospholipid (aPL) antibodies, either lupus anticoagulant or anticardiolipin antibodies

- Primary aPL syndrome
  - No evidence of underlying disease
- Secondary aPL syndrome
  - In rheumatic and connective tissue disorders [systemic lupus erythematosus (SLE), less commonly rheumatoid arthritis, systemic sclerosis]
  - In infections (HIV-1, varicella, hepatitis C), in lymphoproliferative diseases, and in drug exposure
- Cardiac manifestations
  - Valvular disease
  - Nonbacterial vegetations, valvular thickening, mitral (mainly affected) and aortic insufficiency, and fibrocalcific changes
  - Pericardial effusion
  - Myocardial dysfunction
  - Coronary artery disease: Myocardial infarction (MI) in young patients, graft failure after coronary artery bypass grafting
  - Intracardiac thrombosis
  - Pulmonary hypertension

EPIDEMIOLOGY

- Young patients (<45 years)
- aPL antibodies are found in approximately 10% of patients with thromboembolic events.
- Different estimates of aPL antibodies are related to the sensitivity of diverse assays.

RISK FACTORS

Smoking, atherosclerotic disease, hypertension, long-term steroid administration

Pregnancy Considerations

Associated with obstetric complications: Recurrent fetal loss, intrauterine growth retardation, and preeclampsia

Genetics

aPL-positive families exist (association with HLA DR7, DR4, and DQw7 plus DRW53).

ETIOLOGY

- The precise cause of thrombosis is unknown.
- Proposed mechanisms: Inhibition of the protein C pathway, inactivation of factors Va–VIIa, inhibition of antithrombin III activation, impaired fibrinolysis, enhanced platelet activation, factor Xa generation
- Coronary artery disease due to thrombotic occlusion, early atherosclerosis associated with long-term steroid administration and, less frequently, coronary arteritis
- Cardiomyopathy is associated with thrombotic occlusion of myocardial microcirculation.

ASSOCIATED CONDITIONS

- Primary aPL syndrome
  - No evidence of underlying disease
- Secondary aPL syndrome
  - In rheumatic and connective tissue disorders (SLE, less commonly rheumatoid arthritis, systemic sclerosis)
  - In infections (HIV-1, varicella, hepatitis C)
  - In lymphoproliferative diseases
  - In drug exposure (phenothiazine, chlorpromazine, procainamide, quinine, and quinidine)
  - Acute alcoholic intoxication

 DIAGNOSIS

SIGNS AND SYMPTOMS

- Asymptomatic
- Chest pain and/or shortness of breath
- Aortic or mitral murmurs (due to valve involvement)
- If pulmonary hypertension: right ventricle lift, increased pulmonic second sound
- Acute MI
- Venous or arterial thrombosis
- Stroke, transient ischemic attacks, multiple cerebral infarcts (more frequent in patients with valve abnormalities)
- Peripheral arterial disease
- Pulmonary thromboembolism

TESTS

Electrocardiogram (ECG): MI or ischemia

Lab

- Thrombocytopenia (50% of patients)
- Other cytopenias may be associated: Autoimmune hemolytic anemia and leukopenia.
- Platelet dysfunction
- Prothrombin time normal or prolonged
- Activated partial thromboplastin time (aPTT) prolonged
- Plasma clot time prolonged
- Anticardiolipin antibody [immunoglobulin M (IgM) and/or IgG) enzyme-linked immunosorbent assay (ELISA)
- Lupus anticoagulant: Sensitive aPTT, the Russell viper venom time, and the kaolin clotting time
- If prolongation of one of these is observed, confirmation requires demonstration of an inhibitor and demonstration of phospholipid dependence.
- Anticardiolipin antibody (IgM and/or IgG) ELISA
- False-positive Venereal Disease Research Laboratory (VDRL) test result

Imaging
- Echocardiography (two-dimensional and Doppler)
- Valve thickening
- Vegetations (Libman-Sacks): Particularly in the ventricular surface of the mitral valve, typically sessile, wartlike, and small, firmly attached to the valve surface and showing no independent motion
- Atrial thrombi
- Ventricular enlargement, myocardial dysfunction
- Mitral regurgitation, aortic regurgitation (less frequently)
- Pulmonary artery pressure
- Pericardial effusion

DIFFERENTIAL DIAGNOSIS
- Patients with thrombosis also should be evaluated for hypercoagulable conditions: Deficiencies of protein C, protein S, antithrombin III, and plasminogen resistance.
- Coronary artery disease, atherosclerotic MI
- Atrial myxoma
- Infective endocarditis
- Valvular disease

TREATMENT

GENERAL MEASURES
- Avoid or treat any other risk factor, such as hypertension, hypercholesterolemia, and avoidance of smoking and sedentarism.
- Patients with significant thrombotic events are appropriate candidates for long-term treatment with warfarin [international normalized ratio (INR) >3].
- Treatment of asymptomatic patients with aPLS (antiphospholipid antibody syndrome) has not been defined, because only 10–15% will develop life-threatening events.

MEDICATION (DRUGS)

- Anticoagulants
  - Unfractionated heparin
  - Low-molecular-weight heparins, such as enoxaparin (1 mg/kg via subcutaneous injection every 12 hours), obviate the need for laboratory monitoring.
  - Oral anticoagulants (warfarin) on a long-term basis, if INR >3.
- Aspirin
  - Uncertain, but recommended as prophylaxis in asymptomatic patients
- Corticosteroid
  - Uncertain; reserved for treatment of underlying comorbid conditions such as active lupus
- Immunosuppressive agents: Uncertain

SURGERY
Consider valve replacement according to severity and symptoms.

FOLLOW-UP

DISPOSITION
Admission Criteria
Consider hospitalization in life-threatening thromboembolic events.

PROGNOSIS
- Only 10–15% of asymptomatic patients with aPL antibodies will develop life-threatening thromboembolic events.
- Patients receiving oral anticoagulants have had no recurrence over 8 years; patients in whom this drug has been discontinued have had a 50% probability of recurrent thromboembolic episodes after 2 years.
- Catastrophic aPL syndrome has been reported in a small number of cases, including renal dysfunction, cerebrovascular disease, myocardial infarction, and hypertension. This syndrome is fatal.

PATIENT MONITORING
Monitor INR in patients on warfarin regularly (INR goal >3).

REFERENCES
1. Asherson R, Cervera R. Cardiac manifestations of the antiphospholipid syndrome. *Coron Artery Dis*. 1993;4:1137–1143.
2. Greaves M. Antiphospholipid antibodies and thrombosis. *Lancet*. 1999;353:1348–1358.
3. Hughes G. The antiphospholipid syndrome: Ten years on. *Lancet*. 1993;342:341–344.
4. Kaplan S, et al. Cardiac manifestations of the antiphospholipid syndrome. *Am Heart J*. 1992;124:1331–1338.
5. Koopman WJ, ed. *Arthritis and Allied Conditions: A Textbook of Rheumatology*, 13th ed. Philadelphia: Lippincott Williams & Wilkins, 1997.
6. Wendell W, Azzudin G, et al. International consensus statement on preliminary classification criteria for definite antiphospholipid syndrome: Report of an international workshop. *Arthritis Rheum*. 1999;42:1309–1311.

CODES
ICD9-CM
286.5 Hemorrhagic disorder due to circulating anticoagulant

AORTIC REGURGITATION, ADULT

Kevin P. Fitzgerald
Steven C. Herrmann
Bernard R. Chaitman

 BASICS

DESCRIPTION
Aortic regurgitation (AR) is diastolic flow of blood from the aorta through an incompetent aortic valve (AV) into the left ventricle (LV)

GENERAL PREVENTION
Avoidance or treatment of the disease process resulting in AR

EPIDEMIOLOGY
Incidence
Variable by etiology

Prevalence
Prevalence of moderate to severe AR ranges from 0.5% to 2.7% in the Framingham and Strong Heart Studies respectively

RISK FACTORS
Risk factors for AR include: Increasing age, male sex, hypertension, and diseases of the aortic root (Marfan's disease, cystic medial necrosis, syphilis, connective tissue disorders)

Genetics
Can be associated with several genetic diseases (see below)

PATHOPHYSIOLOGY
Chronic diastolic regurgitation of blood into the LV causes LV volume and pressure overload; the LV dilatation, hypertrophy (LVH) and abnormal LV systolic function (LVSF) eventually result in congestive heart failure (CHF)

ETIOLOGY
Diseases involving the aortic root:
- Systemic hypertension (HTN)
- Degenerative aortic dilatation
- Ascending aortic dissection
- Giant cell arteritis
- Ehlers-Danlos syndrome
- Reiter's syndrome
- Cystic medial necrosis
- Marfan's syndrome
- Bechet syndrome
- Syphilitic aortitis
- Osteogenesis imperfecta
- Spondyloarthropathies (psoriasis, ankylosing spondylitis, ulcerative colitis, Reiter's)
- Appetite suppressant medications
- Relapsing polychondritis
Diseases involving the aortic valve:
- Rheumatic disease
- Infective endocarditis (IE)
- Congenital AV abnormalities (unicommissural, bicuspid, quadricuspid)
- Calcific degeneration
- Myxomatous proliferation
- Traumatic injuries to the aortic valve
- Rheumatoid arthritis
- Subaortic stenosis
- Ventricular septal defects (VSD) with prolapse of an aortic cusp
- Takayasu disease

- Systemic lupus erythematous
- Crohn's disease
- Whipple's disease
- Jacoud arthropathy
- Ankylosing spondylitis

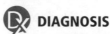 **DIAGNOSIS**

ACUTE SEVERE AR
History
- Most often caused by IE, trauma or aortic dissection
- Symptoms of pulmonary edema or cardiogenic shock

Physical Exam
- Signs of cardiovascular collapse: Tachycardia, marked hypotension vasoconstriction, cyanosis, pulmonary edema
- LV impulse usually normal
Acute AR overloads the normal sized, non-compliant LV resulting in very high filling pressures. Rapidly increasing LV diastolic pressure leads to early mitral valve (MV) closure
- Pulse pressure may not be widened
- Murmur of AR may or may not be present
- Low pitched early diastolic murmur
- Soft or absent first heart sound (S1)
- Soft aortic component (A2) of second heart sound (S2)
- Prominent pulmonary component (P2) of second heart sound due to pulmonary HTN
- Third (S3) heart sound and fourth (S4) are often present

CHRONIC AR
History
- Often asymptomatic until the fourth or fifth decade of life, when cardiac reserve is reduced
- Chronic severe AR may cause:
  - Exertional dyspnea, orthopnea and paroxysmal nocturnal dyspnea
  - Nocturnal angina
  - Splanchnic ischemia and abdominal pain
  - Palpitations due to increased stroke volume

Physical Exam
Murmur
- High pitched holodiastolic descrendo murmur that starts after A2; severity of AI reflected by length of murmur and not intensity
- Third or fourth intercostal space at the left sternal border with AV disease or the right sternal border with aortic root disease
- Auscultate with patient leaning forward at end-expiration
- Austin Flint murmur: Mid to late diastolic apical rumble
- Systolic ejection murmur often present due to the increased forward flow across the AV
Peripheral signs (usually with chronic severe AR)
- Widened pulse pressure
- Apical impulse is hyperdynamic and displaced laterally and inferiorly

- S1 is often normal but it might be muffled if the P-R interval is prolonged
- A2 may be decreased (with valvular disease) or increased (with aortic root disease)
- Ejection clicks are rare in adult patients
- S3 may be present with a dilated LV
- Systolic thrill from augmented stroke volume over the heart base
- De Musset sign: Head bobbing with pulse
- Corrigan pulse: Water hammer pulse
- Bisferiens pulse: Two systolic impulses
- Traube sign: Pistol shot systolic and diastolic sounds over the femoral artery
- Muller sign: Systolic pulsation of the uvula
- Duroziez sign: Femoral artery systolic murmur when it is compressed proximally and diastolic murmur when it is compressed distally
- Quincke sign: Capillary pulsations seen by transmitting light through the patient's fingertips
- Hill sign: Popliteal systolic BP exceeds brachial systolic BP by more than 60 mmHg

TESTS
Lab
Electrocardiogram:
Left axis deviation; left intraventricular conduction delay; T wave inversions; ST segment depressions, Q waves in leads I, aVL, V3-V6 and a small R wave in V1

Imaging
Chest X-ray
- Depending on the acuteness, etiology and severity of the AR there may be cardiomegaly, pulmonary edema, widened mediastinum, ascending aorta dilatation, calcified ascending aortic arch in syphilis aortitis, calcified AV with combined AR and aortic stenosis (AS)
Echocardiography
- Provides reliable evaluation of AV and root
- Frequently identifies the cause of AR
- Doppler echocardiography and color flow Doppler are excellent for evaluating AR severity
- Provides reproducible measurement of LV dimensions, volumes and systolic function
Magnetic Resonance Imaging
- Very accurate at assessing regurgitant volumes, LV mass and LV volumes
Angiography
- Aorta root injections can assess AR severity as well as evaluate the aorta and aortic root
Radionuclide Imaging
- Useful if echocardiography does not provide all the needed information
- Can accurately assess the LVSF, LV function during exercise and regurgitant fraction
- Left ventricle/Right ventricular stroke volume ratio >2 implies severe AR

DIFFERENTIAL DIAGNOSIS
- The AR murmur may be confused with the murmur of pulmonary regurgitation
- Acute severe AR can mimic any disease process causing cardiogenic shock
- Chronic severe AR may be asymptomatic or may mimic other causes of CHF
- Austin Flint murmur may be confused with mitral stenosis

TREATMENT

GENERAL MEASURES
- All patients with AI of any severity should receive antibiotic prophylaxis against IE
- AI due to RF requires continuous antibiotic prophylaxis for ≥10 years, at least until age 40 and sometimes lifelong

MEDICATION (DRUGS)

First Line
- Acute severe AR requires urgent surgery
- Pre-operative medical therapy in acute severe AR includes inotropes and/or vasodilators
- Intra-aortic balloon pumps are contraindicated in the presence of AI
- Patients with chronic severe AR who are not surgical candidates or who do not yet meet the criteria for aortic valve replacement (AVR) may be treated with medical therapy
- Primary medical treatment of chronic severe AR is vasodilator therapy with ACEI, nifedipine, felodipine or hydralazine to improve forward stroke volume and reduce regurgitant volume
- Beta blockers increase the diastolic filling time and are a relative contraindication

Second Line
- Medical therapy should not substitute for AV surgery when indicated
- Patients with abnormal LV size or function who are not surgical candidates should receive the usual therapy for CHF (ACEI, digoxin, diuretics, hydralazine, nitrates, salt and fluid restrictions)

Surgery
AV surgery (± aortic root repair) is indicated for AR in patients with symptoms or with abnormal LV size or function (LVEF<50% or LV end diastolic dimension (LVEDD) >75 mm or LV end systolic dimension (LVESD) >55 mm). Asymptomatic patients with severe AR and normal LV function do not require prophylactic valve replacement.

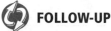

FOLLOW-UP

DISPOSITION
Admission Criteria
- Acute severe AR requires emergent admission to the critical care unit
- Patients with chronic AI may require admission for decompensated heart failure

Discharge Criteria
Patients can be discharged after appropriate surgical or medical interventions have resulted in sufficient clinical improvement

Issues for Referral
- Acute severe AR requires urgent referral to cardiothoracic surgery (CTS) for AVR
- Patients with chronic AR should be monitored by a cardiologist and referred to CTS when surgery is indicated.

PROGNOSIS
Asymptomatic patients with chronic severe AR and normal LV function have an excellent prognosis: <6%/yr progress to symptoms or LV dysfunction; <0.2%/yr have sudden death
Patients with LVESD <40 mm are likely to be stable and can be monitored; when LVESD >50 mm there is a 19% per year risk of developing CHF symptoms; LVESD >55 mm there is a risk of permanent LV dysfunction

COMPLICATIONS
Possible complications of AR include IE, recurrent rheumatic carditis, LV remodeling, angina, CHF, cardiogenic shock and death

PATIENT MONITORING
- Patients with mild to moderate AR and normal LV size and function should be followed by exam and echocardiography every 1 to 2 years.
- Asymptomatic patients with chronic severe AR and normal LV size and function require an exam and echocardiogram every 6 months.
- AVR is indicated if the patient develops symptoms or abnormal LV size or function (LVEF<50% or LVEDD >75 mm or LVESD >55 mm).

Geriatric Considerations
- Usual etiologies of chronic AR in the elderly include HTN, calcific AS, primary aorta disease.
- Usual etiologies of acute AR in the elderly include aortic dissection and IE.
- Limited data on surgical outcomes for AR in elderly patients.
- Symptoms are generally the primary indication for elderly patients ≥80 years old.

Pediatric Considerations
Congenital VSD, IE, RF and aortic dissection (trauma, Marfan's, Ehlers-Danlos) may cause AR in childhood.

Pregnancy Considerations
- Patients with normal LV function and AR usually tolerate pregnancy well. Cardiac output may improve due to the fall in systemic vascular resistance during pregnancy.
- Pregnant patients with severe AR and abnormal LVSF are at risk for developing CHF and should have AV surgery prior to pregnancy.
- May treat with nifedipine (pregnancy class C), hydralazine (C), furosemide (C), digoxin (C)
- To avoid fetal renal agenesis avoid ACEI and angiotensin II receptor blockers.
- Controlled induced vaginal delivery preferred over cesarean delivery
- If AR is due to aortic dilatation (ie Marfan's Syndrome) beware of possible aortic dissection. If the aortic root diameter (ARD) ≥40 mm then discourage pregnancy. If the ARD ≤40 mm then treat with beta blockers and monitor the patient via exams and echocardiograms during gestation.

REFERENCES
1. Bonow RO, Carabello B, de Leon AC Jr, et al. ACC/AHA 2006 guidelines for the management of patients with valvular heart disease: A report of the American College of Cardiology/American Heart Association Task Force on Practice Guidelines (Writing Committee to Revise the 1998 Guidelines for the Management of Patients with Valvular Heart Disease). American College of Cardiology Web Site. Available at: http://content.onlinejacc.org/cgi/reprint/48/3/e1
2. Evangelista A, et al. Long-term vasodilator therapy in patients with severe aortic regurgitation. *N Eng J Med*. 2005;353:1342–1349.
3. Enriquez-Sarano M, et al. Aortic Regurgitation. *N Eng J Med*. 2004;351:15 1539–1546.
4. Zipes DP, et al., *Braunwald's Heart Disease: A Textbook of Cardiovascular Medicine*, 7th ed. Philadelphia: Elsevier Saunders, 2005.
5. Milewicz DM, Dietz HC, Miller DC. Treatment of aortic disease in patients with Marfan syndrome. *Circulation*. 2005;111:e150–e157.
6. Elkayam U, Bitar F. Valvular heart disease and pregnancy part I: Native valves. *J Am Coll Cardiol*. 2005;46:223–230.
7. Bonow RO, Cheitlin MD, Crawford MH, Douglas PS. Task Force 3: Valvular heart disease. *J Am Coll Cardiol*. 2005;45:1334–1340.
8. Rahimtoola SH. The year in valvular heart disease. *J Am Coll Cardiol*. 2005;45:111–122.
9. Carabello BA. Is it ever too late to operate on the patient with valvular heart disease? *J Am Coll Cardiol*. 2004;44:376–383.

CODES
ICD9-CM
424.1

PATIENT TEACHING
Prophylactic antibiotic therapy, patient counseling for symptoms of HF, angina or syncope.

Activity
- Asymptomatic patients with normal LV function can participate in most activities.
- Strenuous isometric exercise should be avoided.

AORTIC REGURGITATION, PEDIATRIC

David Solowiejczyk
Welton M. Gersony

 BASICS

DESCRIPTION
Incompetence of the aortic valve causes leakage of blood into the left ventricle during diastole.

EPIDEMIOLOGY
Sex
Predominant sex is related to the specific etiology.

Incidence
Aortic regurgitation may occur in approximately 5% of whites and up to 50% of Asians with subaortic ventriculoseptal defect (VSD). Aortic incompetence is also associated with various forms of left ventricular outflow abnormalities and numerous other entities.

RISK FACTORS
Genetics
Isolated congenital aortic regurgitation is a rare congenital malformation. May occur with rheumatic fever and this may have a genetic component.

PATHOPHYSIOLOGY
- A regurgitant jet of 20% of the orifice area can double left ventricular output and work.
- In severe cases the diastolic leak can be as much as 60% of the left ventricular stroke volume.
- The increase in left ventricular end-diastolic volume and compensatory reflex peripheral vasodilation results in an increase in total stroke volume.
- With the exhaustion of compensatory mechanisms along with myocardial ischemia, left ventricular failure will ensue.
- Systems Affected
  - Cardiovascular

ETIOLOGY
- Bicuspid aortic valve (congenital)
- Rheumatic
- Other forms of congenitally abnormal aortic valve
- Aneurysm of the sinus of Valsalva
- VSD with prolapsing aortic cusp
- Marfan syndrome
- Ehlers-Danlos syndrome
- Osteogenesis imperfecta
- Aortic regurgitation may also occur in association with discrete subaortic stenosis.
- Aortic regurgitation may also occur following intervention for aortic valve stenosis (catheter or surgical) or other cardiac interventions.

ASSOCIATED CONDITIONS
- VSD
- Rheumatic heart disease
- Connective tissue disease
- Other congenital cardiac defects

DIAGNOSIS

SIGNS AND SYMPTOMS
History
Natural History
- Natural history data are available for adult patients only.
  - In patients who are asymptomatic and have normal left ventricular function, the rate of development of symptoms or left ventricular dysfunction averages 4.3% per year.
  - Average mortality rate is <0.2% per year. Conversely, 25% of the patients who die or develop systolic dysfunction do so before the onset of warning symptoms.
  - Variables identified as being associated with higher risk for the development of future symptoms, systolic dysfunction, or death include age, left ventricular end-diastolic dimension, and end-systolic dimension.
  - On serial longitudinal studies, rate of increase in left ventricular end-systolic dimension and decrease in ejection fraction are reported as independent predictors of outcome.
- Chronic aortic regurgitation is better tolerated than acute and less likely to have symptoms associated with a given amount of regurgitation. Cardiac awareness may result because of the large stroke volume.
- Excessive sweating and heat intolerance due to vasodilation may be an early symptom.
- Chest pain may occur with exertion.
- Symptoms associated with left ventricular failure include dyspnea, shortness of breath, fatigue.

Physical Exam
- Characteristic peripheral signs are produced by a combination of large pulse volume and vasodilation.
  - With more severe disease the systolic pressure increases and the diastolic pressure decreases.
  - A sharp increase in the pulse gives it a "water hammer quality."
- Apical impulse may be displaced inferiorly and laterally with an apical diastolic thrust.
- Systolic thrill may be palpable over the base.
- Heart sounds are usually normal.
- The typical murmur of aortic regurgitation is heard in early diastole, characterized as a high-pitched decrescendo beginning with the second heart sound and maximally along the left and midsternal borders with radiation to the apex.
  - An ejection murmur is often at the base due to increased flow across the aortic valve.
  - With moderate or severe regurgitation a mid-diastolic rumble (Austin-Flint murmur) may be audible over the mitral area. This is due to the regurgitant jet impeding opening of the mitral valve anterior leaflet.

TESTS
- Electrocardiogram (ECG)
- Normal in mild aortic regurgitation and at times in severe disease
- Severe cases display increased QRS voltage in the left precordial leads with tall and upright T waves
- ST and T wave strain pattern
- Left bundle branch block
- Large Q waves in left precordial leads

Exercise Test and Radionuclide Angiography
- In selected patients, exercise and radionuclide studies may be useful.

Imaging
Chest X-ray
- Left ventricle enlargement in an inferior and leftward direction
- Aortic root is dilated.
- Pulmonary venous congestion may be seen in association with left ventricular failure.

Echocardiography
- Two-Dimensional Imaging
  - Useful in assessing potential etiology of aortic regurgitation, including:
  - Acquired A1
  - VSD with aortic cusp prolapse
  - Bicuspid aortic valve
  - Subaortic stenosis
  - Dilation of the aortic root and mitral valve prolapse in Marfan syndrome.

Doppler Imaging
- Assesses the presence and severity of aortic regurgitation
- Holodiastolic reversal of flow can be seen in the descending aorta in patients with moderate severe regurgitation.
- Color Doppler flow mapping of the jet using jet width and area is useful.

M-Mode Imaging
- Useful in the evaluation of secondary changes of the left ventricle resulting from aortic regurgitation, such as dilatation, hypertrophy, and diminished function
- Serial evaluation of left ventricle cavity size and function is important for management decisions.

Diagnostic Procedures/Surgery
Cardiac Catheterization
- No longer indicated for the diagnosis of aortic regurgitation
- Occasionally indicated in the management, when questions remain unanswered regarding severity, hemodynamics, or left ventricular function

DIFFERENTIAL DIAGNOSIS

Other causes of aortic runoff with similar physical findings include:

- Patent ductus arteriosus
- Ruptured sinus of Valsalva
- Coronary arteriovenous fistula
- Aorta to left ventricle tunnel and aorticopulmonary window
- The diastolic murmur of pulmonary regurgitation in the presence of pulmonary hypertension (Graham Steell murmur) is also high pitched, similar to that of aortic regurgitation.

TREATMENT

GENERAL MEASURES

- Endocarditis prophylaxis
- Management depends on the cause, duration, secondary cardiac changes (ventricular dilation and function), and associated symptoms.
- Significant symptoms of preoperative left ventricular systolic dysfunction are major indicators of decreased likelihood for optimal postoperative outcome.
- Ideal timing of surgery for aortic regurgitation balances the risk of surgery with the possible prevention of left ventricular dysfunction.

MEDICATION (DRUGS)

- Digoxin and diuretic therapy for patients in congestive heart failure
- Vasodilator therapy
  - Nipride, hydralazine, nifedipine, and angiotensin-converting enzyme (ACE) inhibitors have been shown to reduce systemic vascular resistance, augment forward stroke volume, and reduce regurgitant volume in adults. Standards for children are not available.
  - Criteria for the use of chronic vasodilator therapy in the pediatric patients with mild to moderate aortic insufficiency have not been established. No specific data exist showing long-term benefit in children.
  - More recent data in asymptomatic patients with severe aortic regurgitation and normal LV function indicated no beneficial effect from nifedipine or enalapril in reduction or delay of surgery, reduction of regurgitant volume, decrease in size of LV or improvement of LV function.

SURGERY

Pulmonary autograft procedure (Ross operation)

- The patient's pulmonary valve replaces the aortic valve in the left ventricular outflow tract.
- A homograft is used on the right side of the heart.
- Intermediate follow-up shows excellent durability of the pulmonary valve in the aortic position in most patients.
- Growth of the pulmonary valve has been demonstrated in children. There is no need for anticoagulation postoperatively.
- Good results demonstrated in a population of infants and toddlers, some of whom had aortic regurgitation prior to the pulmonary autograft procedure following earlier intervention for congenital LV outflow tract obstruction.
- Procedure of choice in this subset of very young pediatric patients.

Aortic valve replacement with a mechanical prosthesis

- Bi-leaflet mechanical valves such as St. Jude or Carbomedics are durable with excellent function but will need replacement when used in pediatric patients.
- Anticoagulation is necessary to minimize the risk of thrombosis.

Aortic valve repair

- In select patients this is preferable.

Aortic valve replacement with bioprosthesis

- A significant risk of valve degeneration and calcification over time requiring replacement
- These complications are more common in children and adolescents.

Asymptomatic patients with normal ventricular function

- Precise timing of surgery in this group of patients is controversial.
- Patients with left ventricular dysfunction require valve replacement with or without symptoms.
- Surgery may be recommended in asymptomatic patients with left ventricular end diastolic dimension >75 mm or left ventricular systolic dimension >55 mm; specific data are not available for infants and children.
- Patients with ventricular dimensions approaching these values should be followed closely with serial studies.
- Because of inherent variability in testing, no decision should be made on a single measurement.

Aortic regurgitation with ventricular septal defect

- Surgery for aortic regurgitation in association with ventricular septal defect and prolapsing aortic cusp is performed earlier than in most other situations.
- Although controversy exists as to the precise timing, all would agree that regurgitation that progresses to moderately severe as assessed by both Doppler echocardiography and physical examination warrants surgical repair.

Aortic regurgitation with Marfan syndrome or bicuspid aortic valve

- Timing of surgery is more likely to be determined by the finding of aortic root dilation.
- Surgery is generally recommended when the aortic root measures >50–55 mm in diameter by echocardiography, at which point the risk of sudden death is thought to outweigh the risk of surgery.

Aortic regurgitation with discrete subaortic stenosis

- Timing of surgery for subaortic stenosis is controversial.
- Aggressive approach is to resect a subaortic membrane when Doppler echocardiographic evidence of severe obstruction.
- Many patients exist in whom there are no signs of progression of left ventricular outflow tract obstruction with conservative management.
- Aortic regurgitation is not a primary indication for surgery since it is rarely severe.

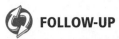

FOLLOW-UP

PATIENT MONITORING

- Serial echocardiograms after surgery to assess surgical results and serve as a baseline for late follow-up
- Approximately 80% of the overall reduction in volume occurs within the first 10–14 days postoperatively.
- The magnitude in reduction correlates with the improvement in function and late postoperative period:
  - Patients with persistent left ventricular dilation should be treated similar to other patients with ventricular dysfunction, including therapy with ACE inhibitors.
  - Repeat clinical evaluation along with echocardiography, if there is significant residual aortic regurgitation, will determine necessity for repeat surgical intervention.

REFERENCES

1. Bonow et al. ACC/AHA Task Force Report. *J Am Coll Cardiol.* 1998;32:1486–1588.
2. Emmanouilides GC, et al., eds. *Moss and Adams' Heart Disease in Infants, Children and Adolescents: Including the Fetus and Young Adult,* 5th ed. Baltimore: Williams & Wilkins,1995.
3. Evangelista A, et al. Long-term vasodilator therapy in patients with severe aortic regurgitation. *N Engl J Med.* 2005;353:1342–1349.
4. Garson A, et al., eds. *The Science and Practice of Pediatric Cardiology,* 2nd ed. Baltimore: Lippincott Williams & Wilkins,1998.
5. Hasaniya N, et al. Outcome of aortic valve repair in children with congenital aortic valve insufficiency. *J Thor Cardiovasc Surg.* 2004;127(4):970–974.
6. Scognamiglio R, et al. Nifedipine in asymptomatic patients with severe aortic regurgitation and normal left ventricular function. *N Engl J Med.* 1994;331:689–694.
7. Solowiejczyk D, et al. Serial echocardiographic measurements of the pulmonary autograft in the aortic valve position following the Ross operation in a pediatric population using normal pulmonary artery dimensions as the reference standard. *Am J Cardiol.* 2000;85:1119–1123.
8. Williams I, et al. Ross procedure in infants and toddlers followed into childhood. *Circulation.* 2005;112[Suppl I]:I-390–I-395.

CODES
ICD9-CM
424.1

AORTIC STENOSIS, ADULT

Michael Forsberg
Steven C. Herrmann
Bernard R. Chaitman

 BASICS

DESCRIPTION
Obstruction to outflow of blood from left ventricle to aorta

GENERAL PREVENTION
Prophylaxis against infective endocarditis and recurrent rheumatic fever, if applicable, is indicated.

EPIDEMIOLOGY
Age
- Calcific aortic valve disease presents clinically at 50–60 years in patients with a bicuspid valve versus age 70–80 years in those with trileaflet valve. However, rheumatic aortic stenosis (AS) presents at an earlier age and is usually associated with aortic regurgitation.
- Aortic valve replacement (AVR) is the only option for treatment of symptomatic AS. However, elderly patients have confounding factors, which make aortic valve surgery more risky than in a younger population. These factors include coronary artery disease, left ventricular (LV) dysfunction, and comorbidities. Therefore, the decision to proceed with the surgery should take the previously mentioned factors as well as the patient's wishes and expectations into consideration.

Incidence
- Affects 5 in 10,000 people
- 80% of adults with symptomatic AS are men.

Prevalence
In adults undergoing surgery for AS in the United States, calcific AS accounts for 51% of cases, bicuspid AS 36%, and rheumatic disease 9%. The prevalence of bicuspid aortic valve in the general population may be as high as 1–2% of the general population.

RISK FACTORS
- Age
- Dyslipidemia
- Male

PATHOPHYSIOLOGY
- Progressive calcification and decreased excursion of the valve leaflets lead to worsening stenosis.
- The progressive aortic valve stenosis causes increased myocardial afterload, LV hypertrophy, and decreased systemic and coronary blood flow.

ETIOLOGY
- Calcific (degenerative): The most common cause of valve lesion that requires replacement
- Congenital
- Rheumatic
- Other rare causes include obstructive infective vegetations, homozygous type II hyperlipoproteinemia, Paget disease of the bone, systemic lupus erythematosus, ochronosis, rheumatoid disease, and radiation to the thorax.

ASSOCIATED CONDITIONS
Bicuspid aortic valve may be associated with coarctation or interrupted aortic arch, Williams syndrome, patent ductus arteriosus (PDA), or Turner syndrome.

 DIAGNOSIS

SIGNS AND SYMPTOMS
Symptoms
- Asymptomatic
  - Patients can remain asymptomatic for a long time despite severe obstruction. The condition is commonly first diagnosed based on detection of a systolic murmur on auscultation.
- Dyspnea
  - The most common initial symptom is exertional dyspnea, which may progress to symptoms of congestive heart failure.
- Exertional angina is a common symptom.
- Exertional presyncope or syncope.

History
Patients may present with complaints of chest pain, shortness of breath, or syncopal episodes.

Physical Exam
- Pulse: The timing and amplitude of the carotid pulse contour reflects central aortic pressure. With severe AS, the peak occurs later in systole (pulsus tardus) and pulse amplitude is decreased (pulsus parvus).
- In elderly patients, the carotid examination may not show the classic findings because of increased peripheral wave transmission.
- Murmur: The second characteristic sign is a crescendo-decrescendo systolic murmur over the right second intercostal space. A late peaking murmur represents more severe AS. The presence of a thrill is specific for severe AS. The murmur radiates to the carotids and to the apex (the latter is referred to as the Gallavardin phenomenon).
- The second heart sound (S_2) is diminished or absent in severe AS and may have paradoxical splitting indicating delayed LV contraction.
- A fourth heart sound (S_4) is common and reflects increased atrial contribution to ventricular filling.

TESTS
Lab
Electrocardiography: The classic finding is LV hypertrophy. Other nonspecific changes are left atrial enlargement, left axis deviation, and left bundle–branch block. Electrocardiographic changes may occur only during exercise despite a normal resting electrocardiogram (ECG).

Imaging
Chest Radiography
May be entirely normal. However, poststenotic dilatation of the ascending aorta may be evident. Calcification of the aortic valve is rarely seen on radiography but may be seen on fluoroscopy.

Echocardiography
- Echocardiography is helpful in assessing the severity of AS, the degree of coexisting aortic regurgitation, LV size and function; estimating pulmonary systolic pressure; and in identifying other cardiac abnormalities.
- Aortic valve area can be estimated, as can the maximum jet velocity, which are the most useful clinical measurements of severity.

Cardiac Catheterization
Indicated for hemodynamic evaluation whenever there is discrepancy between the clinical picture and echocardiography. It is also indicated to evaluate coronary anatomy in patients at risk for coronary artery disease prior to valve replacement.

Dobutamine Echocardiography
Indicated in patients with moderate aortic valve gradient and severe LV dysfunction to assess the severity of the aortic valve lesion and predict the reversibility of LV dysfunction after AVR.

Pathologic Findings
- The aortic valve area must be reduced to one-fourth of its natural size before significant changes in the circulation occur.
- Aortic stenosis is graded based on the aortic valve area into mild (>1.5 cm^2), moderate (1.1–1.5 cm^2), severe (<0.75 to 1 cm^2), and very severe (critical) (<0.75 cm^2).
  - Average rate of decrease of the valve area is 0.12 cm^2 per year.

DIFFERENTIAL DIAGNOSIS
- Supravalvular AS
- Hypertrophic cardiomyopathy
- Subaortic membrane

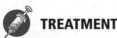 **TREATMENT**

GENERAL MEASURES
Prophylaxis against infective endocarditis and recurrent rheumatic fever, if applicable, is indicated.

MEDICATION (DRUGS)

AS is a mechanical limitation, and medical treatment has little role in preventing the progression of the disease process or in the treatment of the outflow obstruction once symptoms develop. However, with the onset of LV systolic dysfunction, the use of intravenous inotropic agents may be advocated for acute decompensation.

Contraindications

Vasodilators are relatively contraindicated in severe AS.

SURGERY

Indications for Aortic Valve Replacement

- Symptomatic patients
  - AVR improves survival in patients with depressed as well as normal LV function.
  - Depressed LV function is secondary to either afterload mismatch or depressed contractility. In the latter, the improvement in LV function and symptoms may not be complete.
- Asymptomatic patients
  - The risks of surgery and prosthetic valve complications outweigh the benefits of preventing sudden cardiac death and prolonged survival in asymptomatic patients. An exercise test may be useful in these patients to assess functional limitation.
- Prophylactic AVR
  - Patients with severe AS undergoing coronary artery bypass grafting or other valve replacement should undergo AVR as well.
  - Consideration for AVR in patients with moderate AS if undergoing coronary bypass grafting, other valvular surgery, or aortic surgery
  - This issue is controversial in patients with mild AS.

Aortic Balloon Valvotomy

- Percutaneous balloon dilatation offers little benefit for adults with calcific AS or with secondary calcification of a bicuspid aortic valve.
- This procedure is reserved for patients with serious severe comorbidities that are not candidates for AVR, patients requiring urgent noncardiac surgery, and as a bridge to AVR.

 FOLLOW-UP

PROGNOSIS

- Prognosis is similar to that for age-matched normal adults during the asymptomatic period.
- Development of symptoms is associated with a grave prognosis, showing a 2-year survival rate of ~50% without surgical intervention.

COMPLICATIONS

- Congestive heart failure
- Sudden cardiac death
- Atrial arrhythmias
- Infective endocarditis
- Systemic calcium embolism
- It can be associated with intestinal arteriovenous malformation.
- Prosthetic valve–related complications

PATIENT MONITORING

- Mild: Annual history and physical examination and echocardiography every 5 years
- Moderate: More frequent visits and echocardiogram every 2 years
- Severe AS: Yearly echocardiogram
- Echocardiogram should be performed if any change occurs in clinical findings or symptoms.

REFERENCES

1. Aurigemma GP, Gaasch WH. Low flow-low gradient aortic stenosis: The pathologist weighs in. *J Am Coll Cardiol.* 2004;44:1856–1858.
2. Bonow RO, Carabello B, de Leon AC Jr, et al. ACC/AHA 2006 guidelines for the management of patients with valvular heart disease: A report of the American College of Cardiology/American Heart Association Task Force on Practice Guidelines (Writing Committee to Revise the 1998 Guidelines for the Management of Patients With Valvular Heart Disease). American College of Cardiology Web Site. Available at: http://content.onlinejacc.org/cgi/reprint/48/3/e1
3. Roberts WC, Ko JM. Frequency by decades of unicuspid, bicuspid, and tricuspid aortic stenosis, with or without associated aortic regurgitation. *Circulation.* 2005;111:920–925.
4. Sharma UC, Barenbrug P, Pokharel S, et al. Systematic review of the outcome of aortic valve replacement in patients with aortic stenosis. *Ann Thorac Surg.* 2004;78:90–95.

CODES
ICD9-CM

424.1

PATIENT TEACHING

The development of symptoms in patients with AS is one of the cornerstones of the process of decision making. Therefore, asymptomatic patients should report the onset of dyspnea, angina, or syncope.

Diet

Low-salt diet

Activity

Recommendations for physical activity are based on the clinical examination, with special emphasis on the hemodynamic severity of the stenotic lesion.

- Asymptomatic patients with mild AS: Physical activity is not restricted and patients can participate in competitive sports.
- Patients with moderate AS: They should avoid competitive sports that involve high dynamic and static muscular demands. Other forms of exercise can be performed after an exercise test with no ST-segment changes or sustained arrhythmias.
- Patients with severe AS should be advised to limit their activity to relatively low levels.

Prevention

Prophylaxis against infective endocarditis and recurrent rheumatic fever, if applicable, is indicated.

AORTIC STENOSIS, SUPRAVALVULAR

Michael Forsberg
Steven C. Herrmann
Bernard R. Chaitman

 BASICS

DESCRIPTION
Supravalvular aortic stenosis is a congenital narrowing of the ascending aorta originating at the superior border of the sinus of Valsalva above the coronary artery ostia.

Pregnancy Considerations
- Severe supravalvular stenosis may require repair prior to conception.
- Avoid dehydration during pregnancy.
- If symptoms of congestive heart failure develop in the presence of supravalvular stenosis, valvuloplasty or repair may be indicated with possible fetal demise.

EPIDEMIOLOGY
Incidence
0.05% of congenital heart defects.

Prevalence
Rare

Genetics
- Can be non-familial sporadic, familial autosomal dominant, or Williams Syndrome. Williams syndrome is often sporadic, however, autosomal dominant inheritance has been reported.
- Linkage maps suggest the defect is due to a deletion of the tropoelastin gene in chromosome 7q11.

PATHOPHYSIOLOGY
- Supravalvular obstruction leads to progressive hypertrophy of the left ventricle.
- Since the coronary arteries are proximal to the stenosis they become dilated and tortuous predisposing them to premature coronary atherosclerosis.

ETIOLOGY
Congenital defect

ASSOCIATED CONDITIONS
Pulmonic stenosis may be present

DIAGNOSIS

SIGNS AND SYMPTOMS
- Williams syndrome has classic associations with elfin faces (prominent forehead epicanthal folds, small nose bridge and mandible, and dental abnormalities), abnormalities in calcium metabolism, and mental retardation.
- Also associated with failure to thrive in infancy, inguinal hernias, constipation, colic, and hyperacusis, as well as narrowing of peripheral and pulmonary arteries.
- Older children may develop severe joint limitations.
- Adults with Williams syndrome generally have hypertension, urinary tract problems, and gastrointestinal defects.
- The familial forms of supravalvular aortic stenosis are associated with normal intelligence and can be seen with pulmonic stenosis.

Physical Exam
- Physical examination shows an increased aortic valve closure sound secondary to increased pressure proximal to stenosis.
- Ejection murmur is common along the sternal border with thrill radiating to the suprasternal notch. Rarely, a diastolic murmur component may be heard if the supravalvular stenosis causes valvular leaflet fusion.
- Blood pressure is frequently higher in the right arm as opposed to the left arm or carotids due to preferential flow down the brachiocephalic vessels (Coanda effect).
- Continuous systolic murmur may be heard with associated pulmonic stenosis, if present.

TESTS
Lab
- The ECG often shows signs of left ventricular hypertrophy.
- Biventricular hypertrophy may be noted with coexisting pulmonic stenosis.

Imaging
Chest Radiography
- In contrast to both valvular and subvalvular aortic stenosis, post-stenotic dilation is rare on the chest radiograph.
- Sinus of Valsalva is dilated.
- Ascending aorta and arch appear normal on the chest film.

Diagnostic Procedures/Surgery
Echocardiography
- Echocardiography is the most helpful in diagnosis and localization of obstruction.
- The ratio of the measurement of the sinotubular junction to aortic annulus is less than that in supravalvular stenosis.
- Cardiac catheterization is also valuable to measure the degree of hemodynamic abnormalities associated with the supravalvular stenosis.

Pathological Findings
There are three types of supravalvular aortic stenosis:
- The most common form is a marked thickening of the aorta media, with disorganization of the media fibers forming a constricting ridge just proximal to the sinus of Valsalva. This is designated the hourglass type of supravalvular stenosis. Occurs in 50–75% of patients.
- The membranous type results from a fibrous membrane with a small central opening stretched across the aorta lumen.
- Rarely, the ascending aorta has diffuse narrowing of variable length, resulting in hypoplastic supravalvular aortic stenosis.
- There are occasional thoracic aneurysms.

DIFFERENTIAL DIAGNOSIS
Valvular aortic stenosis, subvalvular aortic obstruction, hypertrophic obstructive cardiomyopathy

TREATMENT

GENERAL MEASURES

Prophylaxis against bacterial endocarditis is indicated.

 MEDICATION (DRUGS)

- Precautions
  - Avoid negative inotropic medications. Use diuretics and vasodilators cautiously.

SURGERY

- Surgery should be considered if the patient is symptomatic, has a mean gradient by echo or peak to peak gradient by catheterization of 50 mmHg, or evidence of LVH with strain on ECG.
- Surgical repair of supravalvular aortic stenosis is less favorable than valvular aortic stenosis.
- Aortotomy with excision of the fibrous obstruction is performed, often with a fabric prosthesis inserted into the area of the supravalvular narrowing to expand the lumen.
- The hypoplastic repair may require reconstruction of the aortic arch.
- Transcatheter balloon angioplasty with or without stenting is not effective treatment.

 FOLLOW-UP

PROGNOSIS

Similar to valvular aortic stenosis in respect to sudden cardiac death and risk of endocarditis.

COMPLICATIONS

Arterial hypertension, left ventricular hypertrophy, sudden death.

PATIENT MONITORING

Dependent on the severity of the hemodynamic abnormality:

- Severe obstruction should be monitored every 6–12 months, and mild obstruction every 2–5 years.
- A change in symptomatology demands immediate evaluation.

REFERENCES

1. Kirklin JW, Barratt-Boyes BG: Congenital aortic stenosis. In: *Cardiac Surgery. Vol 2*. 2nd ed. New York, NY: Churchill Livingstone Inc; 1993: 1195–1238.
2. Dridi SM, Foucault Bertaud A, Igondjo Tchen S, et al. Vascular wall remodeling in patients with supravalvular aortic stenosis and Williams Beuren syndrome. *J Vascular Research*, 2005;42:190–201.
3. Pelech AN, Neish SR. Sudden death in congenital heart disease. *Pediatric Clinics of N Am*, 2004;51:1257–1271.
4. Lupinetti FM. Left ventricular outflow tract obstruction. *Seminars in Thoracic & Cardiovasc Surgery*, 2004;7:102–106.

 MISCELLANEOUS

See also:
- Aortic Stenosis
- Congenital Heart Diseases

CODES
ICD9-CM
747.22

PATIENT TEACHING

Endocarditis prophylaxis required.

Activity
- Mild stenosis without symptoms may participate in full activities.
- Moderate stenosis without symptoms may participate in low impact activities.
- Severe stenosis should not participate in vigorous activities.

AORTIC STENOSIS, PEDIATRIC

Daphne T. Hsu
Welton M. Gersony

 BASICS

DESCRIPTION
Congenital aortic stenosis is characterized by narrowing of the aortic valve orifice, leading to left ventricular hypertrophy, and, in the most severe form, predisposing the patient to exercise intolerance and myocardial dysfunction.
- Pathologic abnormalities described include asymmetric malformation of the valve leaflets leading to a unicuspid or bicuspid valve, or, more rarely, fusion of normal tricuspid leaflets.
- The valve leaflets are often thickened due to the turbulence of flow across the area, which may lead to calcification in later life.

EPIDEMIOLOGY
- Aortic valve stenosis is more common among boys, with a male to female ratio of 4:1.
- Aortic stenosis has two modes of presentation:
  - The majority of patients present in infancy or early childhood with an asymptomatic heart murmur.
  - Neonates with critical aortic stenosis present with severe congestive heart failure shortly after birth secondary to severe obstruction and left ventricular dysfunction.

Incidence
2–4 per 10,000 live births

Prevalence
3–6% of all children with congenital heart disease

RISK FACTORS
Genetics
- Aortic stenosis is rarely associated with a chromosomal abnormality.
  - Valvar aortic stenosis has been described in 18% of patients with Turner syndrome (XO).
  - In patients with multiple congenital anomalies, rare reports of associated chromosomal deletions have been described.

PATHOPHYSIOLOGY
Aortic stenosis causes obstruction to blood flow from the left ventricle to the aorta. Left ventricular hypertrophy occurs in response to the increased afterload on the left ventricle.
- Systolic left ventricular dysfunction occurs rarely with severe obstruction and hypertrophy
- Diastolic dysfunction may occur with severe left ventricular hypertrophy and systolic dysfunction, most commonly in the neonate.
- In critical aortic stenosis of the neonate, the patent ductus arteriosus augments cardiac output via flow from the right ventricle to the aorta.

ETIOLOGY
Congenital

ASSOCIATED CONDITIONS
Associated cardiac anomalies occur in approximately 20% of cases. Aortic stenosis is a common finding in association with other left-sided obstructive lesions such as coarctation of the aorta, subaortic stenosis, mitral valve abnormalities, hypoplastic left ventricle, and other complex lesions such as single ventricle. It is rarely associated with other congenital heart defects.

Pregnancy Considerations
The presence of significant aortic stenosis is a risk factor for adverse outcomes during pregnancy due to the increased cardiac demands of the fetus.
- Adequate relief of aortic stenosis should be achieved prior to pregnancy whenever possible.
- Patients with severe aortic stenosis have undergone balloon valvuloplasty during pregnancy, with care to limit radiation exposure.

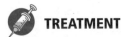 **DIAGNOSIS**

SIGNS AND SYMPTOMS
Aortic stenosis in the older child
- Unlike congenital heart defects characterized by volume overload or cyanosis, significant disease can be present in the absence of symptoms and in general, symptoms are a late manifestation.
- Symptoms are related to decreased cardiac output and/or myocardial ischemia and present only with moderate to severe obstruction.
Critical aortic stenosis of the neonate
- Symptoms are related to congestive heart failure and the presence of a right-to-left shunt via the patent ductus arteriosus

History
- Aortic stenosis in the older child
  - Exercise intolerance
  - Exertional dyspnea
  - Angina
  - Syncope
  - Palpitations
- Critical aortic stenosis in the neonate
  - Tachypnea
  - Tachycardia
  - Cyanosis
  - Poor feeding

Physical Exam
Cardiac examination
- Murmur at the base of the heart, radiating to the jugular notch, carotid vessels, and apex
- Suprasternal notch thrill, even in mild aortic stenosis
- Valve click at the cardiac apex in mild to moderate stenosis
- Left ventricular heave and a thrill at the base of the heart are felt in moderate to severe stenosis.
Heart failure examination
- Failure to thrive
- Tachypnea
- Retractions
- Cyanosis
- Hepatomegaly

TESTS
Electrocardiographic abnormalities including left ventricular hypertrophy, left ventricular strain, and ischemic changes with exercise are an indication of the severity of the obstruction, but occasionally severe stenosis may be associated with a relatively benign electrocardiogram (ECG).

Lab
In the neonate with critical aortic stenosis, evaluation of renal and hepatic function should be performed to assess the adequacy of cardiac output.

Imaging
- Echocardiography
  - Optimal method of evaluating aortic valve anatomy and hemodynamics
  - The instantaneous gradient across the valve can be estimated from the velocity of blood flow measured by continuous-wave Doppler, but overestimation is not unusual. The mean gradient can be more representative of the gradient measured at catheterization.
  - Left ventricular hypertrophy can be quantitatively assessed and aortic insufficiency can be documented by color flow Doppler.

Diagnostic Procedures/Surgery
- Cardiac catheterization
  - Cardiac catheterization is not indicated to establish the diagnosis of valvar aortic stenosis in the majority of patients.
  - Catheter assessment of the aortic valve gradient may be necessary in patients when symptoms are out of proportion to the predicted echocardiographic gradient.
- Exercise testing can be carried out with caution in the patient with moderate aortic stenosis to assess symptomatology and the degree of hemodynamic compromise due to left ventricular outflow obstruction.

Pathologic Findings
Thickened, dysplastic valve leaflets with fusion of one or more of the valve cusps to form a bicuspid or unicuspid valve

DIFFERENTIAL DIAGNOSIS
The differential diagnosis of the asymptomatic child with a murmur of the left ventricular outflow tract obstruction includes subaortic stenosis, valvar aortic stenosis, and supravalvar aortic stenosis.

 TREATMENT

GENERAL MEASURES
Antibiotic prophylaxis against bacterial endocarditis should be administered according to the recommendations of the American Heart Association.

MEDICATION (DRUGS)

- Medical therapy is not indicated in the asymptomatic patient with valvar aortic stenosis.
- In neonates with critical aortic stenosis, aggressive medical therapy is required to stabilize the patient, including mechanical ventilation, correction of acidosis, and inotropic support.
- Prostaglandin E_1 may be used to maintain ductal patency and augment systemic output via the right ventricle prior to intervention.

INDICATIONS FOR INTERVENTION
- Echocardiographic estimation of the gradient across the aortic valve >70 mmHg usually in conjunction with at least moderate left ventricular hypertrophy by echocardiography or electrocardiogram
- In children with lesser echocardiographic findings and symptoms, cardiac catheterization may be indicated to determine hemodynamics.

- If the gradient at catheterization is ≥60 mmHg, balloon valvuloplasty is indicated in infants, children, and young adults.
- Balloon valvuloplasty may be indicated in patients with a gradient <60 mmHg who have significant ventricular hypertrophy or symptoms of exercise intolerance and/or myocardial insufficiency.

Balloon Valvuloplasty
- Procedure of choice for relief of moderate to severe aortic stenosis in infants and children
- Although effective in the majority of patients, balloon valvuloplasty may be complicated by aortic insufficiency.
- Aortic valve replacement may be required following balloon valvuloplasty if severe aortic insufficiency occurs.
- In patients who develop restenosis of the aortic valve following valvuloplasty, repeat valvuloplasty cannot be performed if significant aortic insufficiency is present.

SURGERY
Surgical Valvotomy
- May be performed as a primary procedure in the severely compromised neonate with critical aortic stenosis as circulatory support via cardiopulmonary bypass is provided prior to relieving the obstruction.
- In older children and adults, direct visualization of the aortic valve at surgery also may be necessary to relieve stenosis in certain types of aortic valve morphology, especially calcific, that are unresponsive to balloon valvuloplasty.

Aortic Valve Replacement
Can be performed using a prosthetic mechanical valve, a bioprosthesis, such as an aortic allograft, bovine, or porcine valve, or a pulmonary autograft (the Ross Procedure)
- Ross Procedure
  - Procedure of choice at many centers for aortic valve replacement in children
  - The native aortic and pulmonary valves are excised, and the pulmonary valve is inserted into the aortic root.
  - A pulmonary or aortic homograft is used to reestablish continuity between the right ventricle and the main pulmonary artery.
  - The use of the native pulmonary valve to replace the stenotic aortic valve obviates the need for chronic anticoagulation and affords the potential for growth.
  - The incidence of restenosis of the neoaortic valve is low, although valve replacement has been necessary in the setting of significant neoaortic insufficiency.
  - In patients with right ventricular outflow tract obstruction, replacement of a right ventricular to pulmonary artery homograft usually is necessary within 10 years, but following the Ross Procedure, the homograft may last longer because it is positioned anatomically in a nonhypertrophied right ventricle.
- Mechanical Valve Replacement
  - In adult patients, mechanical valves, such as the St. Jude's prosthetic valve, offer excellent relief of stenosis for up to 15–20 years.
  - Replacement may be necessary for recurrent stenosis or paravalvar leak.
  - Chronic anticoagulation is necessary to prevent complications of thromboembolism.
  - In infants and small children, mechanical valve use is limited by the lack of growth, which necessitates earlier valve replacement.
  - Chronic anticoagulation can be more difficult to regulate in pediatric patients and carries a greater risk of bleeding in children learning to ambulate.
- Bioprosthetic Valve
  - Aortic valve replacement with a bioprosthetic valve is rarely indicated because the failure rate is high.
  - A bioprosthetic valve may be used in patients in whom chronic anticoagulation may be contraindicated, such as young women who are planning pregnancy.

FOLLOW-UP

- Aortic stenosis is a progressive disease that requires close monitoring for signs of increasing obstruction and left ventricular hypertrophy.
- Once intervention has been performed, follow-up may be necessary to:
  - Assess the degree of aortic valve insufficiency post valvotomy
  - Monitor anticoagulation therapy following artificial valve placement

DISPOSITION
Admission Criteria
- Signs and symptoms of heart failure
- Monitoring postcatheterization or postsurgical procedure

Discharge Criteria
- Relief of obstruction
- Resolution of heart failure symptoms

PROGNOSIS
Aortic stenosis in the older child
- Although balloon valvuloplasty and surgical valvotomy result in significant relief of obstruction in 80–90% of patients, valvar aortic stenosis is a progressive disease, with 50% of patients requiring further intervention within 10 years after initial therapy.
- If obstruction recurs, balloon valvuloplasty or valvotomy should be performed, however, if unsuccessful or contraindicated, surgical intervention is indicated.
- Balloon valvuloplasty or valvotomy may be contraindicated for recurrent aortic stenosis in the presence of significant aortic insufficiency. Valve replacement is indicated in the presence of mixed valve disease
Critical aortic stenosis in the neonate
- The mortality rate in newborns with critical aortic stenosis is 12–30%, due to the presence of significant left ventricular systolic and diastolic dysfunction.
- Restenosis is common after surgical or catheter relief of obstruction in the neonatal period, with 20% of survivors requiring further intervention within 5 years of their initial procedure.
- Nevertheless, long-term survival and quality of life has improved markedly in recent years.

COMPLICATIONS
- Left ventricular systolic and diastolic dysfunction if ventricular hypertrophy is long-standing or in the neonate with critical aortic stenosis
- Aortic insufficiency following valvuloplasty or valvotomy
- Right ventricular outflow tract obstruction following the replacement of the pulmonary valve in the Ross procedure
- Complications of anticoagulation therapy following artificial valve replacement

REFERENCES
1. Fyler D, Buckley L, Hellenbrand W, et al. Report of the New England Regional Infant Cardiac Program. *Pediatrics*. 1980;65:375–461.
2. Graham TP, Jr, Driscoll DJ, Gersony WM, et al. Task Force 2: Congenital heart disease. *J Am Coll Cardiol*. 2005;45:1326–1333.
3. Kirklin JW, Barratt-Boyes BG, eds. Chapter 32: Congenital valvar aortic stenosis in Cardiac Surgery, 2nd ed. London: Churchill Livingstone. 1993:1196–1212.
4. McCrindle BW for the VACA registry investigators. Independent predictors of immediate results of percutaneous balloon aortic valvotomy in childhood. *Am J Cardiol*. 1996;77:286–293.
5. Mosca RS, Iannettoni MD, Schwartz S, et al. Critical aortic stenosis in the neonate. *J Thorac Cardiovasc Surg*. 1995;109:147–154.
6. Prevention of bacterial endocarditis: Recommendations by the American Heart Association. *JAMA*. 1997;277:1794–1801.
7. Ross DN. Replacement of aortic and mitral valves with pulmonary autograft. *Lancet*. 1967;2:956–958.
8. Shim D, Lloyd T, Beekman RH. Usefulness of repeat balloon aortic valvuloplasty in children. *Am J Cardiol*. 1997;79:1141–1143.
9. Hoffman JI, Kaplan S. The incidence of congenital heart disease. *J Am Coll Cardiol*. 2002;39:1890–1900.
10. Wessels MW, Berger RM, Frohn-Mulder IM, et al. Autosomal dominant inheritance of left ventricular outflow tract obstruction. *Am J Med Genet A*. 2005;134:171–179.
11. McBride KL, Pignatelli R, Lewin M, et al. Inheritance analysis of congenital left ventricular outflow tract obstruction malformations: Segregation, multiplex relative risk, and heritability. *Am J Med Genet A*. 2005;134:180–186.
12. Siu SC, Colman JM. Heart disease and pregnancy. *Heart*. 2001;85:710–715.
13. Williams IA, Quaegebeur JM, Hsu DT, et al. Ross procedure in infants and toddlers followed into childhood. *Circulation*. 2005;112:I390–395.
14. McElhinney DB, Lock JE, Keane JF, et al. Left heart growth, function, and reintervention after balloon aortic valvuloplasty for neonatal aortic stenosis. *Circulation*. 2005;111:451–458.

CODES
ICD9-CM
746.3 Aortic stenosis

PATIENT TEACHING
Diet
No restrictions
Activity
- Recommendations for participation in recreational and competitive sports are guided by the echocardiographically estimated valve gradient, the degree of left ventricular hypertrophy, and the presence of symptoms such as exertional dyspnea, chest pain, syncope, or exercise intolerance.
- (See the Appendix for the table on Activity Recommendations in Patients with Congenital Aortic Stenosis.)

APOPTOSIS
Joseph L. Bouchard

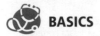 **BASICS**

DESCRIPTION
- Apoptosis is a programmed cell death that is a tightly regulated energy dependent method, in which a specific genetic process leads to activation of a molecular cascade that than causes the destruction of DNA
- Important aspect of normal organ development as well as reaction to cell injury
- It was once thought that terminally differentiated cell lines such as cardiac myocytes did not possess the genetic machinery to undergo apoptosis; however, recent evidence suggests that apoptosis may play an essential role in the cardiovascular diseases.
- Apoptosis versus necrosis
  - Apoptosis
    - Genetically driven cell death
    - Cell membrane remains intact
    - No inflammatory response
    - Segregation of the nuclear chromatin into masses that abut nuclear envelope
    - Cell shrinkage
    - Condensation of the cytoplasm
    - Nuclear fragmentation, then blebbing forming apoptotic bodies
    - Phagocytosis by surrounding cells
  - Necrosis
    - Accidental form of cell death caused by injury to the cell: Ischemia or toxins
    - Cell membrane rupture
    - Inflammation present

PATHOPHYSIOLOGY
- Molecular basis of cardiac apoptotic pathways
  - At least 2 pathways are known to exist: Intrinsic and extrinsic.
  - Both pathways involve the activation of caspases, which are a family of proteases that cleave target proteins resulting in cell death.
  - In the myocyte, the target proteins include: Actin, myosin, tropomyosin, and troponin.
  - Further regulation takes place through complex molecular interactions involving multiple proteins including: Bcl-2 family, BH3, p53, IGF-1, inhibitor of apoptosis proteins (IAPs), and apoptosis regulator with caspase recruitment domain (ARC).
  - Intrinsic pathway
    - Cellular stresses such as hypoxia, ischemia, and oxidative stress activate the intrinsic pathway of the myocyte.
    - Cellular stresses induce the mitochondrial permeability transition pore (MPTP) to open and release cytochrome c and other proteins including apoptosis-inducing factor (AIF) into the cytosol.
    - Cytochrome c activates caspase-9 and caspace-3 resulting in apoptosis.
    - Extrinsic pathway
    - Also called death receptor pathway
    - Death receptors (Fas/CD95 and TRF-α) are activated by ligands
    - Death inducing signaling complex (DISC) is activated
    - DISC activates caspace-8 and caspace-3 resulting in apoptosis.
  - Other pathways
    - Other less well-studied pathways involve the endoplasmic reticulum and caspase-12.

ETIOLOGY
Evidence of apoptosis in cardiovascular diseases
- Ischemic heart disease
  - Studies have demonstrated that apoptosis is present with ischemic heart disease in both the animal and human models.
  - Interestingly, in rat coronary occlusion model a reduction in infarct size and ischemic area were smaller in rats treated with a caspase inhibitor.
- Heart failure
  - It has been proposed that the progressive left ventricular (LV) dysfunction in heart failure may occur secondary to a loss in myocytes from apoptosis.
  - Supporting this argument are numerous animal and human studies showing evidence of apoptosis in heart failure.
- Hypertrophy
  - The process in which there is a transition from a compensated hypertrophic heart to decompensated heart failure is not completely understood.
  - Although not much evidence yet exists to support apoptosis as a cause of this transition, it has been proposed that hypertrophy may make the hypertrophic myocyte more susceptible to apoptosis.

TREATMENT

- Target anti-apoptotic therapies
  - Neurohormonal axis
    - It is well known that the neurohormonal axis is overactive in heart failure patients.
    - There is evidence that both angiotensin II and norepinephrine cause apoptosis, and in animal models angiotensin-converting enzyme (ACE) inhibitors and β-blockers have shown to prevent apoptosis.
    - In effect, the benefits of ACE inhibitors and β-blockers in heart failure patients may be partly explained by their antiapoptosis activity.
  - Caspase
    Caspases are known to be crucial to the apoptotic pathway and thus are a natural target.
  - Endonucleases
    - Endonucleases provoke DNA strand breaks and are in the final process of the apoptotic pathway.
    - Aurintricarboxylic acid is an inhibitor of endonucleases and in animal models has been shown to inhibit apoptosis.
  - Insulin like growth factor-1 (IGF-1)
  - Limiting oxidative stress
- Limitation of anti-apoptotic therapies
  Apoptosis plays a necessary role in cell regulation, specifically in cancer. An important obstacle to overcome in anti-apoptotic therapy would be to selectively deliver treatment to the organ system of interest and avoid adverse effects on other organ systems.

REFERENCES

1. Colucci WS, Braunwald E. Pathophysiology of heart failure. In: Zipe D, et al. ed. *Braundwald's Heart Disease,* 7th ed. Philadelphia: Elsevier Saunders, 2005:509–535.
2. Kang PM, Yue P, Izumo S. New insights into the role of apoptosis in cardiovascular disease. *Circ J.* 2002;66:1–9.
3. Olivetti G, Abbi R, Quaini F, et al. Apoptosis in the failing human heart. *N Engl J Med.* 1997;336: 1131–1141.
4. Sabbah HN, Sharov VG, Goldstein S. Cell death, tissue hypoxia and the progression of heart failure. *Heart Fail Rev.* 2000;5:131–138.
5. Van Empel VP, Bertrand AT, Hofstra L, et al. Myocyte apoptosis in heart failure. *Cardiovasc. Res.* 2005;67:21–29.
6. Yaoita H, Ogawa K, Maehara K, et al. Attenuation of ischemia/reperfusion injury in rats by a caspase inhibitor. *Circulation.* 1998;97:276–281.

FAQ

Q: What is apoptosis?
A: A programmed cell death that is a tightly regulated energy dependent process in which a specific genetic process leads to activation of a molecular cascade that than causes the destruction of DNA.

Q: What role does apoptosis play in cardiovascular disease?
A: Although the extent of the role of apoptosis in cardiovascular disease has not yet been elicited, both human and animal models have shown that apoptosis does play a role in ischemia, heart failure, and hypertrophy.

Q: What are the potential anti-apoptotic targets that are being studied?
A: Potential anti-apoptotic targets include neurohormonal axis, caspases, endonucleases, insulin like growth factor-1 (IGF-1), and the limitation of oxidative stress.

ARRHYTHMIAS, APBs

Peter Ott
Andrew E. Epstein

 BASICS

DESCRIPTION

Atrial premature beats or complexes (APCs) are early atrial systoles identified on the electrocardiogram (ECG) by early P waves.

- The contour of the P wave may resemble sinus P waves, but it is usually different.
- APCs mimic sinus P waves when they arise near the sinus node, or close to it.
- When P waves occur very early, atrioventricular (AV) conduction may remain refractory, such that the impulse is not propagated to the ventricles (blocked APC).
- Sometimes the P wave of an APC is difficult to identify because it falls in the T wave of the preceding QRS complex.
- Synonyms:
  - Atrial premature complexes
  - Atrial premature contractions

Pregnancy Considerations

- Pregnancy may exacerbate frequency of APCs.
- Changes in intravascular volume and subsequent atrial wall stress may trigger stretch-induced atrial arrhythmias.

EPIDEMIOLOGY

APCs increase with aging. In the elderly, APCs are ubiquitous.

RISK FACTORS

Structural heart disease with abnormalities of atrial structure or physiology, such as infiltrative diseases (amyloid), right or left ventricular failure, mitral or tricuspid insufficiency, following cardiac surgery, pericarditis

ETIOLOGY

- Often APCs have no particular cause, and are a function of aging.
- During times of stress and sympathetic stimulation
- Hyperthyroidism
- With myocardial infarction in >50% of patients
- In association with elevated atrial pressure and wall stress, for example left ventricular failure or cor pulmonale
- Alcohol, tobacco, and caffeine consumption
- Drug toxicity, for example, digitalis toxicity

 DIAGNOSIS

SIGNS AND SYMPTOMS

- Usually none, but occasionally can be felt as palpitations.
- They may presage sustained supraventricular tachycardia, atrial fibrillation, and atrial flutter

TESTS

- ECG
- Event recorder; especially useful to correlate symptoms with PACs
- Holter monitor, useful to correlate symptoms and assess number of PACs
- Telemetry in hospital

Lab

- None per se, except to test for hyperthyroidism
- Erythrocyte sedimentation rate if myocarditis or pericarditis suspected

DIFFERENTIAL DIAGNOSIS

- Junctional premature beats
- Wandering atrial pacemaker

TREATMENT

GENERAL MEASURES
Usually no treatment is indicated or required.

 MEDICATION (DRUGS)

- If palpitations are a major complaint, β-blockade may be helpful.
- β-Blockers
  - May decrease catecholamine stimulus, vigor of post-APC ventricular contraction, or timing of ventricular contraction, thereby improving symptoms
  - In otherwise healthy patients, adverse drug effects may be worse than symptoms resulting from the arrhythmia.
- Calcium channel blockers

Second Line
In highly symptomatic patients—not responding to previously described medical therapy, antiarrhythmic drugs (class 1C if no structural heart disease—or class 3) can be tried—either alone or in combination with β-blockers.

SURGERY
In selected patients electrophysiologic mapping and catheter ablation of the PAC focus is needed.

 FOLLOW-UP

DISPOSITION
Admission Criteria
Not applicable; patients are not admitted for APCs

PROGNOSIS
Normal; occasionally APCs may be a harbinger to atrial fibrillation, and may trigger reentrant supraventricular tachycardias.

PATIENT MONITORING
- Virtually never needed
- If monitoring chosen, Holter monitor to quantify daily APC frequency and correlate symptoms with rhythm.
- Because drugs usually are not prescribed, proarrhythmia usually is not an issue.

REFERENCES
1. Braunwald E, ed. *Heart Disease: A Textbook of Cardiovascular Medicine*. Philadelphia: WB Saunders,1997.

 MISCELLANEOUS

See also: Atrial fibrillation, Atrial flutter, Multifocal atrial tachycardia, Supraventricular tachycardia

CODES
ICD9-CM
427.61 Supraventricular premature beats

PATIENT TEACHING
- APCs are common and benign.
- Aggressive treatment with primary antiarrhythmic drugs may lead to morbidity and mortality in excess of that expected from APCs by themselves and can be avoided in most patients.
- Rarely, antiarrhythmic drugs or catheter ablation is required.
- Avoiding caffeine and other precipitating stimuli (alcohol, tobacco) may decrease APC frequency.
- Activity is usually not restricted, but rather encouraged.

ARRHYTHMIAS, ATRIAL FIBRILLATION

Andrew E. Epstein
Peter Ott

 BASICS

DESCRIPTION
Atrial fibrillation (AF) is the rapid, disorganized, and asynchronous contraction of atrial muscle.
- Characterized by the absence of clearly defined atrial complexes on the surface electrocardiogram
- The ventricular rate is typically fast and irregularly irregular.
- AF increases cardiovascular mortality, total mortality following myocardial infarction, and stroke (17-fold if rheumatic heart disease)
- AF may be
  - Paroxysmal: Self terminating episodes (typically hours or days)
  - Persistent: AF does not terminate by itself; however, after cardioversion sinus rhythm can be established
  - Permanent (chronic): AF does not terminate, and, even after cardioversion, AF reoccurs quickly

Pregnancy Considerations
- May exacerbate arrhythmias in young women
- If AF occurs in concert with Wolff-Parkinson-White syndrome, regular reentrant tachycardias may be more frequent and can degenerate to AF.
- If there is underlying heart disease, pregnancy may either be dangerous or contraindicated. Warfarin is associated with congenital birth defects.

EPIDEMIOLOGY
- Dependent on age and presence or underlying heart disease
- AF is increasingly frequent as population ages (0.02% prevalence among those 18–39 years of age; 11.6% among those >75 years of age)

RISK FACTORS
For AF
- Hypertension
- Coronary artery disease
- Valvular heart disease
- Cardiomyopathy
For stroke in association with AF
- Hypertension
- Congestive heart failure
- Diabetes
- Increasing age (>65 years)
- Left ventricular dysfunction, and increased left atrial dimension on echocardiogram
- Prior stroke or transient ischemic attack (TIA)

ETIOLOGY
Usually related to one or more of the following:
- Hypertension
- Coronary artery disease
- Valvular heart disease
- Cardiomyopathy
Rare cases of familial AF have been reported.

 DIAGNOSIS

SIGNS AND SYMPTOMS
- None
- Palpitations
- Dyspnea
- Fatigue
- Congestive heart failure
- Angina
- Syncope
- Stroke

TESTS
- Electrocardiogram (ECG)
- Ambulatory monitor (especially useful if AF paroxysmal) or event monitor
- Echocardiogram to evaluate structural heart disease (myocardial and valvular)
- Rule out hyperthyroidism

Imaging
Cardiac catheterization and angiography if ischemia and/or coronary artery disease are suspected

DIFFERENTIAL DIAGNOSIS
- Atrial flutter (regular and irregular)
- Multifocal atrial tachycardia (irregular)
- Atrial tachycardia (regular)
- Atrioventricular (AV) reentrant and AV nodal reentrant tachycardias (regular)
- Junctional tachycardia (regular)

 TREATMENT

GENERAL MEASURES
- Stroke is significantly reduced by anticoagulation with warfarin.
- All patients >65 years of age, or younger if a risk factor for stroke is present (hypertension, diabetes, left ventricular hypertrophy, prior stroke or TIA, or congestive heart failure), should be anticoagulated.
- Symptoms and quality of life can be improved either by controlling the ventricular response or by restoring sinus rhythm.
- The Atrial Fibrillation Follow-up Investigation of Rhythm Management (AFFIRM) Trial showed no difference in survival in 4,000 patients (mean age 69 years) with AF randomized to either heart rate control or rhythm control.
- The decision to cardiovert depends on an assessment of relative risks and benefits of the procedure.
  - Benefits of restoring sinus rhythm include the possibilities of fewer symptoms related to AF and stopping anticoagulation.
  - Associated with risks of proarrhythmia from antiarrhythmic drugs, bradycardia, and an increased chance for adverse drug reactions

- Rate control strategy may be less costly.
- Patients left in AF with a controlled ventricular response may have more symptoms, and certainly need continued anticoagulation.
- Either drugs or AV node ablation with pacemaker implantation can accomplish the goal of rate control.
- Conversion can be accomplished by drug therapy or by synchronized electrical cardioversion.
- Cardioversion should be immediate when there is hemodynamic instability, ongoing angina, or congestive heart failure.
- Rapid conduction over an accessory pathway in the Wolff-Parkinson-White syndrome is also an indication for emergent cardioversion. Patients with less severe signs or symptoms can be cardioverted electively.
- In the absence of an urgent indication, certain patients should not be cardioverted, including those who are not anticoagulated (at least 3 weeks) when the duration of AF is unknown or >48 hours.
- Patients with an ECG showing left atrial thrombus or a predictor of stroke (such as mitral stenosis) should be therapeutically anticoagulated for at least 3 weeks.
- Patients with frequent recurrences of AF despite multiple prior antiarrhythmic drug trials would not be anticipated to maintain sinus rhythm and therefore should not be converted.
- AF with a slow ventricular response may also have sick sinus syndrome or drug-induced sinus node suppression. They may have significant sinus bradycardia after cardioversion of atrial fibrillation. For these patients rate support should be available at the time of shock delivery; for example, with a temporary or permanent transvenous pacemaker.
- New options for therapy to maintain sinus rhythm include the surgical Maze procedure and the catheter-based Maze procedure. The latter is undergoing intense clinical evaluation.
- Atrial defibrillators are in clinical trials.
- There are usually not restrictions on activity, and dietary recommendations are made as appropriate for underlying disease or syndrome such as diabetes, coronary artery disease, heart failure, and hypertension.

MEDICATION (DRUGS)
Rate Control
- Acutely: Intravenous or oral β-blocker (metoprolol, atenolol, esmolol) or calcium channel blocker (diltiazem, verapamil)
- Chronically: β-Blocker (metoprolol, atenolol, esmolol) or calcium channel blocker (diltiazem, verapamil)
Rhythm Control
- Acutely: Ibutilide, procainamide, oral flecainide, or propafenone
- Chronically: Quinidine, procainamide, disopyramide, propafenone, flecainide, sotalol, dofetilide or amiodarone
- QT-prolonging drugs contraindicated if history of Torsades de Pointes ventricular tachycardia

SURGERY

New, innovative therapies to manage AF include
— AV node ablation (or modification) and implantation of pacemaker (dual-chamber if AF paroxysmal)—especially in patients with fast, difficult to control ventricular rates

— Specialized atrial pacing techniques (dual-site and dual-chamber atrial-based pacing)—especially in patients with a pacing indications (overall benefit appears small)

— Atrial implantable defibrillator—its role remains poorly defined

— Possible cure with a MAZE procedure either surgical (open heart or minimal invasive—mostly performed as adjunct to other heart surgery) or transvenous catheter-based left atrial ablation—highly skilled EP labs have reported very encouraging results particularly in patients with paroxysmal AF

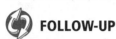 **FOLLOW-UP**

DISPOSITION
Admission Criteria
• Patients can often be treated for AF on a completely outpatient basis.
• Criteria for admission include complications of AF such as:
  – Uncontrolled ventricular response
  – Heart failure or angina as a consequence of AF
  – Initiation of antiarrhythmic drug therapy (especially in patients with structural heart disease at increased risk for proarrhythmia)
• Controversy exists as to who needs to be admitted for drug initiation, with considerations being:
  – Age (and hence drug metabolism)
  – Underlying heart disease
  – Proarrhythmia potential

PROGNOSIS
• Depends on age and population in question
• Young people with "lone" AF (no predisposing cause <65 years of age) have normal prognosis even without anticoagulation.
• Elderly patients with risk factor for stroke have risk ratio of >12 for stroke and death.
• AF can best be prevented by treating and preventing reversible risk factors [i.e., hypertension, congestive heart failure (CHF)].

PATIENT MONITORING
• Anticoagulation followed with international normalized ratio (INR) that should be 2–3 for optimal protection against embolization and minimization of risk for bleeding; start warfarin carefully
• Risk of thromboembolism increases with INR <2.0, risk of central nervous system (CNS) bleed increases with INR >4.0
• Follow ECG and response to antiarrhythmic drugs, especially QT interval. Heart rate (HR) and PR interval. Watch for ventricular proarrhythmia related to antiarrhythmic drug therapy.
• Assess ventricular rate control if left in AF with Holter or ambulatory monitoring. Criteria used in the AFFIRM trial were: rest HR <80 bpm, HR with hall walk <110 bpm)

REFERENCES
1. Cairns JA, Connolly SJ. Nonrheumatic atrial fibrillation—risk of stroke and role of antithrombotic therapy. *Circulation*. 1991;84:469–481.
2. Cox JL, Jaquiss RDB, Schuessler RB, et al. Modification of the maze procedure for atrial flutter and fibrillation. *J Cardiovasc Surg*. 1995;110:485–495.
3. Feinberg WM, Blackshear JL, Laupacis A, et al. Prevalence, age distribution, and gender of patients with atrial fibrillation. *Arch Intern Med*. 1995;155:469–473.
4. Gilligan DM, Ellenbogen KA, Epstein AE. The management of atrial fibrillation. *Am J Med*. 1996;101:413–421.
5. Lêvy S, Maarek M, Coumel P, et al. Characterization of different subsets of atrial fibrillation in general practice in France—the ALFA Study. *Circulation*. 1999;99:3028–3035.
6. Planning and Steering Committees of the -AFFIRM Study for the NHLBI AFFIRM Investigators. Atrial Fibrillation Follow-up Investigation of Rhythm Management—the AFFIRM Study design. *Am J Cardiol*. 1997;79:1198–1202.
7. Prystowsky EN, Benson DW, Fuster V, et al. Management of patients with atrial fibrillation. A statement for health care professionals from the Subcommittee on Electrocardiography and Electrophysiology, American Heart Association. *Circulation*. 1996;93:1262–1277.
8. Wellens HJJ, Lau C-P, Lüderitz B, et al. Atrio-verter: An implantable device for the treatment of atrial fibrillation. *Circulation*. 1998;98:1651–1656.
9. AFFIRM trial. A comparison of rate control and rhythm control in patients with atrial fibrillation. *N Engl J Med*. 2002;347:1825–1833.

CODES
ICD9-CM
427.31 Atrial fibrillation

PATIENT TEACHING
• Importance of anticoagulation and control of INR to prevent stroke
• Be vigilant for bleeding as consequence of anticoagulation, and proarrhythmia from antiarrhythmic drugs.

ARRHYTHMIAS, ATRIAL FLUTTER

Peter Ott
Andrew E. Epstein

 BASICS

DESCRIPTION

Atrial flutter (Afl) is a reentrant tachycardia utilizing a circuit defined by the tricuspid annulus, with the anterior free wall of the right atrium activated in the craniocaudal direction and the septum in the caudocranial direction.

- An isthmus between the inferior vena cava and the tricuspid annulus is the lower turnaround point; because it is narrow, it can be targeted for interruption by radiofrequency energy with subsequent cure of the arrhythmia.
- The Afl circuit around the tricuspid annulus can support reentry in either the clockwise or counterclockwise direction.
  - Counterclockwise reentry around the tricuspid annulus is called typical, usual, or common Afl and is characterized by negative (sawtooth) flutter waves in electrocardiogram (ECG) leads II, III, and aVF. The flutter wave is positive in V1 and negative in V6.
  - Clockwise reentry around the tricuspid annulus is called unusual or uncommon atrial flutter and is characterized by positive flutter waves in ECG leads II, III, and aVF. These flutter waves often have a notch in the upstroke. The flutter wave is negative in V1 and positive in V6.
- The term *atypical Afl* has been used for not only isthmus-dependent clockwise Afl, but also atrial tachycardias not dependent on isthmus conduction.

Pregnancy Considerations

- May exacerbate arrhythmias in young women
- If there is underlying heart disease, pregnancy may be either dangerous or contraindicated.
- Warfarin is associated with congenital birth defects such that risk–benefit ratio weighted against its use for Afl in this situation.

EPIDEMIOLOGY

Incidence

- Increases as the population ages
- Incidence may be up to 30% following open heart surgery.
- Common after surgery for congenital heart disease

Prevalence

Dependent on age and presence of underlying heart disease

RISK FACTORS

- Prior cardiac surgery
- Hypertension
- Treatment with IC antiarrhythmic drugs or amiodarone for atrial fibrillation—20% of patients will have Afl as their recurrent arrhythmia

ETIOLOGY

- Idiopathic
- Structural heart disease (including coronary and valvular heart disease and cardiomyopathy)
- Following open heart surgery
  - In children/young adults atypical Afls may use atrial incisions or prosthetic material (atrial septal defect patch) as an anatomic barrier around which reentry occurs.
- Usual, counterclockwise Afl may occur for the first time in patients treated with class IC antiarrhythmic drugs (i.e., flecainide, propafenone).
- Afls are often slowed by the IC antiarrhythmic drugs such that 1:1 atrioventricular (AV) conduction can occur leading to a faster ventricular response than at baseline when the Afl rate was faster but degree of AV block greater.

 DIAGNOSIS

SIGNS AND SYMPTOMS

- None
- Palpitations
- Dyspnea
- Fatigue
- Congestive heart failure
- Angina
  - History

TESTS

- ECG is essential to establish diagnosis and determine if arrhythmia is amenable to ablative therapy (e.g., dependent on the isthmus discussed previously).
- Ambulatory monitor (especially useful if paroxysmal) and evaluate heart rate (HR) during Afl
- ECG to evaluate structural heart disease (myocardial and valvular)

Lab

Check for hyperthyroidism.

Imaging

Cardiac catheterization and angiography if coronary artery disease suspected ECG if hypertensive or valvular heart disease is suspected

DIFFERENTIAL DIAGNOSIS

- Atrial fibrillation (irregularly irregular, no flutter waves on ECG)
- Atrial tachycardia (regular)
- AV reentrant and AV nodal reentrant tachycardias (regular)
- Junctional tachycardia (rare, regular)
- Multifocal atrial tachycardia (irregular)

TREATMENT

GENERAL MEASURES

- The standard of therapy is slowing of the ventricular rate with drugs that block the AV node, followed by the administration of an antiarrhythmic drug (class I or III) to restore and maintain sinus rhythm.
- Conversion can be accomplished by drug therapy, electrical cardioversion, rapid atrial pacing (performed internally or via the esophagus), and most recently radiofrequency ablation. It is controversial as to the magnitude of risk for stroke attributable to Afl. Hence, the decision to anticoagulate is individual.
- After cardiac surgery the epicardial atrial pacing wire can be used to overdrive pace terminate Afl in the intensive care unit (ICU)

Interventional Measures

- Catheter ablation of Afl isthmus is curative in nearly 100% of patients if done by electrophysiologists skilled in the technique.
- For young patients and those who wish to avoid long-term drug dependency, it is the management of choice.

 ## MEDICATION (DRUGS)

Rate Control
- Acutely: Intravenous or oral β-blocker (metoprolol, atenolol, esmolol) or calcium channel blocker (diltiazem, verapamil)
- Chronically: β-Blocker (metoprolol, atenolol, esmolol) or calcium channel blocker (diltiazem, verapamil)

Rhythm Control
- Acutely: Ibutilide, procainamide, oral flecainide, or propafenone
- Chronically: Quinidine, procainamide, disopyramide, propafenone, flecainide, sotalol, or amiodarone
- QT-prolonging drugs are contraindicated if history of torsade de pointes ventricular tachycardia

 ## FOLLOW-UP

DISPOSITION

Admission Criteria
- Often patients can be treated for Afl on a completely outpatient basis.
- Criteria for admission include complications of Afl such as an uncontrolled ventricular response, heart failure, or angina as a consequence of AFl, and for the initiation of antiarrhythmic drug therapy, especially drugs that are associated with proarrhythmia.
- Controversy exists as to who needs to be admitted for drug initiation, with considerations being:
  - Age (and hence drug metabolism)
  - Underlying heart disease
  - Proarrhythmia potential

PROGNOSIS
- Depends on age and population in question
- Patients with Afl in the absence of other diseases have a normal prognosis, and probably a very low risk for stroke.
- In contrast, patients with structural heart disease will have prognosis determined by their underlying disease.

PATIENT MONITORING
- If anticoagulation chosen
  - Follow INR, which should be 2–3 for optimal protection against embolization and minimization of risk for bleeding.
  - Start warfarin carefully.
- Follow ECG and response to antiarrhythmic drugs.
  - Watch for ventricular proarrhythmia related to antiarrhythmic drug therapy.
- Assess ventricular control if left in Afl with Holter or ambulatory monitoring.
- Bleeding as consequence of anticoagulation

REFERENCES
1. Cosio FG, Arribas F, López-Gil M, et al. Radiofrequency ablation of atrial flutter. *J Cardiovasc Electrophysiol*. 1996;7:60–70.
2. Olshansky B, Wilber DJ, Hariman RJ. Atrial flutter—update on the mechanism and treatment. *PACE*. 1992;15:2308–2335.
3. Windecker S, Kay GN, Epstein AE, et al. Atrial flutter. *Cardiac Electrophysiol Rev*. 1997;1/2:52–60.
4. Wood KA, Eisenberg SJ, Kalman JM, et al. Risk of thromboembolism in chronic atrial flutter. *Am J Cardiol*. 1997;79:1043–1047.

CODES
ICD9-CM
427.32 Atrial flutter

PATIENT TEACHING
- Importance of anticoagulation and control of INR to prevent stroke if anticoagulated
- Be vigilant for bleeding as a consequence of anticoagulation, and for proarrhythmia from antiarrhythmic drugs.

Diet
Appropriate for underlying disease or syndrome such as diabetes, coronary artery disease, heart failure, and hypertension.

ARRHYTHMIAS, AVNRT

Peter Ott
Andrew E. Epstein

 BASICS

DESCRIPTION

Atrioventricular nodal reentrant tachycardia (AVNRT) is the most common paroxysmal, regular supraventricular tachycardia, accounting for greater than half of all cases referred for electrophysiologic study. The substrate for the arrhythmia is dual AV nodal pathway physiology.

Synonym(s): PAT (paroxysmal atrial tachycardia); term now obsolete; Junctional reentrant tachycardia; Junctional reciprocating tachycardia; Junctional tachycardia (this is a misnomer)

Pregnancy Considerations

Pregnancy not contraindicated, but supraventricular tachycardias may be more frequent and precipitated by pregnancy.

EPIDEMIOLOGY

AVNRT is common. There is a 70% female predominance. Any age can be affected, but AVNRT usually presents at ages 30–50 years.

ETIOLOGY

- There are at least two functionally distinct AV nodal conduction pathways:
  - The fast pathway is characterized by fast conduction properties and a long refractory period.
  - The slow pathway is characterized by slow conduction properties and a short refractory period.
- AVNRT usually begins with a premature atrial depolarization that blocks in the fast pathway since the latter has a long refractory period.
- The impulse then conducts through the slow pathway, and if the fast pathway recovers from depolarization, the impulse can reenter the fast pathway and conduct retrogradely to the atria. This completes the reentry circuit, which can repeat.
- Pathologic studies have shown a variety of changes, including entrapment, distortion, and division of the AV node, fibrosis, and even acute necrosis.
- Pathologic findings usually are described in electrical terms. Dual AV nodal pathway physiology is identified at electrophysiologic study.

 DIAGNOSIS

SIGNS AND SYMPTOMS

- Palpitations: These are typically described as sudden onset/abrupt onset ("like switching on a light").
- Pounding in the neck
- Dyspnea
- Dizziness
- Syncope
- Fatigue (sometimes related to drug therapy)
- Chest pain
- Diaphoresis

TESTS

- Electrocardiogram (ECG) during episode is diagnostic
  - Narrow QRS tachycardia either without identifiable P waves, or P waves immediately at the end of the QRS, sometimes seen as pseudo-R wave in lead V1 and/or pseudo-S waves in leads II or III
  - An atypical variety of AVNRT that uses the slow pathway in the retrograde direction has P waves in the second half of the ST segment (so-called long RP tachycardia).
- Electrophysiologic study, required if undergoing catheter ablation

Lab

Slow and fast AV nodal pathways are not clearly identifiable except at electrophysiologic study.

DIFFERENTIAL DIAGNOSIS

- AV reentrant tachycardia that uses an accessory pathway in the retrograde direction
- Atrial tachycardia
- Atrial flutter with 2:1 AV conduction
- Junctional tachycardia

 TREATMENT

GENERAL MEASURES

- Recording of 12-lead ECG during tachycardia is extremely important to help with diagnosis.
- If cured by catheter ablation, there is no long-term follow-up requirement.
- Due to the problems of long-term drug administration (adverse drug reactions, problem of multiple daily doses/noncompliance, and failure at some time over years of treatment), catheter ablation has emerged as one of the treatments, if not the treatment of choice, for recurrent AVNRT.
- The procedure can be performed safely with a low risk of AV block, and long-term is likely cost effective and improves quality of life compared with drug therapy, especially class IA and IC agents.
- For a single episode, a conservative approach may be adopted, including observation without drug therapy.
- If ablation is not performed, general medical follow-up is required. For acute management, cardioversion is almost never required because arrhythmia is very drug responsive.

MEDICATION (DRUGS)

Acute Management
- Adenosine intravenous (IV) rapid bolus injection of 6–12 mg IV, results in abrupt supraventricular tachycardia (SVT) termination—premature ventricular contractions (PVCs) and premature atrial contractions (PACs) can be seen frequently; then sinus rhythm resumes.
- Verapamil (IV)
- Esmolol (β-blocker)

Chronic Management
  - Calcium channel blocker (e.g., verapamil)
  - β-Blocker
  - Class IC antiarrhythmic drugs (e.g., flecainide and propafenone)
  - Digoxin may be helpful.

Precautions
- Watch for atrial fibrillation if adenosine used.
- Class IA drugs (quinidine, procainamide, disopyramide) limited due to adverse drug reactions.

SURGERY
Open heart surgery has been performed in the past, but this has been superseded by catheter ablation for cure.

 FOLLOW-UP

- Patients in general do not need to be admitted for AVNRT.
- If drug therapy is chosen, most antiarrhythmics can be started on an outpatient basis, especially because the risk for proarrhythmia is low in these patients with structurally normal hearts, and because drugs causing torsade de pointes ventricular tachycardia are usually not used for this disorder.
- After being seen by an electrophysiologist, a same-day ablation procedure can be arranged.

PROGNOSIS
Excellent

PATIENT MONITORING
Relates to treatment options, especially opportunity for cure with catheter ablation

REFERENCES
1. Ganz LI, Friedman PL. Supraventricular tachycardia. *N Engl J Med*. 1995;332:162–173.
2. Jackman WM, Beckman KJ, McClelland JH, et al. Treatment of supraventricular tachycardia due to atrioventricular nodal reentry by radiofrequency catheter ablation of slow-pathway conduction. *N Engl J Med*. 1992;327:313–318.
3. Kay GN, Plumb VJ. Selective slow pathway ablation (posterior approach) for treatment for atrioventricular nodal reentrant tachycardia. In: *Radiofrequency Catheter Ablation of Cardiac Arrhythmias: Basic Concepts and Clinical Applications*. Armonk, NY: Futura, 1994:171–203.

CODES
ICD9-CM
427.0 Paroxysmal supraventricular tachycardia

PATIENT TEACHING
- Although AVNRT can sometimes be precipitated by exercise and catecholamine increase, there are no specific recommendations regarding activity.
- Vagal maneuvers may terminate arrhythmia.

Diet
There are usually no dietary restrictions.

ARRHYTHMIAS, HEART BLOCK (1ST, 2ND, AND 3RD DEGREE)
Peter Ott
Andrew E. Epstein

 BASICS

DESCRIPTION
- First-degree block is prolongation of the PR interval (<200 msec).
- Second-degree AV block is classified into two subcategories:
  - Type I or Mobitz I second-degree atrioventricular (AV) block. Progressive prolongation of the PR interval before a blocked beat (Wenckebach block) usually is associated with a narrow QRS complex.
  - Type II or Mobitz II second-degree AV block is the sudden loss of AV conduction without progressive prolongation of the PR interval before the blocked beat. Usually it is associated with a wide QRS complex.
- Advanced AV block refers to the block of two or more consecutive P waves.
- Third-degree AV block (complete heart block) is defined as absence of AV conduction.
  - Patients with abnormalities of AV conduction may be asymptomatic.
  - Patients may experience serious symptoms related to bradycardia, ventricular arrhythmias, or both.
  - Decisions regarding the need for a pacemaker are importantly influenced by the presence or absence of symptoms directly attributable to bradycardia.
- Synonym(s): Heart block

EPIDEMIOLOGY
Prevalence
Prevalence variable, depends on underlying structural heart disease, and increases with increasing age.

RISK FACTORS
Structural heart disease

ETIOLOGY
- Aging and fibrosis of AV conducting system
- No pathology if AV block is functional and related to drug therapy
- AV node and His–Purkinje system may be damaged due to myocardial infarction, impingement by calcium from aortic or mitral valve, or the development of fibrosis (Lev and Lenégre diseases).

- Aortic or mitral stenosis, especially following valve replacement. Because the mitral valve is close to the AV node, impaired AV conduction often is due to inflammation and resolves. The aortic valve, however, is close to the His–Purkinje system, and when AV block occurs as a consequence of aortic valve disease or surgery. AV block is usually permanent and pacing is required.
- Not a genetic disease, except in neuromuscular diseases with AV block such as myotonic muscular dystrophy, Kearns-Sayre syndrome, Erb dystrophy (limb-girdle), and peroneal muscular atrophy

ASSOCIATED CONDITIONS
Structural heart disease

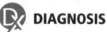 **DIAGNOSIS**

SIGNS AND SYMPTOMS
- None
- Lightheadedness
- Syncope
- Dyspnea, congestive heart failure
- Symptoms may be due to bradycardia itself, or to ventricular arrhythmias precipitated by bradycardia (e.g., torsade de pointes ventricular tachycardia).

TESTS
- Electrocardiogram (ECG) most useful
- Ambulatory monitoring (Holter or telemetry)
  - Event monitoring for intermittent symptoms

Lab
Generally not applicable; drug level measurement (especially digitalis) is indicated if toxicity suspected.

DIFFERENTIAL DIAGNOSIS
- Junctional rhythm
- Concealed junctional extrasystoles
- When 2:1 AV block is present, the differentiation between Mobitz I and Mobitz II block is difficult because there is no progressive change in the PR interval that can be assessed.
  - In general, 2:1 AV block with a narrow QRS is usually due to block in the AV node (e.g., Mobitz I) and 2:1 AV block with a wide QRS is usually due to block below the AV node (e.g., infra-Hissian, Mobitz II).
  - Exceptions to these rules do occur.
  - The importance of this distinction lies in the indication for pacing.

 TREATMENT

GENERAL MEASURES
- For first-degree AV block and second-degree Mobitz type I AV block usually no treatment is recommended. These conduction disturbances are often the result of drug therapy and simply represent drug effects.
- Second-degree Mobitz type II AV block, especially if the QRS is wide, reflects infra-Hissian conduction disease, and permanent pacing is usually indicated.
- High-degree and third-degree AV block may be a consequence of drug therapy/toxicity, and a decision on pacing is made on the etiology.
- If a drug causing AV block is not essential, the drug can be stopped. If the drug is essential, permanent pacing is required to support the rate to allow drug administration.
- If there is drug toxicity, the rhythm should be supported by temporary pacing if needed while the toxicity resolves.

 MEDICATION (DRUGS)

There are no drugs that directly enhance AV conduction. If digitalis is toxic, Digibind antibody is indicated to inhibit digitalis effect on the heart.

SURGERY
The indications for permanent pacing are outlined in the American College of Cardiology/American Heart Association Guidelines referenced below and include the following.
- Third-degree AV block at any anatomic level associated with any one of the following conditions:
  - Bradycardia with symptoms presumed to be due to AV block
  - Arrhythmias and other medical conditions that require drugs that result in symptomatic bradycardia
  - Documented periods of asystole >3.0 seconds or any escape rate <40 bpm in awake, symptom-free patients
  - After catheter ablation of the AV junction
  - Postoperative AV block that is not expected to resolve
  - Neuromuscular diseases with AV block such as myotonic muscular dystrophy, Kearns-Sayre syndrome, Erb dystrophy (limb-girdle), and peroneal muscular atrophy

- Second-degree AV block regardless of type or site of block, with associated symptomatic bradycardia
- Asymptomatic third-degree AV block at any anatomic site with average awake ventricular rates of 40 bpm or faster
- Asymptomatic type II second-degree AV block
- Asymptomatic type I second-degree AV block at intra- or infra-Hissian levels found incidentally at electrophysiologic study for other indications
- First-degree AV block with symptoms suggestive of pacemaker syndrome and documented alleviation of symptoms with temporary AV pacing
- Marked first-degree AV block (>0.30 second) in patients with left ventricular dysfunction and symptoms of congestive heart failure in whom a shorter AV interval results in hemodynamic improvement, presumably by decreasing left atrial filling pressure

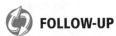 **FOLLOW-UP**

DISPOSITION
Admission Criteria
If a patient has symptomatic AV block (especially third-degree or 2:1 AV block with a wide QRS), admission is warranted, usually for pacemaker implantation or treatment of drug toxicity.

PROGNOSIS
- Variable and depends on underlying heart disease
- Patients with AV block have a worse prognosis than those with sinus node dysfunction, probably because the former have greater degrees of structural heart disease.

COMPLICATIONS
Complications due to the AV block itself or to its treatment include syncope, injury, and occasionally death.

PATIENT MONITORING
- For those without pacemakers, AV conduction should be systematically followed with ECGs or Holter monitors.
- Patients with pacemakers need telephone and intermittent face-to-face follow-up.
- Other than avoiding drug toxicity and preventing coronary artery disease, AV block is not preventable.

REFERENCES
1. Braunwald E, ed. *Heart Disease: A Textbook of Cardiovascular Medicine*. Philadelphia: WB Saunders, 1997.
2. Gregoratos G, Cheitlin MD, Conill A, et al. ACC/AHA guidelines for implantation of cardiac pacemakers and antiarrhythmia devices: A report of the American College of Cardiology/American Heart Association Task Force on Practice Guidelines (Committee on Pacemaker Implantation). *J Am Coll Cardiol*. 1998;31:1175–1206.

CODES
ICD9-CM
- 426.0 Atrioventricular block, complete
- 426.1 Atrioventricular block, other and unspecified
- 426.10 Atrioventricular block, unspecified
- 426.11 First-degree atrioventricular block
- 426.12 Mobitz (type) II atrioventricular block
- 426.13 Other second-degree atrioventricular block

PATIENT TEACHING
- Mostly related pacemaker follow-up in those with pacemakers. If drug toxicity is the cause, counsel to take measures to avoid further toxicity.
- At risk for falls or syncope, counsel to avoid activities that put the patient or others in danger.

Diet
No specific diet

Activity
Depends on hemodynamic consequences and underlying cause of AV block

ARRHYTHMIAS, JUNCTIONAL RHYTHM

Peter Ott
Andrew E. Epstein

 BASICS

DESCRIPTION

Normally the heartbeat is initiated by the sinus node (i.e., sinus rhythm).

- When it originates from the atrioventricular junction, it is called a junctional rhythm.
- A rhythm that is <100 beats per minute is usually considered an escape rhythm, as during sinus bradycardia. If it is faster, it is called junctional tachycardia.

EPIDEMIOLOGY

Depends on patient population, and can be seen in all ages

RISK FACTORS

None specific

ETIOLOGY

- Idiopathic
- Junctional ectopic tachycardia (JET) is a rapid arrhythmia that can be life-threatening, seen in youth after congenital heart disease operations with β-adrenergic stimulation.
- Seen in older individuals in concert with acute myocardial infarction (especially inferior with enhanced vagal tone) and as a manifestation of drug toxicity
- Catecholamine stimulation

 DIAGNOSIS

SIGNS AND SYMPTOMS

- Asymptomatic
- Palpitations
- Dyspnea
- Heart failure (if incessant, causing "tachycardia-associated cardiomyopathy")

TESTS

- Electrocardiogram (ECG) shows narrow QRS tachycardia without discernible P waves. If there is retrograde conduction to the atria, a P wave can be seen following the QRS.
- For the specific arrhythmia JET, there is often atrioventricular (AV) dissociation because the junctional rate is significantly greater than the atrial rate.

Lab

Only to assess drug levels if patient is thought to have toxicity

DIFFERENTIAL DIAGNOSIS

- AV nodal reentry
- AV reentry
- Permanent form of junctional reciprocating tachycardia, which virtually always has a deeply inverted P wave in ECG leads II, III, and aVF with the RP interval longer than the RR interval
- Ectopic atrial tachycardia
- Sinus tachycardia
- Atrial flutter

 TREATMENT

GENERAL MEASURES

Remove precipitating cause (toxic drug, catecholamine stimulation).

 MEDICATION (DRUGS)

- Drugs not often effective
- Sometimes substrate may be abatable, but risk for damage to normal AV conduction is significant (AV node or His bundle)
- For postoperative JET, β-blockers, verapamil, procainamide (with hypothermia), and amiodarone have been used with varying success.
- For accelerated idioventricular rhythm in acute myocardial infarction, administration of antiarrhythmic drugs may suppress this escape pacemaker and lead to asystole.
  - In this setting, observation is indicated because the junctional rhythm usually resolves.
  - Especially common in inferior myocardial infarction. In the uncommon circumstance that it does not resolve, permanent pacemaker implantation may be indicated.

SURGERY

Usually a pacemaker is not needed.

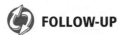

FOLLOW-UP

Admission Criteria
Usually arrhythmia is first recognized in inpatients. Discharge is determined by resolution of other medical problems.

PROGNOSIS
Depends on underlying diseases

PATIENT MONITORING
Usually arrhythmia is transient and corrects during hospitalization for underlying cause.

REFERENCES
1. Hamdan MH, Scheinman MM. Role of invasive EP testing in the evaluation and management of junctional tachycardia. *Cardiol Electrophysiol Rev.* 1997;4:439–442.
2. Walsh EP, Saul P, Sholler GF, et al. Evaluation of a staged treatment protocol for rapid automatic junctional tachycardia after operation for congenital heart disease. *J Am Coll Cardiol.* 1997;29:1046–1053.

CODES
ICD9-CM
427.89 Other, specified conduction disorders

PATIENT TEACHING
- Depending on presentation and underlying disease:
  - If observed in healthy athlete with high vagal tone, no intervention is necessary.
  - Rarely, electrophysiologic study may be considered to identify substrate and perhaps cure with ablation (i.e., AV nodal reentry, AV reentry, ectopic atrial tachycardia).

ARRHYTHMIAS, MAT

Peter Ott
Andrew E. Epstein

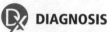 **BASICS**

DESCRIPTION
Multifocal atrial tachycardia (MAT) is characterized by a rate greater than 100 beats per minute and the following:
- Discrete P waves of varying morphology from at least three different foci
- Irregular variation in PP, PR, and RR intervals reflecting absence of dominant pacemaker
- Isoelectric baseline between P waves
- Synonym(s): Chotic atrial rhythm; Chotic atrial tachycardia

EPIDEMIOLOGY
- May occur at any age, but usually in older individuals
- Rarely seen in children and then occurs in the absence of structural heart disease and is usually self-limited (months)
- Although MAT occurs primarily in patients with lung disease in intensive care units, it can occur in critically ill patients in any setting.

Prevalence
Prevalence depends on level of sickness of population and location where assessment is performed.

RISK FACTORS
- Chronic lung disease
- Recent surgery
- Diabetes

ETIOLOGY
MAT usually occurs during critical illness, especially in the setting of chronic lung disease. β-Agonists and methylxanthine derivatives (theophylline) may be contributory.

ASSOCIATED CONDITIONS
See above regarding Etiology.

 DIAGNOSIS

SIGNS AND SYMPTOMS
- None
- Palpitations
- Dyspnea
- Hypotension

TESTS
ECG is the only diagnostic test.
- Discrete P waves of varying morphology from at least three different foci
- Atrial rate greater than 100 beats per minute
- Isoelectric baseline between P waves
- Irregular variation in PP, PR, and RR intervals reflecting absence of dominant pacemaker

DIFFERENTIAL DIAGNOSIS
- Wandering atrial pacemaker (multiple P-wave morphologies, but average atrial rate <100 beats per minute; common in elderly patients who are otherwise well)
- Multiple premature atrial contractions (can identify dominant, e.g., sinus, P waves)
- Atrial fibrillation (no clear P waves)
- Atrial tachycardia (regular with only one morphology P wave)

 TREATMENT

GENERAL MEASURES
- Optimize pulmonary and general care.
- Reverse causes of illness and debility.
- Avoid theophylline.

MEDICATION (DRUGS)

- Verapamil usual drug of choice
- Amiodarone reported to be useful in children with MAT in need of therapy

Precautions
- Use of β-blockers is controversial, and they may be difficult if not impossible to use in patients with serious lung disease.
- Digoxin is not helpful.
- Classic antiarrhythmics are not useful (procainamide, quinidine).

ALTERNATIVE DRUGS
Intravenous magnesium may be helpful.

First Line
Electrical cardioversion is NOT helpful.

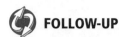 **FOLLOW-UP**

DISPOSITION
Admission Criteria
Usually arrhythmia is first recognized in inpatients. Discharge is determined by resolution of other medical problems.

PROGNOSIS
Depends on underlying disease

PATIENT MONITORING
MAT is usually an acute problem and does not require long-term monitoring following hospital release.
- During the acute phase, there must be vigilance for hypotension, hypoxia, and excessive myocardial demand.
- Caregivers should maintain nutrition, especially in intensive care units.

REFERENCES
1. Kastor JA. Multifocal atrial tachycardia. *N Engl J Med*. 1990;1713–1717.
2. Scher DL, Arsura EL. Multifocal atrial tachycardia: Mechanisms, clinical correlates, and treatment. *Am Heart J*. 1989;118:574–580.
3. Shine KI, Kastor JA, Yurchak PM. Multifocal atrial tachycardia: Clinical and electrocardiographic features in 32 patients. *N Engl J Med*. 1968;279:344–349.

 MISCELLANEOUS

See also: Atrial premature beats, Atrial fibrillation

CODES
ICD9-CM
427.89 Other, specified cardiac dysrhythmias

ARRHYTHMIAS, PVCs

Peter Ott
Andrew E. Epstein

 BASICS

DESCRIPTION

Premature ventricular contractions (PVCs) involve depolarization of the ventricle with inscription of QRS earlier than expected.

- The depolarization is initiated in the ventricles, causing the QRS morphology to be bizarre and not typical of depolarization via the normal conducting system.
- The term premature ventricular contraction is in one respect a misnomer because there can be depolarization without contraction. However, the term is so ingrained in the medical lexicon that its continued use is reasonable.
  Synonym(s): Premature ventricular beats; Premature ventricular depolarizations; Ventricular premature contractions; Ventricular premature beats; Ventricular premature depolarizations

ALERT
Pregnancy Considerations
- Contraindications related to underlying heart disease
- No contraindication if structurally normal heart; symptoms may increase during pregnancy

EPIDEMIOLOGY
- Frequent after myocardial infarction, and ubiquitous as age increases and in setting of cardiomyopathy
- May occur at any age, but prevalence increases with age, and PVCs are ubiquitous in the elderly.
- Can occur in otherwise healthy individuals [idiopathic ventricular tachycardia (VT)]; usually associated with good prognosis. In these patients, PVCs are monomorphic and have a typical right bundle–branch block (RBBB)/superior axis or LBBB/inferior axis pattern

RISK FACTORS
- Increasing age
- Structural heart disease

ETIOLOGY
- Reentry, automaticity, and triggered mechanisms
- Most frequently seen in structural heart disease, especially during acute and after myocardial infarction and cardiomyopathy
- Drug toxicity (digitalis, QT-prolonging agents)
- Sympathetic stimulation (e.g., β-agonists used to treat bronchospasm, caffeine)
- Slow heart rates during which ventricular beats may represent escape rhythms

ASSOCIATED CONDITIONS
Because the frequency of ischemic heart disease and cardiomyopathy increases with age, PVCs are seen in association with these diseases.

 DIAGNOSIS

SIGNS AND SYMPTOMS
- Symptoms may be absent.
- Palpitations
- Dyspnea
- On physical examination, PVCs are associated with early beats followed by a pause that may be either compensatory (depolarization does not change timing of intrinsic rhythm) or not.
  – Giant A waves are seen in the neck veins because with the PVC there is atrial contraction against a closed tricuspid valve.
  – There may be an absent peripheral pulse with the early beat because the heart has not had time to fill in diastole, and the contraction pattern of the ventricles is abnormal.

TESTS
- Electrocardiogram (ECG)
- Ambulatory (Holter) monitor
- Event recorder
- Evaluate for underlying heart disease
  – Ischemia (exercise test)
  – Myocardium [echocardiogram, magnetic resonance imaging (MRI)]
- Pathology: Depends on substrate, but usually scar/fibrosis; sometimes in a structurally normal heart, PVCs arise from triggered activity or automatic focus in normal tissue

Lab
Imaging
- Depends on age and suspicion for heart disease
- Echocardiogram
- Perfusion imaging to evaluate ischemia (e.g., thallium) and ejection fraction
- MRI (also called nuclear magnetic resonance, or NMR)

DIFFERENTIAL DIAGNOSIS
Atrial premature contractions (APCs) with aberrancy

 TREATMENT

GENERAL MEASURES
- Treat underlying heart disease.
- β-Blockers if ischemic heart disease
- Because there is no evidence that treatment of PVCs extends life and that treatment may even increase mortality (Cardiac Arrhythmia Suppression Trial), first therapy should be reassurance and avoidance of therapy if possible.
- The Canadian Amiodarone Myocardial Infarction Arrhythmia Trial and the European Myocardial Infarction Amiodarone Trial showed that prophylactic amiodarone following myocardial infarction does not improve overall survival.
- See chapter on Ventricular Tachycardia for management of nonsustained ventricular tachycardia (PVCs occur in runs of three or more).
  – For patients with ischemic heart disease and low left ventricular ejection fractions, electrophysiologic study can be justified, and if sustained ventricular tachycardia is induced, an implantable defibrillator can be offered (refer to Buxton et al. and Mess et al. in References).
- The best prevention of PVCs is the prevention of heart disease.

MEDICATION (DRUGS)

- No therapy is ideal.
- β-Blocker if ischemic heart disease
  - Even though β-blockers may not suppress PVCs, they will increase survival.
  - In symptomatic patients β-blockers may decrease symptoms by decreasing vigor of post-PVC beat that is usually responsible for the palpitation (increased contraction after pause via Starling principle).
- Lidocaine is usually used in acute settings, such as myocardial infarction.
  - Lidocaine should not be used prophylactically because meta-analyses suggest an increase in mortality due to bradycardic deaths when the drug is used in this manner.
  - If the patient has had ventricular tachycardia or ventricular fibrillation, lidocaine is the usual first antiarrhythmic drug chosen.
- Primary antiarrhythmic drug should be chosen for long-term use if reassurance not satisfactory.
- Amiodarone or sotalol if structural heart disease
- Anxiolytic sometimes helpful if patient worried about palpitations
Contraindications
- Class IC drugs are contraindicated, and all class I drugs are probably inadvisable in ischemic heart disease.
- Proarrhythmia
  - May manifest as increased mortality from class I drugs in ischemic heart disease
  - Torsade de pointes ventricular tachycardia with class IA and class III drugs
  - Avoid class I and III drugs if corrected QT interval prolonged at baseline.

SURGERY

Not applicable; however, in patients with idiopathic PVCs may be "cured" by ablation of arrhythmia focus in right ventricular outflow tract and in fascicles of His-Purkinje system.

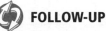

FOLLOW-UP

DISPOSITION
Admission Criteria
All attempts should be made to avoid treating PVCs per se. β-Blockers and anxiolytics can be started on an outpatient basis. For patients with structural heart disease, admission is indicated for loading of drugs with proarrhythmic potential (class I drugs, e.g., quinidine, procainamide, disopyramide, sotalol).

PROGNOSIS
- Normal if structurally normal heart
- Decreased survival if ischemic heart disease
- Controversial if cardiomyopathy

PATIENT MONITORING
- Monitor on-line with telemetry and record ECGs at least daily in acute setting.
- Outpatients may have repeat Holter monitors or event recorders to correlate symptoms with the rhythm if empiric therapy does not decrease symptoms.

REFERENCES
1. Buxton AE, Lec KL, Fisher JD, et al. A randomized study of the prevention of sudden death in patients with coronary artery disease. *N Engl J Med*. 1999;341:1882–1890.
2. Cairns JA, Connolly SJ, Roberts R, et al., for the Canadian Amiodarone Myocardial Infarction Arrhythmia Trial Investigators. Randomised trial of outcome after myocardial infarction in patients with frequent or repetitive ventricular premature depolarisations: CAMIAT. *Lancet*. 1997;349: 675–682.
3. The Cardiac Arrhythmia Suppression Trial II Investigators. Effect of the antiarrhythmic agent moricizine on survival after myocardial infarction. *N Engl J Med*. 1992;327:227–233.
4. Echt DS, Liebson PR, Mitchell LB, et al. Mortality and morbidity in patients receiving encainide, flecainide, or placebo: The Cardiac Arrhythmia Suppression Trial. *N Engl J Med*. 1991;324: 781–788.
5. Epstein AE, Bigger JT, Wyse DG, et al. Events in the Cardiac Arrhythmia Suppression Trial (CAST): Mortality in the entire population enrolled. *J Am Coll Cardiol*. 1991;18:14–19.
6. Julian DG, Camm AJ, Frangin G, et al. Randomised trial of effect of amiodarone on mortality in patients with left-ventricular dysfunction after recent myocardial infarction: EMIAT. *Lancet*. 1997;349:667–674.
7. Moss AJ, Hall WJ, Cannom DS, et al. Improved survival with an implanted defibrillator in patients with coronary disease at high risk for ventricular arrhythmia. *N Engl J Med*. 1996;335:1933–1940.

CODES
ICD9-CM
427.69 Ventricular premature beats, contractions, or systoles

PATIENT TEACHING
- Teach patients that PVCs per se are not a cause for mortality alone, and that antiarrhythmic drug treatment may worsen prognosis.
- In setting of structurally normal heart, prognosis is normal. There is no indication for treatment in the absence of symptoms.
- No specific diet is indicated, although in some individuals caffeine may increase frequency of PVCs.
- Teach that antiarrhythmic drugs may be proarrhythmic.

ARRHYTHMIAS, SICK SINUS SYNDROME

Peter Ott
Andrew E. Epstein

 BASICS

DESCRIPTION

The term sick sinus syndrome (SSS) incorporates a number of disorders involving impulse generation in the atria.

- Included are sinus bradycardia, sinus pauses or arrest, sinoatrial exit block, and the bradycardia–tachycardia syndrome (bradycardia alternating with atrial tachycardias, usually atrial fibrillation, but also atrial flutter and ectopic atrial tachycardia).
- Sinus pauses or arrest implies failure of normal intrinsic cardiac pacemaker function.
- Asymptomatic pauses of >2 seconds have been reported in >10% of patients undergoing ambulatory monitoring.
- Pauses of >3 seconds are uncommon, but frequent enough and asymptomatic such that pauses alone do not constitute evidence for pacemaker implantation.
- Patients may be symptomatic from paroxysmal tachycardia or bradycardia or both.
  Synonym(s):
- Bradycardia–tachycardia syndrome
- Brady–tachy syndrome
- Sinus node dysfunction

Geriatric Considerations
- SSS is typically a disease of the elderly.
- The incidence of AV block is increased, suggesting a global disease of the specialized conduction system.
- The elderly are especially susceptible to drug induced sinus node dysfunction.

Pregnancy Considerations
- There is no specific contraindication to pregnancy.
- Extremely slow heart rates may compromise uterine blood flow, and atrial arrhythmias are more frequent during pregnancy.

EPIDEMIOLOGY
Incidence increases with age.

RISK FACTORS
- Structural heart disease
- Increasing age

PATHOPHYSIOLOGY
Sinus bradycardia and sinus pauses are common during sleep and do not constitute a pacing indication *per se*.

ETIOLOGY
- Any structural heart disease
- Aging process
- Myocardial infarction leading to damage to the sinoatrial node or atria

ASSOCIATED CONDITIONS
Structural heart disease

 DIAGNOSIS

SIGNS AND SYMPTOMS
- None
- Lightheadedness
- Syncope
- Dyspnea, congestive heart failure
- Stroke if atrial fibrillation
- Fatigue
- In older persons, personality and memory changes, nausea, and nonspecific complaints
- Symptoms may be due to bradycardia itself, or to ventricular arrhythmias precipitated by bradycardia (e.g., torsade de pointes ventricular tachycardia).

TESTS
- Electrocardiogram (ECG)
- Ambulatory monitor/event recorder
- Holter monitor/telemetry
- Rarely, invasive electrophysiologic study is needed to assess sinus node dysfunction.
- These studies are associated with a significant number of both false-positive and -negative test results.

Lab
- No laboratory test is needed to diagnose SSS.
- Thyroid function should be assessed because hypothyroidism may cause bradycardia.

DIFFERENTIAL DIAGNOSIS
Symptoms alone are not sufficient to assign a diagnosis of SSS. Symptoms must be correlated with the rhythm. This correlation is especially important when assessing the need and justification for permanent pacing. The differential diagnosis includes:
- Normal sinus arrhythmia
- Reversible causes of sinus node dysfunction such as drug toxicity
- Hypothyroidism

 TREATMENT

GENERAL MEASURES
- If the SSS is due to nonessential drug therapy, those drugs should be stopped.
- When there is not a reversible cause of SSS, pacing is indicated to manage bradycardia and to allow drug therapy of tachycardia when it is present.
- Patients with SSS associated with atrial fibrillation (bradycardia–tachycardia syndrome) should be anticoagulated.
- There is no known way to prevent the development of intrinsic sinus node dysfunction.

MEDICATION (DRUGS)

There are no drugs to treat intrinsic sinus node dysfunction. Permanent pacing is usually required and is very effective to relieve symptoms of sinus node dysfunction.

SURGERY

- The indications for pacemaker implantation are outlined in the American College of Cardiology/American Heart Association Guidelines referenced below and include:
- Sinus node dysfunction correlated with symptomatic bradycardia, including frequent sinus pauses that produce symptoms. In some patients, bradycardia is iatrogenic and will occur as a consequence of essential long-term drug therapy of a type and dose for which there are no acceptable alternatives.
- Symptomatic chronotropic incompetence
- Sinus node dysfunction occurring spontaneously or as a result of necessary drug therapy, with heart rate <40 beats/minute when a clear association between significant symptoms consistent with bradycardia and the actual presence of bradycardia has not been documented.
- In minimally symptomatic patients, chronic heart rate <30 beats/minute while awake

 FOLLOW-UP

DISPOSITION
Admission Criteria

- When patients have extremely slow heart rates, severe symptoms, or ventricular arrhythmias as a result of bradycardia (torsade de pointes ventricular tachycardia), admission is warranted.
- Drug toxicity may be another indication for admission. Patients may be discharged after the arrhythmias have been treated.

PROGNOSIS
Prognosis is governed by underlying heart disease and competing mortality. If SSS is associated with atrioventricular (AV) block, prognosis is worse than if AV block were absent.

PATIENT MONITORING

- Pacemaker follow-up for those with permanent pacemakers
- For patients without pacemakers, systematic ECG and ambulatory monitoring are used to identify disease progression (e.g., longer pauses). This is especially true when new negatively chronotropic drugs are prescribed.

REFERENCES

1. Gregoratos G, Cheitlin MD, Conill A, et al. ACC/AHA guidelines for implantation of cardiac pacemakers and antiarrhythmia devices: A report of the American College of Cardiology/American Heart Association Task Force on Practice Guidelines (Committee on Pacemaker Implantation). *J Am Coll Cardiol*. 1998;31:1175–1206.

 MISCELLANEOUS

See also: Atrial premature beats; Atrial fibrillation; Atrial flutter; AV block; Pacemakers

CODES
ICD9-CM
427.81 Sinoatrial node dysfunction

PATIENT TEACHING

- Mostly related to pacemaker follow-up in those with pacemakers
- If drug toxicity is the cause, counsel to take measures to avoid further toxicity.
- Recommendations regarding activity depend on hemodynamic consequences of bradycardias and tachycardias.

Diet
There is no specific diet.

ARRHYTHMIAS, SVT

Peter Ott
Andrew E. Epstein

 BASICS

DESCRIPTION

Supraventricular tachycardia (SVT) is the generic term for paroxysmal, regular supraventricular tachyarrythmias.

- The tachycardia may be due to atrioventricular nodal reentrant tachycardia (AVNRT), AV reentrant tachycardia (AVRT), junctional tachycardia, or atrial tachycardia.
- The term is not generally used for atrial fibrillation or flutter, even if they are paroxysmal, but rather for other usually regular, narrow QRS arrhythmias that occur paroxysmally.

Synonym(s):

- Paroxysmal atrial tachycardia (PAT): Term now obsolete

Pregnancy Considerations

Pregnancy is not contraindicated, but SVTs may be more frequent and precipitated by pregnancy.

EPIDEMIOLOGY

SVT is common. The prevalence depends on the population studied. SVT is more common in younger groups but can present at any age.

RISK FACTORS

None

ETIOLOGY

Dual AV nodal pathways, accessory pathway, junctional automaticity, atrial reentry, or automaticity

ASSOCIATED CONDITIONS

AVNRT and AVRT are usually isolated conditions. Other atrial tachycardias may be associated with structural heart disease.

 DIAGNOSIS

SIGNS AND SYMPTOMS

- Palpitations
- Dyspnea
- Dizziness
- Syncope
- Fatigue (sometimes related to drug therapy)
- Chest pain
- Diaphoresis
- Polyuria (usually after tachycardia)

TESTS

- Electrocardiogram (ECG): Morphology depends on arrhythmia substrate. See chapters addressing specific SVTs.
- Electrophysiologic study: Required if undergoing catheter ablation

Lab

None

DIFFERENTIAL DIAGNOSIS

- AVNRT
- AVRT
- Junctional tachycardia
- Atrial tachycardia
- Atrial flutter with 2:1 atrioventricular (AV) conduction

 TREATMENT

GENERAL MEASURES

- Recording of 12-lead ECG during tachycardia and during termination of tachycardia extremely important to help with diagnosis
- Due to the problems of long-term drug administration (adverse drug reactions, problem of multiple daily doses/noncompliance, and failure at some time over years of treatment), catheter ablation has emerged as one of the treatments of choice for (recurrent) atrial flutter, atrial tachycardia, AVNRT, and AVRT (Wolff-Parkinson-White syndrome), especially the latter if atrial fibrillation is present.
- The procedure can be performed safely with a low risk of complications; over the long term it improves quality of life compared with drug therapy and is likely cost-effective.
- For a single episode, a conservative approach may be adopted, including observation without drug therapy.
- Patient education about nature of SVT and treatment options is vital.

MEDICATION (DRUGS)

Treatment depends on arrhythmia substrate. See the chapters addressing specific SVTs.

- Watch for atrial fibrillation if adenosine is used and accessory pathway is present because rapid AV conduction over the accessory pathway can occur and lead to cardiac arrest.
- For patients with structurally normal hearts, "bolus" oral doses of flecainide (300 mg) or propafenone (600 mg) can be used to acutely terminate SVTs on an intermittent basis so that daily drug administration can be avoided.

SURGERY

Although surgery has been undertaken in the past for SVTs, it has been superseded by catheter ablation. Surgical treatment of SVTs is now primarily of historical interest.

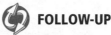 ## FOLLOW-UP

DISPOSITION
Admission Criteria

- Patients with SVT usually do not need to be admitted.
- Admission is warranted if SVT is incessant, or if there is a life-threatening associated problem such as atrial fibrillation with rapid conduction over an accessory pathway (shortest preexcited RR interval 250 msec or less).

PROGNOSIS
Excellent

PATIENT MONITORING

- General medical care if on drugs
- If cured by catheter ablation, none required; SVTs are rarely associated with hypotension
- Cardiac arrest can occur if there is rapid conduction over the accessory pathway during atrial fibrillation.

REFERENCES

1. Ganz LI, Friedman PL. Supraventricular tachycardia. N Engl J Med. 1995;332:162–173.
2. Morady F. Radio-frequency ablation as treatment for cardiac arrhythmias. N Engl J Med. 1999;340:534–544.

CODES
ICD9-CM
427.0 Paroxysmal supraventricular tachycardia

PATIENT TEACHING

- Relates to treatment options, especially opportunity for cure with catheter ablation
- Vagal maneuvers to terminate arrhythmia

ACTIVITY
There are no specific recommendations regarding activity, although SVTs can occasionally be precipitated by exercise and catecholamine increase.

ARRHYTHMIAS, TORSADE DE POINTES VENTRICULAR TACHYCARDIA

Peter Ott
Andrew E. Epstein

 BASICS

DESCRIPTION

Torsade de pointes (translated from French as "twisting of the pointes") ventricular tachycardia (TdP) is a polymorphic ventricular tachycardia that occurs in the setting of a long QT interval.

- It is recognized by the electrocardiographic appearance of nonuniform but organized rotation, or twisting, of the peaks of the QRS around the central axis of the electrocardiographic (ECG) baseline.
- Although polymorphic, there is a distinct progressive increase and decrease in the amplitude of the QRS within each burst.
- The arrhythmia may occur in the congenital long QT syndrome, as an idiosyncratic response to a variety of drugs, as well as in bradycardia and electrolyte abnormalities, specifically hypokalemia and hypomagnesemia.
- The congenital variety is discussed in the chapter on Long QT Syndrome. The short-term management of the acquired and congenital syndromes has many similarities, but the long-term management and prognosis are different.

Synonym(s):
- Torsades
- Polymorphic ventricular tachycardia with QT prolongation
- Atypical ventricular tachycardia
- Ventricular fibrilloflutter
- Paroxysmal ventricular fibrillation
- Transient ventricular fibrillation
- Cardiac ballet

Pregnancy Considerations

There is not a contraindication to pregnancy. However, arrhythmias are sometimes exacerbated by pregnancy, especially if electrolyte disturbances develop.

EPIDEMIOLOGY

Prevalence depends on population studied, especially on what drugs are used in the population. All age groups can be affected, although presentation of the congenital form occurs more often in the younger age group and presentation of the acquired form in older patients after drug administration.

RISK FACTORS

- Female gender
- Length of QT interval

ETIOLOGY

Genetic Abnormality/Predisposition
At least six genes have been identified, as discussed in the chapter on the Long QT Syndrome.

- When TdP occurs independently of the congenital form, it is unknown whether there is genetic predisposition that becomes manifest when a precipitating stimulus is present (i.e., drugs listed below, hypokalemia, hypomagnesemia).
- Drugs that prolong repolarization
  - Hypokalemia
  - Hypomagnesemia
  - Hypocalcemia
  - Bradycardia
  - Hypothyroidism
- Altered nutritional states (liquid protein diet, anorexia nervosa)
- Neurologic catastrophes, such as subarachnoid hemorrhage, that alter myocardial repolarization.

ASSOCIATED CONDITIONS

None are known in the congenital form. For the acquired form, patients are usually being treated with a QT-prolonging drug for a specific medical problem.

 DIAGNOSIS

SIGNS AND SYMPTOMS

- Syncope and presyncope
- Palpitations

TESTS

The electrocardiogram (ECG) is the diagnostic test and shows:

- Polymorphic ventricular tachycardia that varies from beat to beat and appears to rotate around the central axis of the ECG
- Rate variable, usually 160–250 beats/minute
- Long QT interval
- Initiated by long-short coupling interval [e.g., premature ventricular complex (PVC) followed by pause, sinus beat, and late cycle PVC (after peak of T wave)]
- ECG may show T-wave alternans, or variability of T waves before TdP onset.
- Often multiple nonsustained bursts

Lab

None for general use, although genetic screening is done in a research context

DIFFERENTIAL DIAGNOSIS

- Recognition of the characteristic pattern in the setting of a prolonged QT interval on the ECG is the foundation of the diagnosis.
- Polymorphic ventricular tachycardia caused by ischemia, or as an idiopathic arrhythmia, Brugada syndrome, central nervous system injury, that is, disease states that can alter cardiac repolarization, and therefore the QT interval

TREATMENT

GENERAL MEASURES

- See chapter on long QT syndrome for management of TdP in that setting.
- For the idiopathic variety, avoidance of and withdrawal of drugs that cause the syndrome are the mainstays of therapy.
- Correction of hypokalemia, hypomagnesemia, and hypocalcemia are essential.
- Pacing can be used to prevent TdP in the acute setting, especially when it occurs in the setting of bradycardia.
- Treat hypothyroidism, if present.

 MEDICATION (DRUGS)

- Defibrillation if sustained (cardiac arrest)
- Intravenous magnesium (1–2 g acutely)
- Isoproterenol can be used in the acute setting for drug-induced TdP. This is less frequently done today when TdP is acquired because it is frequently ineffective and temporary pacing is so successful.
- Alternatively to isoproterenol, atropine can be used.
- β-Blockers are the pharmacologic mainstay of therapy in the congenital form (see chapter on Long QT syndrome).
- Antiarrhythmic drugs, such as lidocaine, bretylium, and phenytoin, yield inconsistent benefit.
- Isolated reports of successful acute suppression with verapamil

SURGERY

See chapter on Long QT syndrome for congenital variety.

 FOLLOW-UP

DISPOSITION

Admission Criteria

- Admission is virtually always indicated when this arrhythmia is recorded because it can lead to cardiac arrest.
- Discharge is dictated by resolution of the precipitating cause or management of the congenital long QT syndrome.

PROGNOSIS

In the acquired form, outcome is excellent if precipitating causes are avoided. See chapter on Long QT syndrome regarding congenital form.

PATIENT MONITORING

- See chapter on Long QT syndrome for follow-up monitoring in the congenital form.
- For acquired TdP, avoidance of precipitating causes is essential.
- If antiarrhythmic treatment is necessary, use drugs that shorten QT (mexiletine, phenytoin). Note that amiodarone can uncommonly cause TdP.
- When in response to precipitating cause, it is idiosyncratic and therefore cannot be predicted.
- Avoid and prevent bradycardia, hypokalemia, hypomagnesemia, hypocalcemia, hypothyroidism, and drugs described in this chapter.

REFERENCES

1. Dessertenne F. La tachycardie ventriculaire á deux foyers opposé variables. *Arch Mal Coeur*. 1966;59:263–272.
2. Haverkamp W, Shenasa M, Borggrefe et al. Torsades de pointes. In: Zipes DP, Jalife J, eds. *Cardiac Electrophysiology: From Cell to Bedside*. Philadelphia: WB Saunders, 1995:885–899.

CODES
ICD9-CM
427.1 Paroxysmal ventricular tachycardia

PATIENT TEACHING
Contraindications
- Avoid contraindicated drugs, hypokalemia, hypomagnesemia, and hypocalcemia.
- Learn contraindicated drugs.
- See the Appendix for the table on list of QT-prolonging drugs.

ARRHYTHMIAS, VENTRICULAR FIBRILLATION

Peter Ott
Andrew E. Epstein

 BASICS

DESCRIPTION

Ventricular fibrillation (VF) is the rapid, disorganized, and asynchronous contraction of ventricular muscle.

- On the surface electrocardiogram (ECG), it is characterized by the absence of clearly defined QRS complexes.
- VF represents the final common pathway for death in most patients who experience out-of-hospital cardiac arrest.
- Its rate of recurrence is on the order of 30% in the 1st year in successfully resuscitated patients.
- Much of the discussion of ventricular tachycardia (VT; see chapter of that name) is relevant to VF. Synonym(s):
- Cardiac arrest (refers to collapse due to VT or fibrillation)
- Sudden death (VT followed by VF is usual cause of sudden, unexpected death)

ALERT

Pregnancy Considerations

May exacerbate any arrhythmia, and is not uncommon in long QT syndrome

EPIDEMIOLOGY

Approximately 350,000 sudden, unexpected, arrhythmic cardiac deaths occur each year in the United States.

- The prevalence is variable and depends on the presence or absence of structural heart disease.
- Persons of any age can be affected, but the incidence of VF increases with age because structural heart disease, especially coronary artery disease, is the most common substrate and is more frequently present as we age.
- Although VF is not specifically a genetic disease, there is a genetic component, as in congenital long QT syndrome, Brugada syndrome, and arrhythmogenic right ventricular dysplasia.
- Cardiomyopathies, both hypertrophic and dilated, are associated with VT and VF.

RISK FACTORS

- Same as in coronary artery disease (cigarette use, hyperlipidemia, and hypertension)
- Prior myocardial infarction with or without residual ischemia

- Abnormal left ventricular function (i.e., depressed left ventricular ejection fraction, dilated or hypertrophic cardiomyopathy)
- ECG abnormalities
  - ECGs of VF are rarely recorded because efforts are directed at resuscitation during the arrhythmia.
  - Rhythm strips show irregular and disorganized ventricular activity; VF is often preceded by VT.
  - The baseline ECG is often abnormal with nonsustained VT, left ventricular hypertrophy, nonspecific ST-T wave changes, intraventricular conduction delays, increased QT dispersion, T-wave alternans, decreased heart rate variability, and in specific syndromes signature findings (long QT in long QT syndrome, epsilon wave in arrhythmogenic right ventricular dysplasia, incomplete right bundle–branch block with ST elevation in leads V_1 and V_2 in Brugada syndrome).
- Very rarely, VF will spontaneously terminate.
- Increased age
- Glucose intolerance
- Nonsustained ventricular arrhythmias
- Digitalis use
- Inducible VT in a high-risk patient (after myocardial infarction, low left ventricular ejection fraction)

ETIOLOGY

- Coronary artery disease (with or without acute myocardial infarction)
- Myocardial scar from any cause (most commonly coronary artery disease, but also any structural heart disease, and surgical scars)
- Cardiomyopathy (dilated, hypertrophic, arrhythmogenic right ventricular dysplasia)
- Ischemia
- Drug toxicity: Includes traditional antiarrhythmic drugs such as class IC agents in coronary artery disease, QT prolonging drugs (torsade de pointes VT)
- Congenital
  - Diseases involving the ventricles (e.g., tetralogy of Fallot)
  - Long QT syndromes
- Valvular heart disease (e.g., aortic stenosis)
- Wolff-Parkinson-White syndrome with rapid ventricular preexcitation during atrial fibrillation
- Myocarditis
- Electrolyte and acid–base abnormalities (hypokalemia, metabolic acidosis)
- Primary electrical disease (idiopathic, Brugada syndrome, nocturnal death in Asians)

ASSOCIATED CONDITIONS

See list of etiologies and risk factors for VF.

 DIAGNOSIS

SIGNS AND SYMPTOMS

- Cardiac arrest
- Syncope, sometimes with seizure activity

TESTS

- ECG (myocardial infarction)
- Electrophysiologic study
- Pathology: Depends on substrate, including coronary artery disease, any cause of myocardial fibrosis (cardiomyopathy, trauma), fibroadipose infiltration of the myocardium (arrhythmogenic right ventricular dysplasia), or none (Brugada syndrome)

Imaging

- Echocardiogram (to evaluate cardiomyopathy, localized wall motion abnormalities such as in coronary artery disease)
- Coronary and left ventricular angiography
- Cardiac magnetic resonance imaging (useful in diagnosing arrhythmogenic right ventricular dysplasia)
- Exercise test with perfusion imaging (to assess ischemia)

DIFFERENTIAL DIAGNOSIS

ECG/monitor shows rapid and disorganized ventricular electrical activity. There is very little that can be confused with VF, other than artifact (e.g., when ECG leads have become dislodged from their positions).

 TREATMENT

GENERAL MEASURES

- Electrical defibrillation is the only definitive, acute treatment.
- Treat underlying heart disease, especially ischemia.
- Treat reversible causes (withdraw toxic drugs, correct electrolyte disturbances).

MEDICATION (DRUGS)

- Drugs can alter the ease of defibrillation (the defibrillation threshold) by implantable cardioverter defibrillators (ICDs) and the rate of ventricular tachycardia.
- When antiarrhythmic drugs are begun in patients with ICDs, electrophysiologic study should usually be considered to assess the possibility of adverse drug–device interactions.
- Acutely, external electrical defibrillation is required. In concert with resuscitation efforts, the following drugs are used:
  - Lidocaine
  - Amiodarone
  - Bretylium
  - Rarely procainamide
  - Antidigoxin antibodies if digoxin toxicity suspected
  - Drugs to correct electrolyte abnormalities (e.g., potassium for hypokalemia)

- Chronically drug therapy is secondary to ICD therapy, but may be required to treat frequent ventricular arrhythmias or coexisting atrial fibrillation
- Amiodarone
  – Sotalol
- β-Blockers, to treat ischemia, and as prophylaxis in congenital long QT syndrome
- Class I drugs less effective than class III agents and should be avoided in patients with structural heart disease

SURGERY
- VF is not treated by surgery *per se*.
- Surgery can be used to correct and/or treat reversible causes of VF, such as coronary artery disease and aortic stenosis.
- The Antiarrhythmics Versus Implantable Defibrillators (AVID) Trial showed that survivors of cardiac arrest have a greater survival chance when treated with an implantable cardioverter-defibrillator (ICD) compared with an antiarrhythmic drug.
- In the absence of a reversible cause or reasons to not implant an ICD, one should be offered.

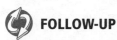 **FOLLOW-UP**

DISPOSITION
Admission Criteria
- The resuscitation rate in the field is usually <10%.
- If a survivor reaches the hospital, admission is obviously the only option. Even survivors to admission still have a high in-hospital mortality rate and often disability if they are discharged.

PROGNOSIS
Outcome depends on underlying heart disease and comorbid conditions. For patients with VF and a structurally normal heart, prognosis is better than if structural heart disease is present. However, the risk for recurrence persists.

PATIENT MONITORING
- Patients are followed according to the needs dictated by the cause of their VF.
- Reversible causes of VF must be treated.
- If drug therapy is chosen, assess compliance, drug levels, effect on ECG, and changes in myocardial substrate.
- Device follow-up if ICD chosen

REFERENCES
1. The AVID Investigators (prepared by the AVID Executive Committee: Zipes DP, Wyse DG, Friedman PL, et al.). A comparison of antiarrhythmic drug therapy with implantable defibrillators in patients resuscitated from near-fatal sustained ventricular arrhythmias. *N Engl J Med*. 1997;337:1576.
2. Belhassen B, Viskin S. Idiopathic ventricular tachycardia and fibrillation. *J Cardiovasc Electrophysiol*. 1993;4:356.
3. Echt DS, Liebson PR, Mitchell LB, et al. Mortality and morbidity in patients receiving encainide, flecainide, or placebo: The Cardiac Arrhythmia Suppression Trial. *N Engl J Med*. 1991;324:781.
4. Emergency Cardiac Care Committee and Subcommittees, American Heart Association. Guidelines for cardiopulmonary resuscitation and emergency cardiac care. *JAMA*. 1992;268:2171.
5. Gillum RF. Sudden coronary death in the United States 1980–1985. *Circulation*. 1989;79:756.
6. Klein GJ, Bashore TM, Sellers TD, et al. Ventricular fibrillation in the Wolff-Parkinson-White syndrome. *N Engl J Med*. 1979;301:1080.
7. Maron BJ, Fananapazir L. Sudden cardiac death in hypertrophic cardiomyopathy. *Circulation* 1992;85(suppl I):57.
8. Viskin S, Belhassen B. Idiopathic ventricular fibrillation. *Am Heart J*. 1990;120:661.

 MISCELLANEOUS

See also: Implantable defibrillators; Premature ventricular contractions; Torsade de pointes ventricular tachycardia; Ventricular tachycardia; Brugada syndrome; Long QT syndrome; Sudden death

CODES
ICD9-CM
427.41 Ventricular fibrillation

PATIENT TEACHING
- For patients with genetic syndromes, inform regarding need for screening of family members.
- For patients with long QT syndrome, educate regarding drugs to avoid, and for those with the congenital form avoidance of precipitating causes of torsade de pointes VT.
- With regard to specific therapies such as the ICD and drugs with potential organ toxicity (e.g., amiodarone), specialized information must be made available.

Diet
Choose diet appropriate for underlying heart disease (low cholesterol if coronary artery disease, low sodium if congestive heart failure, calorie restricted if diabetic).

Activity
For VF related to hypertrophic cardiomyopathy, exercise is restricted. Similarly, patients with aortic stenosis (presumably awaiting valve replacement or repair) should not exercise while awaiting surgery.

ARRHYTHMIAS, VENTRICULAR TACHYCARDIA

Peter Ott
Andrew E. Epstein

BASICS

DESCRIPTION
Ventricular tachycardia (VT) is wide QRS tachycardia originating in the ventricles due to reentry, triggered activity, or automaticity.
Synonym(s): The following have been used interchangeably but are not synonymous.
- Cardiac arrest (refers to collapse due to ventricular tachycardia or fibrillation)
- VT followed by ventricular fibrillation is the usual cause of sudden death.

ALERT
Pregnancy Considerations
Pregnancy may precipitate ventricular arrhythmias in long QT syndrome.

EPIDEMIOLOGY
- Coronary artery disease is the most common cause and is not specifically a genetic disease, although there is a genetic component.
- Prevalence is variable and depends on presence or absence of structural heart disease.
- All ages can be affected, but VT is more common in older individuals because coronary artery disease is more common.
- Cardiomyopathies, both hypertrophic and dilated, are associated with nonsustained and sustained VT.
- Some clear genetic syndromes, such as long QT syndrome, Brugada syndrome, and arrhythmogenic right ventricular dysplasia, are associated with VT.

RISK FACTORS
- Same as in coronary artery disease (cigarette use, hyperlipidemia, and hypertension)
- Electrocardiographic abnormalities, often determined by ambulatory monitoring, including:
  - Premature ventricular contractions and nonsustained ventricular tachycardia, left ventricular hypertrophy, nonspecific ST-T wave changes, intraventricular conduction delays, increased QT dispersion, T-wave alternans, and decreased heart rate variability
- Low left ventricular ejection fraction
- Increased age
- Inducible VT in high-risk patient (after myocardial infarction, low left ventricular ejection fraction)

ETIOLOGY
- Myocardial scar from any cause
- Drug toxicity [digoxin (bidirectional VT) or QT-prolonging drugs (torsade de pointes VT)]
- Electrolyte abnormalities (hypokalemia)
- Ischemia
- Bundle–branch reentry
- Congenital heart disease, especially postoperatively where there has been a ventriculotomy (as in tetralogy of Fallot)
- In structurally normal hearts two VTs can occur:
  - Right ventricular outflow tract VT
  - Idiopathic left VT

ASSOCIATED CONDITIONS
See Etiology and Risk Factors.

DIAGNOSIS

SIGNS AND SYMPTOMS
Signs and symptoms depend on rate and duration of VT, and extent of underlying heart disease, if any.
- None
- Syncope
- Cardiac arrest
- Dyspnea
- Palpitations
- Chest discomfort/angina

TESTS
Electrocardiography is the cornerstone of the diagnosis. When a 12-lead electrocardiogram (ECG) is available, the criteria listed below can be used not only to diagnose VT (to distinguish it from supraventricular tachycardia), but also to help guide therapy when ablation is considered.
- General: Atrioventricular (AV) dissociation, extremely wide QRS (>160 msec), QRS axis −90 to 180 degrees, and fusion (capture) beats all favor VT over supraventricular tachycardia with aberrancy.
- Morphology may be uniform (monomorphic) or variable (polymorphic)
- If left bundle beats all favor VT over supraventricular tachycardiabranch block morphology, VT suggested if:
  - In V_1 or V_2, R wave is >30 msec
  - In V_1 or V_2, there is a notch on the downstroke of the QRS
  - In V_1 or V_2, the interval from the onset of the QRS to the nadir of the S or Q wave is ≥60 msec
  - In V6 there is a Q wave
- If right bundle–branch block morphology, VT suggested if:
  - In V_1, QRS is monophasic or biphasic, especially if R is greater in amplitude than R′
  - In V_6, R to S ratio is <1 by either amplitude or area under the QRS complex
- Also useful to document if prior or new myocardial infarction present
- Electrophysiologic study

Lab
None except to assess electrolytes and drug levels where appropriate

Imaging
- Echocardiogram (to evaluate cardiomyopathy, localized wall-motion abnormalities such as in coronary artery disease, arrhythmogenic right ventricular dysplasia)
- Coronary and left ventricular angiography
- Cardiac magnetic resonance imaging (especially useful in diagnosing arrhythmogenic right ventricular dysplasia)
- Exercise test with perfusion imaging to assess ischemia

Pathologic Findings
Pathology depends on substrate, including coronary artery disease, any cause of myocardial fibrosis (cardiomyopathy, trauma), fibroadipose infiltration of the myocardium (arrhythmogenic right ventricular dysplasia), inflammatory disease (myocarditis, sarcoidosis), or none (right ventricular outflow tract tachycardia, idiopathic left VT, Brugada syndrome).

DIFFERENTIAL DIAGNOSIS
- Supraventricular tachycardia with aberrancy
- Preexcited tachycardia [antidromic reentrant tachycardia, or preexcitation as an innocent bystander such as during atrial flutter with atrioventricular (AV) conduction over a Mahaim accessory pathway]

TREATMENT

GENERAL MEASURES
- Treat underlying heart disease, especially ischemia and left ventricular dysfunction.
- Treat reversible causes (withdraw toxic drugs, correct electrolyte disturbances).
- Be sure to synchronize if performing electrical cardioversion.

MEDICATION (DRUGS)

- Acute
  - Lidocaine is easy to administer and has few hemodynamic effects.
  - Procainamide (but may cause hypotension)
  - Amiodarone is very effective.
  - Bretylium
  - Antidigoxin antibodies if digoxin toxic
  - Drugs to correct electrolyte abnormalities (e.g., potassium for hypokalemia)
  - For most VTs, intravenous calcium channel blockers remove compensatory peripheral vasoconstriction and lead to (life-threatening) hypotension.
- Chronic
  - Amiodarone
  - Sotalol
  - Class IC drugs (flecainide, propafenone) contraindicated if structural heart disease

SURGERY
In selected patients, curative therapy is possible with ablation or surgery.
- Catheter ablation is especially useful and efficacious for right ventricular outflow tract and idiopathic left VTs.
- Sometimes VT in the setting of coronary artery disease is amenable to catheter ablation, but ablation is often combined with drug or implantable cardioverter–defibrillator (ICD) therapy.
- In the past, endocardial resection was often used to treat VTs arising from myocardial infarction scars, and is still used today in highly selected patients (presence of surgical coronary artery disease and an anterior aneurysm).
- Because of the mortality and morbidity associated with this operation, ICDs have been used in recent years as an alternative. This approach is further supported by The Antiarrhythmics Versus Implantable Defibrillators (AVID) Trial, which showed superior survival in patients with hemodynamically unstable VTs when treated with ICDs compared with antiarrhythmic drugs.

- In the absence of a reversible cause or reasons to not implant an ICD, one is usually offered (see chapter on ICDs).
- Finally, surgery is used to correct and/or treat reversible causes of VF, such as coronary artery disease and aortic stenosis.

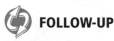

FOLLOW-UP

DISPOSITION

Admission Criteria

Admission criteria are variable and depend on hemodynamics during VT and the underlying substrate.

- VT from the right ventricular outflow tract and idiopathic left ventricular tachycardias occur in patients with otherwise normal hearts. Hemodynamics are usually preserved, and death due to these VTs is extremely uncommon. These patients can be managed in part on an outpatient basis.
- Admission is warranted for radiofrequency ablation of these VTs or the initiation of drug therapy.
- Conversely, VT in patients with coronary artery disease warrants admission because VT can degenerate to cardiac arrest (ventricular fibrillation).

PROGNOSIS

Outcome depends on underlying heart disease and comorbid conditions. For patients with VT and a structurally normal heart, prognosis is excellent (right ventricular outflow tract and idiopathic left ventricular tachycardias).

PATIENT MONITORING

- If drug therapy is chosen, follow to assess compliance, drug levels, effect on ECG, and changes in myocardial substrate.
- Device follow-up ICD chosen
- Drugs can alter the rate of ventricular tachycardias and the ease of defibrillation (defibrillation threshold) such that when antiarrhythmic drugs are begun in patients with ICDs, these potential effects need to be considered and an electrophysiologic study may be necessary

REFERENCES

1. The AVID Investigators (prepared by the AVID Executive Committee: Zipes DP, Wyse DG, Friedman PL, et al.). A comparison of antiarrhythmic drug therapy with implantable defibrillators in patients resuscitated from near-fatal sustained ventricular arrhythmias. *N Engl J Med*. 1997;337:1576.
2. Callans DJ, Schwartzman D, Gottlieb CD, et al. Insights into the electrophysiology of ventricular tachycardia gained by the catheter ablation experience: "Learning while burning." *J Cardiovasc Electrophysiol*. 1994;5:877–894.
3. Kindwall KE, Brown J, Josephson ME. Electrocardiographic criteria for ventricular tachycardia in wide complex left bundle branch block morphology tachycardias. *Am J Cardiol*. 1988;61:1279–1283.
4. Strickberger SA, Man KC, Daoud EG, et al. A prospective evaluation of catheter ablation of ventricular tachycardia as adjuvant therapy in patients with coronary artery disease and an implantable cardioverter-defibrillator. *Circulation*. 1997;96:1525–1531.
5. Wellens HJJ. The electrocardiogram 80 years after Einthoven. *J Am Coll Cardiol*. 1986;7:484–491.

MISCELLANEOUS

See also: Implantable defibrillators; Premature ventricular contractions; Torsade de pointes ventricular tachycardia; Ventricular fibrillation; Brugada syndrome; Long QT syndrome; Sudden death

CODES

ICD9-CM

427.1 Paroxysmal ventricular tachycardia

PATIENT TEACHING

Counseling depends in part on the VT substrate.

- For those with genetic syndromes, genetic screening of family members should be discussed.
- Patients with torsade de pointes VT need to be educated about which drugs to avoid, and for those with congenital long QT syndrome avoidance of precipitating causes of VT (startle reflexes).

Diet

Choose diet appropriate for underlying heart disease (low cholesterol if coronary artery disease, low sodium if congestive heart failure, calorie restricted if diabetic).

Activity

If VT is exercise related, exercise should be restricted.

ARRHYTHMIAS, WOLFF-PARKINSON-WHITE SYNDROME

Peter Ott
Andrew E. Epstein

 BASICS

DESCRIPTION

Wolff-Parkinson-White (WPW) syndrome is defined by the combination of preexcitation on the electrocardiogram (ECG) (delta wave) and supraventricular tachycardia (either atrial fibrillation or reentrant tachycardia using the accessory pathway as part of the circuit). In the purest sense, simple preexcitation without arrhythmias is not the "syndrome."

Synonym(s): Paroxysmal atrial tachycardia (PAT): Term now obsolete

ALERT

Pregnancy Considerations

Pregnancy is not contraindicated, but supraventricular tachycardias may be more frequent and precipitated by pregnancy.

EPIDEMIOLOGY

Supraventricular tachycardia and WPW syndrome can occur at any age. Conversely, accessory pathway conduction may disappear with aging.

- The prevalence of ECG preexcitation has been reported to range from 0.1–3/1,000 population.
- The intermittent nature of preexcitation may have led to underestimation of the true prevalence of the disease.
- Accessory pathway-mediated tachycardia accounts for about 30–40% of paroxysmal supraventricular tachycardias seen in practice.
- WPW syndrome is more frequent in males.

ETIOLOGY

- WPW syndrome results from a developmental abnormality of the atrioventricular (AV) groove.
- During normal cardiogenesis, direct continuity between the atrial and ventricular myocardium is lost by growth of the annulus fibrosis.
- Defects in the annulus leave muscular connection(s) called accessory pathways or Kent bundles between the atrial and ventricular myocardium.
- By bypassing the AV node, these pathways can lead to preexcitation of the ventricles because atrial impulses are not delayed in the AV node.
- Accessory pathways are most often described in electrical terms, with the ECG showing the characteristic delta wave, or they are identified at the electrophysiologic study. The pathways typically have "all or none" conduction properties, or rarely have decremental conduction properties, as does the AV node. They may conduct only from the atria to the ventricles (called anterograde or antegrade conduction), only from the ventricles to the atria (called retrograde conduction), or in both directions.
- The majority of patients with WPW syndrome do not have a familial/genetic disorder. However, there have been case reports of autosomal-dominant inheritance without associated cardiac disorders.
- Right-sided accessory pathways are associated with Ebstein anomaly of the tricuspid valve.
- Other conditions that have been associated with WPW syndrome are hypertrophic cardiomyopathy, mitral valve prolapse, and a variety of congenital heart diseases.

 DIAGNOSIS

SIGNS AND SYMPTOMS

- Palpitations
- Dyspnea
- Dizziness
- Syncope
- Fatigue (sometimes related to drug therapy)
- Chest pain
- Diaphoresis
- Polyuria (usually following tachycardia)

TESTS

- ECG is the cornerstone of diagnosis:
- The ECG may be normal (if AV nodal conduction is faster that accessory pathway conduction to the ventricles) or abnormal, with varying degrees of preexcitation (depending how much of the ventricles are activated via the accessory pathway and how much via the normal AV node–His-Purkinje system).
- The cardinal ECG features in sinus rhythm are (i) a short PR interval (<120 msec), (ii) a QRS duration of >120 msec with a slurred upstroke called a delta wave, and (iii) secondary ST-T wave changes.
- In tachycardia, there may be:
  - A narrow, regular QRS rhythm (orthodromic AV reentrant tachycardia) in which AV conduction is via the AV node. P waves may be buried in the QRS complex and not identifiable, or after the end of the QRS in the ST segment or T wave. In these tachycardias, ventriculoatrial conduction is via the accessory pathway.
  - A wide, regular QRS rhythm due to either orthodromic AV reentry with rate-related bundle-branch block aberrancy, or antidromic AV reentrant tachycardia, in which AV conduction is via the accessory pathway, and ventriculoatrial conduction is via the AV node.
  - An irregular QRS rhythm due to atrial fibrillation; the QRS may be narrow, or wide as a consequence of either rate-related aberrancy or preexcitation of the ventricles via the accessory pathway.
- Electrophysiologic study, required if undergoing catheter ablation

DIFFERENTIAL DIAGNOSIS

- AV nodal reentrant tachycardia
- Atrial tachycardia
- Atrial flutter with 2:1 AV conduction
- Junctional tachycardia
- ECGs may mask or mimic myocardial infarction, bundle-branch block, ventricular hypertrophy, accelerated idioventricular rhythm, ventricular bigeminy, and electrical alternans (the latter two diagnoses when accessory pathway conduction is intermittent).

 TREATMENT

GENERAL MEASURES

- 12-lead ECG is extremely important to secure the diagnosis
- Digoxin: Not desirable drug because if atrial fibrillation occurs, there may be rapid conduction over the accessory pathway and induction of ventricular fibrillation
- Cardioversion is indicated for acute management if atrial fibrillation occurs with rapid conduction over the accessory pathway, or if there is hemodynamic compromise. Cardiac arrest may occur during atrial fibrillation if there is rapid conduction to the ventricles via the accessory pathway.
- Because of the problems of long-term drug administration (adverse drug reactions, problem of multiple daily doses/noncompliance, and failure at some time over years of treatment), catheter ablation has emerged as a (if not "the") treatment of choice for recurrent AV reentrant tachycardia.
  - The procedure can be performed safely with a low risk for complications and a high degree of efficacy.
  - Long-term, ablation is likely cost-effective and improves quality of life compared with drug therapy, especially with class IA and IC agents.
  - Virtually all deaths attributed to accessory pathway conduction have occurred in patients with prior arrhythmia symptoms, and not as a first event.
  - Thus, electrophysiologic study may be performed to determine the anterograde refractory period of the accessory pathway (or pathways) and the risk of rapid AV conduction during atrial fibrillation before chronic drug treatment is prescribed.

 MEDICATION (DRUGS)

- Acute Management
  - To interrupt the reentry circuit:
    - Valsalva, and vagal maneuvers
    - Adenosine (intravenous), but watch for atrial fibrillation because it may lead to rapid conduction over the accessory pathway and precipitate ventricular fibrillation.
    - Although not approved for this indication, ibutilide is effective in blocking conduction in accessory pathways and may have a special place in the treatment strategy of patients with the WPW syndrome and atrial fibrillation.

- Intravenous procainamide may be used acutely because it decreases conduction over the accessory pathway and is safe if anterograde accessory pathway conduction is present in atrial fibrillation. However, intravenous procainamide may cause hypotension.
- Chronic Management
  - See comments regarding catheter ablation.
  - Drugs that shorten accessory pathway refractoriness and facilitate rapid ventricular rates during atrial fibrillation are contraindicated in patients with anterograde conduction over the accessory pathway because in atrial fibrillation conduction over the accessory pathway may be sufficiently rapid that ventricular fibrillation is precipitated.
    - In such patients, class I or class III drugs may be used alone or in combination with an AV nodal blocking agent.
    - Otherwise, a calcium channel blocker such as verapamil or a β-blocker can be used. The class IC antiarrhythmic drugs flecainide and propafenone and the class III antiarrhythmic drug sotalol are effective and well tolerated.
- Amiodarone, a class III antiarrhythmic drug, is potentially effective but its use is limited by adverse drug reactions.
- Class IA drugs (quinidine, procainamide, and disopyramide) are of limited value due to frequent adverse drug reactions during long-term treatment.

SURGERY
Surgery has been performed in the past. This has been superseded by catheter ablation for cure.

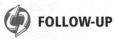 **FOLLOW-UP**

DISPOSITION
Admission Criteria
Admission is usually not required.
- Admission is warranted if supraventricular tachycardia is incessant, or if there is a life-threatening associated problem such as atrial fibrillation with rapid conduction over an accessory pathway (shortest preexcited RR interval 250 msec or less, equivalent to a heart rate of 240 beats/minute or more).
- Radiofrequency catheter ablation of accessory pathways can be undertaken on a same-day admission schedule.

PROGNOSIS
If accessory pathways are ablated and the heart is structurally normal, prognosis is normal. The prognosis is also excellent if accessory pathway has a long anterograde refractory period and cannot preexcite the ventricles rapidly during atrial fibrillation.

PATIENT MONITORING
General medical care if on drugs. If cured by catheter ablation, none. Recurrence can be prevented by either drug therapy or cure by catheter-based radiofrequency ablation.

REFERENCES
1. Al-Khatib SM, Pritchett ELC. Clinical features of Wolff-Parkinson-White syndrome. *Am Heart J.* 1999;138:403–413.
2. Ganz LI, Friedman PL. Supraventricular tachycardia. *N Engl J Med.* 1995;332:162–173.
3. Kay GN, Plumb VJ. Selective slow pathway ablation (posterior approach) for treatment for atrioventricular nodal reentrant tachycardia. In: Radiofrequency Catheter Ablation of Cardiac Arrhythmias: Basic Concepts and Clinical Applications. Armonk, NY: Futura,1994;171–203.
4. Jackman WM, Wang X, Friday KJ, et al. Catheter ablation of accessory atrioventricular pathways (Wolff-Parkinson-White Syndrome) by radiofrequency current. *N Engl J Med.* 1991; 324:1605–1611.
5. Miles WM, Klein LS, Rardon DP, et al. Atrioventricular reentry variants: Mechanisms, clinical features, and management. In: Zipes DP, Jalife J, eds. *Cardiac Electrophysiology: From Cell to Bedside,* 2nd ed. Philadelphia: WB Saunders,1995; 638–655.

 MISCELLANEOUS

See also: AV nodal reentrant tachycardia; Junctional rhythm

CODES
ICD9-CM
426.7 Anomalous atrioventricular excitation

PATIENT TEACHING
There are no specific dietary recommendations. Similarly, there are no specific activity recommendations, although arrhythmias can occasionally be precipitated by exercise and catecholamine increase. Otherwise, counseling relates to treatment options, especially opportunity for cure with catheter ablation. Vagal maneuvers to terminate arrhythmia can be taught.

ARTERIAL EMBOLISM
Carlos A. Roldan

 BASICS

DESCRIPTION
Occlusion of a cerebral artery resulting in stroke or transient ischemic attack (TIA) in 80% of patients, of a peripheral artery in 15%, or a visceral artery in ≤5% of patients.

GENERAL PREVENTION
- Primary prevention
  - Blood pressure (BP) control: <140/90 mmHg; <130/85 mmHg if renal or heart failure; <130/80 mmHg in diabetics
  - Low-density lipoprotein LDL <70 mg/dl in patients with atherosclerosis.
  - Smoking cessation
  - Physical activity 30–60 minutes >3 times/week
  - Weight reduction to body mass index (BMI) 18.5–24.9 kg/m2
  - Diabetes control (glucose <110 mg/dL and HbA1c <7%)
  - Aspirin in those with a >10% 10-year risk of or established atherosclerosis has an up to 48% stroke/TIA risk reduction.
  - In nonvalvular atrial fibrillation, warfarin [international normalized ratio (INR) 2–3] reduces embolism from 5.8% to 2.6% per year (63% relative risk reduction) and aspirin from 6.3–3.6% (42% relative risk reduction).
  - Warfarin (INR 2–3) reduces stroke rate from 3.8–0.8% in patients with anterior infarcts, left ventricular ejection fraction (LVEF) <35%, or left ventricular (LV) thrombus.
  - Warfarin (INR 2 to 3): In rheumatic mitral valve disease and atrial fibrillation; mitral stenosis and left atrial enlargement (>5.5 cm); before mitral valvuloplasty; nonischemic cardiomyopathy and atrial fibrillation, and mechanical heart valves (INR 2.5–3.5)
  - Low-molecular-weight heparin for those at high risk of embolism who require interruption of warfarin.

EPIDEMIOLOGY
Incidence
- Every year, 600,000 Americans develop new or recurrent stroke and >50,000 sustain TIAs.
- Incidence is higher in men >55 years old.

Prevalence
- Stroke prevalence ranges from 1.1–2.2% in men and 0.8–1.9% in women.
- Highest in non-Hispanic whites and increases from 2% for age 50–59 years to 12% for age ≥80 years.
- In women more than men when younger than 30 years old.
- In men more than women after the 4th decade of life.

RISK FACTORS
- Atrial fibrillation: Causes >50% of cases.
- Prosthetic heart valves: 2–4% Embolism per year, highest for mechanical mitral valves.
- Aortic atheromatous disease: 12–33% Embolism over a 1-to-2-year period.
- Anterior myocardial infarction: 30% Incidence of LV thrombus within first week and embolism of 5–27% without anticoagulation.

- Nonischemic cardiomyopathy: Up to 30% prevalence of intracardiac thrombus and 14% embolism in normal sinus rhythm.
- Aortic or cardiac surgery, aortic or arterial angiography, angioplasty, or intraaortic balloon pump insertion: Embolism up to 12% and predominantly due to aortic atheroembolism.
- Infective native or prosthetic valves. Endocarditis: 11–44% Embolism, highest in:
  - Staphylococcus aureus endocarditis or vegetations >10 mm.
- Antiphospholipid syndrome: Up to 30% embolic risk.

ETIOLOGY
- Intra and extracranial atherothrombosis or embolism, most common cause of stroke/TIA.
- Lacunar or small-vessel disease (20%)
- Undefined etiology (20–25%)
- Cardioembolism (15–20%)
  - Patent foramen ovale (PFO) and atrial septal aneurysm in those younger than 40 years
- Aortic atheroembolism, common.
- Coagulopathy, vasculitis, or migraine (< 5%)

ASSOCIATED CONDITIONS
- Atrial fibrillation
- Highly associated coronary, carotid, and peripheral arterial disease
- Myocardial infarction or cardiomyopathy
- Prosthetic heart valves or mitral stenosis
- Infective or noninfective endocarditis
- PFO with or without atrial septal aneurysm
- Large atrial septal aneurysm without PFO
- Coronary or peripheral arteries angiography, angioplasty with or without stenting, or surgery
- Primary or acquired hypercoagulability

 DIAGNOSIS

SIGNS AND SYMPTOMS
- Irregular rhythm; third heart sound or heart murmurs; carotid, abdominal or peripheral bruits; an ankle-brachial index of <0.9
- Acute ischemic stroke
  - Left or right hemisphere—major or branch cortical infarction: Aphasia, spatial neglect, homonymous hemianopsia, impaired conjugated gaze hemiparesis, sensory loss
  - Deep (subcortical) hemisphere or brainstem: Dysarthria–clumsy hand, ataxic hemiparesis, pure motor hemiparesis or sensory loss
  - Brainstem: Motor or sensory loss in all 4 limbs, dysconjugated gaze, dysarthria, nystagmus, ataxia, dysphagia
  - Cerebellum: Gait ataxia, ipsilateral limb ataxia
- Ophthalmic artery occlusion
  - Total or partial monocular blindness
- Cholesterol embolism
  - Purple toe syndrome
  - Acute or subacute nonoliguric renal failure
  - Uncommonly, focal neurologic deficits, amaurosis fugax, or retinal emboli
  - Nonhealing ulcerations or necrosis
  - Refractory hypertension
  - Rarely, mesenteric artery embolism

- Acute aortic occlusion
  - Cold, pale, cyanotic or pulseless extremities, symmetrical weakness, loss of sensation, and areflexia
- Acute limb ischemia
  - Severe pain in extremity, paresthesias, motor dysfunction, pulseless, and gangrene
- Splenic or renal infarct
  - Left upper quadrant abdominal, shoulder pain and left pleural effusion; or flank pain, or gross or microscopic hematuria

HISTORY
- Time of symptoms onset is critical in stroke
- Chronic or recent atrial fibrillation or flutter
- Coronary artery disease (CAD), myocardial, or valvular heart disease
- Carotid or peripheral arterial disease
- Prosthetic valve surgery
- Recent vascular instrumentation or surgery
- Hypercoagulability

Physical Exam
- Neurologic deficit is of prognostic value
  - Patients with a stroke score <10 as compared to those with a score >20 have a 60–70% complete or near-complete recovery and 3% intracranial hemorrhage as compared to 4–16% and 17%, respectively.
- Those corresponding to atrial arrhythmias, myocardial or valvular heart or arterial disease
- Normal with PFO and septal aneurysm

TESTS
Laboratory
- Complete blood and platelet count
- Prothrombin and partial thromboplastin time
- Blood glucose and serum electrolytes
- Renal function tests and fasting lipids
- Antiphospholipid antibodies if primary or secondary antiphospholipid syndrome suspected.

Imaging
- Xenon-enhanced computed tomography (CT) or single proton emission computed tomography (SPECT) or perfusion and diffusion-weighted magnetic resonance imaging/angiography (PWI/ DWI/MRI/MRA)
  - CT is better than MRI for detection of primary or postthrombolysis intracerebral hemorrhage.
  - Xenon-enhanced CT and SPECT can determine cerebral blood flow (CBF).
    - CBF >20 mL/100 g/min indicates tissue viability and reversible neurologic deficits without need for vascular recanalization.
    - CBF<10 mL/100 g/min indicates evolution to infarction, hemorrhage, edema.
  - MR techniques discriminate reversible from nonreversible ischemic brain tissue.
  - MR more sensitive than CT for detecting acute small cortical or subcortical infarcts.
  - DWI and PWI detect ischemic and perfusion abnormalities within minutes of symptoms and distinguish acute from old infarcts.
  - MR detects brain infarctions in 20% of TIAs.
  - MRA detects intracranial and vertebrobasilar or peripheral artery occlusions.

- Electrocardiography to detect arrhythmias
- Color-Doppler ultrasonography with 90% accuracy for carotid/vertebral artery disease
- Transcranial Doppler ultrasonography to detect intra or extracranial arterial occlusions and/or microemboli
- Angiography/aortography for definition of severity/extent of carotid, vertebral, and basilar artery disease in symptomatic patients with <70% carotid stenosis on ultrasonography or MRA
  - Also to assess severity of peripheral arterial disease and confirms aortic occlusion
- Echocardiography
  - Detect major cardioembolic substrates
  - Saline contrast with Valsalva maneuver increases sensitivity for interatrial shunt.
  - Transesophageal echocardiogram (TEE) if equivocal or limited transthoracic echocardiogram or in young patients with embolism of undefined etiology
- Testing for asymptomatic CAD
  - 25–60% of patients with TIA/stroke have asymptomatic CAD, twice more common in those with atheroembolism.
  - Thus, patients with carotid disease or high risk for CAD (10-year risk >20%) should undergo testing for detection of CAD.

Pathologic Findings
- Atherosclerosis, atherothrombosis, thrombotic vascular occlusion, and organ infarction
- Healed/active myocardial or valvular disease
- Vasculitis

DIFFERENTIAL DIAGNOSIS
- Intracranial/subarachnoid hemorrhage
- Hypoglycemia, drug overdose, seizures, or cerebral trauma
- Migraine, brain tumor, or subdural hematoma
- In situ aortic, peripheral, or carotid artery atherothrombosis

 TREATMENT

GENERAL MEASURES
- In stroke patients, assure oxygenation and protect airways
- ECG monitoring for ≥24 hours.
- Keep nothing per oral (NPO) for at least first 24 hours.
- In stroke patients, do not treat hypertension unless systolic or diastolic blood pressure >220/>120 mm Hg), suspected hemorrhagic infarction, myocardial ischemia/infarction, hypertensive nephropathy, or aortic dissection.
- Early mobilization and rehabilitation
- Standard measures to prevent deep venous thrombosis (DVT).

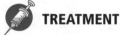 **MEDICATION (DRUGS)**

First Line
- Intravenous (IV) thrombolytics [rtPA (alteplase) at 0.9 mg/kg, maximum dose 90 mg] within 3 hours of onset of stroke (cardioembolic, large artery atherosclerosis, or small artery occlusion) in carefully selected patients without a multilobar infarction (>1/3 cerebral hemisphere) or hemorrhage on CT or MRI.
- IV labetalol or nitroprusside if blood pressure >220/>120 mmHg or end-organ damage.

Secondary Prevention
- Aspirin 325 mg/day or ticlopidine 250 mg b.i.d. or clopidogrel 75 mg/day (if aspirin failure/intolerance) reduces recurrent nonfatal stroke, myocardial infarction, and vascular death by 14–36%
- Clopidogrel 75 mg/day if aspirin failure or aspirin or ticlopidine intolerance
- Early heparin IV and lifelong anticoagulation are indicated after surgical correction of aortic occlusion.
- Antiplatelets or anticoagulants are not beneficial for cholesterol embolism.
- Significant Possible Interactions: Warfarin interacts with many drugs; lipid-lowering drugs to an LDL <70 mg/dL in patients with clinically evident atherosclerosis.

Second Line
IV direct thrombin inhibitors (hirudin, bivalirudin, or argatroban) or oral ximelagatran are safe and effective in patients intolerant to heparin or with heparin-induced thrombocytopenia.

SURGERY
- Primary prevention
  - In ascending aortic atheromatosis, change site of aortic cannulation.
- Secondary prevention
  - Elective carotid endarterectomy for symptomatic >70% carotid stenosis reduces ipsilateral stroke from 13.1–16.8% to 2.5–2.8% over a 2- to 3-year period.
- Immediate thromboembolectomy with aortic reconstruction or aortofemoral/axillofemoral bypass or thrombolysis in aortic or peripheral atherothrombotic occlusion.
- Primary angioplasty/stent for aortoiliac, femoral, popliteal, or infrapopliteal artery occlusion.

 FOLLOW-UP

- Routine follow-up for those on warfarin
- Echocardiography at 3–6 months in those with anterior myocardial infarction and LV thrombus.
- Carotid duplex at 6 months after carotid surgery or stent placement.

PROGNOSIS
- Stroke is the third leading cause of death and the leading cause of long-term disability in the United States.
- Stroke/TIA clinical course
  - The stroke risk after TIA is 4–8% the first month, 12–13% the first year, and 24–29% in 5 years.
  - Patients with stroke/TIA related to carotid stenosis have a 7–12% recurrent rate per year and 30–35% within 5 years.
- Stroke/TIA mortality and morbidity
  - Mortality ranges from 26.8–52% in men and 22.7–39.9% in women.
  - Highest rates in black males and females, and in patients older than 65 years of age.
  - Worst prognosis in those with basilar artery, internal carotid artery, or main stem middle cerebral artery occlusion (50–75% die or have poor neurologic recovery).
  - Patients with cerebral edema or intracranial hypertension have a 10–20% mortality rate during the first week.
  - DVT and pulmonary embolism account for a 10% mortality.

- Peripheral arterial embolism
  - Patients with cholesterol embolism have a 38–80% mortality rate and those with aortic occlusion a 30–40% operative mortality.
- CAD accounts for an independent 0.5–6.2% mortality within 3 months to 2 years and a 10-year mortality of 10.6–21%.

COMPLICATIONS
Incapacitation, dementia, blindness, limb or organ loss, death

REFERENCES
1. Adams H, Adams R, Del Zoppo G, et al. Guidelines for the early management of patients with ischemic stroke. 2005 guidelines update. *Stroke*. 2005;36:916–921.
2. Adams HP, Adams RJ, Brott T, et al. Guidelines for the early management of patients with ischemic stroke. *Stroke*. 2003;34:1056–1083.
3. Cerrato P, Grasso M, Imperiale D, et al. Stroke in young patients: Etiopathogenesis and risk factors in different age classes. *Cerebrovasc Dis*. 2004;18:154–159.
4. Faxon DP, Creager MA, Smith SC, et al. Atherosclerotic vascular disease. Executive summary. *Circulation*. 2004;109:2595–2604.
5. Latchaw RE, Yonas H, Hunter GJ, et al. Guidelines and recommendations for perfusion imaging in cerebral ischemia. *Stroke*. 2003;34:1084–1104.
6. Pearson TA, Blair SN, Daniels SR, et al. AHA guidelines for primary prevention of cardiovascular disease and stroke: 2002 Update. *Circulation*. 2002;106:388–391.

CODES
ICD9-CM
- 434.1 Cerebral embolism
- 444.22 Peripheral artery embolism

FAQ
- What is the rate of complete or near complete neurologic recovery with IV rtPA in acute ischemic stroke?: 31–50% versus 20–38% in those receiving placebo.
- What is the overall rate of brain hemorrhage with rtPA in acute ischemic stroke?: 6.4% versus 0.6% in those receiving placebo.
- What is the consensus on the degree of hypertension that precludes the use of thrombolytics in acute ischemic stroke?: Systolic blood pressure (SBP) >185 mmHg or diastolic blood pressure (DBP) >110 mmHg.
- Are anticoagulant and antiplatelet therapy indicated following IV rtPA in ischemic stroke?: No. They should not be used within 24 hours of IV thrombolytics.
- Does urgent anticoagulant or antiplatelet therapy improve neurologic outcome or prevent recurrent events in acute ischemic stroke?: Current data do not support a benefit.

ARTERIAL HYPERTENSION

Rajesh Dash
Helene Glassberg

 BASICS

DESCRIPTION
New 4 group classification system instituted in 1993 by JNC 7, based upon the level of blood pressure associated with the long-term risk of cardiovascular events:
- Normal = systolic blood pressure <120 mmHg, diastolic blood pressure <80 mmHg
- Pre-Hypertension = systolic blood pressure 120–139 mmHg, diastolic blood pressure 80–89 mmHg
- Stage I Hypertension = systolic blood pressure 140–159 mmHg, diastolic blood pressure 90–99 mmHg or taking antihypertensive medication
- Stage II Hypertension = systolic blood pressure >140 mmHg, Diastolic blood pressure >100 mmHg

EPIDEMIOLOGY
The prevalence of hypertension increases with the age of the population, such that 60% of U.S. adults 65–74 years of age have hypertension, and normotensive patients at age 55 have a 90% lifetime risk of developing hypertension.
- Race
  - The prevalence of hypertension among blacks is greater at every age, they tend to have more severe hypertensive disease with a higher mortality rate than whites.
  - Among Americans 60 years or older: 60% of whites, 71% of blacks, and 61% of Mexican-Americans have hypertension.
- Gender
  - Before menopause, hypertension is less common in women than in men.

RISK FACTORS
- Obesity
- Sleep apnea
- Physical inactivity
- Alcohol intake
- Smoking
- Polycythemia vera or "pseudo-polycythemia vera"
- Hyperuricemia

Genetics
- Familial aggregation and twin studies confirm that hereditary plays a role and that genetic contributions are estimated to range from 30–60%.
- Hypertension appears to be polygenic and multifactorial with involvement of numerous genes, the functions of which span from the renin–angiotensin–aldosterone axis to various ion channels and the subcellular signaling pathways of multiple receptor subtypes.

ETIOLOGY
In nearly 95% of patients with hypertension, there is no recognizable cause and it is referred to as "primary" hypertension.
- Because blood pressure is determined by cardiac output and peripheral resistance, alteration in the factors that influence these parameters may precipitate hypertension, such as excessive sodium intake, stress, obesity, endothelium-derived factors, and genetic alterations.
  Secondary hypertension in which an identifiable secondary process precipitates hypertension includes the following possible causes:
- Renal/renovascular disease
- Endocrine disorders
- Coarctation of the aorta
- Neurologic disorders
- Acute stress
- Ethanol/drug use
- Pregnancy-induced hypertension

ASSOCIATED CONDITIONS
- Coronary artery disease/congestive heart failure, sudden death, arrhythmias
- Left ventricular hypertrophy
- Stroke/transient ischemic attacks
- Renal failure
- Retinopathy
- Carotid atherosclerosis
- Peripheral arterial disease

Pregnancy Considerations
Synonyms include preeclampsia, pregnancy induced hypertension, and gestational hypertension.
- Preeclampsia is hypertension accompanied by proteinuria with or without abnormal coagulation, renal dysfunction, and liver dysfunction, which may progress to a convulsive phase and eclampsia.
- Occurs in 10% of first pregnancies in previously normotensive women
- Usually self-limited, rarely recurs in subsequent pregnancies
- Predisposing factors include increased age, black race, multiple gestations, concomitant renal or cardiac disease, and chronic hypertension.
- Clinical features include young age (<20 years), primigravida, >20 weeks of pregnancy, systolic blood pressure <160 mmHg, edema, spasm and edema on funduscopic examination, proteinuria, and elevated plasma uric acid.
- Treatment includes modified bed rest, normal sodium intake, and antihypertensive medications if diastolic blood pressure exceeds 100 mmHg. Antihypertensive therapy includes methyldopa and hydralazine. Angiotensin-converting enzyme (ACE) inhibitors are contraindicated.
- Cure is achieved with delivery.
- Excellent prognosis; does not cause hypertension and is not a sign of latent hypertension

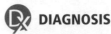 **DIAGNOSIS**

SIGNS AND SYMPTOMS
- Majority of patients are asymptomatic, for as long as 10–20 years
- Can present with symptoms of headache, tinnitus, syncope, angina, and dyspnea
- Common physical findings include prominent left ventricular apical impulse, fourth heart sound, funduscopic signs of arterial narrowing/arterio-venous nicking, hemorrhages, and exudates
- Look for other signs of target organ damage such as atherosclerosis and left ventricular failure.
- In hypertensive crisis: Headache, confusion, somnolence/stupor, visual loss, focal neurologic deficits, seizure, coma, funduscopic hemorrhages/exudates, papilledema, and nausea/vomiting

TESTS
- Electrocardiogram (ECG)
  - Left ventricular hypertrophy, evidence of ischemic heart disease, arrhythmias
- Renin, catecholamines, and aldosterone are not recommended in the initial evaluation unless there are specific clinical clues to indicate them.
- Ambulatory blood pressure monitoring
  - Correlates better with target organ involvement than office blood pressure measurement; may be useful in ruling out "white coat hypertension," assessing abnormal nocturnal patterns in blood pressure, apparent drug resistance, and hypotensive symptoms with antihypertensive medication
  - Not routine procedure in initial evaluation
- Additional studies may be necessary in the following conditions:
  - Patients younger than 15 years of age with hypertension; elderly patients with recent onset of moderate or moderate-severe hypertension
  - Accelerated hypertension
  - Worsening renal dysfunction
  - Spontaneous hypokalemia
  - Hypertension despite triple therapy including a diuretic
  - Hypertension and symptoms of headache, unusual patterns of sweating and palpitations

Lab
- Urinalysis
- Chemical profile including creatinine, blood glucose, potassium, uric acid, and lipids
- Optional tests include creatinine clearance, 24-hour urine protein, blood calcium, glycosylated hemoglobin, and thyroid-stimulating hormone.

Imaging
- Echocardiography
  - Not indicated in routine initial evaluation unless there is another specific indication; more sensitive and specific for identifying left ventricular hypertrophy than the electrocardiogram; too expensive for routine use
- Chest X-ray
  - Not indicated in routine evaluation

DIAGNOSTIC PROCEDURES/SURGERY
Obtain the average of at least two blood pressure measurements taken at each of at least two visits after an initial screening visit, using standardized technique.

DIFFERENTIAL DIAGNOSIS
- Secondary hypertension
  - Because of the low frequency of secondary causes, be selective in screening and diagnostic tests. Reserve testing for the presence of features inappropriate for usual, uncomplicated primary hypertension, including:
  - Onset at <20 or >50 years of age
  - Extreme hypertension, particularly if refractory to standard treatment
  - Accelerated or malignant hypertension
  - Recent elevation of serum creatinine that is unexplained or reversibly induced by an ACE inhibitor
  - Unprovoked hypokalemia
  - Abdominal bruit
  - Labile paroxysms of hypertension with headache, tachycardia, sweating, tremor
  - Abdominal or flank mass
  - Delayed/absent femoral pulses with lower blood pressure in the lower extremities
  - Truncal obesity with purple striae
- Isolated systolic hypertension
  - Defined as an elevated systolic pressure ≥140 mmHg with normal diastolic pressure <90 mmHg
  - Increased pulse pressure indicates reduced vascular compliance in large arteries
  - Accounts for more that half of the cases of hypertension in the elderly
  - Increased risk of stroke, congestive heart failure, and coronary heart disease
  - Elevated systolic blood pressure is a stronger risk factor for cardiovascular morbidity and mortality than elevated diastolic blood pressure
- White coat hypertension
  - An excessive increase in blood pressure in response to the stress of being in the physician's office
  - Particularly affects the systolic blood pressure
  - Common in older women
  - In the absence of target organ damage, if suspected, should obtain readings outside of the office with self-measurement or ambulatory monitoring
- Pseudohypertension
  - Due to excessive vascular stiffness in which markedly calcified, sclerotic arteries do not collapse under the cuff, leading to spuriously high readings
- Hypertensive crisis
  - Involves clinical circumstances that require rapid blood pressure reduction to prevent or limit target organ damage, including encephalopathy, intracranial hemorrhage, unstable angina, acute myocardial infarction, acute left ventricular failure with pulmonary edema, acute aortic dissection, acute renal failure, and eclampsia. Hypertensive crisis can be categorized as follows:
  - Hypertensive emergency that requires immediate reduction of blood pressure within 1 hour (e.g., encephalopathy, acute myocardial infarction, acute pulmonary edema, eclampsia)
  - Hypertensive urgency in which blood pressure reduction is desirable within a few hours (e.g., optic disc edema, severe perioperative hypertension)

TREATMENT

GENERAL MEASURES
- Risk stratify patients according to severity of hypertension and presence of target organ damage, clinical cardiovascular disease, or cardiovascular risk factors in order to determine treatment strategy (see the Appendix for the table on Risk Stratification in Hypertensive Patients) as follows:
- Target organ damage includes those with:
  - Heart diseases
    - Left ventricular hypertrophy
    - Angina or prior myocardial infarction
    - Prior coronary revascularization
    - Heart failure
  - Stroke or transient ischemic attacks
  - Nephropathy
  - Peripheral arterial disease
  - Retinopathy
- Lifestyle modification includes weight loss, sodium restriction, moderation of alcohol intake, cessation of smoking, physical activity, adequate intake of calcium/potassium, and magnesium.

MEDICATION (DRUGS)

Initial medical drug therapy for hypertension should be determined by the patient's blood pressure classification and other compelling medical indications.
- Lifestyle modification is recommended to all patients, regardless of hypertensive classification.
- For stage I hypertension, a thiazide-type diuretic should be chosen as the initial line of treatment. Additional agents (β-blockers, ACE inhibitors, angiotensin receptor blockers, calcium channel blockers, and vasodilators) should be employed as first-line therapy or in combination with thiazide-type diuretics if indicated (see below).
- For stage II hypertension, a two-drug combination is recommended as initial therapy (usually involving as thiazide-type diuretic).
- Thiazide-type diuretics have been shown to increase the response rates to all other antihypertensive agents.
- In certain clinical conditions, there are compelling indications for specific agents as initial treatment, such as β-blockers in patients with coronary artery disease or heart failure, and ACE inhibitors in patients with diabetes with proteinuria or heart failure.
- A second or third agent may be necessary if the response is inadequate after the full dose is given. An inadequate response is defined as a blood pressure persistently 20/10 mmHg higher than goal blood pressure.
- Black patients have a somewhat reduced response to monotherapy with β-blockers, ACE inhibitors, and angiotensin receptor blockers, compared with diuretics and calcium channel blockers.

FOLLOW-UP

PROGNOSIS
- Several trials have shown a 38% reduction in stroke morbidity/mortality, a 16% reduction in coronary heart disease events, and a 52% reduction in congestive heart failure occurrence with adequate control of hypertension.
- Lowering blood pressure in elderly hypertensive patients has resulted in a 37% reduction in stroke, a 25% reduction in transient ischemic attacks, a 30% reduction in myocardial infarctions, and a 54% reduction in occurrence of congestive heart failure

PATIENT MONITORING
- Goal blood pressure is <130/80 mmHg for all diabetic and chronic renal disease patients.
- Most patients should be seen within 1–2 months after initiation of treatment to determine adequacy of blood pressure control.
- Once blood pressure stabilized, follow up at 3- to 6-month intervals.
- Consider secondary causes of hypertension in patients who fail to respond to 3 or more anti-hypertensive agents.

REFERENCES
1. Joint National Committee on Prevention, Detection, Evaluation and Treatment of High Blood Pressure the JNC 7 report. *JAMA*. 2003;21;289:2560–2572.
2. Kaplan NM. System hypertension: Mechanism and diagnosis. In: Braunwald E, ed. *Heart Disease*, 5th ed. Philadelphia: WB Saunders,1997;807–839.
3. Moser M. *Clinical Management of Hypertension*, 3rd ed. Professional Communication,1998.
4. Tanira MO, Al Balushi KA. Genetic variations related to hypertension: A review. *J Hum Hypertens*. 2005;19:7–19.

CODES
ICD9-CM
- 401.9 Unspecified
- 401.1 Malignant

PATIENT TEACHING
- Lifestyle modification as discussed in the preceding text
- Medication compliance

ATHEROSCLEROSIS

James H. Chesebro

 BASICS

DESCRIPTION
- Lipid-induced monocyte/macrophage infiltration (inflammation) aggravated by risk factors (RFs) and lifestyle produce fibroproliferation, foam-cells, apoptosis, plaque disruption with thrombosis and endothelial dysfunction.
- Synonym(s): Coronary artery disease (CAD); Peripheral arterial disease (PAD); Cerebral vascular disease (CVD)
  - Coronary artery disease (CAD)
  - Peripheral arterial disease (PAD)
  - Cerebral vascular disease (CVD)

ALERT
Geriatric Considerations
Increasing prevalence, worse prognosis, and more events with age
Pediatric Considerations
Rare; consider homozygous familial hyperlipidemia or homocystinuria; worse if diabetes mellitus with metabolic syndrome or more RF
Pregnancy Considerations
Rare; consider other causes of coronary obstruction: Spasm, emboli, dissection, and vasculitis.

EPIDEMIOLOGY
- Leading cause of death in U.S. and other developed countries (>50%)
- Risk is potentiated by number of RFs and degree of uncontrol.
- Poor lifestyle increases risk and early age onset via obesity, especially via metabolic syndrome (see RF).
- Genetic risk (e.g., low high-density lipoprotein-cholesterol [HDL-C]) minimized by aggressive risk reduction (especially lowering LDL-C) and lifestyle control.

Incidence
Men have higher absolute risk than women at any age (4:1).

RISK FACTORS
- Traditional/independent
  - Age: men >45 years, women >55 years (postmenopausal)
  - Hypertension (worse with increasing blood pressure [BP] >120 mmHg)
  - Diabetes mellitus (worse with poor control)
  - Family history of atherosclerosis in primary relative, especially in men <55 years, women <65 years
  - Increased low-density lipoprotein-cholesterol (LDL-C) (1% risk for each mg% rise)
  - Low HDL-C (risk 3% less for each mg% rise)
  - Cigarette smoking
- Nontraditional
  - Metabolic syndrome, ≥3/5
    - Abdominal obesity, low HDL-C, hyperglycemia, hypertriglyceridemia, hypertension
  - Physical inactivity
  - Increased lipoprotein (a)
  - Increased homocysteine
  - Increased C-reactive protein (reflects multiple RF and life style)
  - Secondary tobacco smoke
  - Renal insufficiency, especially with anemia

- Increased fibrinogen, plasminogen activator inhibitor type-1, thrombin, factors VIII or VII
- Angiotensin-converting enzyme DD genotype
- Increased oxidized LDL-C
- Increased small dense LDL (pattern B)
- Increased soluble CD 40 ligand
- Increased interlukin-6

Genetics
- Mutations in *PCSK9* gene cause autosomal-dominant hypercholesterolemia.
- Haplotype 3 with the E670G variant is an independent determinant of LDL-C levels and the severity of CAD.
- Tangier disease (absent HDL and apoA-1) with LDL-C 40% of normal causes premature CAD due to mutations in *ABCA-1* gene—autosomal recessive.
- Normal or increased LDL-C with *ABCA1* mutations may markedly enhance atherosclerosis, whereas LDL-C reduction can reduce adverse gene expression.

PATHOPHYSIOLOGY
LDL-C initiates "fat-induced inflammation by chemoattraction of macrophages (see description).

ETIOLOGY
See pathophysiology. Highly associated with risk factors, lifestyle, and polygenic inheritance with clustering of these within families.

ASSOCIATED CONDITIONS
Diffuse disease—CAD, PAD, and CVD often occur together

 DIAGNOSIS

SIGNS AND SYMPTOMS
- CAD: Long silent period until angina, dyspnea, or acute coronary syndrome (ACS—unstable angina, myocardial infarction [MI] or sudden death).
- PAD: Bruit, claudication, arterial ischemia, aneurysm, renal failure
- CVD: Carotid bruit, transient ischemic attack, stroke, dementia

TESTS
- Risk stratification by number of risk factors and their control for prevention, prognosis, and treatment.
- Resting ECG usually normal; use continuous ST-segment monitoring for acute chest pain evaluation for high-risk (2/3 ischemias asymptomatic), left ventricular (LV) hypertrophy false + and unreliable in left bundle-branch block (LBBB), Wolff-Parkinson-White (WPW) syndrome, or delayed intraventricular conduction.
- Stress testing: Exercise (Ex) or pharmacologic (Pharm); (e.g., adenosine, dipyridamole, or dobutamine) if unable to exercise or β-blocked; exercise ECG detects ischemia (not location) if analyzable; all indirectly detect stenosis > 50% and define ischemic severity to guide management.
- Myocardial imaging with stress:
  - Stress echocardiogram provides regional wall motion and global function assessment of coronary stenoses; difficult with ventricular pacing or LBBB (Ex or Pharm).

- Technetium-99m/thallium 201 myocardial perfusion location and severity; perfusion imaging may miss three-vessel or left main coronary stenoses (Ex or Pharm).
- MRI of myocardial perfusion with gadolinium also detects myocardial viability with presence and extent of old MI (Pharm only); <1 hour procedure.

Lab
Complete blood count, creatinine, blood urea nitrogen (BUN), hemoglobin A1C, fasting glucose and lipid profile; also serum lipoprotein (a), homocysteine, and C-reactive protein

Imaging
- Noninvasive
  - Radiograph: Detects calcification of coronary or peripheral arteries or aorta as indicator of atherosclerosis.
  - Doppler ultrasound: Evaluates peripheral arteries for plaque, wall thickness, aneurysms, stenoses by Doppler flow velocity (e.g., carotids, aorta, renal, iliac, femoral, or popliteal arteries).
  - Electron-beam CT: Quantifies coronary artery calcification for plaque location and extent but is age-, gender-, and/or diabetes-dependent.
  - MRI: Detects arterial plaque presence, thickness, and composition (e.g., fat and fibrous cap thickness).
  - MRA: Quantitates arterial lumen and stenosis in three dimensions (3D) with gadolinium; coronary size and motion still a problem due to motion/small artery size.
  - Computed tomography angiogram: Quantitates arterial lumen and stenosis in 3D with x-ray contrast; best in proximal half of coronary arteries; calcification, metal clips, and small arteries still a problem.
- Invasive
  - Angiography: Gold standard
  - Intravascular ultrasound: Quantitates arterial lumen and stenoses and arterial wall thickness and density characteristics.
  - Transesophageal echocardiography: Identifies aortic atherosclerotic plaque and its thickness.

Pathological Findings
- Initiated in arterial wall by entry of lipid droplets that initiate chemoattraction of macrophages.
- Macrophages and smooth muscle cells (SMC) engulf lipid droplets, promote inflammation, cell and fibrous tissue proliferation, vascular destruction, and thrombosis.
- Apoptosis of lipid-containing cells contributes to confluence of extracellular lipid (especially oxidized LDL-C) in arterial wall, surrounded by collagen, macrophages, and SMC, with release of growth factors and cytokines, SMC migration from media to intima, and SMC proliferation; collagen forms fibrous cap between fat pool and arterial lumen.
- Plaque disruption of fibrous cap in 95% leads to mural thrombus and plaque growth.
- Plaque erosion or disruption in 5% leads to larger mural thrombus with ACS (subtotal >total occlusion).

TREATMENT

GENERAL MEASURES

- Maximal risk-factor reduction prevents disease, arrests progression, and prevents clinical events.
- Optimize lifestyle with reduction of obesity to BMI ≤25, Mediterranean-style diet, stop smoking and eliminate secondary smoke, and exercise continuously for 30 min 3–6 days per week.
- Assess CAD status by angina class, stress testing for exercise capacity, stress myocardial imaging or wall motion for location and extent of ischemia (useful to assess cause of exertional dyspnea), and need for revascularization for class III + angina or severe ischemia.
  - Medical management of mild angina/ischemia
  - Revascularize for symptom-limiting or severe ischemia
    - Drug-eluting stenting (DES) possible in 2/3 of cases
    - Coronary artery bypass graft (CABG) in about 1/3 with multivessel/left main disease
- Assess PAD by severity of claudication and ankle/brachial index at rest and exercise to check need for angiography and revascularization.
- Assess aneurysms by ultrasound and remote or larger sizes, especially presurgical, by MRA or CTA.
- Assess cerebrovascular disease (CVD) by carotid ultrasound, MRA or CTA, and MRI of thoracic aorta to detect atherothromboembolic disease.

 MEDICATION (DRUGS)

- Patients with atherosclerosis (CAD, PAD, or CVD), diabetes mellitus, or metabolic syndrome:
  - Antithrombotic: Aspirin 80–325 mg daily
  - Hypertension control to <130/85 (left ventricular hypertrophy by echocardiogram present in 30–40% of hypertensives, indirectly predicts poor control and risk of heart failure)
  - Decrease LDL-C <70 mg% (e.g., statin; risk 1% lower for each mg% decrease)
  - Raise HDL-C: Niacin, fish oil, or fibrate (if elevated triglycerides)(risk 3% less for each mg% rise)
  - Angiotensin-converting enzyme (ACE) inhibitor (CAD or diabetes and probably metabolic syndrome)
  - β-Blocker (CAD or diabetes and probably metabolic syndrome)

 FOLLOW-UP

PROGNOSIS

Age, sex, and number and control of RFs predict prognosis; reduced RF reduces clinical events.

COMPLICATIONS

Unstable angina, MI, sudden death, congestive heart failure, renal failure, aortic aneurysm or dissection, claudication, amputation, transient ischemic attack (TIA) or stroke

PATIENT MONITORING

Patient symptoms, exercise capacity, aggressive reduction of risk factors including normalization of body weight (BMI ≤25)

REFERENCES

1. Chesebro JH. Acute coronary syndromes: pathogenesis, acute diagnosis with risk stratification, and treatment. *Am Heart Hosp J.* 2004;2:21–30.
2. Davies MJ. Stability and instability: Two faces of coronary atherosclerosis. The Paul Dudley White Lecture 1995. *Circulation.* 1996;94:2013–2020.
3. Fuster V, Badimon L, Badimon JJ, Chesebro JH. The pathogenesis of coronary artery disease and the acute coronary syndromes. *N Engl J Med.* 1992; 326:242–50 (1);310–318 (2).
4. Fuster V, Fayad ZA, Moreno PA, et al. Atherothrombosis and high-risk plaque. Part II: Approaches by noninvasive computed tomographic/magnetic resonance imaging. *J Am Coll Cardiol.* 2005;46:1209–1218.
5. Fuster V, Moreno PR, Fayad ZA, et al. Atherothrombosis and high–risk plaque. Part I: Evolving Concepts. *J Am Coll Cardiol.* 2005;46: 937–954.
6. Ross R. Atherosclerosisan inflammatory disease. *N Engl J Med.* 1999;340:115–126.

 MISCELLANEOUS

- Organizations
  - American Heart Association; 1-800-242-8721; http: www.americanheart.org
  - American College of Cardiology; http:www.acc.org
  - National Institutes of Health; http:www.nih.gov
- See also:
  - Myocardial Infarct
  - Angina
  - Peripheral Vascular Disease
  - Renal Failure
  - Arrhythmia (Atrial And Ventricular)
  - Congestive Heart Failure
  - Stroke
  - Hypertension
  - Coronary Artery Disease
  - Aortic Aneurysm
  - Dissecting Aneurysm

CODES
ICD9-CM

- 414.01 Coronary artery disease
- 414.00 CASHD, unspecified vessel
- 437.0 Cerebrovascular disease
- 443.9 Peripheral vascular disease, unspecified

PATIENT TEACHING
Diet

Low-cholesterol, low-saturated fat, <2,000 mg sodium, AHA step I & step II diets; two saltwater fish meals/week, ≥25 gm fiber/day, Mediterranean-type diet, Ω-3 fatty acids, antioxidants interfered with lipid drugs in HATS study

Activity

Exercise minimum 30 min × 3/week, ideally 30 min x 6/week; post MI or revascularization, start cardiac rehabilitation program; cardiac fitness is inversely related to incidence of the metabolic syndrome.

Prevention

- Primary prevention: Eliminate/minimize RFs to arrest progression and prevent clinical events
  - Aspirin 81–325 mg PO daily
  - Hypertension control: <130/85, see Medication
  - Stop smoking: Reduces MI, limb loss (PAD), endothelial dysfunction, and arterial thrombus
  - Weight reduction to BMI ≤25, 500 fewer calories/day reduces weight by 1 lb/week; see Diet and Activity
  - Hyperlipidemia: Treatment depends on LDL-C and RF per National Cholesterol Education Program: Target LDL-C <160 if 0–1 RF; LDL-C,130 if >2 RF; diabetic patients or those with metabolic syndrome are high risk, thus target LDL-C <70 with statin ± Zetia (ezetimibe) or resin; raise HDL-C if <40 (men) and <50 (women); see Medication and Diet
  - Eliminate glycemia: Any elevation, even subdiabetic, increases risk of cardiovascular disease and events.
- Secondary prevention: Eliminate/minimize RF to arrest progression and prevent clinical events.
  - Aspirin 81–325 mg PO daily; if allergic, use clopidogrel or warfarin to INR 2.0–3.0
  - Hypertension control: <130/85, continuous increased risks as BP >120; see Medication
  - Stop smoking: Reduces MI, limb loss (PAD), endothelial dysfunction, and arterial thrombus
  - Weight reduction to BMI ≤25, 500 fewer calories/day reduces weight by 1 lb/week; see Diet and Activity
  - Hyperlipidemia: Pursue aggressive treatment for existing atherosclerosis, diabetes, or metabolic syndrome because of high risk; thus target LDL-C <70 with statin ± Zetia (ezetimibe) or resin; raise HDL-C if <40 (men) and <50 (women); see Medication and Diet
  - β-Blocker decreases ischemia, mortality, blood pressure/hypertension, arrhythmia, and LV failure.
  - ACE inhibitors decrease mortality post MI, hypertension, heart failure, and complications of diabetes.
  - Diabetes mellitus: Eliminating metabolic syndrome reduces risk to that of nondiabetic. The better the control, the greater the risk reduction. Thus, ESC and NIH advise hemoglobin A1c ≤6.1% and <6.05%, respectively

FAQ

- Q: How is atherosclerosis initiated?
  - A: In the arterial wall by entry of lipid droplets which initiates chemoattraction of macrophages
- Q: In patient monitoring, what level of BMI should be considered normal?
  - A: ≤25

ARTERIOVENOUS FISTULAS

Thomas J. Starc
Welton M. Gersony

BASICS

DESCRIPTION

Arteriovenous fistulas or malformations (AVM) are direct connections between the arterial and venous blood supplies, bypassing the capillary bed.

- They may be found in the systemic, pulmonary, and coronary circulation, and are a rare cause of congestive heart failure and myocardial ischemia.
- They also can cause a variety of clinical problems, including cutaneous lesions, disfigurement, and a mass effect causing local compression.

EPIDEMIOLOGY

- The majority of arteriovenous fistulas are congenital. Fistulas also may occur after surgery or trauma.
- Reported incidence depends on varying definitions and local referral patterns
- Large arteriovenous fistulas (Knudson, $n = 157$)
  - Central nervous system: 52%
  - Hepatic vascular tumors: 39%
  - Pulmonary arteriovenous fistulas: 9%
- Boston Children's Series 1973–1987 (Fyler, $n = 31$)
  - Coronary: 45%
  - Cerebral: 16%
  - Systemic: 16%
  - Pulmonary: 13%
  - Hepatic: 10%

PATHOPHYSIOLOGY

Direct arterial-to-venous shunt; If large, results in high output cardiac failure, or other manifestations depending on location

ETIOLOGY

The causes of the congenital fistulas are unknown.

ASSOCIATED CONDITIONS

- Hereditary hemorrhagic telangiectasias
- Capillary–cavernous hemangiomas
- Klippel-Trenaunay-Weber syndrome

DIAGNOSIS

SIGNS AND SYMPTOMS

Intracranial Arteriovenous Fistulas

- These are commonly aneurysms of the vein of Galen but may be found in any vessel in the central nervous system.
- Clinical manifestations depend on the age of presentation.
- Birth to 1 month of age
  - Heart failure is the most common presenting sign and may be associated with a cranial bruit and rarely with hydrocephalus.
  - Severe symptoms may present in the first few hours after birth.
  - Because the shunt is mandatory and not dependent on pulmonary vascular resistance, right and left heart failure occur early.
  - Right ventricular failure is secondary to both volume loading from the arteriovenous malformation and pressure loading from the high pulmonary vascular resistance of the newborn period.
  - The early onset of heart failure seen in this lesion is in sharp contrast to intracardiac left-to-right shunts such as a ventricular septal defect, in which manifestations of heart failure are not seen until the pulmonary vascular resistance decreases associated with an increase in left-to-right shunting.
  - Rarely an AVM can be the cause of fetal hydrops.
- 1–12 months of age, or later
  - Hydrocephalus is the most common presenting sign at this age. Heart failure (33%) and seizures (33%) also can occur.

Coronary Artery Fistulas

- Can occur between the coronary arteries and the atria, ventricles, and pulmonary artery; the right ventricle is most common, followed by the right atrium, pulmonary artery, and left ventricle.
- Small fistulas
  - Usually asymptomatic but can present with a heart murmur, endocarditis, or ischemia later in life secondary to coronary steal
- Large fistulas
  - Can rarely present with congestive heart failure in the newborn period

Pulmonary Arteriovenous Fistulas

- Congenital
  - Hereditary hemorrhagic telangiectasia
- Acquired
  - Severe liver disease and cirrhosis
  - Following cardiopulmonary anastomosis (Glenn shunts)
- Clinical manifestations include dyspnea, cyanosis, clubbing, polycythemia, hemoptysis, and signs of embolic phenomenon including transient ischemic attacks, strokes, and cerebral abscesses.
- The heart examination is usually normal.

Hemangiomas

Hemangiomas are not true AVMs, but rather are vascular tumors of proliferating endothelial cells with capillary channels. These tumors are common in the first year of life and then usually undergo spontaneous involution. Occasionally they require treatment because of their unusual size or location.

- Small hemangiomas often are visible in the skin, usually follow a benign course, and resolve spontaneously.
- Large capillary cavernous hemangioma can present with serious or life-threatening complications secondary to:
  - Congestive heart failure due to increased volume
  - Respiratory compromise due to tracheal compression
  - Loss of vision due to invasion of the orbit
  - Kassbach-Merritt syndrome (rapidly enlarging hemangioma, thrombocytopenia, acute or chronic consumption coagulopathy)
- Hepatic hemangiomas most commonly are hemangioendotheliomas or cavernous hemangiomas. These may present in infancy, causing congestive heart failure or hepatomegaly and are often associated with hemangiomas of the skin.

History
Depends on location

Physical Exam
Intracranial Arteriovenous Fistulas
- Tachypnea, tachycardia, and congestive heart failure
- Pulses are usually bounding, especially in the upper extremities.
- In patients with an intracranial aneurysm, bounding pulses in the arms and neck with decreased pulses in the lower extremities simulating a coarctation of the aorta have been reported.
- A bruit is typically heard over the fistula; therefore, auscultation of the head should be part of the physical examination in all newborns.

Imaging
- Intracranial arteriovenous fistulas
  - Chest radiographs
    - Demonstrate cardiomegaly and increased pulmonary markings
  - Echocardiography
    - Demonstrates normal intracardiac anatomy in most children
    - The degree of cardiac enlargement is proportional to the size of the fistula.
    - The presence of a large cerebral AVM can be suspected on echocardiography because of the increased size of the aorta, pulmonary artery, and superior vena cava.
    - The great vessels leading to the AVM are enlarged.
    - Doppler flow studies demonstrate abnormal retrograde diastolic flow patterns in the descending aorta.
    - Cranial ultrasonography will demonstrate the abnormal vessels in the majority of patients.
  - Cardiac catheterization is not the usual method to establish the diagnosis of a cerebral AVM.
- Coronary artery fistulas
  - Echocardiography
    - Can localize the size and location
    - More precise localization by angiography is usually necessary to determine the extent of the lesion.
- Pulmonary arteriovenous fistulas
  - Echocardiography utilizing peripheral venous contrast techniques may be useful by identifying abnormal appearance of pulmonary arteries and veins.
  - Catheterization demonstrates pulmonary venous desaturation in the affected segment.
  - Angiography demonstrates the rapid filling of the pulmonary vein in the affected segment.

DIFFERENTIAL DIAGNOSIS
- Large cerebral, hepatic, or peripheral AVMs can present shortly after birth with signs and symptoms of congestive heart failure. Tachycardia, tachypnea, hepatomegaly, and severe respiratory distress mimic heart failure due to other causes such as cardiomyopathy, and congenital heart lesions with large left-to-right shunts.
- Pulses are bounding, especially in the upper extremities, similar to findings in a patent ductus arteriosus, and often there is a differential in blood pressures between the arms and the legs, simulating a coarctation of the aorta.

TREATMENT

GENERAL MEASURES
- Intracranial arteriovenous fistulas
  - Treatment consists of medical control of congestive heart failure and occlusion of the arteriovenous fistulas with embolization. Surgical techniques may be utilized depending on the size and location of the lesion.
  - A variety of catheterization techniques using liquid adhesives, particulate agents, balloons, and coils can be used to achieve closure of the AVM.
  - Optimal management uses a team approach combining neurosurgical, interventional, and pediatric disciplines.
  - The use of these catheterization procedures can sometimes obviate or delay the need for neurosurgical procedures. Despite all measures, the prognosis is often poor.
- Coronary artery fistulas
  - Because the majority of these remain open, surgical treatment is usually required and may be lifesaving in those children with heart failure.
  - Small to moderate fistulas are closed to prevent endocarditis and late myocardial ischemia.
  - Tiny fistulas may close spontaneously.
- Pulmonary arteriovenous fistulas
  - Pulmonary AVMs often can be treated successfully by coil embolization.
- Hemangiomas
  - Small hemangiomas usually require no treatment and undergo spontaneous regression.
  - Large hemangiomas have been treated with steroids, cyclophosphamide, laser therapy, and interferon with variable rates of success.
  - Surgical excision is difficult because of the lack of clear lines of demarcation between normal and abnormal tissue. Fortunately, these lesions often regress with age.

SURGERY
May be useful in selected patients depending on location and size (see individual lesions)

PROGNOSIS
Variable (see individual lesions)

COMPLICATIONS
Variable (see individual lesions)

PATIENT MONITORING
- Patient follow-up depends on the size of the fistulas and the response to treatment.
- Children in heart failure require hospitalization to initiate management of heart failure and undergo closure of the fistulas.
- These children uniformly do poorly without treatment, and the success of treatment is dependent on the degree of closure of the AVM.
- Complete closure of the lesion is sometimes not possible, and partial closure can significantly decrease the degree of heart failure and allow the infant to grow and develop.
- Repeat attempts at closure can be undertaken when the child is older. In general, the overall prognosis for large AVMs in the central nervous system is guarded, although new catheter closure techniques are promising.
- The prognosis for hepatic hemangiomas most often is favorable, depending on the type of hemangioma. The prognosis for cardiac AVMs is usually excellent with optimal management.

REFERENCES
1. Burrows PE, Dubois J, Kassarjian A. Pediatric hepatic vascular anomalies. *Pediatr Radiol*. 2001; 31:533–545.
2. Fyler DC. Aortopulmonary fistulas. In: Fyler DC, ed. *Nadas' Pediatric Cardiology*. Baltimore: Hanely & Belfus, 1992;707–714.
3. Grifka RG, Preminger TJ. Vascular anomalies, In: Allen HD, Clark EB, Gutgesell HP, Driscoll DJ, eds. *Moss and Adams, Heart Disease in Infants, Children, and Adolescents Including the Fetus and Young Adult*, 6th ed. Baltimore: Lippincott Williams & Wilkins, 2001;689–706.
4. Holzer R, Johnson R, Ciotti G, Piozzi M, Kitchiner D. Review of an institutional experience of coronary arterial fistulas in childhood set in context of review of the literature. *Cardiol Young*. 2004;14:380–385.
5. Knudson RP, Alden ER. Symptomatic arteriovenous malformations in infants less than 6 months of age. *Pediatrics*. 1979;45:81–102.
6. McMahon WS. Arteriovenous fistulas. In: Garson A, Bricker JT, Fisher DJ, Neish SR, eds. The Science and Practice of Pediatric Cardiology, 2nd ed. Baltimore: Lippincott Williams & Wilkins, 1998;1677–1688.
7. Musewe NN, Burrows PE, Culham JAG, Freedom RM. Arteriovenous fistulae: A consideration of extracardiac causes of congestive heart failure. In: Freedom RM, Benson LN, Smallhorn JF, eds. *Neonatal Heart Disease*. London: Springer Verlag, 1992;759–772.
8. Preminger TJ, Perry SB, Burrows PE. Vascular anomalies. In: Emmanouilides GC, Riemenschneider TA, Allen HD, Gutgessel HP, eds. *Moss and Adams' Heart Disease in Infants, Children, and Adolescents Including the Fetus and Young Adult*, 5th ed. Baltimore: Williams & Wilkins, 1995.

CODES
ICD9-CM
- 747.81
- 746.85

ATHLETIC HEART SYNDROME

Michael H. Crawford

 BASICS

DESCRIPTION

Sustained exercise training induces adaptive changes in the cardiovascular system that allow for greater athletic performance. The major adaptations involve the heart, blood, and peripheral vascular system.

Heart
- Cardiac hypertrophy that is eccentric with predominant isotonic exercise and concentric with predominant isometric exercise
- Resting sinus bradycardia

Blood
- Total blood volume increases due to proportional increases in red cells and plasma.

Peripheral Vascular System
- Peripheral vascular capacitance increases, resulting in relative decreases in peripheral vascular resistance, allowing movement of a greater stroke volume without increases in systolic pressure.

Systems Affected
- Cardiovascular
- Hematopoietic

GENERAL PREVENTION

Exercise training does not eliminate heart disease. Risk-factor control is still necessary to avoid coronary artery disease.

EPIDEMIOLOGY

- Predominant Age: Late adolescence to middle aged
- Predominant Sex: Male more than female

Age-Related Factors
- Pediatric: Congenital heart disease predominates
- Middle aged: Coronary artery disease dominates

Incidence

Sudden death in athletes is rare.

RISK FACTORS

Underlying heart disease

Genetics

Adaptations to exercise and athletic ability may be partially determined by heredity.

PATHOPHYSIOLOGY

The ability to increase cardiac output largely determines exercise ability.

ETIOLOGY

Regular, vigorous exercise training

ASSOCIATED CONDITIONS

Cardiac hypertrophy

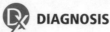 **DIAGNOSIS**

History
- History of athletic training and prowess
- Orthostatic symptoms

Physical Exam
- Athletic physique
- Sinus bradycardia
- Sinus arrhythmia
- Enlarged apical impulse
- Right ventricular lift
- Diastolic gallop sounds
- Systolic flow murmurs

TESTS
- Electrocardiogram (ECG): Ventricular hypertrophy patterns (may mimic myocardial infarction), bradyarrhythmias
- Exercise: Maximum oxygen uptake will identify exercise-trained individuals.

Lab

No specific abnormalities

Imaging
- Chest X-ray: Cardiac enlargement
- Echocardiography: Distinguish physiologic versus pathologic ventricular hypertrophy; identify valvular disease and cardiomyopathy

Diagnostic Procedures/Surgery
- If coronary artery disease is suspected, exercise testing with echo or radionuclide imaging may be indicated, or in some cases coronary angiography.
- Electrophysiologic testing may be required to distinguish pathologic rhythm disturbances from benign ones.
  - Tilt table testing may help elucidate the cause of dizziness or syncope encountered in an athlete.

Pathological Findings

Ventricular hypertrophy

DIFFERENTIAL DIAGNOSIS
- Abnormal bradyarrhythmias
- Pathologic ventricular hypertrophy
- Valvular heart disease
- Cardiomyopathy
- Coronary artery disease

 TREATMENT

GENERAL MEASURES
- Outpatient evaluation
- Distinguish normal physiologic changes from disease
- Many cardiac diseases increase the risk of athletic activity:
  - Hypertrophic cardiomyopathy
  - Coronary artery anomalies or disease
  - Marfan syndrome
  - Aortic valve disease
  - Complex congenital heart disease
  - Pulmonary hypertension
  - Mitral stenosis
  - Pulmonic stenosis

MEDICATION (DRUGS)

First Line
- Depends on cardiac diseases
- Some performance-enhancing drugs have potential adverse effects on the heart, such as anabolic steroids and catecholamines.

Contraindications
- Refer to manufacturer's profile of each drug.

Precautions
- Athletically trained individuals are especially susceptible to drugs with vasodilator or heart rate-slowing properties such as α and β-blockers.

Significant Possible Interactions
- Refer to manufacturer's literature.

Second Line

Occasionally athletic training will need to be stopped temporarily until a specific disease is treated with drugs that affect a response in the patient.

SURGERY

Corrective surgery for cardiac conditions may permit athletic activity.

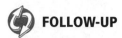 **FOLLOW-UP**

Depends on the cardiac condition

DISPOSITION
Admission Criteria
- Syncope
- Heart failure
- Severe chest pain
- Cardiac arrest

Discharge Criteria
Resolution of the problem

Issues for Referral
Suspected cardiac disease in an athlete

PROGNOSIS
- Exercise-trained individuals are usually healthier and live longer than sedentary individuals in the absence of significant cardiovascular disease.
- The combination of athletic activities and certain cardiovascular diseases can shorten life.

COMPLICATIONS
- Sudden arrhythmic death
- Aortic dissection
- Precipitation of heart failure
- Syncope

PATIENT MONITORING
- Occasionally the only way to distinguish normal physiology from disease is to cease exercise training and observe the patient.
  - Sinus bradycardia and chamber enlargement usually regress significantly within weeks.

REFERENCES
1. Maron BJ, Zipes DP. 36th Bethesda conference: Eligibility recommendations for competitive athletes with cardiovascular abnormalities. *J Am Coll Cardiol*. 2005;45:1312–1375.
2. Pellica A, et al. Clinical Significance of abnormal electrocardiographic patterns in trained athletes. *Circulation*. 2000;102:278.

ADDITIONAL READING
Maron BJ, et al. Recommendations for preparticipation screening and the assessment of cardiovascular disease in master's athletes. *Circulation*. 2001;103:327.

CODES
ICD9-CM
429.3 Athlete's heart

PATIENT TEACHING
Important to describe risks of cardiac disease if patient desires participation in athletic activities.

Diet
Depends on cardiac conditions and training requirements

Activity
Based on type of cardiac abnormality and the desired physical activity/sport

Prevention
Patients with certain cardiac diseases should have exercise activities limited to avoid sudden death or other serious consequences. Occasionally athletic competition can be allowed with successful drug, surgery, or device therapy (i.e., implantable defibrillator).

FAQ
Does chronic heavy exercise damage the heart? No, there is no evidence that physiologic cardiac hypertrophy is deleterious.

ATRIAL SEPTAL DEFECT, SECUNDUM

William E. Hellenbrand
Welton M. Gersony

 BASICS

DESCRIPTION
A secundum atrial septal defect (ASD 2°) is defined as the absence of septal tissue in the septum secundum, allowing for a free communication between the left and right atrium at or near the level of the fossa ovalis. A spectrum of defect size occurs, from a large fossa defect to multiple small perforations within the septum. The foramen ovale may or may not be included in the defect. A significant left-to-right shunt across the atrial septal defect causes enlargement of the right atrium and right ventricle, usually associated with normal pulmonary artery pressures.

EPIDEMIOLOGY
- Secundum atrial septal defects are common, reported to occur in 7–10% of children with congenital cardiac anomalies as the predominant cardiac lesion.
- The defect is more common in females, F:M ratio = 2:1.
- The condition is associated with a lack of early symptoms and the subtlety of the physical examination, which may delay the diagnosis into adult life. Thus, ASD 2° is the most common form of congenital heart disease to present in the adult population.

ETIOLOGY
Isolated secundum atrial septal defects are almost never associated with specific chromosomal abnormalities. However, certain skeletal malformations exist, such as Holt-Oram syndrome, with a reported incidence of atrial septal defects as high as 50%.

RISK FACTORS
None

PATHOPHYSIOLOGY
The presence of an atrial septal defect results in left-to-right shunting of blood from left to right atrium. The degree of shunting depends on the size of the defect and diastolic compliance of the right or left ventricles. The shunt is left to right because the right ventricle is more compliant. On this basis, the left-to-right shunts can be over 3:1, and right ventricular volume is markedly increased. The left-to-right shunt is tolerated well, because pulmonary pressure is almost always normal. Pulmonary vascular resistance is extremely low.

ASSOCIATED CONDITIONS
- Atrial septal defects may be associated with pulmonary valve stenosis, as well as with ventricular septal defects.
- The incidence of partial anomalous pulmonary venous return is 3% in patients with secundum defects, compared with 83% of those with a sinus venosus atrial septal defect.
- Pulmonary vascular obstructive disease with right-to-left shunting may develop in patients with large ASDs that have been left unrepaired into middle age.

 DIAGNOSIS

SIGNS AND SYMPTOMS
- Usually, no symptoms are related to an ASD in the pediatric age group. In the presence of a very large defect, mild dyspnea on exertion and/or easy fatigability may be seen, but often only appreciated in retrospect after repair of the ASD.
- Symptoms become more common in the fourth or fifth decade and include:
  - Dyspnea on exertion
  - Easy fatigability
  - Congestive heart failure (CHF)
  - Atrial arrhythmias

History
Most often asymptomatic

Physical Exam
- An abnormal second heart sound that either is split widely and fixed, or is persistently split, but varies somewhat with respirations.
- A medium-pitched short systolic ejection murmur is audible at the upper left sternal border, related to increased blood flow across the pulmonary valve.
- The murmur may be prominent at the base and throughout the lung fields due to increased flow over the distal pulmonary vessels.
- A soft, early diastolic murmur may be heard at the mid left sternal border related to increased flow across the tricuspid valve.

TESTS
Lab
- ECG
  - Usually shows right-axis deviation and a right bundle-branch block pattern over the right precordial leads. A left superior axis is consistent with an ASD 1°.

Imaging
- Chest radiograph may show mild to moderate cardiomegaly with a large right atrium, right ventricle, and pulmonary artery segment, and pulmonary vascular markings are increased. Enlargement of the right ventricle is often only manifested on lateral view. Many patients have a relatively normal radiograph.
- Echocardiography is the optimal method of evaluating the anatomy of ASD 2°. It is also essential to rule out associated abnormalities. The exact location and size of the ASD is visualized, and enlargement of the right atrium and right ventricle are defined. Visualization of the margins of the defect is important in determining plans for interventional/surgical management.

DIAGNOSTIC PROCEDURES/SURGERY
Cardiac catheterization is not necessary to establish a diagnosis of ASD 2° in any age group. It is indicated only to evaluate suspected pulmonary hypertension, or when interventional procedures are utilized as a form of therapy.

DIFFERENTIAL DIAGNOSIS
The differential diagnosis for ASD includes mild pulmonary stenosis, because of similarities in the physical examination. Partial anomalous pulmonary venous connections without an associated ASD, although unusual, can be confused with an ASD 2° because both result in a right-heart volume load. The straight back syndrome, with a systolic ejection murmur at the upper left sternal border and a prominent pulmonary artery on chest radiograph, may superficially suggest the presence of an ASD.

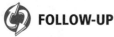 **TREATMENT**

GENERAL MEASURES
- Most children with an ASD 2° are asymptomatic.
- No indication exists for drug therapy for this condition.
- Patients with evidence of volume overload of the right ventricle on echocardiography should be evaluated for definitive closure.
- Some small to moderate ASDs may close spontaneously in the first 1–2 years of life; for uncomplicated patients, all approaches to closure should be delayed until patients are at least 2 years of age.
- Antibiotic prophylaxis is not required.

SURGERY
- The most common form of ASD repair has been surgical closure using the standard technique of open heart surgery.
- More recently, methods of transcatheter closure of ASD 2° have undergone investigation; device repair has become an alternative to surgical closure of this defect. The recent results of transcatheter technique are excellent, with complete closure rates of 90–95%. The complication rate is low, comparable to that of open heart surgery.
- Transcatheter closure has become the procedure of choice at many medical centers.

FOLLOW-UP

PROGNOSIS
- Patients repaired in the pediatric age require minimal follow-up.
- A rare patient develops atrial arrhythmia, but this is a very unusual event when ASD closure has been performed within the first two decades of life.
- In older patients who have CHF and/or pulmonary hypertension, continue to follow after surgery for evidence of progressive pulmonary hypertension and/or arrhythmia.
- The rare unoperated patient who develops pulmonary vascular obstruction later in life receives symptomatic therapy. ASD closure is not indicated in this group of patients, and the prognosis is guarded.
- Long-term prognosis for children with a repaired ASD is excellent; a normal lifespan is expected. In the older patient, who presents with symptoms, the lifespan may be shortened despite successful surgical closure.
- Antibiotic prophylaxis is not required.

Pregnancy Considerations

- The presence of a large ASD does not adversely affect the outcome of pregnancy, but occasionally, patients have signs of mild CHF and, rarely, severe decompensation. An infrequent complication associated with ASD during pregnancy is paradoxical embolization across the ASD into the systemic circulation.
- Pregnancy is not associated with increased risk after closure.

REFERENCES

1. Kirklin JW, Barratt-Boyes BG: Atrial Septal Defect and Partial Anomalous Pulmonary Venous Connection, *Cardiac Surgery*, Second Edition, Volume I, 15:609–644.
2. Chessa M, Carminati M, Butera G, et al. Early and late complications associated with transcatheter occlusion of secundum atrial septal defect. *J Am Coll Cardiol*. 2002;39:1061–1065.
3. Hessling G, Hyca S, Brockmeier K, Ulmer HE. Cardiac dysrhythmias in pediatric patients before and 1 year after transcatheter closure of atrial septal defects using the Amplatzer septal occluder. *Pediatr Cardiol*. 2003;24:259–262; Epub 2003 Jan. 15.
4. Mandell V, Nimkin K, Hoffer FA, Bridges ND. Devices for transcatheter closure of intracardiac defects. *Am J Roentgen*. 1993;160:179–184.
5. Mandell V, Nimkin K, Hoffer FA, Bridges ND. Devices for transcatheter closure of intracardiac defects. *Am J Roentgen*. 1993;160:179–184.
6. *Moss and Adams' heart disease in infants, children, and adolescents*, 6th ed. 2005 Atrial Septal Defects.

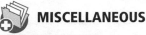

MISCELLANEOUS

PATIENT TEACHING

Diet

No dietary restrictions

Activity

Normal activity is recommended.

BRUGADA SYNDROME

Peter Ott
Andrew E. Epstein

 BASICS

DESCRIPTION
- RBBB (right bundle branch block) and ST elevation in leads V_1 and V_2
- Risk of sudden death due to polymorphic ventricular tachycardia
- Half have inducible ventricular arrhythmia
- Synonym(s): none
- Sudden unexpected death in Asian immigrants (also called pokkuri in Japan, bangungot in the Philippines, and lai tai in Thailand) are probably related.

Pregnancy Considerations
There is no contraindication to pregnancy. However, genetic counseling is recommended in view of the genetic cause and transmission of this disease.

EPIDEMIOLOGY
The incidence and prevalence are unknown. It can be recognized in patients of any age.

RISK FACTORS
None

ETIOLOGY
- Genetic abnormality of *SCN5A* and other genes
- Missense mutation: Channel recovers from inactivation more rapidly than normal.
- Frameshift mutation renders channel nonfunctional, which increases dispersion of refractoriness and repolarization.
- Splice-donor mutation: Consequences unknown

 DIAGNOSIS

SIGNS AND SYMPTOMS
- Syncope
- Cardiac arrest
- Asymptomatic

TESTS
- Electrocardiogram (ECG) shows RBBB and ST elevation in leads V_1 and V_2.
- ECG abnormalities may be unmasked by flecainide or intravenous procainamide.
- Signal averaged ECG often shows late potentials, even in absence of r' waves in right precordial leads.
- Ventricular arrhythmias provokable by programmed stimulation at electrophysiologic study
- Endomyocardial biopsies have been done to exclude arrhythmogenic right ventricular dysplasia.

Lab
No test available

Imaging
- Echocardiography to exclude cardiomyopathy
- Coronary angiography to exclude ischemia
- Ventriculography to exclude cardiomyopathy
- Cardiac magnetic resonance imaging (MRI) to exclude arrhythmogenic right ventricular dysplasia

Diagnostic Procedures/Surgery
Electrophysiologic study: Role in diagnosis and risk stratification remains controversial

DIFFERENTIAL DIAGNOSIS
- Simple RBBB—typically does not have ST elevation (present in Brugada syndrome), and has wide slurred S wave in V_6 and lead I (not present in Brugada syndrome)
- Acute myocardial infarction (because of ST elevation)
- Left ventricular aneurysm
- Myocarditis
- Right ventricular infarction
- Duchenne muscular dystrophy
- Long QT syndrome (because of polymorphic ventricular tachycardia)
- Hypercalcemia
- Hyperkalemia
- Central and autonomic system abnormalities

 TREATMENT

GENERAL MEASURES
Because drug therapy is thought to be ineffective, implantation of an implantable cardioverter–defibrillator (ICD) is usually recommended, in symptomatic patients. The management of asymptomatic patients is controversial.

 MEDICATION (DRUGS)

- Drug therapy is apparently ineffective, including β-blockers.
- Drugs that block transient outward current (Ito) current (i.e., quinidine and disopyramide) may be efficacious.

SURGERY
None except implantation of an ICD

FOLLOW-UP

DISPOSITION
Admission Criteria
- If the presentation of the Brugada syndrome is cardiac arrest, ICD implantation is recommended.
- If the syndrome is diagnosed incidentally, risk of disease (cardiac arrest) must be discussed. If ICD is desired, admission is then planned.
- If the patient presents with syncope and the ECG pattern of the Brugada syndrome is recognized, he or she should be hospitalized because recurrence of ventricular arrhythmia may result in sudden death.

PROGNOSIS
Guarded

PATIENT MONITORING
- Once diagnosis is established, the patient should be seen by an electrophysiologist knowledgeable about Brugada syndrome.
- Syncope would be indication to initiate treatment (i.e., ICD).
- Avoid class I antiarrhythmic drugs that block INa more than Ito (i.e., procainamide and flecainide).

REFERENCES
1. Alings M, Wilde A. "Brugada" syndrome: Clinical data and suggested pathophysiological mechanism. *Circulation*. 1999;99:666–673.
2. Brugada J, Brugada P. Further characterization of the syndrome of right bundle branch block, ST segment elevation, and sudden cardiac death. *J Cardiovasc Electrophysiol*. 1997;8:325–331.
3. Gussak I, Antzelevitch C, Bjerregaard P, et al. The Brugada syndrome: Clinical, electrophysiologic and genetic aspects. *J Am Coll Cardiol*. 1999;33:5–15.

MISCELLANEOUS

- See also: Implantable cardioverter–Defibrillator, Ventricular Fribrillation, Ventricular Tachycardia, Long QT Syndrome, Sudden Death
- Internet Resources: http://www.netvision.be/brugada

CODES
ICD9-CM
427.9 Cardiac dysrhythmia, unspecified

PATIENT TEACHING
- No intervention is known to prevent cardiac arrest. New drugs that selectively block Ito may be effective.
- Sudden death is a major risk of disease.
- Unknown if mental stress and alcohol are provocative factors

CARCINOID HEART DISEASE

Kevin P. Fitzgerald
Steven C. Herrmann
Bernard R. Chaitman

 BASICS

DESCRIPTION

Carcinoid heart disease (CHD) is predominantly a valvular heart disease (VHD) of the tricuspid valve (TV) and pulmonary valve (PV). It results as a sequelae of metastatic carcinoid, which is a neuroendocrine secreting tumor producing vasoactive compounds.

Incidence
Yearly incidence of carcinoid tumors in the United States is 1–2 per 100,000.

Prevalence
- About 10% of patients with carcinoid tumors develop the carcinoid syndrome.
- About 50% of patients with carcinoid syndrome develop CHD.

RISK FACTORS
- Serotonin is related to the development of CHD but does not correlate with the risk for progressive CHD.
- Patients who have received cytotoxic chemotherapy may have the highest risk for progressive CHD.

PATHOPHYSIOLOGY
- Carcinoid tumors arise from the enterochromaffin cells typically of the gastrointestinal (GI) tract (midgut carcinoids) or the lungs (foregut carcinoids).
- 90% of carcinoid tumors are located in the GI tract, most commonly the appendix and ileum.
- These tumors release serotonin and other vasoactive substances, which cause the signs and symptoms of carcinoid syndrome.
- The vasoactive substances include serotonin (5-hydroxytryptamine), bradykinin, histamine, 5-hydroxytryptophan, and prostaglandins.
- Primary midgut carcinoid tumors metastasize to the liver and regional lymph nodes.
- Ordinarily, the vasoactive substances are metabolized by the liver, lung, and brain.
- Liver metastases cause the right heart to be exposed to high levels of vasoactive substances, ultimately resulting in right-sided endothelial deposition of carcinoid plaques.
- The precise cause for plaque formation is not clear but may be due to the direct actions of serotonin and bradykinin.
- Most CHD only involves the TV and PV due to lung deactivation of the vasoactive substances.
- There may be left-sided valvular involvement with right-to-left cardiac shunts, bronchial carcinoids, or pulmonary metastases (5–10% cases).
- Plaques are preferentially deposited on the ventricular rather then the atrial side of the TV.
- In progressive CHD, the TV and PV leaflets become thickened, retracted, and fixed, causing right-sided VHD and right heart failure.

ASSOCIATED CONDITIONS
Carcinoid tumors may be associated with elevated levels of gastrin, glucagons, insulin, adrenocorticotropic hormone (ACTH).

 DIAGNOSIS

SIGNS AND SYMPTOMS
- One half of the patients with carcinoid syndrome will have CHD.
- The syndrome consists of cutaneous vasomotor flushing, GI hypermotility, secretory diarrhea, bronchospasm, and hypotension.
- Patients with CHD may have symptoms attributable to tricuspid regurgitation (TR), tricuspid stenosis (TS), pulmonary regurgitation (PR), and pulmonary stenosis (PS).
- Serotonin can lead to tachycardia and hypertensive crisis refractory to traditional therapy.
- Patients may have labile blood pressure (BP), with high or low BP depending on the relative amounts of vasoactive substances in the blood.

History
- Carcinoid symptoms typically occur at a mean age of 55–60 years.
- The time-period between the onset of carcinoid syndrome and the diagnosis of CHD averages 24–28 months.
- Patients may have complaints of flushing, diarrhea, and wheezing suggestive of carcinoid syndrome.
- There may be symptoms of right heart failure: Lower extremity swelling, abdominal pain and bloating, constipation, anorexia, and early satiety.
- Patients who have had chemotherapy for carcinoid may be at risk for progression of CHD.

Physical Exam
Many of the patients with CHD will present with signs of right heart failure: Edema, hepatomegaly, ascites, hepatojugular reflux, and elevated jugular venous pressure and a systolic murmur of TR. Pulmonic stenosis or regurgitant murmurs may also be present.

TESTS
Lab
- Carcinoid tumors convert tryptophan to serotonin.
- Serotonin is metabolized to 5-hydroxyindole acetic acid (5-HIAA).
- Elevated levels of urinary 5-HIAA have a 75% sensitivity and a 100% specificity for carcinoid.
- Levodopa, ethanol, imipramine, aspirin, and phenothiazines may falsely lower urinary 5-HIAA levels.
- Acetaminophen, guaifenesin, ephedrine, nicotine, caffeine, and phenobarbital may falsely increase urinary 5-HIAA levels.
- Diets rich in banana, kiwi, eggplant, nuts, pineapple, and avocado may falsely increase urinary 5-HIAA levels.
- Right heart failure may cause elevated liver function tests due to passive hepatic congestion.

Imaging
Electrocardiogram
- In advanced CHD the QRS has low voltage.
- May see p-pulmonale or right bundle–branch block, or nonspecific ST-T wave changes.

Chest x-ray
- May see right ventricle enlargement (RVE) and right atrium enlargement (RAE) (~50% cases)
- Pleural effusions and metastatic pleural plaques are late findings.

Echocardiography
- CHD is diagnosed by the characteristic right-sided cardiac lesions in patients with histologically proven carcinoid disease.
- CHD usually produces diffuse thickening and immobility of the right heart valves (TV>PV).
- RAE and RVE are present in >90% of cases of CHD.
- Abnormal ventricular septal motion is present in 50% of CHD.
- Calcification of the valves is not associated with CHD.

Diagnostic Procedures/Surgery
In a surgical series, nearly all patients had moderate to severe TR, 80% had PR, 50% had PS, and 7% had left-sided VHD.

Pathologic Findings
- Histologically, carcinoid plaques consist of smooth muscle cells with sparse collagen embedded in an acid mucopolysaccharide matrix with no elastic fibers.
- Grossly, plaques are focal or diffuse, white, shiny, and fibrous.
- Plaques are deposited on the endocardium of the valvular leaflets, subvalvular apparatus, cardiac chambers, vena cava, pulmonary artery, and coronary sinus.
- Plaques preferentially involve the ventricular surface of tricuspid valve leaflets and the arterial aspect of the pulmonic valve.

DIFFERENTIAL DIAGNOSIS
- Pheochromocytoma
- Panic attacks
- Cocaine abuse
- Causes of isolated right-sided heart failure (e.g., restrictive cardiomyopathy, primary pulmonary hypertension, etc.)

 TREATMENT

GENERAL MEASURES
- Most patients with carcinoid syndrome have metastatic disease and treatment is usually palliative
- CHD therapies focus on the treatment of right heart failure, VHD, and reduction of neuroendocrine secretions
- Right heart failure should be managed with salt and fluid restrictions and lower extremity compression stockings
- Hepatic artery embolization or ligation may reduce the hepatic metastatic tumor burden and reduce the carcinoid syndrome symptoms.
- The changes from CHD are not usually reversible despite reductions in the levels of vasoactive substances.

MEDICATION (DRUGS)

- Right heart failure is managed with diuretics and possibly digoxin.
- Somatostatin analogs, octreotide and lanreotide, provide symptomatic relief by reducing the vasoactive peptides.
- Interferon-α alone or in combination with somatostatin has been used to reduce tumor size and relieve symptoms.
- Chemotherapy has not shown any benefit.

SURGERY
- Surgical resection of a localized carcinoid tumor can be curative.
- Surgery is the only effective therapy for CHD.
- It is preferable to operate on the valves earlier before the right heart failure worsens and increases the surgical risk.
- Surgical options are palliative and not curative.
- Indications for surgery are poor exercise tolerance, worsening fatigue, or a reduction in ventricular function, despite an otherwise indolent course of metastatic carcinoid syndrome.
- Balloon angioplasty can produce improvement in right heart failure, but symptoms may recur.
- Mechanical valves in the TV position are not affected by the vasoactive peptides but are complicated by the need for chronic anticoagulation with coexisting liver metastases.
- Bioprosthetic valve durability will likely outlast the patient's lifespan and are generally preferable, but the valves can be affected by the CHD.
- TV repair is not usually an option due to underlying leaflet damage.
- The pulmonary valve may be managed with a valvectomy or a valve replacement.
- Pulmonary valve replacement may reduce postoperative right heart dilatation.

 ## FOLLOW-UP

Admission Criteria
Patients with right-sided heart failure exacerbations may require hospital admission.

Discharge Criteria
Patients can be discharged once they have adequate resolution of their admission symptoms.

Issues for Referral
- Patients with carcinoid tumors should be monitored regularly for evidence of metastatic disease and CHD.
- Once CHD is diagnosed, referral to cardiology and cardiothoracic surgery is prudent.

PROGNOSIS
- Carcinoid tumors are slow growing.
- Localized carcinoid has a 94% 5-year survival.
- Carcinoid syndrome portends a worse prognosis with a median survival of 1–3 years.
- CHD signals a further decline in survival with a mean 3-year survival of approximately 30%.
- Patients with CHD usually die of severe TR and right heart failure rather than carcinomatosis.

REFERENCES
1. Bonow RO, Carabello B, de Leon AC Jr, et al. ACC/AHA 2006 guidelines for the management of patients with valvular heart disease: A report of the American College of Cardiology/American Heart Association Task Force on Practice Guidelines (Writing Committee to Revise the 1998 Guidelines for the Management of Patients with Valvular Heart Disease). American College of Cardiology Web Site. Available at: http://content.onlinejacc.org/cgi/reprint/48/3/el.
2. Connolly M, et al. Outcome of cardiac surgery for carcinoid heart disease. *J Am Coll Cardiol*. 1995;25:410–416.
3. Fox DJ, Khattar RS. Carcinoid heart disease: Presentation, diagnosis and management. *Heart*. 2004;90:1224–1228.
4. Knott-Craig CJ, Schaff HV, Mullany CJ, et al. Carcinoid disease of the heart: Surgical management of ten patients. *J Thorac Cardiovasc Surg*. 1992;104:475–481.
5. Moller JE, et al. Factors associated with the progression of carcinoid heart disease. *N Engl J Med*. 2003;348:1005–1015.

 ## MISCELLANEOUS

CODES
ICD9-CM
259.2

CARDIAC SURGERY, IMMEDIATE POSTOPERATIVE MANAGEMENT

Patrick Whalen
*Richard Chen**
*Jerre Lutz**
Nanette K. Wenger

 BASICS

DESCRIPTION
Pathophysiologic effects of cardiopulmonary bypass

- Fluid, electrolytes: Increased extracellular fluid, total exchangeable sodium; decreased exchangeable potassium, elevated glucose levels
- Inflammatory response: From blood contact with synthetic surface of bypass equipment; inflammatory state results in platelet–endothelial cell interactions, vasospastic responses causing low-flow states in coronary circulation, and capillary leak syndrome
- Transient depression ventricular function: From oxygen free radical production in response to reperfusion injury; depressed by 2 hours after cardiopulmonary bypass, worse at 4–5 hours, significant recovery by 8–10 hours, full recovery by 24–48 hours
- Hypothermia: Predisposes to dysrhythmias, increases systemic vascular resistance (SVR), causes shivering, which increases oxygen consumption, impairs coagulation
- Respiratory insufficiency: Secondary to alveolar dysfunction (atelectasis), decreased central respiratory drive (anesthetics), decreased respiratory muscle function (incisional pain), exacerbation underlying chronic obstructive pulmonary disease

See also the following tables in the Appendix:

- Risk Stratification Scoring System for Patients Undergoing Coronary Bypass Surgery
- Intravenous Drugs for Cardiac Surgical Patients: Pharmacologic Therapy
- Interpretation of Hemodynamic Patterns in Cardiac Patients
- Intravenous Positive Inotropic Agents

 TREATMENT

GENERAL MEASURES
Postoperative Complications
Hypertension

- Present in most patients without left ventricular dysfunction secondary to increased peripheral vascular resistance from hypothermia

Low-Output Syndrome
Clinical features include:

- Cold extremities
- Systolic blood pressure (SBP) <90 mmHg
  - Low output may be present with SBP >100 mmHg when SVR is increased (>1,500 dyne-sec/cm^{-5}).
- Urine output <30 mL/h
- Cardiac index <2.0 L/min/m^2 (except in sepsis)
  - Strong relationship between early postoperative low cardiac index and probability of cardiac surgery death
  - Mixed venous O2 saturation <50 (except in sepsis)
  - Acidosis
- Obtain hemodynamic data with Swan-Ganz catheter, echocardiogram
- Categorize etiology: Decreased preload, cardiogenic, sepsis, etc.

Perioperative Myocardial Infarction

- Symptoms unreliable
- Diagnose by ECG, creatine kinase-MB, troponin levels. Echocardiogram may be confirmatory, not routinely performed.

- No routine cardiac enzymes postoperatively unless hemodynamically unstable intraoperatively, new ECG changes

Dysrhythmias Reactivate ICD /Interrogate PM

- Supraventricular
  - Sinus tachycardia most common
  - Atrial fibrillation
    - 10%–30% occurrence postoperatively
    - Advanced age most important associated factor
    - Most common postoperative day 2
    - 80% return to sinus rhythm within 1–3 days following digoxin or β-blocker
    - IV diltiazem, esmolol for rate control
    - 10% require cardioversion
  - Atrial flutter
    - May convert to normal sinus rhythm using atrial epicardial pacing wires
    - Burst pacing: 15–30 seconds of 300–600 beats/min atrial rate
- Ventricular
  - Frequent ectopy (>6 beats/min) in first 12 hours postoperatively suggests ischemia.
    - Lidocaine for suppression often recommended by some (bolus 75 mg followed by 50 mg every 5 minutes for total of 225 mg or bolus 75 mg followed by 150 mg over 20 minutes)
  - Ventricular tachycardia
    - Most commonly due to revascularization in nonviable myocardium leading to reentry
    - Usually requires amiodarone to suppress or eliminate
    - Note: Wide complex tachycardia with rates of 250–300 beats/min suggests accessory pathway. Procainamide drug of choice for accessory pathway tachycardias with very fast rates.

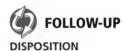

- Bradyarrhythmias/conduction defects
  - Conduction defects in up to 45% of patients
  - Majority transient
  - Right bundle branch block most common conduction defect
  - Atrial fibrillation with slow ventricular response, sinus bradycardia, junctional rhythm less common
  - May support bradycardia with temporary atrial pacing (85–100 beats/min)
- Pulmonary
  - Most significant cause of morbidity after cardiopulmonary bypass
    - Atelectasis: Common, 70% of patients
  - Decreased chest wall movement due to incisional pain
  - Decreased diaphragmatic excursion due to phrenic nerve damage may require up to 6 weeks for recovery, may be permanent.
  - Decreased central respiratory drive: Anesthetics, analgesics
  - Exacerbation underlying chronic obstructive pulmonary disease
  - Pleural effusions, if large, may require repeat thoracentesis after chest tubes removed.
  - Postpump syndrome/capillary leak/adult respiratory distress syndrome
    - Early clues include diminished pulmonary compliance (determined from ventilator), increased arterial-alveolar gradient, clear chest x-ray, and increasing difficulty maintaining oxygenation
    - Supportive management includes positive end expiratory pressure, minimization of wedge pressure with diuretics, and nutritional support

Infection
- Incisional
  - Leg
    - 1% of patients
    - More common in obese women
  - Sternal/mediastinitis
    - 2% of patients
    - Diabetics with bilateral IMA grafts at greatest risk
- Infective endocarditis
  - Perioperative antibiotic prophylaxis beneficial
  - CABG does not increase infection risk of abnormal native valves
  - Prosthetic valve endocarditis rare, but serious

Neurologic
- Altered mental status
  - Approximately 30% of patients
  - Some patients note mild long-term cognitive disorders (may be decreased with off pump CABG)
- Major cerebrovascular accident: 1%–2%
- Brachial plexopathy, ulnar nerve dysfunction
  - Usually temporary
  - May require up to 6 months for recovery

Hematologic
- Blood loss anemia
  - Transfuse as needed to keep HCT > 30 (no evidence that lowering Hgb threshold worsens outcomes)
- Monitor for heparin induced thrombocytopenia

Anticoagulation: Prosthetic Valves
- Risk considerations for thromboembolism
  - Type of valve (greater risk with mechanical than bioprosthetic)
  - Valve location (greater risk with mitral than aortic)
  - Presence of atrial fibrillation
  - Left atrial size
  - History of thromboembolism
  - Presence of intracardiac thrombi
- Goal INR 2.5–3.5

MEDICATION (DRUGS)

- Reinstitute medications for comorbid diseases
- Aspirin, lipid-lowering agents for CABG patients
- Infective endocarditis prophylaxis with valve disease
- β-Blockers for atrial fibrillation prophylaxis
- Amiodarone may be of benefit in select populations
- Diltiazem for 1 month if radial artery graft used to prevent spasm
- Diuretics transiently if volume overloaded
- DVT prophylaxis
- Insulin infusion if hyperglycemic

SURGERY

Reexploration may be necessary with persistent, uncontrolled bleeding; suspected tamponade is secondary to thrombus formation.

FOLLOW-UP

DISPOSITION

Discharge Criteria
Hemodynamically stable, normal sinus rhythm or rate-controlled atrial fibrillation, able to ambulate and eat, adequate family support to provide basic needs

PROGNOSIS
6 weeks to several months required to regain or improve exercise tolerance if postoperative course uncomplicated. No driving and no lifting above 20 pounds are allowed for 4–6 weeks after sternotomy.

PATIENT MONITORING
First few weeks to months after discharge, physicians include cardiac surgeon, cardiologist, and primary care provider. Patients are monitored for:
- Emotional/mental well being, attitude
- Healing at sternal, extremity wound sites
- Activity level/physical reconditioning
- Return of CBC indices to baseline

REFERENCES
1. Antman E. Medical management of the patient undergoing cardiac surgery. In: Braunwald E, ed. *Heart disease: A textbook of cardiovascular medicine*, 7th ed. Philadelphia: WB Saunders, 2005;1993–2020.
2. Higgins TL, Estafanous FG, Loop FD, et al. Stratification of morbidity and mortality outcome by preoperative risk factors in coronary artery bypass patients. *JAMA*. 1992;267:2344–2348.
3. Reich DL, Mittnacht A, Kaplan JA. Anesthesia and the Management of patients with Cardiac Disease. In: Alexander RW, Schlant RC, Fuster V, eds. *Hurst's the heart*, 11th ed. New York: McGraw-Hill, 2004; 2051–2062.
4. Morris DC, St. Claire D Jr. Management of patients after cardiac surgery. *Curr Probl Cardiol* 1999;24: 161–228.
5. Morris DC, Clements SD, Bailey JM. Management of the patient after cardiac surgery. In: Alexander RW, Schlant RC, Fuster V. eds. *Hurst's the heart*, 11th ed. New York: McGraw-Hill, 2004;1509–1516.

PATIENT TEACHING
- Modify cardiac risk factors.
- Proper diet, types of activity, coping with stress
- Educate regarding anticoagulation as appropriate.

C

CARDIAC SURGERY, PREOPERATIVE ASSESSMENT

Patrick Whalen
Richard Chen*
Jerre Lutz*
Nanette K. Wenger

 BASICS

DESCRIPTION
Evaluation before coronary artery bypass graft (CABG) surgery, valve repair or replacement, repair of congenital heart disease, or other procedures, including surgical procedures on or off cardiopulmonary bypass, minimally invasive or robotic approach, or classic median sternotomy.

EPIDEMIOLOGY
515,000 cardiac surgical procedures in the United States in 2001 (373,000 men, 142,000 women). According to the American Heart Association 95,000 patients underwent valve surgery.

RISK FACTORS
Clinical severity score based on 13 clinical variables can help predict mortality risk: Low-risk score <3; high risk score ≥6.

Emergency surgery	6
Serum creatinine 1.6–1.8	1
≥1.9	4
Severe LV dysfunction (LVEF <35%)	3
Reoperation	3
Mitral regurgitation	3
Age 65–74 years	1
≥75	2
Prior vascular surgery	2
COPD	2
Anemia (Hct <35)	2
Aortic stenosis	1
Weight ≤65 kg	1
Diabetes not diet controlled	1
Cerebrovascular disease	1

LV, left ventricular; LVEF, left ventricular ejection fraction; COPD, chronic obstructive pulmonary disease; Hct, hematocrit.
Adapted from Higgins, et al. Stratification of morbidity and mortality outcome by preoperative risk factors in coronary artery bypass patients. *JAMA*. 1992;267:2344–2348.

ETIOLOGY
Pending underlying illness

ASSOCIATED CONDITIONS
Potentially increase morbidity/mortality (see chart in preceding text)

 DIAGNOSIS

SIGNS AND SYMPTOMS
History
Pertinent findings include:

Underlying pulmonary disease, dysrhythmias, renal insufficiency, liver dysfunction, peripheral vascular disease, previous cerebrovascular accident/baseline neurologic deficits, poor nutritional status, underlying infection, anemia/bleeding, poor family support

Physical Exam
Pertinent findings:
- Dental caries, active upper respiratory tract infection (increase risk of endocarditis)
- Prior radical mastectomy contraindicates use of internal mammary artery (compromised thoracic blood supply).
- Aortic regurgitation worsens with cardiopulmonary bypass due to aortic jet.
- Intraaortic balloon pump contraindicated with significant abdominal aortic aneurysm. Use is complicated by arterial insufficiency.
- Lower extremity venous varicosities may necessitate use of arm veins or only arterial conduits for bypass. No intravenous lines in veins to be harvested.
- Tinea pedis increases risk local cellulitis.
- Carotid bruits increase risk of perioperative cerebrovascular accident. Stenoses >75% diameter narrowed require staged or combined procedure.
- Baseline neurologic deficits may worsen postoperatively.

TESTS
- Carotid Doppler for carotid bruits or diffuse atherosclerosis
- Intraoperative transesophageal echocardiogram used to safely cannulate aorta with aortic atherosclerotic disease
- Pulmonary function testing if clinically indicated

Lab
- Routine complete blood count, platelet count, prothrombin time/partial thromboplastin time, blood urea nitrogen, creatinine, potassium, magnesium, calcium, albumin, liver function tests, stool for occult blood, and urinalysis
- Thyroid function tests if clinically indicated

Imaging
Pertinent data from cardiac catheterization and echocardiography include:
- Elevated left ventricular end-diastolic pressure
  - May remain elevated postoperatively
  - Requires adequate preload postoperatively
- Elevated right atrial pressure
  - May reflect tricuspid valve disease or right ventricular dysfunction
  - May require aggressive volume expansion postoperatively
- Elevated pulmonary artery diastolic pressure greater than pulmonary capillary wedge pressure
  - Suspect fixed pulmonary vascular resistance
  - May require vigorous oxygenation and pulmonary vasodilator therapy
- Ventricular systolic dysfunction
  - Right ventricle: Digoxin; perioperative supplemental oxygen to decrease pulmonary vascular resistance
  - Left ventricle: Digoxin; afterload reduction with angiotensin-converting enzyme (ACE) inhibitors/angiotensin receptor blockers (ARBs) aldo receptor blockade
- Mitral regurgitation: Afterload reduction with ACE inhibitors or intravenous Nipride to maintain systolic pressure of 90–100 mmHg (possible contraindications to Nipride include severe aortic stenosis, significant cerebral or renal vascular disease). Left ventricular failure may occur postoperatively because left ventricle is conditioned to a low afterload state preoperatively.

DIFFERENTIAL DIAGNOSIS
None; diagnosis established prior to surgery

TREATMENT

GENERAL MEASURES

Dysrhythmia Prophylaxis
Correct electrolyte abnormalities (potassium 4.0–5.0 mEq/L and magnesium ≥2.0 mEq/L).
- Supraventricular tachyarrhythmias
- β-Blocker prophylaxis recommended by some in absence of severe bronchospastic pulmonary disease, bradyarrhythmias
- Atrial fibrillation (A-fib)
- In normal sinus rhythm before surgery, continue antiarrhythmics until surgery.
  – A-fib, controlled ventricular response: Hold anticoagulation and continue other medications until surgery.
  – A-fib, uncontrolled rate: Control with β-blockers or digoxin prior to surgery.

Ventricular Tachyarrhythmias
- Continue previous antiarrhythmics until surgery.
- Chronic amiodarone with lung disease: Consider discontinuation drug 3 months preoperatively if no life-threatening rhythm.

- Automatic implantable cardioverter–defibrillators: Disable unit prior to surgery to minimize unnecessary shocks.

Bradyarrhythmias
- High-grade atrioventricular block (third-degree or type II second-degree): Temporary transvenous pacer
- Permanent pacemaker

Document specifications, pacemaker dependency (magnet mode intraoperatively Removal of Telectronics AccuFIX atrial J lead at atriotomy recommended due to history of retention wire fracture, protrusion)

Tricuspid valve replacement with mechanical prosthesis: Lead may be placed at the time of surgery (epicardial or endocardial) or in the coronary sinus at a later date.

  – Intraoperatively: Transvenous pacer wires contraindicated through tricuspid prosthesis

FOLLOW-UP

PROGNOSIS

Operative mortality rates: Isolated CABG 1–2%, isolated aortic valve replacement 2%, isolated mitral valve replacement 6%

PATIENT MONITORING

Not indicated preoperatively unless unstable

REFERENCES

1. Antman E. Medical management of the patient undergoing cardiac surgery. In: Braunwald E, ed. *Heart Disease: A Textbook of Cardiovascular Medicine,* 7th ed. Philadelphia: WB Saunders, 1997–2005;1993–2020.
2. Reich DL, Mittnacht A, Kaplan JA, et al. Anesthesia and the Management of patients with cardiac disease. In: Fuster V, Alexander RW, ORourke RA, eds. *Hurst's the Heart,* 11th ed. New York: McGraw-Hill, 2004;2051–2062.
3. Higgins TL, Estafanous FG, Loop FD, et al. Stratification of morbidity and mortality outcome by preoperative risk factors in coronary artery bypass patients. *JAMA.* 1992;267:2344–2348.
4. Morris DC, St. Claire D Jr. Management of patients after cardiac surgery. *Curr Prob Cardiol.* 1999;24:161–228.

CODES

ICD9-CM
- 414.0 Coronary artery disease
- 424.1 Aortic valve disease
- 394.9 Mitral valve disease, etc.

CARDIAC TRAUMA
Duy Nguyen

 BASICS

DESCRIPTION
Cardiac trauma is direct injury to the heart as the result of a violent injury. Injury can be classified as penetrating or nonpenetrating. This discussion will be limited to nonpenetrating injury.
- Nonpenetrating injury may involve:
  - Contusion of myocardium
  - Laceration of any cardiac structure
  - Septal perforation
  - Pericarditis
  - Postpericardiotomy syndrome
  - Constrictive pericarditis
  - Pericardial laceration
  - Hemorrhage with tamponade
  - Cardiac herniation
  - Rupture of a papillary muscle
  - Rupture of chordae tendineae
  - Rupture of atrioventricular and semilunar valves
  - Coronary artery thrombosis
  - Great vessel injury
  - Electrical/rhythm disturbances
  - Commotio cordis

Pregnancy Considerations
- May be injurious to the fetus if cardiac function is significantly compromised
- Cardiac surgery often results in fetal loss.

EPIDEMIOLOGY
- In persons younger than the age of 40, violent or traumatic injury accounts for majority of deaths in the United States.
- Injury is frequently secondary to a motor vehicle accident, work related (e.g., using heavy machinery), or as a result of acts of violence.
- Among these victims, cardiac trauma accounts for 30–50% of 150,000 total annual deaths from trauma.
- Young adult males are the most common sufferers of cardiac trauma because they are most likely to be involved in acts of violence.
- Predominant Age: Young more affected than elderly
- Predominant Sex: Men affected more than women

Pediatric Considerations
Unusual

ETIOLOGY
Mechanism of Injury
- Direct force against the chest, either unidirectional or multidirectional, compresses the heart between the sternum and spine.
- Indirect forces produce increased intravascular hydrostatic pressure and predispose to rupture of fluid-filled cavities.
- Deceleration forces, blast forces, and fractures of the ribs or sternum may lead to cardiac trauma.
- Commotio cordis refers to a fatal cardiac arrest without detectable structural cardiac damage as a result of blunt thoracic trauma. Ventricular fibrillation, among other mechanisms, has been postulated as the etiology.

ASSOCIATED CONDITIONS
Trauma to other parts of the body often influences surgical decisions and prognosis.

 DIAGNOSIS

SIGNS AND SYMPTOMS
- Presentation can range from asymptomatic to cardiogenic shock with rapid progression to death.
- Chest pain that is often similar to that of acute coronary syndromes, frequently precordial, may have a pleuritic component.
- Pain may be difficult to assess secondary to simultaneous musculoskeletal trauma, such as rib fractures.
- Congestive heart failure, which may manifest acutely or over several days

History
- Recent blunt trauma to the chest wall, including vehicular impact, either directly or indirectly
- Direct blows to the chest wall, direct cardiac compression (e.g., during cardiopulmonary resuscitation, kicks from animals, falls)
- The injury pattern in a motor vehicle accident is dependent on the location of the victim in the automobile, the use of seatbelts, and deployment of airbags.
- The use of airbags may be associated with rupture of the right atrium.

Physical Exam
- Hypovolemia, which may present as hypotension and tachycardia
- Pericardial involvement: Hypotension, oliguria, anuria, distant heart sounds, elevated jugular venous pressure, pulsus paradoxus, pericardial friction rub, narrow pulse pressure
- Myocardial contusion: Chest wall tenderness or traumatic lesions
- Other: Holosystolic murmur, which may represent mitral regurgitation or ventricular septal defect, third heart sound (S3), rales
- Electrocardiogram (ECG) with nonspecific ST-T wave changes or classic findings of pericarditis; ST elevation in coronary thrombosis; pathologic Q waves may represent deep myocardial injury, conduction disorders, arrhythmias
- Chest X-ray: May show an enlarged cardiac silhouette with pericardial effusion; evidence of congestive heart failure, pericardial tears with visceral herniation; may reveal air bubbles in the pericardium

TESTS
Lab
- Serum enzymes: Creatinine kinase (CK) and CK-MB fraction are elevated in patients with blunt cardiac trauma, but this is often related to skeletal muscle damage.
- Troponin I and T are more specific cardiac markers and may increase the sensitivity in detecting myocardial damage.
- Serial cardiac markers with CK-MB fraction should be routinely drawn in patients admitted to the hospital with cardiac contusion or trauma.

Imaging
- Radionuclide imaging: Technetium pyrophosphate scan can label infarcted myocardium and can be useful in the diagnosis of myocardial necrosis.
  - Not sufficiently sensitive to identify nontransmural and right ventricular damage

- Gated biventricular radionuclide scans can be done at the bedside and can accurately assess wall motion.
  - Thallium with single-photon computed tomography (CT) has been used for the diagnosis of myocardial damage but does not adequately assess the right ventricle.
- Echocardiography can identify contused myocardium by the appearance of increased echogenicity, wall motion abnormality, myocardial edema, and impaired systolic function.
  - The most common echocardiographic finding in cardiac contusion is right ventricular wall motion abnormality with some dilation.
  - Presence of wall motion abnormality does not signify a worse outcome if the patient has a normal ECG and cardiac markers.
  - A transesophageal echocardiogram is the modality of choice if visualization of the great vessels is necessary, if patients have painful chest wall injuries, or if surface transthoracic echocardiogram (TTE) is suboptimal.
  - ECG can also be useful in identifying pericardial effusions in patients with pericarditis, postpericardiotomy syndrome, and pericardial tamponade.
- Angiography can be considered if the patient has evidence of coronary artery involvement or thrombosis.
  - It is useful in defining left ventricular function and coronary artery anatomy.

Diagnostic Procedures/Surgery
- Subxiphoid pericardial window, pericardiocentesis may be required to treat tamponade.
- Finding a bloody effusion may confirm the diagnosis of traumatic cardiac/great vessel rupture.

Pathologic Findings
- Anatomic considerations
  - Anterior right ventricular wall is most commonly involved, followed by the anterior interventricular septum and anterior apical left ventricle.
  - May also involve the conduction system, resulting in bundle branch block

DIFFERENTIAL DIAGNOSIS
Differential includes acute coronary syndromes, chest wall trauma, musculoskeletal pain, pericarditis, aortic injury, and congestive heart failure.

TREATMENT

GENERAL MEASURES
- Patients with suspected cardiac trauma are usually admitted to a monitored bed or intensive care unit (ICU) if at high risk for hemodynamic instability.
- Any patient with hemodynamic instability should undergo emergent thoracotomy.
- On arrival, if hemodynamically stable, the patient should give a complete history and undergo a detailed physical examination, ECG, and chest X-ray.
- If no abnormalities are detected and patient is mildly injured or asymptomatic, the patient can be observed in the emergency room for 12 hours and then discharged if the observation period is uneventful and patient has a normal follow up ECG.

- If the ECG reveals nonspecific ST-T wave changes, the patient should be observed for 24 hours and be assessed for serial cardiac markers.
- If ECG reveals specific abnormalities, if patient clinically deteriorates, or if there is a discrepancy between clinical status and clinical data, proceed to TTE or transesophageal echocardiography (TEE).
- Depending on the findings, patients should be monitored or have an urgent thoracotomy.
- If the chest X-ray is abnormal, an echocardiogram should be performed.
- If other emergent surgery is indicated requiring general anesthesia, preoperative cardiac assessment including echocardiography should be performed.
- Intraoperative hemodynamic monitoring is prudent. Patients with marked cardiac risk or known coronary/cardiac disease should be monitored closely.

MEDICATION (DRUGS)

- Cardiac contusion
  - Chest pain is best treated with analgesics; nonsteroidal antiinflammatory drugs (NSAIDs) are not advised because they interfere with myocardial healing and may contribute to increased bleeding.
- Pericardial effusion/postpericardiotomy syndrome
  - Pericarditis generally resolves spontaneously.
  - Recurrent effusions with associated fever and chest pain are classified as the postpericardiotomy syndrome.
  - Usually respond to aspirin or NSAIDs, but steroids are occasionally necessary. Colchicine may be an alternative.
    - Treatment with anticoagulants and thrombolytics is generally contraindicated because it can predispose to bleeding and myocardial rupture.

SURGERY

- Patients with rupture of the cardiac chamber, interventricular septum, or interatrial septum require emergent surgery.
- Myocardial rupture results in sudden death in most patients: atria involved > ventricles, right-side chambers involved > left-sided chambers.
- Intracardiac fistulas include ventriculoseptal defects (VSDs), atrial septal defects, and atrioventricular fistulas. Patients with VSDs occasionally present late with heart failure and a holosystolic murmur.
  - A small defect can be treated conservatively with supportive measures and subsequent repair if necessary.
- With myocardial rupture, there are often concurrent pericardial tears.
  - Tears most often occur on the left.
  - Tears also may involve the diaphragmatic pericardium, anterior pericardium, or left pleuropericardium.
  - Any of these sites will predispose the patient to cardiac herniation and strangulation.

FOLLOW-UP

DISPOSITION

Triage depends on acuity of trauma and suspicion for hemodynamic compromise secondary to cardiac trauma.

Admission Criteria

Patients with suspected cardiac trauma are usually admitted to a monitored bed or ICU if at high risk for hemodynamic instability. If the ECG reveals nonspecific ST-T wave changes, the patient should be observed for 24 hours and assessed for serial cardiac markers.

Discharge Criteria

If no abnormalities are detected and patient is mildly injured or asymptomatic, the patient can be observed in the emergency room for 12 hours and then discharged if the observation period is uneventful and patient has a normal follow-up ECG.

Issues for Referral

- Any patient with hemodynamic instability should be referred for emergent thoracotomy.
- Referral to cardiac rehabilitation is often useful, especially in the elderly population and those patients with other comorbidities.

PROGNOSIS

- Young patients who sustain myocardial contusion have an excellent prognosis.
- Although there are similarities between cardiac necrosis caused by trauma and that caused by coronary artery disease, the pathophysiology is different.
- Patients with coronary artery disease generally have other comorbidities and are much older. Both of these considerations markedly influence outcomes.

COMPLICATIONS

Late complications such as arrhythmia, heart failure, aneurysm, valvular regurgitation, pericardial constriction or tamponade, late VSD, or free wall rupture have been reported but are rare.

PATIENT MONITORING

- If patients are evaluated and discharged, they should have follow-up within a week.
- Those admitted should have follow-up geared to the severity of their injuries.

REFERENCES

1. Mattox K. 5760 cardiovascular injuries in 4459 patients: Epidemiologic evolution 1958 to 1987. *Ann Surg.* 1989;209:698.
2. Sybrandy KC, et al. Diagnosing cardiac contusion: Old wisdom and new insights. *Heart.* 2003;89: 485.

CODES
ICD9-CM
- 861.01 Contusion
- 861.02 Laceration
- 861.03 Rupture
- 860.2 Hemopericardium

PATIENT TEACHING

- Young patients with minor blunt trauma/myocardial contusion should be treated similarly to those with myocardial infarction with a similar amount of myocardium at risk.
- Patients with severe injury requiring surgery should undergo a recovery similar to that of a postoperative coronary bypass patient.
- Cardiac rehabilitation is often useful, especially in the elderly population and those patients with other comorbidities.

Activity

Bed rest until diagnosis and necessary surgery completed

Prevention

Practical measures include protection during contact sports, seatbelts while driving, and enforcing safety regulations in high-risk occupations.

FAQ

- When should an echocardiogram be obtained when a patient has sustained a chest-wall trauma? An echocardiogram should be obtained if there is hemodynamic compromise thought to be cardiac in origin, if the ECG reveals specific abnormalities, if the patient deteriorates clinically, or if there is a discrepancy between clinical status and clinical data.
- When should surgical consultation be obtained? Surgery consultation should be obtained when there is hemodynamic compromise or when the ECG reveals new structural cardiac abnormalities such as intracardiac fistulas or pericardial tears.

C

CARDIAC NEOPLASMS

Christopher K. Dyke

 BASICS

DESCRIPTION

Tumors and cysts of the heart or pericardium are relatively rare but have been detected more frequently since the introduction of echocardiography.

- Cardiac tumors secondary to metastatic disease are 16–40 times more common than primary cardiac tumors. However, identification of primary cardiac tumors is important because resection is likely to result in a cure.
- In contrast, resection of metastatic cardiac tumors is palliative at best.

Metastatic Cardiac Tumors

- 10% of malignant neoplasms metastasize to the heart; 10% of these metastases are clinically evident.
- Epicardium is the most common location.
- Carcinomatous invasion is more common than sarcomatous invasion.
- 85–90% of clinical dysfunction is related to pericardial involvement (effusion, neoplastic thickening).
- Tumors have been reported from every organ and of every tissue type except the central nervous system.
- Lung, breast, leukemia, and lymphoma are the most common metastatic malignancies.
- The highest percentages of cardiac metastases are melanomas (70%), leukemia, and lymphoma.
- Extension is via direct (lung, breast, esophagus), retrograde lymphatic drainage (most carcinomas), venous extension (renal cell, hepatoma), and hematogenous (sarcoma, leukemia, lymphoma, melanoma).

Benign Cardiac Tumors

- Intracavitary neoplasms have the potential of producing a triad of obstruction, embolization, and constitutional symptoms.
- Myxoma most common, distribution as follows: left atrium (75%), right atrium (23%), and ventricular (2%)
- Rhabdomyoma most common in infants and children and usually multiple, ventricular, pedunculated masses
- Fibromas are most common in children; these are usually solitary and located in the intramural ventricular septum, and calcific deposits can be seen. Sudden death occurs in up to 1/3 due to conduction abnormalities.
- Lipomas may be extremely small or massive, may be located on valves, and sometimes are mistaken for pericardial cysts.
- Hemangiomas give tumor blush on angiography and may resolve spontaneously.

Malignant Cardiac Tumors

- Primary malignant cardiac neoplasms are almost always sarcomas.
- Local relapse in PCS (primary cardiac sarcoma) is relatively rare, and most patients die because of metastatic recurrence.

- Most frequent is angiosarcoma, which usually originates from right atrium and forms large quantity of vascular channels. Metastases occur in 66–89% of cases, most commonly to the lung.
- Rhabdomyosarcoma is the second most common primary malignancy and has no chamber predilection.
- Infrequent: Fibrosarcoma, liposarcoma, and primary malignant lymphoma

Carcinoid Heart Disease

- Never primary and rarely metastasize, but distinctive lesions often seen in the right heart
- Fibrous tissue deposits lacking elastic fibers seen on the ventricular aspect of the tricuspid valve leaflets and on the arterial aspect of the pulmonic valve leaflets, and to a lesser extent on the ventricular aspects of the mitral valve
- The development of carcinoid heart disease is not related to duration of carcinoid symptoms.
- Only condition to uniformly involve both tricuspid and pulmonic valve, most commonly tricuspid regurgitation and pulmonic stenosis

EPIDEMIOLOGY

Metastatic cardiac tumors are 16–40 times more common than primary tumors.
Primary tumors of heart and pericardium have an incidence of 0.0001–0.28% in autopsy series.
In adults, almost half of all benign tumors are myxomas.

In infants and children, the most common cardiac tumor is the rhabdomyoma. Angiosarcoma and rhabdomyosarcoma are more frequent in men. Malignant tumors are rare in the pediatric age group, comprising less than 10% of all cardiac and pericardial neoplasms.

Incidence

The peak incidence for myxomas is in the sixth decade of life, and women account for 70% of cases. Malignant primary tumors comprise 25% and consist of angiosarcomas (33%), rhabdomyosarcomas (20%), mesotheliomas (15%), and fibrosarcomas (10%).

RISK FACTORS

- 10% of cardiac myxomas are familial (autosomal dominant) and are more likely to be multiple and located in the ventricular cavity.
- Carcinoid heart disease results from hepatic metastases from ileal, bronchial, or ovarian carcinoid.

ASSOCIATED CONDITIONS

- Familial myxomas associated with NAME (nevi, atrial myxoma, myxoid neurofibroma, and ephelides) and LAMB (lentigines, atrial myxoma, and ephelides) syndromes
- Rhabdomyoma associated with tuberous sclerosis in 1/3 of patients
- Fibromas may be associated with Gorlin syndrome (basal cell nevus syndrome).
- Patients with cardiac hemangiomas also may have skin hemangiomas.

 DIAGNOSIS

SIGNS AND SYMPTOMS

- All cardiac tumors can simulate more common types of cardiac disease.
- The various signs and symptoms relate to tumor location.
- Pericardial involvement is most common with metastatic disease, often presenting with signs and symptoms of tamponade.
- Intramyocardial neoplasms are often silent unless conduction disturbances present.
- Left atrial masses often mimic mitral stenosis, including dyspnea, orthopnea, PND (paroxysmal nocturnal dyspnea), pulmonary edema, and hemoptysis.
- Right atrial or ventricular masses may produce right-sided congestive heart failure signs and symptoms, including peripheral edema, ascites, hepatomegaly, and prominent jugular venous *a* waves.
- A protodiastolic tumor plop murmur may result from right atrial tumors.
- Left ventricular masses frequently occur at the apex and are often clinically silent, but if large enough, can cause systolic murmur, chest pain, syncope, or heart failure.
- Myxomatous constitutional symptoms include fever, weight loss, Raynaud syndrome, digital clubbing, and anemia.
- Rhabdomyomas may mimic pulmonic valve stenosis or present with ventricular obstruction, arrhythmias [including ventricular tachycardia (VT)], atrioventricular (AV) block, pericardial effusion, and sudden death.
- Angiosarcoma may produce a continuous precordial murmur due to vascular channels.

TESTS

- Pericardiocentesis may provide a definitive cytologic analysis in addition to symptomatic relief of tamponade.
- Only in rare cases may an endomyocardial biopsy contribute to the diagnosis.

Lab

Elevated erythrocyte sedimentation rate, elevated white blood cell count, thrombocytopenia, and increased gamma globulins can be seen with myxomas.

Imaging

- Chest radiography is occasionally helpful (mostly for epicardial neoplasms, detection of calcified masses, or complications due to obstructive masses (i.e., pulmonary edema).
- Electrocardiography most common initial diagnostic modality
- TEE (transesophageal echocardiography) more sensitive than TTE (transthoracic echocardiography) and better approximates size, shape, and location as well as stalk attachment for intracardiac masses as well as mediastinal or extracardiac structures.

- Echocardiography is very useful in serial monitoring.
- Computed tomography (CT) is useful for diagnosis and often helpful in defining intramyocardial extension, but magnetic resonance imaging (MRI) provides clearer definition of tumor characteristics.
- Selective angiography techniques have been largely supplanted by noninvasive imaging, but can be useful in detecting intracavitary filling defects as well as in defining the vascular supply of the neoplasm.

Pathologic Findings
- Carcinomatous metastases are usually visible on gross inspection, appearing as multiple small, discrete, firm nodules.
- Sarcomatous metastases are characterized by diffuse infiltration.
- Myxoma cell origin is unclear in endothelial-like cells that are elongated and spindle shaped with round nuclei and prominent nucleoli. Attachment usually atrial septum with stalk smaller than mass diameter. Microscopically, the myxoid matrix is composed of mucopolysaccharide.
- Rhabdomyomas are white to yellow–tan; microscopically they are circumscribed but not encapsulated and contain abundant glycogen.
- Calcific deposits are often seen in fibromas.
- Intramyocardial lipomas are encapsulated and usually small.
- Carcinoid tumors contain fibroblasts, myofibroblasts, and smooth muscle cells in collagen, not elastin.

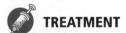 ## TREATMENT

GENERAL MEASURES
- Excision should be made early in primary tumors to prevent complications such as embolization or metastases.
- Treatment of secondary neoplasms is generally directed at underlying malignancy but may require surgical intervention if symptomatic.

 ## MEDICATION (DRUGS)

- The role of adjuvant treatment in resected primary neoplasms (sarcomas) is controversial. In several series, the use of postoperative chemotherapy did not appear to improve survival, but isolated reports show prolonged survival after resection followed by adjuvant chemotherapy and radiation.
- Adjuvant chemotherapy seems advisable in a subset of patients with high mitotic rate tumors and adjuvant radiation with high-grade tumors at risk for metastases.

SURGERY
- Pericardial tumor operative measures include biopsy, drainage, window, or resection.
- Intrapericardial tumors can sometimes be resected without cardiopulmonary bypass.
- Primary therapy for atrial myxoma, rhabdomyoma, fibroma, and lipoma is surgical resection.
- Partial excision should be considered only when it compromises valvular structure, coronary arteries, or the conduction system.
- Surgeon should be very careful regarding potential embolization.
- Total excision of hemangioma is usually not possible.
- Surgery for angiosarcoma and rhabdomyosarcoma is usually futile. After surgical excision, local relapse is relatively rare, but prognosis is poor due to metastatic disease.
- Right-sided valvular excision or replacement or valve commissurotomy or annuloplasty has been performed in some patients with carcinoid heart disease.

 ## FOLLOW-UP

PROGNOSIS
- Recurrences of atrial myxomas are rare, but if they occur, it is usually within a 4-year period
- Angiosarcoma and rhabdomyosarcoma carry extremely poor prognoses because their clinical course is rapid with diffuse metastases. Median survival ranges from 5–11 months in the different series.
- Patients with carcinoid heart disease have a similar lifespan following diagnosis compared with patients with metastatic carcinoid without myocardial involvement.

PATIENT MONITORING
Noninvasive imaging is used to perform serial monitoring to determine size progression or detect recurrence following excision, most often with echocardiography.

REFERENCES
1. Ceresoli G, Passoni P, Benussi S, et al. Primary cardiac sarcoma in pregnancy: A case report and review of the literature. *Am J Clin Oncol*. 1999;22:460–465.
2. Majano-Lainez RA. Cardiac tumors: A current clinical and pathological perspective. *Crit Rev Oncog*. 1997;8:293–303.
3. McAllister HA Jr, Hall RJ, Cooley DA. Tumors of the heart and pericardium. *Curr Prob Cardiol*. 1999;24:57–116.
4. Topol EJ. *Cardiovascular Medicine*. Philadelphia: Lippincott Williams & Wilkins,1998;912–915.

CODES
ICD9-CM
Primary Neoplasms
- 215.9 Neoplasm, connective tissue, benign (myxoma, fibroma, lipoma, rhabdomyoma)
- 228.09 Heart hemangioma
- 171.9 Neoplasm, connective tissue, malignant, primary (angiosarcoma, rhabdomyosarcoma, others)
Secondary Neoplasms
- Refer to ICD for specific primary neoplasm.

CARDIAC TRANSPLANTATION, PEDIATRIC

Linda J. Addonizio
Welton M. Gersony

 BASICS

DESCRIPTION
Cardiac transplantation has become a common and rapidly expanding surgical option for children with end-stage heart disease.

GENERAL PREVENTION
Transplantation is a therapy of last resort when heart disease has become refractory to maximal medical therapy, and when no other surgical procedure can reasonably restore a productive life.

EPIDEMIOLOGY
- Children comprise 12% of total cardiac transplantations performed annually.
- By January 2005, the International Society for Heart and Lung Transplantation (ISHLT) Registry had recorded more than 6,000 heart transplantations in children between birth and 18 years (average 350 children yearly).
- More than 1/2 of children receiving transplants in the past 10 years were younger than 5 years of age.

ETIOLOGY
The 2 main indications for transplantation in pediatrics are cardiomyopathies and complex congenital heart disease (CHD).
- The predominant indication varies by age.
  - In infants undergoing transplantation at <1 year of age, 65% have CHD.
  - In the transition age (1–10 years), 37% of recipients have CHD and 52% myopathies.
  - Cardiomyopathy is the indication for transplantation in 62% of adolescent recipients.
- Cardiomyopathies (in decreasing order of frequency)
  - Dilated: Idiopathic, Adriamycin, familial, postmyocarditis
  - Hypertrophic
  - Restrictive
- CHD: 10–20% of children with CHD might eventually benefit from transplantation in their lifetime; 2% of adult transplantations are now for CHD.
  - Primary operation: For example, hypoplastic left heart syndrome, pulmonary atresia with intact septum and coronary sinusoids, and complex inoperable heterotaxy
  - Previous biventricular repairs: Poor function and/or valvar regurgitation when further repair too risky

- Palliated single ventricle: Failed Fontan procedure or if palliation untenable; patients with failed Fontan physiology constitute a significantly expanding pretransplantation population
- Death while waiting for transplantation still approximates 30% in children, secondary to lack of donors.

ASSOCIATED CONDITIONS
Orthotopic cardiac transplantation is contraindicated in the presence of:
- Inadequate pulmonary arteries
- Degenerative neurologic disease
- Pulmonary hypertension with pulmonary vascular resistance index >6 despite maximal therapy
- HIV infection
- End-stage renal, hepatic, or pulmonary disease, unless listed for the concomitant failed organ

DIAGNOSIS

SIGNS AND SYMPTOMS
- Rejection: Usually no significant cardiovascular symptoms, unless severe, presenting as heart failure and/or shock. Mild to moderate rejection may be accompanied by:
  - Tachycardia or arrhythmia
  - Gallop rhythm
  - Enlarged tender liver
  - Pericardial effusion
  - Fever
  - Malaise in older children, irritability in infants
  - Abdominal complaints resembling gastroenteritis or "flu"
- Graft vasculopathy: Usually presenting late, may occur within first year; a form of chronic rejection; symptoms depend upon severity and distribution of coronary obliteration; patients will not experience angina; common signs are:
  - Congestive heart failure (CHF) in absence of rejection
  - CHF persisting following adequate rejection treatment
  - Arrhythmia: Atrial, ventricular, or progressive heart block
  - Syncope
  - Sudden death

History
- Have immunosuppressants been weaned prior to symptoms?
- Elicit history of noncompliance with immunosuppressant medications.
- Has patient been vomiting medications routinely?
- History of multiple rejection episodes or refractory rejection.

Physical Exam
Varies according to severity of cardiac compromise but may include:
- Third heart sound (S_3) gallop rhythm
- Tachycardia
- Soft heart tones
- Rales
- Enlarged liver
- Poor perfusion and peripheral pulses

TESTS
- Electrocardiogram (ECG): Usually ECG shows sinus rhythm and residual nonconducted, native P waves from recipient sinus node; findings indicative of rejection or coronary disease may or may not be present, including:
  - Tachycardia
  - Atrial or ventricular arrhythmias or progressive heart block
  - Low voltage
  - New Q waves or ST-segment changes
- Endomyocardial biopsy: Right heart catheterization with endomyocardial biopsy is used by many centers on a routine decremental schedule postoperatively to evaluate for acute rejection.
  - Abnormal hemodynamics may be first indication of rejection or coronary disease.
  - Tissue diagnosis of rejection, however, often seen with normal hemodynamics.

Lab
Common laboratory tests include monitoring of immunosuppressant levels, and potential toxic effects on bone marrow, kidney, and liver.

Imaging
The cardiac evaluation of recipients may include:
- Chest x-ray: A change in size of the cardiac silhouette may be the first objective evidence of rejection or pericardial effusion, particularly in long-term survivors. Hilar adenopathy can lead to suspicion of posttransplantation lymphoproliferative disease (PTLD).
- 2D echocardiogram: Function is usually normal in transplanted hearts unless rejection or severe coronary disease.
  - Decreased fractional shortening
  - Pericardial effusion
  - New-onset myocardial hypertrophy or diastolic dysfunction
- Coronary angiograms: Serial angiograms are performed annually or biannually to evaluate graft vasculopathy. It is important to compare serial studies.
- Dobutamine stress echocardiogram: This modality is used to help define the presence of subtle graft vasculopathy not seen on angiography and to assess the functional severity of visible coronary disease.

Diagnostic Procedures/Surgery
Serial cardiac catheterizations are required for myocardial biopsy, hemodynamics, and coronary angiography.

Pathologic Findings
- Cellular rejection is graded by presence and density of lymphocytic infiltrate in the myocardium with or without myocyte necrosis. Edema and hemorrhage can also be seen when severe.
- Humoral rejection usually lacks a cellular infiltrate but immunofluorescent antibody staining can be seen in the myocardium, and frequently edema.
- Coronary disease consists of intimal hyperplasia in the vessels of the graft that can become obliterative.

DIFFERENTIAL DIAGNOSIS
The differential of complications in pediatric heart recipients relates to the cumulative side effects of immunosuppression or from ineffective immunosuppressive protection of the graft. Because symptoms are nonspecific, must differentiate between the most common major complications:
- Rejection
- Infection
- Graft vasculopathy
- PTLD
- End-organ toxicity of immunosuppressants

 TREATMENT

GENERAL MEASURES
Medical management of heart recipients involves assessment of health of the graft and complications from immunosuppressant medications.
- Patients should receive endocarditis prophylaxis prior to dental work or invasive procedures that would normally require prophylaxis.
- Care must be taken to avoid undue exposure to infectious diseases because the patient is on lifelong immunosuppression.
- Live viral vaccines are contraindicated.

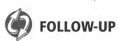 MEDICATION (DRUGS)

Cardiac recipients are on multiple medications.
- Single-, double-, or triple-drug immunosuppression using combinations of:
  - Cyclosporine
  - Tacrolimus (FK506)
  - Azathioprine
  - Prednisone
  - Mycophenolate mofetil
  - Rapamycin
- Antihypertensive therapy (20–65%)
  - Calcium channel blockers
  - Angiotensin-converting enzyme (ACE) inhibitors
  - Angiotensin receptor blockers (ARBs)
  - Possible beneficial effect of these three classes of antihypertensives in preventing graft vasculopathy.
  - β blockers
- Cardiotonic therapy (digoxin, ACE inhibitors, diuretics) may be necessary transiently, at times following transplantation.
  - During recovery from prolonged rejection
  - CHF from coronary disease
  - Perioperative right heart failure
- Lipid-altering drugs (statins) are used by some centers.
  - Treatment of immunosuppressant-induced hyperlipidemia
  - Possible additional immunosuppressant effect, which may retard development of graft vasculopathy or prevent rejection

- 2 classes of drugs should be used with caution in transplant patients. It is vital that patients and their primary care physicians speak with the transplant team prior to use of these medications (includes antibiotics):
  - Any liver-metabolized or long-acting medication can have profound effect on metabolism and levels of immunosuppressant drugs.
  - Drugs cleared by, or affecting, the kidney: Immunosuppressants can potentiate the nephrotoxicity of commonly used medications.

First Line Rejection Treatment
- Steroid boost, either intravenous (IV) or oral (PO) is the first-line treatment of rejection. Other strategies include:
  - Change the main immunosuppressant drug or secondary drugs
  - Add a 3rd or 4th drug

Second-Line Rejection Treatment
- Treatment for steroid-resistant rejection
  - Antilymphocyte globulin, OKT3, daclizumab, methotrexate; total lymphoid irradiation, photopheresis

SURGERY
Posttransplantation surgical intervention would include retransplantation, the only alternative for advanced transplant coronary disease. Indications for retransplantation include:
- Rapidly progressive graft arteriopathy with or without ischemia
- Stable arteriopathy with severe CHF
- Severe acute rejection unresponsive to therapy (outcome poor in this group, considered by most to be a contraindication)

 FOLLOW-UP

DISPOSITION
Transplant recipients must be followed lifelong by transplantation specialists who are familiar with the care and complications seen with this disease.

C

Admission Criteria

Posttransplantation admissions are usually for complications of immunosuppressant medications.

- Inadequate immunosuppression results in rejection or coronary artery disease.
- Overimmunosuppression may occur early postoperatively or following treatment for rejection and can result in admissions for infections or PTLD.

Discharge Criteria

Discharge criteria vary by diagnosis and treatment.

- During the 1st year of follow-up, 51% of pediatric cardiac recipients did not require rehospitalization for illness.
  - Rejection hospitalization: 13%
  - Infection hospitalization: 20%
- During the 4th posttransplantation year, 75% of children did not require hospitalization.
  - Rejection hospitalization: 5%
  - Infection hospitalization: 10%

PROGNOSIS

- The postoperative course in transplant recipients varies with degree of pretransplantation debilitation and morbidity. More stable children recover quickly with the addition of normal heart function.
  - Risk factors for 1-year mortality include diagnosis of CHD, use of extracorporeal membrane oxygenation (ECMO), and being hospitalized, or on a ventilator.
  - Continuous risk factors for 1-year mortality include donor age, weight ratio, serum creatinine, and bilirubin.
- Actuarial survival in children has steadily improved with optimized therapy, making survival for decades likely. The Pediatric Registry of the ISHLT shows excellent survival rates:
  - 86% at 1 year and 80% at 3 years in children who underwent transplantation between 1999 and 2003
  - The conditional survival (survival after the 1st year posttransplantation) is 85% at 5 years and 70% at 10 years for all pediatric recipients since 1982; infants had 80% 10-year survival. The half life is now >14 years for children, and not yet calculable for infants.

- Quality of life in ISHLT Pediatric Registry
  - For pediatric recipients who underwent transplantation between 1994 and 1998, >90% had no activity restrictions at 1 and 3 years of follow-up.
  - Growth spurts were reported in all age groups in the 1st year posttransplantation, with the exception of adolescents.
  - Growth appeared to be sustained in subsequent years in younger age groups.
  - All data show that children have a remarkable ability for rehabilitation to pursue a normal lifestyle following transplantation.

Pregnancy Considerations

Female heart transplant recipients can have successful pregnancies without apparent risk to the newborn from immunosuppressants.

- Hemodynamically the transplanted heart can tolerate pregnancy.
- There is some increased risk for rejection at the time of delivery.

COMPLICATIONS

- End-organ toxicity of immunosuppressants:
  - Cyclosporine can cause systemic hypertension and hyperlipidemia in 20–65% of children.
  - Tacrolimus (FK-506) can also cause hypertension as well as diabetes.
  - With both drugs, renal toxicity is main long-term side effect, occurring in 11% of children at 7 years.
- Causes of death in ISHLT Pediatric Registry:
  - Increased perioperative mortality (25%) in infants transplanted for CHD compared with older children with CHD or other infants with cardiomyopathy (10%).
  - Most common causes of death during the 1st year posttransplantation were acute rejection then infection.
  - Acute then chronic rejection (coronary disease) is the most common cause from 1–3 years posttransplantation.
  - Beyond 3 years posttransplantation, coronary disease is responsible for almost 1/2 of the deaths.
  - Malignancy remains an infrequent cause of death.

- Incidence of coronary disease in ISHLT
- Pediatric registry:
  - 7% at 2 years, 15% incidence within 7 years
  - Rejection episodes in 1st year appear to be an indicator for subsequent events such as coronary disease and late mortality.

PATIENT MONITORING

Close routine outpatient follow-up is necessary at decreasing intervals for optimal survival. Transplant patients require lifelong monitoring of the graft and the chronic effects of the medications.

- Early postoperatively, the patient is seen frequently the first 3 months to adjust medications and monitor for infections, rejections, and rehabilitation.
- Later follow-up visits are centered on weaning immunosuppression to low maintenance levels, preventative care, and monitoring for complications.

REFERENCES

1. Boucek MM, Edwards LB, Keck BM, et al. The Registry of the International Society of Heart and Lung Transplantation: Eighth Official Pediatric Report. *J Heart Lung Transplant*. 2005;24:968–982.
2. Chen JM, Davies RR, Mital SR, et al. Trends and outcomes in transplantation for complex congenital heart disease: 1984–2004. *Ann Thorac Surg*. 2004;78:1352–1361.
3. Harmon WE, McDonald RA, Beyes JD, et al. Pediatric transplantation, 1994–2003. *Am J Transplant*. 2005;5(Part 2):887–903.
4. Lamour JM, Addonizio LJ. Pediatric heart transplantation. In: Edwards N, Chen J, Mazzeo P, eds. *Cardiac Transplantation: The Columbia University Medical Center/ New York-Presbyterian Hospital Manual*. Totowa, NJ: Humana Press, Totowa, 2004.
5. Smith RR, Wray J, Khaghari A, et al. 10 year survival after paediatric heart transplantation: A single centre experience. *Eur J of Cardiothoracic Surg*. 2005;27:790–794.
6. Ross M, Kouretas P, Gamberg P, et al. 10- and 20-year survivors of pediatric orthotopic heart transplantation. *J Heart Lung Transplant*. 2006;25:261–270.
7. Webber SA. The current state of, and future prospects for, cardiac transplantation in children. *Cardiol Young*. 2003;13:64–83.

MISCELLANEOUS

CODES
ICD9-CM
V42.1 Cardiac transplantation

PATIENT TEACHING
- Continuing education about the necessity for strict compliance with immunosuppressant medications is required throughout patients' lives.
  - Significant, chronic noncompliance carries a 60% mortality risk.
  - Adolescent patients have a high incidence of noncompliance.
  - Previous compliance may wane with time from transplantation and age, so continued vigilance is required.
- The family and patient should be educated about signs and symptoms of rejection as well as infection precautions.

Diet
A low-fat healthful diet is recommended.
Activity
There are no activity restrictions for transplant recipients; regular physical activity and exercise is advisable for rehabilitation.
Prevention
- Prevention of many complications can occur with maintenance of a healthy lifestyle and strict adherence to the medical regimen and follow-up care.
- Close collaboration and cooperation between multiple physicians that are caring for a transplant recipient can further minimize posttransplant complications.

FAQ
There are numerous websites and support organizations for transplant recipients:
- The United Network of Organ Sharing, which manages donor allocation in the U.S., has extensive information available on transplantation programs across the United States.
- The ISHLT website provides comprehensive data about the patient registry and heart transplantation issues.
- The Journal of Heart and Lung Transplantation provides extensive information about transplantation research.

C

CARDIOMYOPATHY, DILATED OR CONGESTIVE

Apur R. Kamdar
Deepak L. Bhatt
Gary S. Francis

 BASICS

DESCRIPTION
Dilatation of the ventricles with associated contractile dysfunction due to a variety of causes
When an underlying disorder cannot be identified, dilated cardiomyopathy is referred to as idiopathic, often presumed to be of a viral etiology or on a genetic basis.

EPIDEMIOLOGY
- More common in men, African Americans
- Second most common type of cardiomyopathy after ischemic cardiomyopathy
- Also common etiology of end-stage heart failure leading to eventual cardiac transplantation

Incidence
- Approximately 5/100,000 new cases per year
- The incidence may be increasing.

RISK FACTORS
- Alcohol
- Family history of dilated cardiomyopathy
- Multiparity, advanced maternal age, African American (for peripartum cardiomyopathy)

Pregnancy Considerations
- Peripartum cardiomyopathy is a dilated cardiomyopathy that occurs in the last trimester of pregnancy or in the 6 months following pregnancy.
- Repeat pregnancy is not advised, particularly if left ventricular function has not normalized since the initial pregnancy.
- Women with peripartum cardiomyopathy whose ejection fractions have returned to normal have subsequently had successful pregnancies without development of clinical heart failure.
- Dobutamine echocardiography of women with recovered resting ventricular function often still shows impaired contractile reserve.

ETIOLOGY
- Familial transmission occurs in 30% of cases.
- Usually autosomal dominant, although autosomal-recessive, X-linked recessive, and mitochondrial inheritance patterns have all been identified.
- Muscular dystrophies, such as Duchenne
- Alcohol is another major cause, perhaps accounting for 30% of cases.
- Cocaine
- Infectious etiologies, particularly viral infections, are postulated to cause dilated cardiomyopathy. Coxsackie virus B has been linked with several cases of idiopathic dilated cardiomyopathy. HIV can cause such a cardiomyopathy.
- Peripartum cardiomyopathy occurs in about 1/4,000 births; autoimmune factors may be responsible.
- Uncontrolled tachycardia, such as atrial fibrillation or ventricular tachycardia

- Pheochromocytoma
- Thyroid disease (either hypo- or hyperthyroidism)
- Hemochromatosis and sarcoidosis are infiltrative cardiomyopathies, typically classified as restrictive, although in later stages, both can present as dilated cardiomyopathy.
- Acromegaly
- Chemotherapy with doxorubicin, bleomycin
- Hypertensive, ischemic, and valvular cardiomyopathies may present as dilated cardiomyopathy.
- Nutritional deficiencies (carnitine, selenium, thiamine)

ASSOCIATED CONDITIONS
- Depends on the etiology
- Pulmonary or systemic emboli

 DIAGNOSIS

SIGNS AND SYMPTOMS
- Dyspnea on exertion, at rest
- Paroxysmal nocturnal dyspnea
- Orthopnea
- Cough
- Fatigue
- Chest pain
- Lower extremity edema
- Hepatomegaly, pulsatile liver
- Ascites
- Palpitations
- Pulmonary rales
- S3 (third heart sound)
- S4 (fourth heart sound)
- Apical impulse laterally displaced
- Jugular venous distention
- Murmur of mitral and/or tricuspid regurgitation
- Pulsus alternans

TESTS
- Coronary arteriography
  - Typically would be normal, other than in ischemic cardiomyopathy
  - This test should be performed if there is clinical suspicion of coronary artery disease
- Right heart catheterization
  - In the decompensated patient, reveals a high wedge pressure, an elevated systemic vascular resistance, and a low cardiac output
- Endomyocardial biopsy
  - Formerly a popular procedure for routine diagnosis of dilated cardiomyopathy, but is now discouraged unless a specific etiology is being considered
  - In cases with a high suspicion of giant cell myocarditis, biopsy is generally performed prior to initiation of empiric immunosuppressive therapy.
- Cardiopulmonary exercise stress testing
  - Can objectively assess a patient's functional capacity and can be used to determine the need for heart transplantation

Lab
- Hyponatremia is common in advanced heart failure.
- Thyroid function tests
- Iron, ferritin, and iron saturation levels (for hemochromatosis)
- Urine and serum protein electrophoresis (for amyloidosis)
- Electrocardiogram (ECG) may show sinus tachycardia. Left bundle branch block is not unusual. Ventricular arrhythmias, especially nonsustained ventricular tachycardia, are common.

Imaging
- Chest X-ray reveals cardiomegaly.
  - Pulmonary congestion may be present.
- Echocardiography reveals a dilated left ventricle with global hypokinesis.
  - Segmental wall motion abnormalities can be present and do not necessarily imply the presence of coronary artery disease.
  - Usually all four cardiac chambers are enlarged in systolic heart failure.
  - Mural thrombi may be observed in the ventricles.
  - Atrioventricular regurgitation secondary to annular dilatation is common.

DIFFERENTIAL DIAGNOSIS
Other causes of congestive heart failure

 TREATMENT

GENERAL MEASURES
- Low-salt diet
- Free water restriction
- Cardiac rehabilitation to strengthen peripheral muscles

 MEDICATION (DRUGS)

- Angiotensin-converting enzyme (ACE) inhibitors at adequate doses; contraindicated in pregnancy
- Hydralazine and nitrates for patients intolerant to ACE inhibitors and as add-on therapy, especially in African American patients.
- Angiotensin receptor blockers for patients intolerant to ACE inhibitors or in addition to ACE inhibitors; contraindicated in pregnancy
- β-Blockers unless in pulmonary edema
- Diuretics for symptoms of edema or pulmonary congestion
- Digoxin for symptom control, especially if atrial fibrillation is present
- Warfarin for treatment of thrombi or atrial fibrillation; contraindicated in pregnancy
- Intravenous immune globulin may have a role in peripartum cardiomyopathy, although it does not appear to be beneficial in idiopathic dilated cardiomyopathy.

SURGERY

- Transplantation is an option for end-stage disease, with symptoms refractory to medical therapy.
- Implantable cardioverter–defibrillator is recommended for primary prevention of sudden cardiac death in patients with left ventricular ejection fraction (LVEF) less than 30%.
- Cardiac resynchronization therapy is indicated in patients with LVEF less than 35%, NYHA Class III symptoms, and QRS >120 msec.
- Implantable left ventricular assist devices appear to have a role as a bridge to transplantation, and are occasionally used as destination therapy.

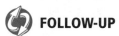 FOLLOW-UP

DISPOSITION

Admission Criteria

- Some exacerbations of congestive heart failure can be managed as an outpatient with frequent telephone contact.
- Intravenous diuresis is possible on an outpatient basis in certain circumstances.
- Admission is advisable for any sudden change in symptomatology or for aggressive diuresis.

Discharge Criteria

- Discharge is possible once a patient is converted to oral medications.
- Home intravenous inotropic therapy is possible for relief of symptoms, but may be associated with worse outcomes.

PROGNOSIS

- Symptomatic patients who are referred to a tertiary care center have a 50% 5-year mortality rate.
- Right ventricular dilatation portends a more ominous prognosis.
- A lower ejection fraction is associated with a higher risk of mortality in populations of patients with heart failure; it is less predictive of outcome in an individual.
- Peripartum cardiomyopathies show significant improvement within 6 months in almost half of all women who develop this disorder.
- Heart transplantation has been successfully used in peripartum cardiomyopathy that does not improve with time or medical measures, although the risk of early rejection episodes may be higher.
- Alcoholic cardiomyopathy is sometimes reversible with complete abstinence.
- Arrhythmias are common.
- Thromboembolic events may occur.

PATIENT MONITORING

- Some have recommended echocardiographic screening of family members with idiopathic dilated cardiomyopathy, even in the absence of symptoms, given the high incidence of familial cardiomyopathy.
- Routine echocardiography, in the absence of worsening symptoms, although frequently performed, is not recommended.

REFERENCES

1. Bozkurt B, Villanueva FS, Holubkov R, et al. Intravenous immune globulin in the therapy of peripartum cardiomyopathy. *J Am Coll Cardiol*. 1999;34:177–180.
2. Dec GW, Fuster V. Idiopathic dilated cardiomyopathy. *N Engl J Med*. 1994;331:1564–1575.
3. Homans DC. Peripartum cardiomyopathy. *N Engl J Med*. 1985;312:1432–1437.
4. Lampert MB, Lang RM. Peripartum cardiomyopathy. *Am Heart J*. 1995;130:860–870.
5. Rickenbacher PR, Rizeq MN, Hunt SA, et al. Long-term outcome after heart transplantation for peripartum cardiomyopathy. *Am Heart J*. 1994;127:1318–1323.
6. Rodkey SM, Ratliff NB, Young JB. Cardiomyopathy and myocardial failure. In: Topol EJ, ed. *Comprehensive Cardiovascular Medicine*. Philadelphia: Lippincott Williams & Wilkins, 1998; 2591–2593.
7. Sun JP, James KB, Yang XS, et al. Comparison of mortality rates and progression of left ventricular dysfunction in patients with idiopathic dilated cardiomyopathy and dilated versus nondilated right ventricular cavities. *Am J Cardiol*. 1997;80:1583–1587.
8. Tajik AJ, Murphy JG. Dilated cardiomyopathy. In: Murphy JG, ed. *Mayo Clinic Cardiology Review*. Philadelphia: Lippincott Williams & Wilkins, 2000; 445–454.
9. Topol EJ, ed. *Textbook of Cardiovascular Medicine*. Philadelphia: Lippincott Williams & Wilkins, 2002.
10. Zipes DP. *Braunwald's Heart Disease: A Textbook of Cardiovascular Medicine*, 7th ed. Philadelphia: Elsevier Saunders, 2005.

CODES

ICD9-CM

- 428.0 Failure, heart, congestive
- 425.4 Cardiomyopathy, dilated
- 674.8 Cardiomyopathy, postpartum

PATIENT TEACHING

Patients should weigh themselves daily and report any sudden increase to their doctor.

Diet

- Avoid alcohol and tobacco.
- Restrict sodium intake.

CARDIOMYOPATHY, HYPERTROPHIC

Deepak L. Bhatt
Gary S. Francis
Apur R. Kamdar

 ## BASICS

DESCRIPTION
Massive hypertrophy of the ventricle results in a dynamic outflow tract obstruction.
Also called idiopathic hypertrophic subaortic stenosis and hypertrophic obstructive cardiomyopathy (HOCM)

EPIDEMIOLOGY
- Familial hypertrophic cardiomyopathy is inherited as an autosomal-dominant trait with variable penetrance.
- Apical HOCM is a variant that is found more often in Japan than in other parts of the world.
- Most common cause of sudden death in young athletes

RISK FACTORS
Family history of HOCM

Pregnancy Considerations
High risk, especially in the postpartum period, where blood and fluid loss can lead to exacerbation of the outflow tract gradient

ETIOLOGY
- Numerous chromosomal abnormalities due to multiple mutations have been identified that are responsible for hypertrophic cardiomyopathy.
- Mutations in the genes for cardiac myosin heavy chain, troponin T, and α-tropomyosin are some that have been discovered, and there will likely be more.

ASSOCIATED CONDITIONS
Arrhythmias

 ## DIAGNOSIS

SIGNS AND SYMPTOMS
- "Spike and dome" contour of the carotid pulse
- S2 (second heart sound) paradoxically split
- Harsh systolic murmur along the left sternal border, increases with Valsalva maneuver or in beat after a premature ventricular contraction
- Systolic thrill
- Pulmonary rales
- Mitral regurgitation murmur
- S4 (fourth heart sound)
- S3 (third heart sound)
- Double or triple apical impulse
- Dyspnea on exertion, and at rest
- Syncope
- Chest pain
- Palpitations

TESTS
- Left ventriculography shows cavity obliteration.
  - In midventricular obstruction, a spade-shaped left ventricle is classic.
- Coronary arteriography typically reveals normal coronary arteries in young patients. Older patients may have coexistent coronary artery disease. Prominent septal perforators may be present, which may display systolic compression from the thickened septum.
- Genetic testing is not routinely recommended; many different mutations have been identified, with varying natural histories.

Lab
- Electrocardiogram (ECG) reveals a large amount of voltage across the precordium.
- T-wave inversion also may be present in the precordial leads.
- Atrial and ventricular arrhythmias may be present, as may septal Q waves.

Imaging
- Chest X-ray may reveal cardiac enlargement.
- Two-dimensional (2D) echocardiography is the cornerstone of diagnosis.
  - Left ventricular hypertrophy is present, classically asymmetric septal hypertrophy
  - However, other patterns of hypertrophy exist, such as predominant apical hypertrophy.
  - There is systolic anterior motion of the mitral valve and associated mitral regurgitation.
  - Left ventricular systolic function is hyperdynamic.
  - The cavity size is not enlarged.
- Doppler interrogation reveals a gradient across the outflow tract that increases with the Valsalva maneuver or inhalation of amyl nitrate.

DIFFERENTIAL DIAGNOSIS
- Athlete's heart
- Hypertensive cardiomyopathy, especially in the elderly
- Amyloid
- Aortic stenosis

 ## TREATMENT

GENERAL MEASURES
Adequate hydration; avoid volume depletion

MEDICATION (DRUGS)

- Antibiotic prophylaxis for procedures that may lead to bacterial endocarditis
- Avoid positive inotropes such as digoxin.
- β-Blockers are first-line therapy.
- Calcium channel blockers such as verapamil and diltiazem can be useful; watch for excessive vasodilation, which can be detrimental.
- Disopyramide, due to its negative inotropic effects, can be useful, but anticholinergic side effects, such as urinary retention in men, can limit its tolerability.

SURGERY

- Septal myectomy can successfully reduce the outflow tract gradient and improve symptoms.
- More recently, percutaneous transluminal septal ablation has been accomplished with localized alcohol injection into the first or second septal perforator in order to selectively destroy septal tissue.
- Implantable defibrillators are highly effective for primary and secondary prevention of sudden cardiac death (SCD) by ventricular arrhythmias in these patients.

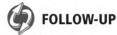 **FOLLOW-UP**

DISPOSITION
Admission Criteria
As for heart failure of any etiology

PROGNOSIS

- Earlier reports of these patients were from referral centers and suggested a high incidence of sudden death.
- More contemporary analyses suggest that the risk of sudden death, while elevated, is not as high as previously believed.
- Risk of sudden death is increased in patients with malignant ventricular arrhythmias or a family history of sudden death, and is more common in children.
- Risk of sudden death also significantly higher in patients with severe left ventricular hypertrophy (>30 mm).
- Hypertrophic cardiomyopathy is the most common identified cause of sudden cardiac death in the young athlete. Competitive sports participation is contraindicated.

PATIENT MONITORING
As for heart failure of any etiology

REFERENCES
1. Maron B, et al. Efficacy of implantable cardioverter-defibrillators for the prevention of sudden death in patients with hypertrophic cardiomyopathy. *N Engl J Med.* 2000;342:365–373.
2. Maron B. Sudden death in young athletes. *N Engl J Med.* 2003;349:1064–1075.
3. Miller DH, Borer JS. The cardiomyopathies: A pathophysiologic approach to therapeutic management. *Arch Intern Med.* 1983;143:2157–2162.
4. Rodkey SM, Ratliff NB, Young JB. Cardiomyopathy and myocardial failure. In: Topol EJ, ed. *Comprehensive Cardiovascular Medicine.* Philadelphia: Lippincott Williams & Wilkins, 1998;2593–2594.
5. Spirito P, et al. Magnitude of left ventricular hypertrophy and risk of sudden death in hypertrophic cardiomyopathy. *N Engl J Med.* 2000;342:1778–1785.
6. Tajik AJ, Murphy JG. Hypertrophic and restrictive cardiomyopathies. In: Murphy JG, ed. *Mayo Clinic Cardiology Review.* Philadelphia: Lippincott Williams & Wilkins, 2000;455–482.
7. Wynne J, Braunwald E. The cardiomyopathies and myocarditides. In: Braunwald E, ed. *Heart Disease: A Textbook of Cardiovascular Medicine,* 5th ed. Philadelphia: WB Saunders, 1997;1414–1426.

CODES
ICD9-CM
- 428.0 Failure, heart, congestive
- 425.1 Cardiomyopathy, hypertrophic obstructive

PATIENT TEACHING
Avoid dehydration; maintain adequate volume intake

Activity
No participation in competitive sports

CARDIOMYOPATHY, PEDIATRIC

Linda J. Addonizio
Welton M. Gersony

 BASICS

DESCRIPTION

- Cardiomyopathy (CM) is defined as disease of the heart muscle with histologic or morphologic myocardial abnormality resulting in myocardial dysfunction. The left ventricle is usually affected, or there may be biventricular involvement. There are primary CMs of unknown origin or secondary, when disease is a result of another known systemic disorder. The World Health Organization/International Society and Federation of Cardiologists (WHO/ISFC) adopted this empiric division in 1995. The three main types of primary CM are classified morphologically:
- Dilated: Left ventricular (LV) dilation; poor systolic function; disproportionately thin free wall and septal thickness; loss of myocytes, fibrosis
- Hypertrophic: Left and/or right ventricular hypertrophy, concentric or asymmetric, involving septum; LV volume normal or reduced; normal systolic, abnormal diastolic function; massive myocyte hypertrophy and fiber disarray with increased connective tissue
- Restrictive: Restrictive filling, low diastolic volume of either ventricle; near-normal systolic function and wall thickness; fibrosis of myocardium, endocardial rigidity

EPIDEMIOLOGY

Estimates of incidence of CM vary widely according to type and age group. The overall incidence from one current report is 1.13–1.24 cases/100,000 children. Variability has been reported according to race, sex, and type of disease.

Incidence

- Idiopathic dilated CM accounts for the majority of all cardiomyopathies seen in childhood:
  - National Heart, Lung, and Blood Institute Workshop: 2–8 cases/100,000 over all age groups
  - Baltimore–Washington Infant Study: 1/10,000 live births (this incidence includes all forms of neonatal CM)
  - Pediatric Cardiomyopathy Registry: .5–.74 cases/100,000 children with infant cases much higher at 4.58/100,000. They found a higher incidence in boys and in black race.
- Hypertrophic CM: About 30% of pediatric cases
  - Mayo Clinic Study: 2.5 cases/100,000
  - Australian Study: .32 cases/100,000
  - Pediatric Cardiomyopathy Registry: .41–.61 cases/100,000 children; infant incidence higher at 3.2/100,000, and a higher incidence in boys and in black race.
- Restrictive CM: Rare 2–5% of cardiomyopathies; includes contracted form of endocardial fibroelastosis (EFE).

RISK FACTORS

None for idiopathic; some risk factors for specific etiologies are listed in subsequent text

Genetics

- It is believed that overall 30% of cardiomyopathies are genetic in origin.
  - Hypertrophic CM are 50–60% genetic, with 35% of these familial (autosomal dominant) and 26% inborn errors of metabolism (autosomal recessive).
  - Dilated CM are 20–30% genetic in origin; 39% of these are associated with neuromuscular disorders and 27% post myocarditis

PATHOPHYSIOLOGY

- Dilated CM is a disease affecting the cytoskeleton and sarcolemma of the myocardium that causes a disruption of systolic function, thought a failure of "force transmission," whether on a genetic or secondary basis
- Hypertrophic CM (also some restrictive CM) is a disease of the sarcomeric proteins, which are responsible for impaired "force generation," and contraction of the muscle.

ETIOLOGY

Cardiomyopathies are a result of damage to the heart muscle.

- Dilated CM may be idiopathic (unknown etiology), familial/genetic, viral and/or autoimmune, alcoholic/toxic, or associated with other disease.
- Hypertrophic CM may be sporadic, associated with syndromes or more commonly familial, with autosomal-dominant pattern and wide variability of penetrance.
  - 60% of families have more than one case.
  - The 14q1 chromosome is a major locus.
- Restrictive CM may be idiopathic, familial, or associated with infiltrative disease (amyloidosis, sarcoidosis, glycogen, and hypereosinophilia).

ASSOCIATED CONDITIONS

Primary CMs, by definition, have no associated conditions. In the specific CMs, >100 associated diseases have been identified.

 DIAGNOSIS

SIGNS AND SYMPTOMS

Symptoms depend on the morphologic type of CM and the degree of impairment of ventricular muscle and function.
Dilated CM
Initial symptoms range from exercise intolerance to overt congestive heart failure (CHF) as a consequence of poor systolic function.

- Respiratory distress, chronic cough, frequent "upper respiratory infections," shortness of breath
- Palpitations/arrhythmias, tachycardia
- Easy fatigability (during feeding with infants)
- Abdominal complaints, pain, nausea, vomiting
- Failure to thrive, growth failure

Hypertrophic CM
Termed "the great masquerader," because signs and symptoms usually result in a false diagnosis of other diseases. Symptoms vary in intensity, depending on the extent and distribution of the hypertrophy. They result from high filling pressures (diastolic dysfunction), low cardiac output from LV outflow tract (LVOT) obstruction, or angina. Obstruction may occur at rest or with provocation.

- Increased fatigability, exercise intolerance
- Cough, breathlessness, "asthma"
- Chest pain
- Syncope or dizziness
- Palpitations: atrial or ventricular arrhythmias
- Sudden death

Restrictive CM
Presentation varies with age and degree of diastolic impairment:

- In newborn, CHF common with respiratory distress and low output
- Pronounced growth retardation in young children
- Abdominal pain or gastrointestinal (GI) complaints
- Dyspnea on exertion, dry cough, and "asthma" are seen in older children.
- Symptoms may progress faster than other forms of cardiomyopathy.
- Hepatomegaly, ascites, and peripheral edema in older children with more chronic course.
- Palpitations: Atrial arrhythmias, predominantly fibrillation and flutter
- Thromboembolism secondary to

History

- A careful attention to history for both symptoms, and family screening is important.
  - Familial cases can often be silent with variable expression of the disease (all types of CM) until the index case is diagnosed.

Physical Exam

- Dilated CM
  - Signs of CHF: Tachycardia, tachypnea, rales, gallop rhythm, hepatomegaly, diminished perfusion, edema
  - Murmur of mitral incompetence may be heard with severe LV dilatation
- Hypertrophic CM: The murmur and examination are related to hemodynamic state:
  - Outflow obstruction: Double or triple apical LV impulse and medium pitch systolic ejection murmur (increases with Valsalva maneuver)
  - Nonobstructive form: Only nonspecific ejection murmur
- Restrictive CM depending on the degree of diastolic dysfunction may have no physical findings or those following.
  - Third heart sound, prominent apical impulse, increased jugular venous pressure
  - Hepatomegaly, ascites, edema
  - Rales, wheezing

TESTS

- Electrocardiogram (ECG): Varying patterns of LV hypertrophy with nonspecific left precordial inversion or flattening of T waves and sometimes deep Q waves. Abnormalities specific to each form:
  - Dilated: Ventricular, atrial arrhythmias; in EFE very tall QRS voltage present in all precordial and limb leads
  - Hypertrophic: 90% abnormal ECG with a wide variety of patterns; infants often have paradoxic right ventricular hypertrophy; cannot discriminate LVOT obstruction or risk for sudden death by ECG; atrial fibrillation or ventricular tachycardia

– Restrictive: Bi-atrial enlargement, right ventricular enlargement in infants, atrial arrhythmias or progressive heart block

Lab
- Blood and urine tests can help to determine etiology in some cases, especially if CM is secondary to other diseases.
  – Metabolic causes such as carnitine deficiency, thyroid disorders, or fatty acid oxidation defects
  – Genetic testing can be performed to rule out known causes.
  – Exposure to viruses that may have caused myocarditis and/or ongoing inflammation or autoimmune causes of CM.

Imaging
Evaluations establish diagnosis and monitor treatment effectiveness.
- Chest x-ray: Enlarged heart
  – Dilated CM: Larger, more globular shape, pulmonary edema or congestion, left atrium dilated
  – Hypertrophic CM: Cardiomegaly greater in infants than older children, unless end-stage
  – Restrictive CM: Bi-atrial dilatation, pulmonary venous pattern, ventricular enlargement not prominent
- Echocardiography: Provides definitive diagnosis of three morphologic types, rules out other abnormalities
  – Dilated CM: Thin-walled, globular LV, low fractional shortening, mitral insufficiency and/or mural thrombi in late stages, both ventricles can be affected
  – Hypertrophic CM: Very thick septum, free wall, near obliteration of LV cavity, normal to hyperdynamic function, systolic anterior motion of mitral leaflet, and/or LVOT obstruction with measurable Doppler gradient, in some cases may only have concentric hypertrophy
  – Restrictive CM: Massive bi-atrial enlargement, normal to small-sized somewhat hypertrophied ventricles, normal systolic function with abnormal diastolic function
- Angiography: Only indicated if unable to visualize coronary arteries by echocardiography or to rule out discrete aortic obstruction
- MRI: Useful to rule out constrictive pericarditis

Diagnostic Procedures/Surgery
- Cardiac catheterization
  – Dilated CM: Rule out myocarditis by endomyocardial biopsy, evaluate hemodynamic efficacy of medical therapy and need for transplantation.
  – Hypertrophic CM: Evaluation for arrhythmias and possible surgical relief of obstruction
  – Restrictive CM: Rule out constrictive pericarditis (dip and plateau pressure tracing present in both, LV end-diastolic pressure greater than right ventricular end-diastolic pressure favors restrictive). Pulmonary hypertension with rapidly increasing resistance is seen frequently and earlier in restrictive types but not in hypertrophic type.
- Skeletal muscle biopsy sometimes is needed for diagnosis of myopathies associated with systemic or neuromuscular disorders

Pathologic Findings
- Dilated CM from all causes
  – Loss of myocytes with some hypertrophy of remaining myocytes and fibrosis, myocardium generally thinned
- Hypertrophic CM
  – Massive myocyte hypertrophy and fiber disarray with increased connective tissue and thickness of the myocardium
- Restrictive CM
  – May have interstitial fibrosis and some myocyte disarray along with hypertrophy; endocardial thickening can also be seen in affected ventricles and atria
  – In secondary restrictive cases, abnormal deposits can be seen such as amyloid and iron.

DIFFERENTIAL DIAGNOSIS
The differential diagnosis of idiopathic CM is one of exclusion.
- Diagnostic focus should center on establishing an etiology that might be curable.
  – Myocarditis
  – Rule out anomalous coronary and coarctation of the aorta in dilated CM
  – Other examples of treatable causes of dilated CM are carnitine deficiency, arrhythmia, toxic reactions, and inflammatory diseases.
  – A treatable cause of hypertrophic CM is subaortic membrane
  – Constrictive pericarditis must be ruled out in cases of restrictive CM.
- Usually there is no difficulty diagnostically in distinguishing dilated CM from either hypertrophic or restrictive forms.

TREATMENT
GENERAL MEASURES
Medical management involves control of CHF and arrhythmias and potential prevention of progression of disease. In asymptomatic patients continued reevaluation is warranted.
- A tailored cardiotonic regimen for patients with CHF is optimal.
- Use of medications to modulate the neuroendocrine system in asymptomatic patients may prevent progression of disease.
- To prevent thromboembolism, warfarin anticoagulation is advised if atrial fibrillation, ejection fraction <20%, and/or mural thrombus is present.
- Endocarditis prophylaxis is only necessary with concomitant valvular abnormality.
- Influenza and pneumococcal vaccines are advisable with significant cardiovascular compromise, and respiratory syncytial viral prophylaxis in infants less than 2 years old.

MEDICATION (DRUGS)
Presentation can vary from asymptomatic, to mild CHF, to shock. Treatment and medications will vary accordingly from outpatient to intensive care unit.

First Line
Dilated CM
CHF treatment should be tailored and maximized. Some of these agents may be needed in other types of CM in later stages.
- Digoxin
- Angiotensin-converting enzyme (ACE) inhibitors
- Diuretics such as furosemide, thiazides
- Spironolactone may be added to maintain potassium levels (caution when adding to ACE inhibitor).
- β-Adrenergic blockers may result in significant improvement, but should only be administered cautiously, under direct care of experienced cardiologist and never in decompensated CHF.
- If outpatient management is unsuccessful, or if patient is unstable on presentation, intravenous inotropic agents and vasodilators may be necessary for stabilization; in extreme cases, ventilatory support or LV assist devices may be needed.
- Arrhythmia management: Isolated or even frequent premature ventricular beats do not warrant the addition of an antiarrhythmic unless:
  – Episodes of ventricular tachycardia with syncope are featured: Amiodarone
  – Implantable defibrillator may be a better option for malignant rhythms
Hypertrophic CM
Treatment usually is focused on minimizing outflow obstruction, myocardial relaxation, and arrhythmia control (see preceding).
- Calcium channel blockers may alleviate symptoms and questionably prevent progression of disease.
- β-Blocker therapy may decrease ectopic beats while controlling heart rate and LV compliance.
- If CHF occurs, cardiotonics may be necessary but may increase chance of ischemia. Caution is needed when using diuretics in hypertrophic or restrictive CM where cardiac output is dependent on preload.
Restrictive CM
No specific medications. Children most often need anticongestive measures which can share the same danger as with hypertrophic patients. Rarely atrial arrhythmias may arise and require treatment.

Second Line
- Angiotensin receptor blockers (ARBs) can be substituted when ACE inhibitors are not tolerated.
- Other vasodilators such as hydralazine may be used when first line drugs are ineffective or not tolerated.

C

SURGERY

- Hypertrophic CM: Excision of muscular LVOT or right ventricular outflow tract obstruction can relieve symptoms.
- Hypertrophic CM: Resolution of symptoms may occur with release of coronary stenosis by myocardial bridging.
- Implantable defibrillators help prevent outpatient sudden death when ventricular arrhythmias are significant in hypertrophic CM.
- When maximal medical therapy fails, cardiac transplantation should be considered.
- The use of mitral valvuloplasty or replacement and/ or ventricular reduction therapy in dilated CM has not been proven efficacious.

 FOLLOW-UP

The frequency of follow-up will be dictated not only by the type of CM but by the severity of symptoms. Since these diseases do progress with time, follow-up by a qualified pediatric cardiologist is essential.

Admission Criteria

- Children can present with mild to severe CHF or shock at time of diagnosis with dilated CM.
  - With significant CHF symptoms patients might initially need to be placed on bed rest with supplemental oxygen and fluid restriction until stabilized.
  - Patients in shock should be stabilized in the intensive care setting and transitioned to oral medicines and an nonintensic setting for teaching.
  - After stabilization and discharge, repeat admissions usually are for acute pulmonary edema or transient low output or progression of disease.
- Patients with hypertrophic CM usually do not require admission except for life-threatening arrhythmia or if end stage.
  - Patients who have syncope should be admitted for observation for acute arrhythmia or ischemia.
- Restrictive patients can have episodic increase in CHF symptoms, and with rising pulmonary vascular resistance index cardio will need transplantation sooner than dilated patients to avoid need for concomitant lung transplantation. Symptoms may progress rapidly in this form of cardiomyopathy.

Discharge Criteria

- Patients whose CHF is stabilized and are able to take their medications and tolerate activities of daily living can be discharged to be followed as an outpatient.
  - In infants, the ability to take and/or tolerate feeding is critical to their CHF management.

Issues for Referral

- A new diagnosis of CM warrants evaluation for etiology and management which may include:
  - Pediatric heart failure/transplant specialists
  - Geneticist
  - Neurologist specializing in neuromuscular disorders
  - Pediatric electrophysiologist

PROGNOSIS

The prognosis varies with the type of CM:
Dilated CM
The course is highly variable, with some children surviving many years but a significant number lost in the first year after diagnosis.

- Survival ranges from 40–90% at 1 year and 40–50% at 5 years.
- Symptoms of CHF despite therapy are a poor prognostic sign.
- LV ejection fraction most often is not predictive of clinical course.
- Elevated LV end-diastolic pressure >25 mmHg: Mortality 46% at 1 year, 68% at 5 years
- Low serum sodium correlated with poor outcome
- Use of cardiac transplantation has improved survival with dilated CM to 90% at 1 year and 83% at 5 years.

Hypertrophic CM
Course depends on age at presentation.

- Infant survival dismal with CHF; transplantation should be considered
- Most diagnosed after age 12 years are stable for many years.
- 3%–6% annual mortality rate; 5-year survival 80%
- Progressive disease, especially during rapid somatic growth
- Sudden death during exercise most common in adolescents.
- No predictive variables for sudden death in children, but sudden death of first-degree relative can be an important prognostic sign.

- If late CHF or unmanageable symptoms develop, transplantation is indicated.

Restrictive CM
Rare, but course is accelerated, with most deaths occurring in young childhood, either sudden or from advancing CHF. May have a period of well-being after initial CHF symptoms, when pulmonary resistance increases. Transplantation should be considered early.

Pregnancy Considerations

- Risk for pregnancy depends on degree of ventricular dysfunction and/or heart failure.
- Symptomatic patients with dilated CM and all patients with hypertrophic CM are at increased risk for mortality and for cardiovascular decompensation during pregnancy.

COMPLICATIONS

- Complications relate to the progression of heart failure and its effects on other organ systems, either from low output or chronic congestion.
  - Cirrhosis, renal dysfunction, cachexia, recurrent pulmonary infections, pulmonary hypertension, and decreased mentation may all occur with severe chronic CHF.
  - Other circulatory complications such as stroke and peripheral vascular abnormalities can also result.

PATIENT MONITORING

- Close outpatient follow-up of all patients with CM is necessary to detect progression of disease and to tailor their medications.
- Frequency of visits will depend on cardiac disability and instability. Progress can be evaluated by periodic:
  - Exercise testing: To determine VO_{2max} in dilated patients, and level of inducible ischemia in hypertrophic CM
  - Holter monitoring: To detect malignant arrhythmias or progressive heart block
  - Use of brain natriuretic peptide (BNP) measurements may help in following progression of CHF
  - Cardiac catheterization: Pretransplantation hemodynamic testing and progression of pulmonary vascular resistance index (PVRI)

REFERENCES

1. Addonizio LJ. Cardiac transplantation in childhood cardiomyopathies. *Prog Pediatr Cardiol*. 1992;1:72–80.
2. Benson LN, Freedom RM, et al. Cardiomyopathies of childhood: Part II. *Prog Pediatr Cardiol*. 1992;14:1–80.
3. Lipshultz SE, Sleeper LA, et al. The incidence of pediatric cardiomyopathy in two regions of the United States. *N Engl J Med*. 2003;348:1647–1655.
4. Lewis AB, Chabot M. Outcome of infants and children with dilated cardiomyopathy. *Am J Cardiol*. 1991;68:365–369.
5. Tsirka AE, et al. Improved outcomes of pediatric dilated cardiomyopathy with utilization of heart transplantation. *J Am Coll Cardiol*. 2004;44:391–397.
6. Thiene G, et al. Twenty years of progress and beckoning frontiers in cardiovascular pathology: Cardiomyopathies. *Cardiovasc Pathol*. 2005;14:165–169.

MISCELLANEOUS

CODES

ICD9-CM
- 425.4 Primary cardiomyopathy
- 425.8 Secondary cardiomyopathy
- 425.1 Hypertrophic cardiomyopathy
- 425.4 Restrictive cardiomyopathy
- 746.84 Hypertrophic cardiomyopathy, congenital

PATIENT TEACHING
- Patients with CM and/or CHF and their family should be educated about:
- Importance of low-salt diet and fluid restriction when necessary
- Adequate rest, but graded regular exercise important (cardiac rehabilitation based on the severity of compromise) in dilated CM.
- Patients with hypertrophic CM must not pursue vigorous exercise, or competitive sports.
- Importance of routine follow-up and compliance with medications.
- Signs and symptoms of disease progression and arrhythmias.
  There are numerous websites and support organizations for patients with heart failure and CM. Many American Heart Association (AHA) sites exist, but most are geared to older adolescents or adults.
- www.healthlinkusa.com
- www.searchwebmd.com
- www.americanheart.org
- www.childrenscardiomyopathy.org

Diet
- Children with CM usually have trouble taking in enough calories secondary to the disease or CHF symptoms and often have a higher caloric requirement.
  – Higher calorie diet or supplements for children with failure to thrive
  – Infants may need tube feeding and older children small frequent meals.
- Low-salt foods when symptomatic CHF or fluid retention
- Foods high in potassium and magnesium are good to help maintain adequate levels when on diuretics.
- Certain metabolic cardiomyopathies may require special diets to prevent disease progression.

Activity
- Hypertrophic CM: Strenuous physical exercise and stress should be avoided, and more sedentary recreation advocated.
- Dilated and restrictive CM: Recommendations for activity according to the degree of ventricular dysfunction and symptomatology

CARDIOMYOPATHY, RESTRICTIVE

Deepak L. Bhatt
Gary S. Francis
Apur R. Kamdar

 BASICS

DESCRIPTION
Infiltration of the myocardium by one of several disease processes leads to severe impairment of diastolic filling of the ventricle.
- Rarely is any specific cause found
- Needs to be distinguished from constrictive pericarditis (not easy), which may respond to pericardiectomy
- Even a small increase in ventricular volume can lead to a substantial increase in intracavitary pressures.
- Systolic function is normal until the terminal stages of the disease.

EPIDEMIOLOGY
- Most forms are uncommon in the United States.
- Least common class of cardiomyopathy
- There are certain rare familial forms of restrictive cardiomyopathy.

RISK FACTORS
Depends on etiology

Pregnancy Considerations
Not advisable in symptomatic restrictive cardiomyopathy

ETIOLOGY
- Amyloidosis
- Sarcoidosis
- Hemochromatosis
- Scleroderma
- Fabry disease
- Glycogen storage disorders
- Gaucher disease
- Hurler disease
- Endomyocardial fibrosis
- Loffler endocarditis
- Endocardial fibroelastosis
- Carcinoid
- Radiation
- Metastatic cancer
- After heart transplantation; also, with rejection
- Idiopathic

ASSOCIATED CONDITIONS
- Atrial fibrillation
- Pleural effusions
- Thromboembolism
- Hypercalcemia, kidney stones (in sarcoid)
- Diabetes (in hemochromatosis)

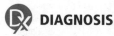 DIAGNOSIS

SIGNS AND SYMPTOMS
- Exertional dyspnea
- Fatigue
- Edema
- Hepatomegaly, pulsatile liver
- Ascites
- JVD (jugular venous distension), with rapid X and Y descents
- Kussmaul sign [increase in JVP (jugular venous pressure) with inspiration]
- Third heart sound (S3), right- or left-sided
- Fourth heart sound (S4) (uncommon)
- Cutaneous flushing, diarrhea, bronchoconstriction (with carcinoid syndrome)
- Anterior uveitis (sarcoid)
- Erythema nodosum (tender red nodules in sarcoid)

TESTS
- Right heart catheterization usually reveals a dip and plateau (square root sign) in ventricular pressure.
- Left and right ventricular pressures are not interdependent, unlike constrictive pericarditis (in which right ventricular pressure increases with inspiration while left ventricular pressure decreases).
- The atrial pressure tracing may have an M or W waveform, due to rapid X and Y descents.
- Endomyocardial biopsy can point to the specific cause, and it can reliably diagnose anthracycline toxicity.
- Computed tomographic (CT) scanning and magnetic resonance imaging (MRI) can help differentiate restrictive cardiomyopathy from constrictive pericarditis, although both entities can coexist.

Lab
- In hemochromatosis, serum ferritin levels are markedly elevated, along with iron levels and transferrin saturation.
- The angiotensin-converting enzyme level may be elevated with sarcoidosis, although it can be within the normal range.
- Eosinophilia is associated with eosinophilic heart disease.
- Urinary 5-hydroxyindoleacetic acid levels are elevated in carcinoid.
- Electrocardiogram (ECG) may show various degrees of conduction block.

Imaging
- Chest X-ray is notable for absence of cardiomegaly
  - Pulmonary congestion and pleural effusions may be present.
  - Bilateral hilar lymphadenopathy may be seen with sarcoid.
- Doppler tracings reveal marked impairment of diastolic function.
  - In contrast to constrictive pericarditis, there is no significant respiratory variation in mitral and tricuspid inflow patterns.
  - The mitral inflow pattern shows a high E-to-A ratio and a short deceleration time. The pulmonary venous flow reveals a blunted systolic waveform.
  - Systolic function may be well-preserved, except at terminal stages.
  - Atria are dilated; the ventricles are of normal size.
  - Apparent hypertrophy, due to infiltration, may occur.
  - Left ventricular aneurysms may be seen in sarcoid.
- Thallium-201 imaging may show patchy perfusion defects in sarcoidosis.
- Gallium-67 scanning may show abnormal uptake in sarcoidosis, although the test is rather nonspecific.

DIFFERENTIAL DIAGNOSIS
- Constrictive pericarditis, which can appear clinically identical in terms of symptoms and physical examination findings
- Other causes of right-sided heart failure

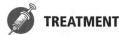

TREATMENT

GENERAL MEASURES

As for heart failure of any cause

MEDICATION (DRUGS)

- Diuretics are useful to treat pulmonary congestion, but overly aggressive diuresis can lead to a marked decline in cardiac output.
- β-Blockers and calcium channel blockers can both be deleterious.
- Digoxin is useful to treat any coexistent atrial fibrillation. It can lead to toxicity at lower than usual doses in amyloidosis.
- Amiodarone can be used for treatment of atrial fibrillation.
- Chelation therapy with desferrioxamine or phlebotomy may be useful in restrictive cardiomyopathy due to hemochromatosis.
- Steroid therapy can treat sarcoidosis successfully.
- Warfarin therapy is indicated in the presence of thrombi or atrial fibrillation.

SURGERY

- Heart transplantation is the only effective long-term therapy for most restrictive cardiomyopathies.
- Sarcoid and amyloid can recur in the transplanted heart.
- Electrical cardioversion can be used for atrial fibrillation.
- Permanent pacemakers may be implanted for advanced heart block or symptomatic bradyarrhythmias.
- Implantable cardioverter–defibrillators may be used for ventricular arrhythmias.

FOLLOW-UP

DISPOSITION

Admission Criteria

Same as for other etiologies of congestive heart failure

PROGNOSIS

- The prognosis is generally poor.
- Involvement of the conduction system can lead to advanced heart block and sudden death or to ventricular arrhythmias. This is of particular concern in amyloid and sarcoid.

PATIENT MONITORING

As for other etiologies of heart failure

REFERENCES

1. Klein AL, Scalia GM. Diseases of the pericardium, restrictive cardiomyopathy and diastolic dysfunction. In: Topol EJ, ed. *Comprehensive Cardiovascular Medicine*. Philadelphia: Lippincott Williams & Wilkins,1998;669–735.
2. Kushwaha SS, Fallon JT, Fuster V. Restrictive cardiomyopathy. *N Engl J Med*. 1997;336:267–276.
3. Newman LS, Rose CS, Maier LA. Sarcoidosis. *N Engl J Med*. 1997;336:1224–1234.
4. Shammas RL, Movahed A. Sarcoidosis of the heart. *Clin Cardiol*. 1993;16:462–472.
5. Sharma OP, Maheshwari A, Thaker K. Myocardial sarcoidosis. *Chest*. 1993;103:253–258.
6. Tajik AJ, Murphy JG. Hypertrophic and restrictive cardiomyopathies. In: Murphy JG, ed. *Mayo Clinic Cardiology Review*. Philadelphia: Lippincott Williams & Wilkins, 2000;455–482.
7. Zipes DP. *Braunwald's Heart Disease: A Textbook of Cardiovascular Medicine*, 7th ed. Philadelphia: Elsevier Saunders, 2005.

CODES

ICD9-CM

- 428.0 Failure, heart, congestive
- 425.4 Cardiomyopathy, restrictive
- 135 [425.8] Cardiomyopathy, sarcoidosis

PATIENT TEACHING

Daily weights with reporting of any significant increase or loss

C

CARDIOVASCULAR PREVENTIVE CARE (PRIMARY PREVENTION)

Jorge F. Trejo
Jorge Alegria

 BASICS

DESCRIPTION
- Primary prevention focuses on individuals who have not had any clinical manifestation of disease in the coronary, cerebrovascular, and peripheral artery territories.
- Primary prevention of cardiovascular disease (CVD) has public health priority as first cause of disability adjusted years of life lost (DALYs) and associated impact on society.
- Primary prevention aims to avoid the presence or harmful level of modifiable causal risk factors (also called primordial prevention) as well as their management once present.

Geriatric Considerations
Appropriate risk-factor modification significantly reduces risk for CVD in the older population (>65 years).

Pediatric Considerations
- Primary prevention in children and youth:
  - Low-saturated fat diet for all children older than 2 years (less than 10% of total calories per day)
  - Favor less sodium consumption from early life
  - Limit TV time and sedentary activities (video games).
  - Encourage at least 1 hour of playtime daily.
  - Give a clear message to abstain from any tobacco use.

Pregnancy Considerations
Management of hyperlipidemia and hypertension in pregnancy should avoid medications harmful to fetus: Statins, angiotensin-converting enzyme inhibitors (ACE-I), angiotensin-2 receptor blockers (ARBs). Aspirin should be avoided in first trimester of pregnancy. In general, any cardiovascular medication in pregnancy should be used cautiously, with a careful individual risk–benefit assessment.

GENERAL PREVENTION
- Atherosclerotic vascular disease accounts for the largest burden of CVD.
- At least 80% of CVD at middle and older age is potentially preventable with a desirable risk-factor profile in earlier life.
- Intensity of preventive effort should be commensurate with the individual's risk for CVD. The management of individuals with high risk for CVD approaches that of patients who have had clinical manifestations of the disease (secondary prevention).
- Physicians should lead in a societal effort to curb this epidemic by promoting:
  - Public areas free of smoking
  - Wide nutrient labeling in restaurants
  - Greater public access to space for exercise

EPIDEMIOLOGY
- In 2003, CVDs accounted for 29% of worldwide mortality. This true, chronic pandemic arises from changes in societal lifestyles.
- Men have a higher absolute risk for CVD at any age than do women. Conversely, risk from dying (case fatality) once disease manifests is higher for women until older age.
- CVDs have well-identified causal risk factors (see below) that permit effective prevention.

Incidence
At age 40, lifetime risk to develop clinical manifestations of coronary heart disease (CHD) is 1 in 2 for men and 1 in 3 for women. At age 70, it is 1 in 3 for men and 1 in 4 for women.

Prevalence
- Atherosclerotic plaque is present in most individuals in Westernized societies.
- Significant coronary intraluminal obstruction in asymptomatic individuals is higher with male gender and increasing age.
- Diabetes erases female advantage, increases plaque burden and risk for complications.

RISK FACTORS
- Major modifiable risk factors:
  - Smoking
  - Elevated low-density lipoprotein (LDL) cholesterol
  - Low high-density lipoprotein (HDL) cholesterol
  - Hypertension
  - Physical inactivity
  - Type 2 Diabetes (CHD risk equivalent)
  - Obesity, particularly abdominal
- Other risk factors:
  - Age: Male >50, Female >60
  - Early CHD onset in first-degree relatives: Males <55, females <65
  - Metabolic syndrome
  - Male gender
  - Low socioeconomic status
  - Diet high in saturated fat and sodium
  - Psychosocial factors (stress)
  - Left ventricular hypertrophy (LVH)
  - Hypertriglyceridemia
- Emerging risk factors:
  - Lipid: Lipoprotein(a); lipoprotein-associated phospholipase A_2; small and dense LDL; HDL subspecies; apolipoproteins B and A1; lipoprotein remnant particles; oxidized LDL
  - Thrombogenic: Fibrinogen; homocysteine; tPA-PAI-1; D-dimer
  - Inflammatory markers: High-sensitivity C-reactive protein (hsCRP) and others

Genetics
Atherosclerotic vascular disease is mostly the result of adverse lifestyle (largely determined by society trends) with variable individual susceptibility that can have some contribution from genetic disorders through specific risk factors (dyslipidemia, thrombogenesis). The contribution from genetic disorders to the whole burden of CV atherosclerotic disease is small.

PATHOPHYSIOLOGY
- The relation of blood pressure, LDL cholesterol, HDL cholesterol, and glucose with CVD is continuous and linear. The level at which risk appears in large observational studies is 115 mmHg for systolic blood pressure (BP), 150–160 mg/dL for total cholesterol, HbA_{1C} of 5%, body mass index (BMI) of 25.
- The basic pathophysiologic mechanism is atherothrombosis: A complex interaction of causal risk factors that leads to the formation of atheromatous plaque and its eventual rupture/erosion, with accompanying thrombotic occlusion of the involved artery. The acute/chronic manifestations of disease vary according to the location of the artery predominantly involved.
  - The threshold and goal for management of risk factors depends critically on overall individual cardiovascular risk.
  - The desirable risk-factor profile for asymptomatic young adults is a nonsmoking status; BP <120/80; total cholesterol <200 mg/dL; nondiabetic status, and BMI <25

ETIOLOGY
Atherosclerotic CVD is a multifactorial disorder that requires a comprehensive approach in its evaluation and management (see Risk Factors).

ASSOCIATED CONDITIONS
- Atherosclerotic CVD shares common risk factors with other chronic diseases such as type 2 diabetes, certain cancers (breast, prostate, esophagus, colon), and Alzheimer dementia
- Erectile dysfunction
- Chronic kidney dysfunction
- Nonalcoholic steatohepatitis

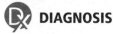 **DIAGNOSIS**

SIGNS AND SYMPTOMS
Asymptomatic in primary prevention

History
- Premature CVD in first-degree relatives
- Nutritional and physical activity habits
- Tobacco products exposure
- Weight fluctuation

Physical Exam
- BMI; waist measurement
- BP in both arms
- Xanthomas, xanthelasma, lipemia retinalis, arcus senilis
- Funduscopic exam: Retinal arteriolar narrowing, hypertensive or diabetic changes
- Carotid, abdominal, or femoral bruits

TESTS
Lab
- In all adults 20 years or older, a fasting lipoprotein profile: Total cholesterol, LDL-C, HDL-C, and triglycerides should be obtained once every 5 years.
- Fasting blood glucose, serum creatinine
- Microalbumin in urine
- Additional tests under validation:
  - Lipoprotein (a); apolipoproteins B and A1 (individuals with family history of early CHD)
  - hsCRP (individuals with intermediate risk category at 10 years; see below)
- Resting ECG
- Calculation of global CVD risk in 10 years with use of standardized formulas is paramount to determine candidacy and intensity of risk-factor management (see Framingham risk calculator reference).
  - High risk: >20%
  - Intermediate risk: 6–20%
  - Low risk: <6%

Imaging

- Individuals with intermediate risk by a global score can be tested for measures of subclinical atherosclerosis or evidence of inflammation to stratify further their risk (strategy currently under validation):
  - Coronary calcium score
  - B-Mode carotid ultrasonography for intima-media thickening
  - Ankle-brachial index (ABI)
  - Stress tests for myocardial ischemia and functional capacity

TREATMENT

GENERAL MEASURES

- Effective primary prevention of CVD requires both a whole-population approach as well as evaluation of the risk of individuals to tailor the intensity of preventive effort. Cost-effective analyses point to a greater number of DALYs prevented with the latter strategy. Instead of focusing on isolated levels of risk factors, the calculation of a global risk at 10 years is most appropriate to classify the person's candidacy and intensity of therapy.
  - Low risk (<6% at 10 years): Advice on a low-saturated fat, low-sodium, low-simple sugar, and high-fiber nutrition conducive to proper BMI; advice on 30 or more minutes of daily physical activity; avoidance of any tobacco exposure; counseling on stress management (therapeutic lifestyle changes, TLC).
  - Intermediate risk (6–20% at 10 years): In addition to TLC, current trend suggests further risk stratification with measures of subclinical atherosclerosis (see above) that could classify the presence of coronary calcium or IMT in the percentile for age and gender. This strategy (to be validated) could provide a "vascular age" indicator that would put individuals in a more accurate low- or high-risk group.
  - High risk (> 20% at 10 years): With emphasis on TLC, intense risk factor modification is pursued, with the use of medications to lower the level of risk factors to the range demonstrated in clinical trials to provide benefit. The benefit of medical therapy in this primary prevention group approximates that of secondary prevention patients, which underscores an arbitrary distinction in the continuous spectrum of risk in these groups of individuals.
- Therapeutic goals
  - Optimal levels of continuous risk factors (BP, LDL cholesterol, HDL cholesterol, glucose, BMI) have shifted recently toward lower (higher HDL-C) values in the normal distribution. The implication is that more individuals now occupy the borderline range, making them candidates for TLC. Simultaneously, evidence suggests that, in high-risk groups, achieving lower targets of the risk factor using TLC and medications has a superior preventive effect for CVD.
  - High risk (global risk >20%/10 years; diabetes; chronic kidney disease)
    - Nonsmoking status
    - BP <130/80
    - LDL-C <100 mg/dL (optional <70 ?)
    - HDL-C >40 mg/dL (optional >60 ?)
    - Triglycerides <150 mg/dL (optional <100 ?)

- Glucose <100 mg/dL (diabetics <120)
- HbA$_{1C}$ <6% (diabetics <7%)
- BMI <25
  - Intermediate risk (global risk 6–20%/10 years)
    - Nonsmoking status
    - BP <135/85
    - LDL-C <130 mg/dL
    - HDL-C, triglycerides, glucose, HbA$_{1C}$, BMI same goals as high-risk group
  - Low risk (global risk <6%/10 years)
    - Nonsmoking status
    - BP <140/90
    - LDL-C <160 mg/dL
    - HDL-C, triglycerides, glucose, HbA$_{1C}$, BMI same goals as high-risk group
- The use of medications in the intermediate- and low-risk groups is recommended when TLC does not achieve the risk-factor therapeutic goals after a reasonable interval (3–6 months in middle-aged and older individuals, 1–2 years in younger ages). Conversely, in high-risk individuals, consider starting medications earlier in management.

MEDICATION (DRUGS)

(First line *, second line **)
- Smoking cessation
  - First line
    - Nicotine replacement therapy
  - Second line
    - Bupropion
- Lipid management
  - First line
    - Statins
    - Fibrates
    - Nicotinic acid
  - Second line
    - Ezetimibe
    - Colesevelam
    - Cholestyramine
    - Cholestid
- Blood pressure management
  - First line
    - Thiazide diuretics
    - β-Blockers
    - ACE inhibitors
    - ARBs
    - Calcium channel blockers
  - Second line
    - Vasodilators (hydralazine, minoxidil)
    - Antiadrenergic drugs (clonidine, guanabenz, guanfacine, reserpine, α-methyl-dopa)
- Antiplatelet therapy (high- and intermediate-risk groups)
  - First line
    - Aspirin
  - Second line
    - Clopidogrel
    - Ticlopidine
- Omega 3-fatty acid supplementation (high-risk group needs further validation)

SURGERY

Surgery is only indicated in carefully selected individuals with obesity stage IV (BMI >40 or >35 with associated diseases).

 FOLLOW-UP

Periodic visits to monitor achievement of therapeutic goals in behavioral and physiological risk factors.

DISPOSITION
Issues for Referral
Refractory management of hypertension, dyslipidemia, obesity, and tobacco addiction should be referred to specialists.

PROGNOSIS
Global risk score calculation provides an effective tool to communicate individualized prognosis and potential for preventive action.

COMPLICATIONS
Periodically inquire for the development of angina, claudication, transient ischemic attacks, stroke, MI (especially intermediate- and high-risk groups).

PATIENT MONITORING
Home blood pressure monitoring with calibrated equipment can help in decision making for initiation and adjustment of medication.

REFERENCES
1. Framingham risk calculator: http://hp2010.nhlbihin.net/atpiii/calculator.asp
2. Grundy SM, et al. Primary prevention of CHD. *Circulation.* 1998;97:1876–1887.
3. Pasternak RC, et al. Identification of CHD risk: Is there a detection gap? *JACC.* 2003;41:1863–1874.
4. Pearson TA, et al. AHA guidelines for primary prevention of CV disease and stroke: 2002 update. *Circulation.* 2002;106:388–391.

CODES
ICD9-CM
- 401.0: Hypertension
- 272.0: Hypercholesterolemia
- 250.0: Diabetes
- 305.1: Tobacco abuse
- 278.0: Obesity

PATIENT TEACHING
TLC has greater impact when adopted by the whole family, particularly children, adolescents, and young adults.
Diet
Less consumption of red meat, high-fat dairy products, and fast food; higher intake of whole-grain cereals and breads, whole fruits, vegetables, and nuts
Activity
30-minute walk or similar most days of the week
Prevention
Optimal risk-factor profile in young adulthood can prevent more than 80% of CVDs and a substantial proportion of other chronic diseases.

FAQ
Q: If I start medications, will I have to take them forever?
A: Frequently, weight loss through appropriate nutrition and physical activity can decrease the dosage needed for BP medication or lipid-lowering drugs and possible discontinuation in some individuals.

Q: Is aspirin good for everybody in the prevention of CVD?
A: It is only appropriate when the global risk is intermediate or higher (≥6%/10 years). This is especially important in women, who often reach middle age with a low-risk status.

CARDIOVASCULAR PREVENTIVE CARE (SECONDARY PREVENTION)

Efrain Gaxiola
Jorge F. Trejo

 BASICS

DESCRIPTION
Secondary prevention aims to delay or avoid fatal and nonfatal cardiovascular (CV) events in those individuals that have previous clinical manifestations of CV disease.

GENERAL PREVENTION
- Patients with established coronary heart disease (CHD) have a high risk of subsequent CV events.
- Secondary prevention can extend overall survival, improve quality of life, decrease need for interventional procedures and reduce the incidence of subsequent CV events.
- Risk factor modification by therapeutic lifestyle changes (TLC) as well as drug therapy and revascularization can decrease morbidity and mortality in such patients.

ALERT
- Secondary prevention interventions remain underutilized despite compelling evidence and large magnitude of their benefit.
- The American College of Cardiology (ACC) and American Heart Association (AHA) urge all healthcare providers to implement systems that ensure the reliable identification of patients who can benefit from secondary prevention interventions and to ensure that these interventions occur.

Geriatric Considerations
Secondary prevention is effective in the elderly (>65 years old).

Pediatric Considerations
In those rare instances of children and adolescents with coronary artery disease it is critical to implement secondary prevention measures according to etiology (atherosclerosis, vasculitis, etc.).

Pregnancy Considerations
Medications used for secondary prevention that are contraindicated in pregnancy include:
- Angiotensin-converting enzyme (ACE) inhibitors
- Angiotensin-II receptor blockers (ARBs)
- Statins
- β-Blockers (not contraindicated, but caution is advised because they can depress vital signs in neonate and cause uterine vasoconstriction)
- Aspirin (potential risk of birth defect and bleeding risk in the first trimester safe in second and third trimester)
- Warfarin (embryopathy, especially between 6 and 12 weeks; central nervous system malformations during any time of gestation)

EPIDEMIOLOGY
- CV disease was the leading cause of death (29%) of the estimated 56 million people who died in 2000 worldwide.
- 12.6 million Americans have a history of myocardial infarction (MI) and/or angina.
- CV disease was the cause of 960,000 deaths in 1999, 47% male and 53% female
- $330 billion of total health care cost, $214 billion for heart disease

Incidence
- The annual incidence of MI in the United States is 650,000; annual incidence of stroke is 500,000.

- Less is known about the incidence of peripheral arterial disease (PAD). Many patients are asymptomatic and are recognized only once their disease has progressed to a severe state.

Prevalence
- It is estimated that overall prevalence of MI and stroke in the United States is 7.5 million and 4.6 million, respectively.
- The prevalence of PAD in the U.S. population older than 55 years is 10.5 million.

RISK FACTORS
Please see subsequent text under Etiology

Genetics
Single gene disorders have a small contribution in the pathogenesis of atherosclerosis, the predominant cause of CV disease.

PATHOPHYSIOLOGY
- Atherosclerosis leading to obstruction of the arterial lumen by plaque, thrombosis/hemorrhage on plaque rupture/erosion and arterial vasomotor abnormalities
- Imbalance in the blood supply-demand in the arterial territory affected by atherosclerotic plaque

ETIOLOGY
- Atherothrombosis is the fundamental disease process that accounts for most of CV disease burden. This chronic disorder is the result of the interaction of multiple factors that operate since early life in the womb. The causal risk factors that are susceptible to modification and capable of offering benefit in secondary prevention include:
  - Cigarette smoking
  - Hypertension
  - Dyslipidemia
  - Type 2 diabetes
  - Physical inactivity
  - Obesity (particularly abdominal)
  - Psychosocial factors (stress)
- Clinical factors that increase the risk for subsequent CV events
  - Left ventricular hypertrophy (LVH)
  - Systolic dysfunction (ejection fraction <50%)
  - Diastolic dysfunction
  - Myocardial ischemia
  - Ventricular arrhythmias

ASSOCIATED CONDITIONS
- Erectile dysfunction
- Chronic kidney dysfunction
- Obesity and related disorders
  - Obstructive sleep apnea
  - Nonalcoholic steatohepatitis/liver cirrhosis

 DIAGNOSIS

SIGNS AND SYMPTOMS
- Coronary: Shortness of breath; chest pain on effort or at rest; syncope
- Peripheral: Upper and lower extremity pain on effort; postprandial abdominal pain; acute onset of painful and cold extremity
- Cerebrovascular: Sudden onset of paresthesia or weakness, particularly unilateral; headache; aphasia; diplopia; amaurosis fugax; ataxia; progressive cognitive dysfunction

History
- Any symptom related to physical activity should be suspected to have CV origin
  - Periodic inquiry regarding angina, dyspnea, claudication, and TIA-related symptoms/signs
- Assessment of functional capacity (New York Heart or Canadian Heart Classification)

Physical Exam
- Waist circumference, body mass index
- Blood pressure and pulses in both arms (asymmetry can indicate subclavian/humeral arterial obstruction)
- Carotid palpation and auscultation (carotid sinus hypersensitivity, bruits, quality of upstroke)
- Jugular vein examination: Central venous pressure (CHF); wave-type predominance
- Precordial exam: Apical and left lower sternal border (LLSB) palpation; intensity of first and second heart sounds; type of second sound splitting; presence of third heart sound (S3) (LV or RV systolic dysfunction) and fourth heart sound (S4) (LV or RV diastolic dysfunction)
- Lung exam: Crackles, pleural effusion
- Abdomen: Pulsatile mass, bruits
- Peripheral pulse amplitude, bruits

TESTS
Lab
- Fasting lipid profile: Total cholesterol, HDL cholesterol (HDL-C), triglycerides, and calculated LDL cholesterol (LDL-C)
- Fasting blood glucose, HbA1c
- Microalbumin in urine
- Blood cell count, creatinine, potassium, thyroid stimulating hormone (TSH)
- Periodic resting electrocardiogram (ECG) [monitoring of silent myocardial infarction (MI)]

Imaging
- Chest x-ray to determine heart size, pulmonary venous hypertension, pleural effusion
- Echocardiography for evaluation of systolic and diastolic function evolution; LVH
- Stress echocardiography, myocardial perfusion imaging or stress magnetic resonance imaging (MRI) when there is clinical indication (angina; unexplained deterioration of functional capacity)
- Computed tomographic, cardiac angiography to investigate patency of coronary artery bypass grafts; presence and degree of coronary artery intraluminal obstructions in patients with noncoronary vascular disease (strategy under validation)

Diagnostic Procedures/Surgery
- Left-sided heart catheterization with coronary angiography in those patients with angina on maximal medical therapy, especially with LV systolic dysfunction
- Myocardial revascularization via percutaneous or surgical approach can improve angina/survival in selected patients with myocardial ischemia
- Automatic implantable cardiac defibrillator improves survival in patients post-MI with ejection fraction $\leq$30%
- Cardiac resynchronization therapy improves functional capacity and survival in patients with CHF stages III–IV of New York Heart Association classification on maximal medical therapy

TREATMENT

GENERAL MEASURES
Aggressive modification of risk factors in high-risk patients produces risk reductions of up to 50%.

Goals for Secondary Prevention (AHA/ACC Guidelines):
- Complete smoking cessation
- Physical activity:
  - A symptom-limited exercise test in selected patients before starting an exercise program
  - Exercise: >30 minutes per day, >3–4 times per week
  - Exercise should involve an aerobic activity such as walking, jogging, or cycling.
- Weight management:
  - Body mass index (BMI) 18.5 to 24.9 kg/m^2
  - Waist <40 inches (102 cm) in men and <35 inches (89 cm) in women
- Dietary
  - Total caloric intake must be balanced with energy expenditure
  - Minimize intake of saturated and *trans* fats as well as rapidly digested carbohydrates. Instead, select monosaturated and polyunsaturated fats and whole grains
  - Maximize fruit and vegetable intake
  - Adequate intake of omega-3 fatty acids appears to reduce the incidence of CV disease and especially sudden death in patients postmyocardial infarction. Inclusion of 2 or 3 servings of fish per week, particularly fatty fish, may help prevent cardiovascular events.
- Hypertension
  - <130/80 mmHg: Diabetics
  - <130/85 mmHg: Heart failure or renal insufficiency
  - <140/90 mmHg: All others
  - The choice of antihypertensive therapy is determined in part by coexisting features:
    - Previous MI: β-Blocker and, in most cases, an ACE inhibitor or ARBs
    - Stable angina: β-Blocker or calcium channel blocker
- Hyperlipidemia
  - LDL-C: <100 mg/dL; (optional <70 mg/dL for "very high risk")
  - HDL-C: >40 mg/dL (optional >60)
  - Triglycerides: <150 mg/dL (optional <100)
  - Non-HDL-C: <130 mgl/dL
- Diabetes mellitus
- Fasting blood glucose <126 mg/dL and HbA1c <7%

MEDICATION (DRUGS)

- Aspirin: 75 to 325 mg per day
  - Reduces CV risk by approximately 22%
- Clopidogrel: 75 mg per day is an alternative to aspirin
  - Clopidogrel in addition to aspirin is beneficial in patients with a non-ST elevation acute coronary syndrome; postcoronary artery stent implantation, and probably in most patients with an ST-elevation MI.
- Warfarin: Dose needed to achieve international normalized ratio (INR) 2–3

- Although more effective than antiplatelet therapy to prevent recurrent CV events, the higher bleeding rate precludes its routine use in CHD unless patient has:
  - Atrial fibrillation
  - Left ventricular thrombus
  - Extensive regional wall motion abnormality
- Statins: Dose usually needed to achieve LDL-C goal:
  - Atorvastatin = ≥10 mg
  - Lovastatin = ≥40 mg
  - Pravastatin = ≥40 mg
  - Simvastatin = ≥20 mg
  - Fluvastatin = ≥40 mg
  - Rosuvastatin = ≥5 mg
  - Combination of a statin with ezetimibe, 10 mg daily can help achieve target LDL-C
- β-Blockers
  - Improve survival; start in all post-MI and acute ischemic syndrome patients or heart failure due to systolic dysfunction
  - Continue indefinitely; observe usual contraindications
  - Use as needed to manage angina, rhythm, or blood pressure in all other patients.
- ACE inhibitors or ARBs:
  - Treat indefinitely in post-MI patients; use in stable high-risk patients (anterior MI, previous MI, Killip class II [S$_3$ gallop, rales, radiographic CHF]; consider chronic therapy for all other patients with coronary or other vascular disease unless contraindicated
  - Slow the rate of progression of chronic kidney dysfunction

FOLLOW-UP

It is important to implement systems that ensure the reliable identification of patients who can benefit from secondary prevention interventions and to ensure, with proper follow-up, that these interventions occur.

Issues for Referral
Patients with lipid disorders that are complex or refractory to treatment should be referred to a specialist.

PROGNOSIS
- Patients with a history of MI have 5- to 7-fold greater risk of MI or CV death, a 3- to 4-fold greater risk of stroke or transient ischemic attack (TIA), and 4- to 6-fold risk of sudden cardiac death.
- Patients with a history of stroke have a 2- to 3-fold greater risk of MI, angina or CV death, and a 9-fold greater risk of stroke.
- Patients with a history of PAD have a 4-fold greater risk of experiencing a fatal MI or other CV death, and a 2- to 3-fold greater risk of experiencing a stroke or TIA.
- Male patients with symptomatic PAD have mortality rates of 62% after 10 years, compared with 16.9% in general population. The mortality rates for women are 33.3% and 11.6%, respectively.

COMPLICATIONS
- Coronary
  - Angina: Congestive heart failure; myocardial infarction; sudden cardiac death
- Peripheral vascular
  - Claudication; abdominal angina; embolism
- Cerebrovascular
  - Stroke; TIA; dementia

PATIENT MONITORING
Home monitoring of the following variables can help substantially in the proper management of risk factors that have impact on recurrent CV events:
Weight; waist size; blood pressure; glucose; number of steps per day (pedometer); calories, total fat, carbohydrate, protein consumption (point system of Weight Watchers)

REFERENCES
1. Smith SC Jr, Blair SN, Bonow RO, et al. AHA/ACC Scientific Statement: AHA/ACC guidelines for preventing heart attack and death in patients with atherosclerotic cardiovascular disease: 2001 update: A statement for healthcare professionals from the American Heart Association and the American College of Cardiology. *Circulation*. 2001;104:1577.
2. Grundy SM, Cleeman JI, Merz CN, et al. Implications of recent clinical trials for the National Cholesterol Education Program Adult Treatment Panel III guidelines. *Circulation*. 2004;110:227.
3. Eng-Ceceña L, Gaxiola-López E. Secondary prevention. In: *Treatment of Q-wave Acute Myocardial Infarction*, 1st ed. Plac Cardio-3, Sociedad Mexicana de Cardiología-Soc. Interamericana de Cardiología. México, Intersistemas SA de CV. 2001;153–178.

MISCELLANEOUS

- Internet sites:
  - www.americanheart.org
  - www.acc.org and www.cardiosource.com
  - www.nhlbi.nih.gov

CODES
ICD9-CM
- 413.9 Stable Angina
- 410.72 Acute non–ST subsequent care MI
- 434.91 Stroke
- 435.3 TIA vertebrobasilar
- 362.34 TIA retinal
- 443.9 Claudication
- 433.10 Carotid artery disease
- 441.4 Abdominal aortic aneurysm
- 290.40 Vascular dementia

PATIENT TEACHING
See Goals of Secondary Prevention

FAQ
Q. What are the most cost-effective measures in secondary prevention?
A. Aspirin and off-patent β-blocker, ACE-I, and statin therapy
Q. Is moderate alcohol drinking a good measure for secondary prevention?
A. Available data do not support encouraging individuals, with or without CHD, who abstain or who drink only occasionally to initiate regular drinking. The presumed benefit of moderate alcohol intake (20% reduction in mortality) is observational evidence that has a widespread study design flaw: The mix of abstainers with previous alcohol users in risk analysis, potentially producing a biased benefit of alcohol use.

CAROTID SINUS SYNDROME

Priya Pillutla
Benoy J. Zachariah

 BASICS

DESCRIPTION
One of the neurally mediated syncopal syndromes characterized by bradycardia and/or hypotension in response to carotid sinus pressure

EPIDEMIOLOGY
• More common in the elderly
• Males > females
• Accounts for 10–20% of presyncopal and syncopal episodes

PATHOPHYSIOLOGY
• Possible mechanisms
  – Abnormalities of the carotid sinus receptors and the medullary cardiovascular centers have all been suggested as possible mechanisms
  – Increased acetylcholine release
  – Increased responsiveness to acetycholine
  – Hypersensitive baroreceptors
  – Failure of baroreceptor feedback mechanisms
  – Dissociation between the afferent signals arising from the sternomastoid muscles and the carotid sinus

ASSOCIATED CONDITIONS
• Coronary and carotid atherosclerosis
• Head and neck cancer

 DIAGNOSIS

SIGNS AND SYMPTOMS
• Dizziness
• Lightheadedness
• Falls
• Syncope; sometimes associated with head turning or with tight collars

TESTS
Carotid Sinus Pressure (CSP)
• Check for carotid bruits first; pressure should not be applied in patient with prior carotid endarterectomy, transient ischemic attack, or stroke.
• Gentle pressure applied to the carotid sinus region for 3–5 seconds.
• A *cardioinhibitory* response is defined as ventricular asystole of >3 seconds and a *vasodepressor* response as ≥50 mmHg in systolic blood pressure without associated bradycardia, or a ≥30 mmHg or more decrease with reproduced symptoms. Most patients have varying combinations of both responses.
• Correlating asystole with the patient's symptoms is important because carotid sinus hypersensitivity (>3-second pause) can be present in about 4% of the healthy elderly population.
• CSP should be determined both supine and upright with continuous electrocardiogram (ECG) and blood pressure monitoring.
• The bradycardia may be only relatively inappropriate to the severity of hypotension.
  Tilt table testing, ambulatory ECG monitoring, electroencephalography, vascular studies, and electrophysiologic studies may be required to exclude other causes of syncope.

DIFFERENTIAL DIAGNOSIS
• Sick sinus syndrome
• Atrioventricular block secondary to conduction tissue disease
• Tachyarrhythmias
• Vasovagal syndromes
• Postural hypotension
• Aortic stenosis
• Seizure disorders
• Transient ischemic attacks
• Falls due to neuromuscular or musculoskeletal disorders

 TREATMENT

GENERAL MEASURES
• Avoid tight collars, neckties, and sudden head turning.
• Avoid vasodilator (e.g., calcium channel blockers) and vagomimetic (e.g., digoxin) medications.
• Elastic support hose may help.
• Tilt training
• Volume expansion, salt intake
Pacing
• Dual-chamber pacing prevents bradycardia in the cardioinhibitory form of the disorder.
• Patients often remain symptomatic from the vasodilatory component, which is more difficult to treat. Rate-drop response pacing (bradycardia triggers relatively rapid pacing for a few minutes) may blunt the hypotensive response.
• Cardiac pacing is of no benefit in the vasodepressor forms of carotid sinus syndrome

MEDICATION (DRUGS)

- β-Blockers, disopyramide, serotonin reuptake inhibitors (fluoxetine, sertraline), vasoconstrictors (midodrine), and sodium-retaining drugs (fludrocortisone) have been tried.
- Response varies and large-scale clinical trials are lacking.

FOLLOW-UP

PROGNOSIS

- Frequency of symptoms is variable, and the severity will depend on the extent of the vasodilatory response.
- In severe cases not responding to pacing or pharmacologic measures, radiation therapy or surgical denervation of the carotid sinus may be required.

COMPLICATIONS

- Injuries related to syncope/falls
- Rarely, sudden death from asystole

PATIENT MONITORING

- If a pacemaker is implanted, evaluate after 1 week, then at 1 month, and every 6 months thereafter.
- Many patients have associated carotid and coronary atherosclerosis, which require monitoring.
- Consider driving restrictions

REFERENCES

1. Benditt DG. Neurally mediated syncopal syndromes: pathophysiological concepts and clinical evaluation. *Pacing Clin Electrophysiol*. 1997;20:572–584.
2. Benditt DG, Fahy GJ, Lurie KG, et al. Pharmacotherapy of neurally mediated syncope. *Circulation*. 1999;100:1242–1248.
3. Benditt DG, Sutton R, Gammage MD, et al. Clinical experience with Thera DR rate-drop response pacing algorithm in carotid sinus syndrome and vasovagal syncope. The International Rate-Drop Investigators Group. *Pacing Clin Electrophysiol*. 1997;20:832–839.
4. Braunwald E, ed. *Heart Disease: A Textbook of Cardiovascular Medicine*, 5th ed. Philadelphia: WB Saunders,1997.
5. Jeffreys M, Wood DA, Lampe F, et al. The heart rate response to carotid artery massage in a sample of healthy elderly people. *Pacing Clin Electrophysiol*. 1996;19:1488–1492.

CODES
ICD9-CM
337.0 Carotid body or sinus syndrome

C

CEREBROVASCULAR DISEASE

Sanjiv J. Shah
Benoy J. Zachariah

 BASICS

DESCRIPTION

- Stroke: The sudden onset of focal neurologic deficit resulting from either infarction or hemorrhage within the brain.
- Transient ischemic attack (TIA): The sudden onset of focal neurologic deficit, usually resulting from atherothrombosis or embolism, which resolves completely within 24 hours.

EPIDEMIOLOGY

- Cerebrovascular disease affects 0.2–0.3% of the U.S. population each year.
- 731,000 strokes occur annually in the United States; there are 4 million stroke survivors.
- Cerebrovascular disease is the third leading cause of death in the United States.
Predominant Age: older than 65 years
Predominant Sex: Men are affected more than women.

RISK FACTORS

- Ischemic Stroke
- Age
- Hypertension
- Smoking
- Diabetes mellitus
- Hyperlipidemia
- Hyperhomocysteinemia
- Family history
- Coronary artery disease

ETIOLOGY

Ischemic Stroke

- Carotid atherosclerosis with *in situ* thrombosis or artery-to-artery embolism
- Cardiogenic embolus: Mitral valve disease (especially stenosis), atrial fibrillation, myocardial infarction (MI), left ventricular (LV) aneurysm, cardiomyopathy, prosthetic valves, endocarditis
- Hypercoagulable states: Antiphospholipid antibodies; oral contraceptives; factor V Leiden mutation; deficiency of protein C, protein S, and antithrombin III
- Hemoglobinopathies
- Carotid dissection
- Cerebral venous thrombosis
- Vasculitis
- Drugs: Cocaine, amphetamines
Intracranial Hemorrhage
- Hypertension
- Anticoagulation, antiplatelet, and fibrinolytic treatment
- Vascular malformations: Atrioventricular (AV) malformation, angiomas, berry aneurysm, Moya Moya disease
- Amyloid angiopathy
- Trauma

ASSOCIATED CONDITIONS

- Coronary artery disease
- Peripheral vascular disease

 DIAGNOSIS

SIGNS AND SYMPTOMS

- Headache, seizures, altered sensorium
- Carotid territory: Aphasia; hemiplegia; hemianesthesia; hemianopia; neglect; confusion; amnesia; monocular blindness; paralysis of gaze; and difficulty in reading, writing, and calculating
- Vertebrobasilar territory: Vertigo, ataxia, diplopia, nystagmus, quadrantanopia, dysarthria, facial weakness, dysphagia, Horner syndrome, hemiplegia, hemianesthesia
- The finding of ≥1 of the following: Acute facial paralysis, arm drift, and/or abnormal speech, has a likelihood ratio of 5.5 for the diagnosis of stroke. The absence of all three has a likelihood ratio of 0.39.

TESTS

- Anticardiolipin antibodies and lupus anticoagulant
- Assays for protein C and S
- Antithrombin III
- Factor V Leiden mutation
- Hemoglobin electrophoresis
- Holter monitor

Lab

CBC, glucose, electrolytes, urinalysis, ABG (atrial blood gas), international normalized ratio (INR), partial thromboplastin time (PTT), electrocardiogram (ECG), chest X-ray

Imaging

- Computed tomographic (CT) scan (emergent study of choice)
- Magnetic resonance imaging (MRI)/magnetic resonance angiography
- Carotid ultrasonography
- Transthoracic or transesophageal echocardiography
- Cerebral and vertebral angiography

DIFFERENTIAL DIAGNOSIS

- Demyelinating disease
- Postictal paralysis
- Tumor
- Abscess
- Encephalitis
- Metabolic disturbances (especially hypoglycemia)
- Migraine
- Psychogenic weakness

 TREATMENT

GENERAL MEASURES

Ischemic Stroke

- Rapid evaluation for possible thrombolysis is essential.
  - Intravenous tissue plasminogen activator (t-PA 0.9 mg/kg, 10% as a bolus and the remainder over 1 hour) administered within 3 hours of ischemic stroke onset improves functional outcome without an increase in overall mortality, despite an increase in the incidence of intracerebral hemorrhage.
  - A large infarct, as evidenced by extensive neurologic deficits or early changes on CT scan, predict an increased risk of bleeding.
  - A CT scan to exclude hemorrhage is mandatory prior to treatment.
  - Strict inclusion and exclusion criteria have been defined.
  - Intravenous thrombolysis more than 3 hours after symptom onset is not beneficial and is probably harmful.
  - Intraarterial thrombolysis might be an option up to 6 hours after symptom onset; research studies are ongoing.
  - Patients who have received t-PA should not be given intravenous heparin, aspirin, ticlopidine, clopidogrel, or Coumadin for 24 hours.
  - Aspirin (ASA) therapy at presentation is not a contraindication for thrombolysis. Thrombolysis is contraindicated if INR >1.7.
- Heparin: Intravenous heparin use is controversial, and although widely used, it does not decrease stroke severity. It may prevent recurrent embolic strokes and may be useful in hypercoagulable states, but it should not be used outside of these settings. If used, heparin should be started without a bolus at 15–18 U/kg/hour; target PTT is 1.5 times control. Massive hemispheric stroke and PTT more than twice control predispose to hemorrhagic transformation. Heparinoids have not shown any benefit.
- Antiplatelet agents: ASA 300–325 mg/day provides a modest benefit in preventing early stroke recurrence when used in acute ischemic stroke; whether it decreases stroke severity is uncertain. Studies of other antiplatelet agents are ongoing.
- Cerebral edema (peaks 3–5 days after onset) should be treated with mannitol or intubation with hyperventilation.
- Seizure prophylaxis with phenytoin for patients with large infarcts
- Admit patient to stroke unit if possible: Patients have fewer complications and better outcomes.
- Monitor cardiac rhythm for 48 hours.
- Blood pressure is often elevated at presentation; most experts recommend against acutely lowering the blood pressure because autoregulation is often defective and stroke severity may be worsened.

– Hypertension should be treated if there is ongoing cardiac ischemia, severe (systolic blood pressure >220 mmHg, diastolic >120 mmHg) or malignant hypertension, aortic dissection, or in those receiving t-PA. Blood pressure should be gradually lowered to 170–180 mmHg systolic and 95–100 mmHg diastolic.

– Angiotensin-converting enzyme inhibitors and β-blockers (including labetalol) are the preferred agents.

• If patients are immobile, they should have deep venous thrombosis (DVT)/PE (pulmonary embolism) prophylaxis.

• Institute feeding early. Patients with dysphagia should be fed through a soft feeding tube and should have gastrostomy early if dysphagia persists.

• Hyperglycemia and fever worsen outcome and should be treated aggressively.

Intracranial Hemorrhage

• Admit to intensive care.

• Ensure airway protection and adequate oxygenation.

• Hypertension should be treated aggressively.

• Intracranial pressure (ICP) monitoring for patients with suspected elevated ICP, deteriorating level of consciousness, Glasgow coma score <9.

• Reduce elevated ICP with mannitol or hyperventilation. Neuromuscular paralysis and barbiturate coma are other options; keep ICP <20 mmHg and cerebral perfusion pressure >70 mmHg.

• Ventricular drains for patients with hydrocephalus

• Seizure prevention with phenytoin

• Surgical evacuation of the hematoma for patients with cerebellar hemorrhage (emergent), subdural or epidural hemorrhages, associated structural lesions such as an aneurysm, AV malformations (if surgically accessible and likely to have a good outcome), and in young patients with large lobar hemorrhage who are deteriorating.

– DVT prophylaxis with compression boots
– Early institution of feeding
– Physical therapy, speech therapy, and occupational therapy as soon as possible

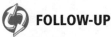 **FOLLOW-UP**

PROGNOSIS

• Ischemic stroke: 1/3 die within a year, 1/3 remain permanently disabled, and 1/3 make a reasonable recovery.

• Intracranial hemorrhage: 35–50% die within a month (half of them in the first 2 days); 20% live independently at 6 months.

COMPLICATIONS

• Death
• DVT/PE
• Hemorrhagic transformation of ischemic strokes
• Pneumonia
• Decubital ulcers
• Residual neurologic deficits
• Contractures

PATIENT MONITORING

• Should be individualized
• Concomitant coronary artery disease (CAD) and PVD (peripheral vascular disease) are common and should be addressed.

REFERENCES

1. Adams H, Adams R, Del Zoppo G, et al. Guidelines for the early management of patients with ischemic stroke: 2005 guidelines update. A scientific statement from the Stroke Council of the American Heart Association/American Stroke Association. *Stroke*. 2005;36:916–923.
2. Broderick JP, Adams HP Jr, Barsan W, et al. Guidelines for the management of spontaneous intracerebral hemorrhage: A statement for healthcare professionals from a special writing group of the Stroke Council, American Heart Association. *Stroke*. 1999;30:905–915.
3. Brott T, Bogousslavsky J. Treatment of acute ischemic stroke. *N Engl J Med*. 2000;343:710–722.
4. Coull BM, Williams LS, Goldstein LB, et al. Anticoagulants and antiplatelet agents in acute ischemic stroke: Report of the Joint Stroke Guideline Development Committee of the American Academy of Neurology and the American Stroke Association (a division of the American Heart Association). *Stroke*. 2002;33:1934–1942.
5. Goldstein LB, Simel DL. Is this patient having a stroke? *JAMA*. 2005;293:2391–2402.
6. Johnston SC. Clinical practice. Transient ischemic attack. *N Engl J Med*. 2002;347:1687–1692.
7. Qureshi AI, Tuhrim S, Broderick JP, et al. Spontaneous intracerebral hemorrhage. *N Engl J Med*. 2001;344:1450–1460.
8. Warlow C, Sudlow C, Dennis M, et al. Stroke. *Lancet*. 2003;362:1211–1224.

CODES

ICD9-CM

• 436 Disease, cerebrovascular acute
• 431 Hemorrhage, cerebral
• 435.9 TIA

PATIENT TEACHING

Organization
National Stroke Association, 96 Inverness Drive, E # I, Englewood, CO 80112

Prevention

• Ischemic Stroke

– Control hypertension: Target blood pressure is <140/90 mmHg.

– Nonvalvular atrial fibrillation: Warfarin for those at high risk (history of hypertension, diabetes, heart failure, prior TIA or stroke, age >60 years); ASA 325 mg/day for low-risk patients

– Hyperlipidemia: For those with CAD and hyperlipidemia and no prior stroke, lipid lowering with statins reduces stroke risk. Treatment is also recommended for stroke patients with hyperlipidemia and following carotid endarterectomy, even if they do not have a history of CAD. Whether lipid lowering should be attempted for stroke prevention in patients without a history of CAD or stroke is unclear; these patients may need to be treated for CAD prevention anyway.

– Smoking is a significant risk factor for a first stroke, recurrent stroke, and restenosis following carotid endarterectomy. Cessation reduces risk of recurrent stroke by about half.

– Diabetes: Tight control reduces the risk of microvascular complications. A beneficial effect on ischemic stroke has not been conclusively demonstrated.

– Antiplatelet agents

• ASA reduces stroke risk following TIA, ischemic stroke, and carotid endarterectomy; 81 mg/day is as effective as higher doses.

• Clopidogrel 75 mg/day is indicated for those who cannot take ASA.

• The optimal treatment for recurrent stroke despite ASA is unclear; options include the addition of warfarin, clopidogrel, or dipyridamole. A recent study found combined ASA 325 mg and sustained-release dipyridamole 200 mg b.i.d. to be better than ASA or dipyridamole alone. ASA does not offer significant protection against a first ischemic stroke in low-risk patients. A recent meta-analysis found that dipyridamole with or without aspirin reduced the risk of recurrent stroke.

– Warfarin reduces stroke risk following MI or a first ischemic stroke; it is recommended for patients who cannot have an antiplatelet agent and for 3–6 months following a large anterior wall MI.

– Carotid endarterectomy (CEA): Indicated for patients with TIAs or nondisabling stroke and 70–99% ipsilateral stenosis. Symptomatic patients with 50–69% stenosis and asymptomatic patients with a life expectancy of >5 years who have >60% stenosis have a modest reduction in stroke incidence.

– Carotid angioplasty/stenting: According to the recent SAPPHIRE trial, stenting was noninferior to CEA in patients with severe carotid artery stenosis and comorbid conditions that made CEA high-risk.

– The optimal preventive strategy for symptomatic patients with ascending aortic arch atheroma or patent foramen ovale is uncertain. Most experts recommend anticoagulation with warfarin.

– Postmenopausal hormone replacement probably does not reduce risk of stroke.

• Intracranial Hemorrhage

– Control hypertension.

– Careful monitoring of anticoagulated patients

– Careful selection of patients for anticoagulation and thrombolytic therapy when these are indicated.

– Avoid heavy alcohol use.

– Increase consumption of fruits and vegetables (recommendation based on epidemiologic data).

CHAGAS DISEASE AND THE HEART

Chandan Devireddy

 BASICS

DESCRIPTION

Multiple clinical syndromes including acute Chagas disease and chronic Chagas disease, both resulting from infection with the protozoan parasite *Trypanosoma cruzi*

- Multiple presentations including acute and chronic myocarditis with potentially devastating effects on conduction, myocyte function, and myocardial architecture
- Acute Chagas myocarditis demonstrates focal myocytolytic necrosis and degeneration with an intense mononuclear infiltrate and parasitism of myofibers.
- An intermediate clinically silent phase of up to 10–30 years
- Chronic Chagas heart disease, however, presents with focal and diffuse chronic fibrosing myocarditis with accompanied lymphomononuclear infiltrate and no evidence of active parasitism.
- Destruction of the parasympathetic nervous system and loss of cardiac innervation is always seen.

Case Definition Criteria for Diagnosis
- History of residence where Chagas disease is endemic, unequivocally positive serologic test for *T. cruzi*, clinical syndrome compatible with Chagas heart disease, no evidence of another cardiac disorder to account for findings.

EPIDEMIOLOGY

Natural reservoirs of *T. cruzi* from the central United States to southern Argentina are thought to be the source.

- Estimated 15–20 million people infected worldwide with >65 million people at risk of infection
- Countries with highest incidence: Brazil, Argentina, Chile, Bolivia, and Venezuela
- Most common cause of dilated cardiomyopathy and significant cause of cardiovascular death in endemic countries, *T. cruzi* infection acquired in the United States is almost nonexistent. However, it is estimated that approximately 400,000 infected immigrants reside in the United States.

RISK FACTORS

Geographic prevalence, rural substandard housing secondary to facilitation of Reduviid breeding

ETIOLOGY

- The parasite is transmitted to humans via bloodsucking insects of the Reduviidae family (assassin bugs) through contaminated feces at the site of the blood meal.
- It is also possibly congenitally transmitted in chronic maternal infection or through blood transfusion.

ASSOCIATED CONDITIONS

Chronic manifestations include megadisease of the esophagus or colon.

 DIAGNOSIS

SIGNS AND SYMPTOMS

Acute Chagas Disease and Myocarditis
- Only 1% develop clinically evident acute myocarditis.
- Incubation period lasts at least 1 week.
- Localized erythema and induration at site of bite (chagoma), fever, generalized lymphadenopathy, hepatosplenomegaly, chest pain/discomfort (ischemic or atypical in quality), tachycardia, arrhythmia/palpitations, local periorbital swelling (Romaña sign)

Chronic Chagas Disease and Cardiomyopathy
- Chronic cardiac involvement in 30–60%
- Fatigue, arrhythmia/palpitations, sudden death, dizziness/presyncope, chest pain/discomfort (ischemic or atypical in quality), shortness of breath, dyspnea on exertion, orthopnea, paroxysmal nocturnal dyspnea, lower extremity edema, transient ischemic attacks/stroke, thromboembolic phenomena, chagasic megaesophagus (dysphagia, regurgitation), chagasic megacolon (constipation, abdominal pain, obstruction)

TESTS

- Electrocardiogram (ECG)
  - Traditional mainstay of diagnosis of chagasic cardiac involvement
  - Involvement of conduction system ubiquitous with cardiac involvement
  - Characteristically right bundle branch block or left anterior fascicular block signifies underlying myocarditis.
  - Complete heart block, atrioventricular conduction abnormalities, and ectopy can be seen. Left bundle branch block is uncommon.
  - Abnormalities resembling myocardial infarction or ischemia may be prominent in advanced disease.

Lab
- Gold standard is xenodiagnosis (culture using actual insect vector), not commonly used.
  - Examine buffy coat of blood for motile trypanosomes in acute disease.
- Serologic testing mainstay of chronic clinical diagnosis
  - Immunoglobulin G (IgG) antibodies to *T. cruzi* trypomastigote antigens
  - Antibodies appear within 3–6 weeks of infection and remain for life.
  - Titer does not correlate with severity of infection.

Imaging
- Two-dimensional (2D) Doppler echocardiography or angiography
  - Hallmark finding of marked segmental ventricular wall motion abnormalities (hypokinesis or akinesis)
  - Narrow neck aneurysm involving localized area of left ventricular (LV) apex with normal surroundings (50% of patients)
  - May resemble segmental changes of ischemic cardiac disease; LV or apical thrombus

DIFFERENTIAL DIAGNOSIS

Toxoplasmosis, viral myocarditis (Coxsackie virus, HIV, cytomegalovirus), postpartum cardiomyopathy, alcoholic cardiomyopathy, endomyocardial fibrosis, ischemic cardiomyopathy, idiopathic cardiomyopathy, toxic cardiomyopathy (anthracycline, cobalt, etc.), neuromuscular dystrophies, hemochromatosis, amyloidosis, sarcoidosis, Kawasaki disease, arrhythmogenic cardiomyopathy, Lyme carditis, eosinophilic myocarditis

 ## TREATMENT

GENERAL MEASURES

- Antitrypanosomal therapy exists for acute Chagas disease (active parasitemia) with evidence for cure and prevention of development of sequelae of chronic manifestations.
- Patients with negative serology after treatment of acute disease can be considered cured.
- Management of chronic cardiomyopathy primarily supportive to treat and prevent complications of congestive heart failure, thromboembolism, arrhythmogenic events, and cardiac conduction abnormalities

 ## MEDICATION (DRUGS)

First Line

- Nifurtimox 10 mg/kg/day in 3 doses for up to 60–120 days and benzimidazole 5 mg/kg/day for up to 60 days act as trypanosomal antimetabolic agents.
  - Drugs available from U.S. Centers for Disease Control and Prevention
  - For use only in acute Chagas disease; transfusion-acquired disease; reactivation in immunosuppressed patients
- Supportive regimens identical to those for congestive heart failure, arrhythmic events, and thromboembolism

Contraindications

- Potential mutagenicity in children

Precautions

- Refer to manufacturer's profile.
- Gastrointestinal toxicity for nifurtimox
- Leukopenia and polyneuritis side effects for both regimens

SURGERY

No specific measures exist for Chagas disease.

 ## FOLLOW-UP

DISPOSITION

Admission Criteria

No specific indications

PROGNOSIS

- No treatment proven to halt progressive myocardial damage in chronic Chagasic cardiomyopathy
- Overall mortality best predicted by LV function
- Strong predictors for mortality include LV dilatation, presence of aneurysm, and development of heart disease at an early age.

PATIENT MONITORING

Periodic clinical evaluation in addition to relevant testing (ECG, echocardiography) to monitor for signs of cardiac disease

REFERENCES

Alexander RW, et al., eds. *Hurst's the Heart,* 9th ed. New York: McGraw-Hill,1998.

Hagar JM, Rahimtoola SH. Chagas heart disease. *Curr Probl Cardiol*. 1995;20:827–924.

Rossi MA, Bestetti RB. The challenge of chagasic cardiomyopathy. *Cardiology*. 1995;86:1–7.

CODES

ICD9-CM

- 422.90 Acute myocarditis, unspecified
- 425.4 Idiopathic cardiomyopathy
- 429.0 Myocarditis, unspecified

C

CHEMOTHERAPY AND THE HEART

Sanjiv J. Shah

 BASICS

DESCRIPTION
- Cardiomyopathy:
  - Cardiomyopathy secondary to chemotherapy is most commonly associated with doxorubicin (Adriamycin), but also has been reported with other anthracycline agents such as daunorubicin and epirubicin, the anthraquinone agent mitoxantrone, and trastuzumab (Herceptin).
- Myocardial ischemia:
  - Abnormal vasoreactivity and spasm have been reported primarily with 5-fluorouracil therapy, but also with vinblastine, vincristine, cisplatin, bleomycin, and interleukin-2 administration.
- Dysrhythmia
  - Rhythm disturbances may occur in the context of anthracycline-induced cardiomyopathy, but ventricular and supraventricular tachycardias also have been described with interferon and rituximab. Taxol has been associated with ventricular tachycardia, sinus bradycardia, and heart block. Arsenic trioxide can cause QT prolongation.
- Other:
  - Cisplatin commonly causes hypertension. Hemorrhagic myopericarditis has been associated with high-dose cyclophosphamide. Imatinib (Gleevec) has been associated with pericardial effusion, heart failure, and edema/fluid retention.

GENERAL PREVENTION
- Care should be taken in dosing strategies for patients with baseline left ventricular (LV) dysfunction and for patients with other risk factors for cardiotoxicity.
- Patients with severely reduced baseline left ventricular ejection fraction (LVEF, <30%) should not receive doxorubicin chemotherapy.
- Dexrazoxane, an iron-chelating agent that reduces free radical production, has been approved for use in patients with metastatic breast cancer receiving >300 mg/m^2 of doxorubicin.

EPIDEMIOLOGY
- Predominant Age: Rates are higher at extremes of patient age, in elderly patients older than 70 years of age, and in pediatric patients younger than 15 years of age.
- Predominant Sex: Men are affected as often as women.

Incidence
The overall incidence of anthracycline-induced cardiomyopathy in the United States is approximately 2.2%.

RISK FACTORS
- In addition to age, the following risk factors increase the incidence of anthracycline-induced cardiomyopathy by as much as 8- to 10-fold:
- Increased cumulative dose
  - The incidence of cardiomyopathy with doxorubicin administration at doses <400 mg/m^2 is approximately 0.12%.
  - The incidence increases to 7% at 550 mg/m^2, and escalates sharply at higher doses.
  - It has been reported at 18–30% at doses >700 mg/m^2.

- Therefore, 550 mg/m^2 is considered to be the upper limit for doxorubicin administration in most clinical scenarios.
- Rapid schedule of administration
  - Less cardiotoxicity has been reported when doxorubicin infusion is prolonged over 48–96 hours than when compared with standard 1- to 2-hour infusions.
  - This may be due to lower peak plasma concentration of drug.
- Other underlying heart disease
  - Anthracycline-induced cardiomyopathy is more common in the presence of preexisting heart diseases, particularly those that increase LV wall stress.
  - These include hypertensive heart disease, hypertensive obstructive cardiomyopathy, aortic stenosis, or other forms of underlying cardiomyopathy.
- Concomitant therapy for malignancy
  - Radiation therapy through a portal that includes the heart (such as mediastinum, breast, or lung) has been shown to substantially increase the risk of developing anthracycline-induced cardiomyopathy.
- Other chemotherapeutic agents, such as concomitant administration of cyclophosphamide, trastuzumab, or mitomycin C chemotherapy, may increase the risk of developing cardiomyopathy, although available data are somewhat variable.

PATHOPHYSIOLOGY
Anthracycline-induced myocardial necrosis is due to direct membrane lipid damage and local free radical production. Vasospasm can occur with 5-fluorouracil and other agents.

ETIOLOGY
Chemotherapeutic agent induced myocardial and vascular inflammation, disease, and damage.

ASSOCIATED CONDITIONS
Anemia

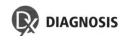 **DIAGNOSIS**

SIGNS AND SYMPTOMS
Heart failure due to anthracycline-induced cardiotoxicity is clinically indistinguishable from other etiologies of biventricular heart failure.
- Symptoms
  - Fatigue
  - Exercise intolerance
  - Dyspnea
  - Paroxysmal nocturnal dyspnea
  - Orthopnea
  - Edema
  - Palpitation, syncope, or presyncope
- Physical findings
  - Resting tachycardia
  - Jugular venous distention
  - S3 (third heart sound) gallop
  - Pulmonary congestion
  - Peripheral edema
- Electrocardiographic abnormalities are nonspecific and may be transient.
  - Sinus tachycardia
  - ST- or T-wave changes

  - Premature ventricular contractions or other dysrhythmias
  - Decreased voltage
  - QT-interval prolongation
- Chest X-ray
  - Cardiac enlargement
  - Pulmonary vascular plethora
  - Kerley B lines
  - Pleural effusions

Clinical Manifestations
- Acute toxicity occurs either during or immediately after treatment (even a single cycle of drug).
  - Acute toxicity is rare and is most commonly manifested as a transient electrocardiographic abnormality or dysrhythmia.
  - However, it can present as myocarditis, pericarditis, fulminant cardiac failure, or even sudden death.
- Chronic toxicity most commonly occurs within 1 year of treatment but also may occur after a prolonged asymptomatic interval, sometimes even years later.
- Asymptomatic reduction in LV systolic function is the most common manifestation of chronic anthracycline-induced cardiomyopathy.
  - The criteria for asymptomatic cardiomyopathy are an absolute decrease in LVEF of >10% or a decline in LVEF to 50% when previously normal.
- Less commonly, anthracycline-induced cardiomyopathy may present as overt clinical congestive heart failure.

TESTS
Lab
Complete blood count (CBC) may show anemia

Imaging
- Radionuclide ventriculography
  - Reduced LVEF
- Echocardiography
  - Biventricular enlargement
  - Abnormal systolic function: Reduced LVEF and fractional shortening, most commonly without segmental wall motion abnormality
  - Abnormal diastolic function: Endocardial thickening and Doppler evidence of prolonged isovolumic relaxation
  - Stress imaging to assess enhancement of LV contractility with exercise may add sensitivity to either radionuclide or echocardiographic imaging.

Diagnostic Procedures/Surgery
- Endomyocardial biopsy
  - Best method for absolute quantitation of cardiac damage and may be used to guide decisions about subsequent anthracycline dosing
  - Cardiac muscle involvement may be patchy, so multiple right ventricular specimens should be obtained when possible.
  - Pathology reveals swelling of sarcoplasmic reticulum and mitochondria, myofibrillar dropout, vacuole formation, and frank myocyte necrosis.
  - Pathologic severity is graded on a scale of 0–3, with biopsy grade >1.5 considered a contraindication to continuing anthracycline therapy.

Pathologic Findings
Cardiac necrosis

DIFFERENTIAL DIAGNOSIS

At presentation, anthracycline-induced cardiomyopathy may be clinically indistinguishable from other etiologies of cardiac dysfunction in the cancer patient, including:

- Underlying cardiovascular disease, which may have been previously subclinical, including atherosclerosis, hypertensive heart disease, valvular heart disease, myocarditis or viral, and alcoholic or idiopathic cardiomyopathy
- Other cardiac complications of malignancy
  - Metastatic or primary tumor involvement of the pericardium or myocardium.
  - Obstruction of venous inflow [SVC or IVC (superior or inferior vena cava) syndrome]
- Radiation-induced pericardial, myocardial, or coronary artery disease
- Dysrhythmia secondary to other drugs or metabolic abnormalities
- Other adverse drug effects

 TREATMENT

GENERAL MEASURES
- Unless overt congestive heart failure occurs, patients can be managed as outpatients.
- Treatment for documented anthracycline-induced cardiomyopathy
  - Anthracycline administration should be discontinued
- Baseline screening should include:
  - History and physical examination
  - Electrocardiogram (ECG)
  - Chest X-ray
  - Assessment of LV function by echocardiography or radionuclide ventriculography

 MEDICATION (DRUGS)

- There is no specific therapy for anthracycline-induced cardiomyopathy.
- Treatment of heart failure, myocardial ischemia, and arrhythmias would be the same as for other etiologies of these conditions.
- Anthracycline dose limitation
  - Total cumulative doxorubicin dose should be limited to less than 550 mg/m^2.
  - Total cumulative doxorubicin dose should be limited to less than 350 mg/m^2 for patients receiving radiation therapy.

SURGERY
Selected patients with severe anthracycline-induced cardiomyopathy who have achieved cure from malignancy might be considered acceptable candidates for cardiac transplantation.

 FOLLOW-UP

Admission Criteria
Standard admission for acute heart failure, ischemia, or arrhythmia.

Discharge Criteria
Resolution of symptoms of heart failure, ischemia, or arrhythmia.

Issues for Referral
Consider referral for severe heart failure that fails to respond to standard therapy. Cardiac assist devices and/or cardiac transplantation are potential therapies.

PROGNOSIS
- Prognosis is poorer in patients who develop overt congestive heart failure, with reported mortality rates as high as 43%.
- Outcomes in patients with congestive heart failure are improved with conventional medical therapy.
- Reversal of even severe cardiac dysfunction has been reported.

COMPLICATIONS
Cardiac death, persistent heart failure

PATIENT MONITORING
- Serial monitoring for patients receiving doxorubicin chemotherapy can be performed using radionuclide ventriculography or echocardiographic assessment of LV systolic function.
- Elevated B-type natriuretic peptide (BNP) during anthracycline therapy may predict onset of LV dysfunction.
- Follow-up LVEF assessment should be performed at least 3 weeks after a given dose, before consideration of subsequent dose administration.
- Guidelines for the frequency of follow-up are as follows:
  - Patients with normal baseline LVEF (>50%)
  - Repeat assessment of LV function after 200–300 mg/m^2 and again after 450 mg/m^2 or after 400 mg/m^2 in patients with other risk factors for cardiomyopathy.
  - Repeat assessment before every dose after 400–450 mg/m^2
  - Discontinue doxorubicin when LVEF falls by >10% or absolute LVEF is less than 50%.
- Patients with moderately reduced baseline LVEF (30–50%)
  - Repeat assessment of LVEF before every dose
  - Discontinue doxorubicin when LVEF falls by >10% or absolute LVEF is less than 30%.

REFERENCES
1. Gharib MI, Burnett AK. Chemotherapy-induced cardiotoxicity: Current practice and prospects of prophylaxis. *Eur J Heart Fail*. 2002;4:235–252.
2. Pai VB, Nahata MC. Cardiotoxicity of chemotherapeutic agents: Incidence, treatment, and prevention. *Drug Saf*. 2000;22:263–302.
3. Yeh ETH, et al. Cardiovascular complications of cancer therapy. *Circulation*. 2004;109: 3122–3131.

 MISCELLANEOUS

See also: Heart failure, Myocardial ischemia

CODES
ICD9-CM
425.4 and 909.5 Cardiomyopathy

PATIENT TEACHING
American Cancer Society

Diet
Low-sodium diet for patients with heart failure

Activity
No specific restrictions. Cardiac rehabilitation may be beneficial.

Prevention
Patients should speak to their doctor about the cardiac toxicities specific to their chemotherapy regimen and how to prevent cardiac complications.

FAQ
Q: How long after chemotherapy is cardiac toxicity no longer a possibility?
A: Although the risk of cardiac toxicity differs with each specific chemotherapeutic agent, and the risk of toxicity decreases with time, anthracycline-induced cardiomyopathy may occur several months to years after initial exposure.

C

CHEYNE-STOKES RESPIRATION

Richard Mascolo
Gerard P. Aurigemma

 BASICS

DESCRIPTION

- Characterized by cyclic variations in minute ventilation
- Periods of hyperpnea alternate with periods of hypopnea and apnea. Sleep is interrupted with frequent arousals. These arousals usually occur during early non-REM sleep (stages 1 and 2), resulting in reduced REM sleep.
- Commonly occurs in patients with congestive heart failure (CHF) and neurologic disorders (cerebral hemorrhage infarct or embolism, meningitis, trauma, tumor)
- Also can be seen with lactic acidosis, diabetic ketoacidosis, and uremic coma
- Mechanism responsible is unclear: However, several theories have been proposed.
- System(s) affected: Respiratory; Cardiovascular
- Synonym(s): Cyclic respiration; Periodic breathing

Pediatric Considerations
Can be seen in premature and full-term infants.

EPIDEMIOLOGY
Predominant sex: Males > Females

Incidence
40–50% of patients with chronic CHF, 25% of cases of cerebral embolism, and 10% of cerebral infarcts

RISK FACTORS
- Predisposing disorders such as:
  - CHF
  - Neurologic disorders
  - Renal failure
  - High altitude
  - Narcotics

ETIOLOGY
- The mechanism responsible is unknown. Cheyne-Stokes respirations may be due to instability in ventilatory control and feedback systems. Factors contributing to this may include:
  - Hypoxemia
  - Circulatory delay
  - Reduced blood gas buffering capacity
  - Abnormal central and peripheral receptors
  - Increased sympathetic activity

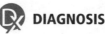 **DIAGNOSIS**

SIGNS AND SYMPTOMS
- History of one of the following:
  - CHF
  - Neurologic disorder (cerebral hemorrhage, infarct or embolism, meningitis, tumor, trauma)
  - Renal failure/uremic coma
  - Acidosis (lactic acidosis, diabetic ketoacidosis)
- Most common signs and symptoms
  - Daytime sleepiness
  - Fatigue
  - Paroxysmal nocturnal dyspnea
  - Snoring
  - Witnessed apnea
  - Dyspnea
  - Orthopnea

TESTS
Polysomnography can verify diagnosis and rule out obstructive sleep apnea.

Lab
Blood gas may reveal a respiratory alkalosis.

Diagnostic Procedures/Surgery
Polysomnogram can verify diagnosis and rule out obstructive sleep apnea.

DIFFERENTIAL DIAGNOSIS
- Obstructive sleep apnea
- Ataxic breathing
- Neurogenic hyperventilation
- Neurogenic hypoventilation

 TREATMENT

GENERAL MEASURES
- The severity of the patient's underlying disorder (i.e., CHF, stroke) usually determines the level of care required.
- Treatment includes treatment of any associated disorder, particularly treatment of CHF.
- Other beneficial therapy may include:
  - Oxygen or continuous positive airway pressure (CPAP)
  - Respiratory stimulants, such as theophylline and acetazolamide, have been used.

 MEDICATION (DRUGS)

- Possible benefit from respiratory stimulants, such as theophylline and acetazolamide
- Contraindications: Narcotics
- Precautions: Refer to manufacturer's profile of each drug.
  - Theophylline: May increase risk of arrhythmias
  - Acetazolamide: Causes a metabolic acidosis
- Significant possible interactions: Many drugs can affect theophylline levels.

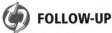

FOLLOW-UP

DISPOSITION

Issues for Referral

- Patients with Cheyne-Stokes respiration have increased mortality if a respiratory alkalosis exists.
- In patients with CHF, the development of Cheyne-Stokes respiration is associated with increased mortality independent of left ventricular function.

REFERENCES

1. Baum GL, Crapo JD, Celli BR, et al. *Textbook of pulmonary medicine*, 6th ed. Philadelphia: Lippincott-Raven, 1998.
2. Crystal RG, West JB, Weibel ER, et al. *The lung*. Philadelphia: Lippincott Raven, 1997.
3. George RB, Matthay MA, Light RW, et al. *Chest medicine: Essentials of pulmonary and critical care medicine*, 3rd ed. Baltimore: Williams & Wilkins, 1995.
4. Piepoli MF, et al. Aetiology and pathophysiological implications of oscillatory ventilation at rest and during exercise in chronic heart failure. Do Cheyne and Stokes have an important message for modern-day patients with heart failure? *Eur Heart J*. 1999;20:946–953.
5. Quaranta AJ, D'Alonzo GE, Krachman SL. Cheyne-Stokes respiration during sleep in congestive heart failure. *Chest*. 1997;111: 467–473.
6. Wilcox I, McNamara SG, Wessendorf T, et al. Prognosis and sleep disordered breathing in heart failure. *Thorax*. 1998;53(Suppl 3):33–36.

MISCELLANEOUS

PATIENT TEACHING

Activity

Physical training may increase exercise tolerance and decrease abnormal ventilation.

C

CLUBBING

Peter Kringstein
Mary Frisella
Gerard P. Aurigemma

 BASICS

DESCRIPTION

Clubbing is a bulbous enlargement of the distal phalanges due to connective tissue proliferation. Concurrent with this proliferation is an increase in the number of capillaries and formation of arteriovenous aneurysms in these regions. These changes occur largely in the dorsal aspect of the fingers and toes and usually are painless.

EPIDEMIOLOGY

- Clubbing may be idiopathic, hereditary, or acquired and is associated with a number of conditions. Among cardiac causes are those associated with central cyanosis such as congenital heart disease with right-to-left shunting. Examples include:
  - Tetralogy of Fallot
  - Tricuspid atresia
  - Transposition of the great vessels
- In these patients, clubbing typically develops after 2 or 3 years of central cyanosis. Pulmonary diseases associated with clubbing include:
  - Cystic fibrosis
  - Pulmonary arteriovenous shunts
  - Bronchiectasis
  - Primary or metastatic lung cancer
  - Lung abscess
  - Mesothelioma
- Clubbing is relatively rare in chronic obstructive pulmonary disease (COPD) and suggests the presence of bronchiectasis or bronchogenic carcinoma.
- Clubbing without cyanosis may be seen in patients with endocarditis, a number of gastrointestinal diseases including inflammatory bowel disease (both Crohn disease and ulcerative colitis), and end-stage liver disease.
- Usually clubbing is symmetric, although occasionally unilateral clubbing has been associated with aneurysms of the subclavian or innominate arteries.
- Rarely, clubbing may be associated with hyperthyroidism and periostitis of the long bones (thyroid acropachy).
- This association occurs in approximately 1% of patient's with Grave disease, and may develop months to years after the resolution of the hyperthyroidism.

ASSOCIATED CONDITIONS

- Clubbing may occur as part of a spectrum of musculoskeletal manifestations referred to as hypertrophic osteoarthropathy (HOA).
  - HOA is characterized by digital clubbing, periosteal bone formation, arthritis, and neurovascular changes of the hands and feet, including chronic erythema, paresthesias, and increased sweating.
  - HOA may occur as a familial form beginning in childhood or as a secondary form, related to any of the diseases previously mentioned.
  - HOA is most frequently diagnosed after the patient presents with persistent pain in the extremities. Bony tenderness due to periostitis may be elicited on palpation of the shafts of the long bones.
  - The skeletal findings in HOA consist of periosteal elevation and new bone formation, seen primarily in the distal phalanges and long bones.
  - Synovial involvement also may lead to pain and swelling of the knees, ankles, wrists, and elbows.
  - Occasionally, other joints such as the shoulders, clavicles, and temporomandibular joints also may be involved.
  - There may be mononuclear infiltration in adjacent soft tissue. Connective tissue proliferation occurs in the nail bed, giving rise to clubbing, which is seen in virtually all patients.
- The etiology and pathogenesis of HOA remain unclear.
  - Neurogenic and humoral theories have both been advanced.
  - The neurogenic theory postulates that bony and soft tissue proliferation may somehow be related to increased vagal tone because many of the conditions associated with HOA involve organs innervated by the vagus.
  - In support of this theory is the observation that vagotomy sometimes leads to a resolution of symptoms.
  - The humoral theory states that a circulating substance normally removed by the lungs is allowed into systemic circulation, causing the manifestations of HOA.
  - A number of mediators have been suggested, but none have been proved.

- Primary HOA (Touraine-Soulente-Gole syndrome) develops slowly in puberty, is inherited in an autosomal-dominant fashion with variable expression, and is more common in boys than in girls.
  - There is marked thickening of the distal extremities as well as clubbing, leading to a spadelike appearance to the hands.
  - The face often has a leonine appearance that may mimic acromegaly. Symptoms of bone and joint pain may not occur until 20–30 years from the onset of the disease.
- Secondary HOA is more common than primary HOA and accompanies many of the cardiac and pulmonary diseases discussed in the preceding text.
  - HOA may precede the accompanying manifestations of the primary disorder by several months.
  - Joint manifestations may be very painful and most commonly involve the metacarpophalangeal and metatarsophalangeal joints, as well as the wrists, ankles, and knees.
  - HOA may occur in as many as 5–10% of pulmonary-related malignancies and may progress particularly rapidly in cases of bronchogenic carcinoma.
  - Symptoms of HOA may precede pulmonary manifestations when there is underlying lung cancer. Full-blown HOA may occur with cyanotic congenital heart disease, but is less common than clubbing alone.
  - Blood tests are normal in patients with HOA, with the exception of a mild increase in the erythrocyte sedimentation rate.
  - Joint effusions are small and most commonly noninflammatory when they occur. Periosteal elevation that occurs in the disease produces a characteristic appearance on radiographs of long bones.
  - Bone scan imaging detects areas of increased osteoblastic activity and may identify periostitis before it is apparent clinically or on plain films.
  - HOA is frequently confused with rheumatoid arthritis.
  - The presence of clubbing is an important clue to the diagnosis. HOA-associated effusions are noninflammatory, as attested to by the absence of rheumatoid factor or antinuclear antibodies.

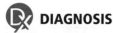 DIAGNOSIS

SIGNS AND SYMPTOMS

- The normal angle between the fingernail and the nail base is approximately 160 degrees and has a firm feeling on palpation. As clubbing progresses, the angle between the nail and its base increases to 180 degrees (and sometimes more) as the nail base becomes swollen and edematous.
- The nail base in the individual with clubbing has a spongy or swollen feeling on palpation. The nail itself may have a convex appearance in advanced clubbing, although this should not be confused with the curved nails sometimes seen in normal individuals. An important distinguishing feature is that the normal nail will have a preserved angle between the nail and its base, whereas the truly clubbed individual will not.
- The diagnosis of clubbing is made solely by physical examination. The softening of tissue at the nail base can be felt on palpation. The skin around the cuticle is noted to take on a smooth and shiny appearance. Although quantification of clubbing has been accomplished using various techniques, including plaster casts and "shadowgrams" of the digital profile, the methods have not replaced bedside diagnosis in standard clinical practice.

 TREATMENT

GENERAL MEASURES

- Vagotomy has provided relief of symptoms in some patients with HOA.
- Nonsteroidal antiinflammatory agents also have shown some benefit.
- Most fundamental to the treatment of both clubbing and HOA, however, is the identification and care of the underlying disorder with which they are associated.
- Both may regress or resolve with identification and proper therapy of the related condition.

REFERENCES

1. Braunwald E, Gilliland B. In: *Harrison's Principles and Practice of Internal Medicine*, 13th ed. New York: McGraw-Hill, 1994;182–183, 1705–1706.
2. Braunwald E. In: *Heart Disease*. Philadelphia: WB Saunders, 1997.
3. Fishman A. In: *Pulmonary Diseases and Disorders*. New York: McGraw-Hill, 1988;352–354.
4. Hansen-Flaschen J, Nordberg J. Clubbing and hypertrophic osteoarthropathy. *Clin Chest Med*. 1987;8:287–299.

C

COARCTATION OF THE AORTA

Ashwin Prakash
Welton M. Gersony

    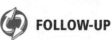

BASICS

DESCRIPTION
- This condition is characterized by a narrowing of the proximal thoracic aorta, resulting in obstruction to systemic blood flow.
- Typically discrete narrowing in the proximal descending aorta opposite to the insertion of the ductus arteriosus, although it may involve a longer segment or be associated with tubular hypoplasia of the aortic transverse arch. Rarely, involves the abdominal descending aorta

EPIDEMIOLOGY
- Age: Severe cases present in the newborn period. Significant proportion of less severe forms diagnosed in childhood or adolescence
- Male:Female ratio 1.3–1.7

Incidence
6–8% of patients with congenital heart disease, Occurs in 1/3,000–4,000 live births

RISK FACTORS
None

Genetics
- Most cases sporadic with multifactorial genetic influence
- Increased incidence in Turner syndrome, with 35% affected

PATHOPHYSIOLOGY
- Increased left ventricular afterload may cause systolic and diastolic left ventricular dysfunction.
- "Critical" coarctation causes left ventricular systolic dysfunction, congestive heart failure, hypotension, and metabolic acidosis in the first month of life
- In less severe forms with later diagnosis, collateral circulation bypassing the narrowing often develops, masking degree of obstruction. Mild coarctation without collaterals is also common.
- Abnormal vascular physiology is common with systemic hypertension.

ETIOLOGY
- Unclear, but discrete forms of coarctation may occur due to migration of smooth muscle cells from the ductus arteriosus into the juxtaductal aorta with constriction and narrowing of the aortic lumen associated with postnatal ductal constriction.
- Intracardiac defects that diminish fetal left ventricular output may promote coarctation.

ASSOCIATED CONDITIONS
- Cardiac: Bicuspid aortic valve, ventricular septal defect, congenital mitral valve stenosis. May be a component of complex congenital heart disease.
- Extracardiac: Turner syndrome; abnormalities of musculoskeletal, genitourinary, gastrointestinal or respiratory systems; berry aneurysms in the circle of Willis

DIAGNOSIS

SIGNS AND SYMPTOMS
Depend on severity of aortic narrowing

History
Newborn infants with critical coarctation: Often catastrophic illness with rapid or labored breathing, poor feeding, lethargy. A ventricular septal defect is often present. Children or adolescents are often asymptomatic.

Physical Exam
- Absent or feeble femoral pulse with normal upper extremity pulses, upper extremity hypertension with normal or low blood pressure of the lower extremities. With critical coarctation, tachycardia, hypotension, poor peripheral perfusion, gallop rhythm
- Simultaneous measurement of upper and lower extremity blood pressure is mandatory when coarctation is suspected.

TESTS
Electrocardiography in newborn infants shows prominent right ventricular forces. In longstanding coarctation, left ventricular hypertrophy or strain may be noted. Normal electrocardiogram does not exclude the diagnosis of coarctation.

Lab
Metabolic acidosis with critical coarctation and low cardiac output

Imaging
- Chest X-ray in infancy may show cardiomegaly. In older children, localized indentation of the aorta (3 sign) and rib notching may be seen.
- Echocardiography diagnostic in most cases, especially infants and young children
- Magnetic resonance imaging useful if evaluation incomplete by echocardiography, especially in older children or adolescents.

Diagnostic Procedures/Surgery
Cardiac catheterization, although rarely needed, is the gold standard for diagnosis

DIFFERENTIAL DIAGNOSIS
Abdominal coarctation: A complex lesion often associated with renal artery stenosis

TREATMENT

GENERAL MEASURES
Treatment is surgical or transcatheter and depends on severity and age of presentation

MEDICATION (DRUGS)

- Continuous intravenous infusion of prostaglandin E_1 to reestablish patency of ductus arteriosus should be started emergently with "critical" coarctation in newborn infants. Intravenous inotropes for left ventricular dysfunction in critically ill infants
- Medical treatment of hypertension, which might persist despite definitive treatment, especially in longstanding cases

SURGERY
- Indicated for significant obstruction to flow. Usually involves resection of involved aortic segment with end-to-end anastomosis
- Percutaneous transcatheter stenting of narrowed segment possible in older children and adolescents for discrete coarctation. Limited long-term data available for this new therapy
- Transcatheter balloon angioplasty has been attempted but is associated with a higher incidence of aortic aneurysms.

FOLLOW-UP

- Lifelong follow-up with a cardiologist with experience in congenital heart defects
- Follow-up includes measurement of upper and lower extremity blood pressure and evaluation of associated cardiac defects.

DISPOSITION
Admission Criteria
Low cardiac output, congestive heart failure

Discharge Criteria
Recovery after surgical or transcatheter treatment

Issues for Referral
An infant or child with diminished femoral pulses or upper extremity hypertension with low or normal lower extremity blood pressure should be referred to a pediatric cardiologist.

PROGNOSIS

- Excellent with normal expected growth and development and minimal or no restrictions to activity
- Follow-up required right arm blood pressure, upper and lower extremity blood pressure gradient, mitral and aortic valve status, and other conditions.

COMPLICATIONS

- Recurrent coarctation in 6–20%, mostly following repair in infancy and is treatable with balloon angioplasty or surgery
- Risk of persistent or late hypertension in 10%, especially when repair delayed
- Aortic aneurysms at site of repair may develop, usually following use of prosthetic material for repair or following balloon angioplasty for native coarctation
- Risk of bacterial endocarditis persists following repair and antibiotic prophylaxis is indicated life long

PATIENT MONITORING

Upper and lower extremity blood pressure monitored periodically following repair for persistent systemic hypertension and recurrent coarctation

REFERENCES

1. Campbell M, Polani PE. The aetiology of coarctation of the aorta. *Lancet*. 1961;1:463–468.
2. Hamdan MA, Maheshwari S, Fahey JT, et al. Endovascular stents for coarctation of the aorta: Initial results and intermediate-term follow-up. *J Am Coll Cardiol*. 2001;38:1518–1523.
3. Nielsen JC, Powell AJ, Gauvreau K, et al. Magnetic resonance imaging predictors of coarctation severity. *Circulation*. 2005;111:622–628.
4. Quaegebeur JM, Jonas RA, Weinberg AD, et al. Outcomes in seriously ill neonates with coarctation of the aorta: A multiinstitutional study. *J Thorac Cardiovasc Surg*. 1994;108:841–851.
5. Strafford MA, Griffiths SP, Gersony WM. Coarctation of the aorta: A study in delayed detection. *Pediatrics*. 1982;69:159–163.

ADDITIONAL READING

Allen HD, Gutgessel HP, Clark EB, et al., eds. *Moss and Adams' Heart Disease in Infants, Children, and Adolescents: Including the Fetus and Young Adult*, 6th ed. Philadelphia: Lippincott Williams & Wilkins, 2002.

CODES

ICD9-CM

747.10 Coarctation of the aorta

Snomed

- D4-32030

PATIENT TEACHING

Diet

Regular. Salt-restriction for significant persistent hypertension

Activity

Unrestricted following successful repair

COLLATERAL BLOOD VESSELS

Joseph L. Bouchard

 BASICS

DESCRIPTION
- Collateral blood vessels are anastomotic connections that offer an important source of blood supply when original vessels fail to provide sufficient blood, and are extremely important in the coronary circulation.
- Coronary collateral vessels limit myocardial ischemia during coronary occlusion and may minimize the infarct area.
- Two types of coronary collateral vessels include:
  - Capillary size collaterals: These vessels do not have vascular smooth muscle, are observed in all layers of the ventricular muscle (but have a predilection for the subendocardium where they form a plexus), and develop via angiogenesis.
  - Larger muscular collaterals: These vessels are located epicardially, develop from preexisting arterioles (arteriogenesis), and can be angiographically classified into 4 types: Septal, atrial, branch–branch in ventricular free walls, and bridging across lesions.

EPIDEMIOLOGY
A reduction in coronary collaterals has been reported in the elderly and diabetics and is associated with a reduction in the expression of angiogenic factors.

PATHOPHYSIOLOGY
- Angiogenesis
  - Stimulated by hypoxia via biochemical signals including vascular endothelial growth factor (VEGF), transforming growth factor (TGF)-β, and basic fibroblast growth factor (b-FGF).
- Arteriogenesis
  - Not stimulated by hypoxia
  - Stimulated by an increase in shear stress
  - That is, hemodynamically relevant stenosis of coronary artery creates a decrease in arterial pressure distal to the stenosis, and blood flow is redistributed through preexistent arterioles from high pressure to low-pressure area. This creates increase in flow velocity and shear stress, which leads to morphologic changes and vascular remodeling.
  - Major biochemical factors include: Granulocyte macrophage colony-stimulating factor (GM-CSF), monocyte chemoattractant protein-1 (MCP-1), TGF-β

ETIOLOGY
- Ischemia
- Pressure gradients and shear stress

ASSOCIATED CONDITIONS
- Coronary artery disease
- Peripheral vascular disease

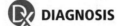 **DIAGNOSIS**

TESTS
Imaging
- Coronary angiography
- Myocardial contrast echocardiography
- Spiral computed tomographic (CT) scan
- Magnetic resonance imaging (MRI)
- Positron emission tomographic (PET) scan

Diagnostic Procedures/Surgery
- Coronary angiography reveals grades of collateral filling
  - 1 = filling of side branches of the artery without visualization of the epicardial segment
  - 2 = partial filling of the epicardial segment
  - 3 = complete filling of the epicardial segment

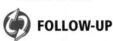 **TREATMENT**

GENERAL MEASURES
- Therapeutic angiogenesis
  - Exogenous growth factors or genes encoding growth factors are administered to stimulate angiogenesis of ischemic tissues.
  - Recent trial administered growth factor plasmid via angioplasty balloon to popliteal artery and showed evidence of angiogenesis in a patient with limb ischemia.

FOLLOW-UP

PROGNOSIS
- Beneficial effects of collaterals include:
  - Decrease severity of myocardial ischemia
  - Decrease infarct size
  - Improve left ventricular function
  - Reduce the likelihood of left ventricular aneurysm formation
  - Improve survival
- Only rarely provide blood flow increases adequate to meet maximal physical exercise

REFERENCES

1. Cohen M, Rentrop KP. Limitation of myocardial ischemia by collateral circulation during sudden controlled coronary artery occlusion in human subjects: A prospective study. *Circulation*. 1986;74:469–476.

2. Fukai M, Ii M, Nakakoji T, et al. Angiographically demonstrated coronary collaterals predict residual viable myocardium in patients with chronic myocardial infarction: A regional metabolic study. *J Cardiol*. 2000;35:103–111.

3. Isner JM, Pieczek A, Schainfeld R, et al. Clinical evidence of angiogenesis after arterial gene transfer of phVEGF165 in patients with ischemic limbs. *Lancet*. 1996;348:370–374.

4. Kern M. Atherosclerotic cardiovascular disease: Coronary blood flow and myocardial ischemia. In: Zipe D, et al. ed. *Braunwald's Heart Disease,* 7th ed. Philadelphia: Elsevier Saunders, 2005; 1103–1127.

5. Koerselman J, van der Graaf Y, de Jaegere PP, et al. Coronary collaterals: An important and underexposed aspect of coronary artery disease. *Circulation*. 2003;107:2507–2511.

6. Rentrop KP, Cohen M, Blanke H, et al. Changes in collateral channel filling immediately after controlled coronary artery occlusion by angioplasty balloon in human subjects. *J Am Coll Cardiol*. 1985;5:587–592.

7. Rockstroh J, Brown G. Coronary collateral size, flow capacity, and growth. Estimates from the angiogram in patients with obstructive coronary disease. *Circulation*. 2002;105:168–173.

8. Schaper W. Collateral vessel growth in the human heart. Role of fibroblast growth factor-2 editorial. *Circulation*. 1996;94:600–601.

FAQ

Q: Where are the coronary collateral vessels located?
A: The capillary-sized vessels are observed in all layers of the ventricular muscle, but have a predilection for the subendocardium where they form a plexus. The larger muscular collaterals are found epicardially.

Q: How do collateral blood vessels form?
A: There are two main types of collateral blood vessels: Capillary-sized vessels without smooth muscle and larger muscular vessels. The capillary-sized vessels form through angiogenesis-stimulated hypoxia via biochemical signals including: VGEF, TGF-β, and b-FGF. The larger muscular vessels are nonfunctional preexisting conduits that become functional in the setting of a hemodynamically significant stenosis. These larger vessels then undergo vascular remodeling in the setting of shear stress.

Q: What are the implications of collateral coronary vessels?
A: Studies have found a decrease in the severity of myocardial ischemia, a decreased infarct size, improved left ventricular function, a reduction in the likelihood of left ventricular aneurysm formation, and improved survival.

C

CONGENITAL HEART DISEASE IN ADULTS

Deborah R. Gersony
Welton M. Gersony

 BASICS

DESCRIPTION

Congenital cardiac lesions are categorized into cyanotic and acyanotic types. These groups are subdivided into patients who have had palliative or corrective cardiac surgery or interventional cardiac catheterization, and those who have never had intervention. The most common defects among patients who are most likely to survive to adulthood are:

- Adult patients with cyanotic heart disease who have survived without corrective surgery/interventional catheterization
  - Eisenmenger syndrome
  - Ebstein anomaly
  - Balanced complex lesions with adequate pulmonary blood flow and normal pulmonary artery pressure (e.g., tetralogy of Fallot with moderate pulmonary stenosis)
- Adult patients with cyanotic heart disease who have had surgery/interventional catheterization and who may remain cyanotic
  - Status post fenestrated Fontan procedure with right-to-left shunt
  - Glenn alone
  - Arterial shunt
- Adult patients with acyanotic congenital heart disease who have not had surgery/interventional catheterization
  - Atrial septal defect (ASD)
  - Small, medium-sized ventricular septal defect (VSD) with left-to-right shunt
  - Bicuspid or quadricuspid aortic valve
  - Coronary artery fistula
  - Sinus of Valsalva aneurysm
  - Partial anomalous pulmonary venous return
  - Mild pulmonary stenosis
  - Idiopathic dilatation of the pulmonary trunk
  - Primary pulmonary hypertension
  - Congenitally corrected transposition
  - Mild subaortic stenosis
  - Mild supraaortic stenosis
  - Mitral valve prolapse
  - Marfan syndrome
  - Situs inversus and dextrocardia

- Adult patients with acyanotic congenital heart disease who have had surgery/interventional catheterization
  - Aortic valve disease, valvotomy or replacement, Ross procedure
  - Pulmonary stenosis, valvotomy
  - ASD
  - VSD
  - Fontan palliation for single ventricle anatomy
  - D-transposition of great arteries, atrial redirection, or arterial switch
  - Tetralogy of Fallot
  - Aortopulmonary window
  - Anomalous origin of left coronary artery from the pulmonary trunk
  - Vascular ring
  - Patent ductus arteriosus, surgical division, or transcatheter occlusion
  - Total anomalous pulmonary venous connection
  - Truncus arteriosus, right ventricular to pulmonary artery conduit, right ventricular outflow tract patch
  - Ebstein anomaly, tricuspid valve repair or replacement, accessory pathway ablation, foramen closure
  - Cor triatriatum
  - Coarctation of the aorta
  - Mitral valve disease, valvotomy or replacement
  - Hypoplastic left heart syndrome, Norwood procedure

Prevalence
The prevalence of adults with residual congenital heart defects requiring follow-up is increasing as the number of patients who have had corrective or palliative surgery has increased and survival improves. It is estimated that there are more than 1,000,000 adults with congenital heart disease in the United States.

PATHOPHYSIOLOGY
Varied

ETIOLOGY
- The cause of most congenital heart disease is unknown; thought to be multifactorial
- An increasing number of cases are known to be genetic, among the most common: Holt-Oram syndrome with autosomal-dominant transmission of an ASD; Williams syndrome with supravalvular aortic stenosis; and Down syndrome with atrioventricular (AV) canal defects.
- 22q11 deletion is associated with conotruncal abnormalities such as interrupted aortic arch, truncus arteriosus, pulmonary atresia with VSD, and tetralogy of Fallot
- Approximately 2% of cases are environmental (e.g., maternal diabetes, infection, and therapeutic or elicit drugs).
- Genetic counseling should be provided for all potential parents with congenital heart disease, both male and female.

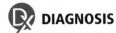 **DIAGNOSIS**

SIGNS AND SYMPTOMS
Varied/dependent on type of defect and severity

History
Depending on the underlying lesion, patients may have one or more of the following:
- History of murmur in childhood
- History of palliative surgery in early infancy
- History of corrective surgery in early infancy or childhood
- History of arrhythmia
- History of endocarditis

Cyanotic Secondary to Uncorrected Cardiac Defect
- Effort-induced dyspnea
- Increased cyanosis with exercise
- Effort induced fatigue

Cyanotic Secondary to Pulmonary Vascular Disease (Eisenmenger Syndrome)
- Decrease in intensity of childhood murmur
- Palpable P2, right ventricular heave
- Clubbing of fingers and toes, perioral cyanosis, hypertrophic osteopathy
- Hemoptysis (late)

Acyanotic
- Range from asymptomatic to significant limitation of activities of daily living with symptoms at rest secondary to heart failure.

Physical Exam

- Depends on type of congenital heart disease (CHD); some examples:
- Jugular venous pressure
  - Elevated in right-sided heart failure
  - Prominent V wave in patients with significant tricuspid regurgitation (TR)
- Carotid artery
  - Prominent upstroke and rapid descent in patients with severe aortic regurgitation (AR)
  - Referred murmur from valvar, supravalvar and aortic obstruction; also suprasternal thrill
- Cardiovascular exam
  - Eisenmenger syndrome/primary pulmonary hypertension (PPH): right ventricular (RV) heave, loud +/− palpable P2, pansystolic murmur of TR
  - D-TGV status post atrial redirection: RV heave, loud second heart sound (S2)
  - ASD patients have a fixed split S2, systolic ejection murmur of increased flow across the pulmonary valve, +/− RV heave
  - Small VSDs will have a loud pansystolic murmur and often a thrill
  - Postoperative tetralogy of Fallot patients will often have harsh systolic ejection murmur and low-pitched diastolic murmur due to significant PR and right ventricular outflow tract turbulence

TESTS

- Cardiovascular/pulmonary anatomy
  - Magnetic resonance imaging (MRI)
  - Magnetic resonance angiography (MRA)
- Arrhythmia
  - Holter
  - Event monitor
  - Electrophysiology study
- Functional capacity and cardiac ischemia
  - Standard Bruce protocol exercise stress testing
  - Thallium and sestamibi nuclear stress testing
  - Cardiopulmonary stress testing

Lab

Cyanotic

- Hemoglobin/hematocrit elevated secondary to elevated erythropoietin levels (hemoglobin 16–23 g/dl, hematocrit 55–80%)
- Platelet count low to markedly reduced
- Blood urea nitrogen/creatinine may be elevated.
- Uric acid elevated secondary to inappropriately low renal excretion

Acyanotic

- Depends on the nature of the underlying lesion

Imaging

Chest X-ray

- Cyanotic secondary to pulmonary vascular disease
  - Decreased pulmonary blood flow
  - Prominent pulmonary arteries at the hilum with rapid tapering
  - Enlarged right ventricular silhouette
- Acyanotic
  - Depends on the underlying lesion

Transthoracic Echocardiogram

- 2D/3D imaging
  - Delineation of segmental anatomy (situs, ventricular looping, great-vessel orientation)
  - Evaluation of ventricular systolic function
  - Valve thickness, morphology, prolapse
  - Anatomic findings such as membranes, pulmonary artery disease, aortic aneurysm, etc.
- Color flow imaging
  - Following the course of arteries and veins
  - Detecting small atrial or ventricular septal defects
  - Detecting small aortic-to-pulmonary connections
  - Delineating stenotic and regurgitant lesions
- Doppler studies for identification and quantification of:
  - Valvular, supravalvular, and subvalvular stenosis
  - Valvular regurgitation
  - Extracardiac and intracardiac conduit obstructions
  - Pulmonary and systemic venous stenoses
  - Septal defects
  - Surgical shunts
  - Diastolic function
  - Dp/dt
- Magnetic resonance imaging/angiography
  - Quantitative measure of systemic ventricular volume and ejection fraction
  - Evaluation of pulmonary anatomy
  - Evaluation of conduit and atrial baffle patency
  - Evaluation of pulmonary venous drainage

Transesophageal Echocardiogram

- Evaluate anatomic areas not easily demonstrated by transthoracic echo.
- Monitor therapeutic interventions in the cardiac catheterization laboratory.
- Prior to cardioversion to exclude intracardiac thrombus
- Intraoperative imaging during cardiac surgery

Diagnostic Procedures/Surgery

Cardiac Catheterization

- Evaluation of coronary artery atherosclerotic disease
- Evaluate ventricular filling pressures.
- Delineate patterns of collateral blood flow.
- Delineate pulmonary anatomy

Percutaneous interventions include coil occlusion of arto-pulmonary coil aterals, peripheral pulmonary stenosis stenting, atral baffle stenting ASD/PFD device closure.

TREATMENT

GENERAL MEASURES

- Nonchemotherapeutic prophylaxis for endocarditis
- Meticulous oral hygiene, skin, and nail care

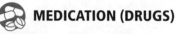

MEDICATION (DRUGS)

First Line

- Patients with left-sided ventricular dysfunction benefit from established medical therapy for congestive heart failure (digoxin, angiotensin-converting enzyme inhibitor, diuretic, β-blockade).
- Prior to dental work or invasive procedures moderate and high risk patients must receive endocarditis prophylaxis.
- Phlebotomy recommended for secondary erythrocytosis only if patient is significantly symptomatic with hematocrit of >65% and no evidence of volume depletion.
- Iron repletion in cyanotic patients who are iron deficient (close monitoring of hematocrit required as blood counts may increase quickly with iron therapy)
- Colchicine for treatment of gouty arthritis in cyanotic patients
- Anticoagulation and chronic pulmonary vasodilator therapy for primary pulmonary hypertension
- Use of aspirin and other antithrombotic medications in patients with Eisenmenger's syndrome is controversial because these patients are at an increased risk for bleeding and thrombosis. Coumadin should be considered if a history of atrial fibrillation, cardiovascular accident, deep venous thrombosis, or pulmonary embolism.
- Antiarrhythmic therapy

SURGERY

Indications for operation in adults with congenital heart disease include:

- Repair of primary congenital heart defect: ASD, aortic stenosis, pulmonary stenosis, Ebstein anomaly, coarctation of the aorta, tetralogy of Fallot, etc.
- Inevitable reoperation: Bioprosthetic heart valve, extracardiac conduit
- Residual defects after repair: Mitral valve regurgitation and/or subvalvular aortic stenosis after atrio-ventricular (AV) canal defect repair
- New/recurrent defects after corrective surgery: Subaortic stenosis recurrence, pulmonary regurgitation after repair of tetralogy of Fallot
- Staged repair of complex defect: Fontan procedure
- Late complications: Infective endocarditis
- Patient with acquired heart disease: Coronary atherosclerotic disease
- Uncorrectable congenital heart disease: Heart or heart/lung transplant
- Insertion of permanent pacemaker and/or defibrillator
- Mapping and ablation of arrhythmias

 FOLLOW-UP

- Adult Congenital Heart Disease Center with multidisciplinary approach
- Noninvasive and invasive cardiologists
- Cardiac surgeon with experience in ACHD
- Electrophysiology
- Availability of cardiac MRI, computed tomography (CT)
- High risk OB-GYN
- Hematology
- Nutritionist
- Psychiatry/social work support

Pregnancy Considerations

- Patients with cyanosis are at high risk of early spontaneous abortion.
- Elevated pulmonary vascular resistance from Eisenmenger syndrome or primary pulmonary hypertension is a contraindication to pregnancy.
- Patients with Marfan syndrome and some patients with bicuspid aortic valve and associated with ascending aortic aneurysm are at risk for aortic dissection/rupture.
- Patients with severe obstructive lesions (aortic stenosis, mitral stenosis, hypertrophic obstruction cardiomyopathy, pulmonary stenosis) are at high risk for complications.
- Patients with moderate/severe native or recurrent aortic coarctation are at risk for aortic dissection/rupture as well as increased fetal risk of compromised placental blood supply. If Berry aneurysms present, the risk of cerebral hemorrhage is increased.
- Management of pregnant women with prosthetic valves is a difficult issue. The 2006 AHA/ACC have described using one of three reasonable anticoagulation regimens with informed consent: 1) low molecular weight heparain (LMWH) or unfractionated heparin (UFH) between 6 and 12 weeks gestation and close to term with warfarin at other times, 2) careful dose-adjusted UFH throughout pregnancy, or 3) adjusted dose LMWH throughout pregnancy. The risk of warfarin embryopathy is approximately 4–10% and may be related to maternal dose with the lowest risk at <5 mg/day.

Admission Criteria
- Symptomatic arrhythmia for drug treatment or electrophysiology study (ablation or intracardiac defibrillator placement)
- Exacerbation of congestive heart failure
- Surgery or interventional/diagnostic cardiac catheterization
- Endocarditis
- Cerebral abscess or stroke in cyanotic patient

PROGNOSIS
Depends on the severity of the underlying lesion

PATIENT MONITORING
Close regular visits with both primary care physician and a cardiologist trained in congenital heart disease. The frequency of visits would depend on the functional class of the patient and the expected natural history of the congenital cardiac lesion.

REFERENCES
1. Bonnow RO, Carabello B, de Leon AC Jr, et al. ACC/AHA guidelines for the management of patients with valvular heart disease: A report of the American College of Cardiology/American Heart Association Task Force on Practice Guidelines (Committee on the Management of Patients with Valvular Heart Disease). *J Am Coll Cardiol.* 2006:e1–e148.
2. Deanfield JE, Gersh BJ, Warnes CA, et al. Congenital heart disease in adults. In: Alexander RW, Schlant RC, Fuster V, eds. *The Heart.* New York: McGraw-Hill,1998;1995–2031.
3. Gatzoulis MA, Webb GD, Daubeney PEF, eds. *Diagnosis and Management of Adult Congenital Heart Disease.* Elsevier, 2003.
4. Perloff JK, Child JS. *Congenital Heart Disease in Adults,* 2nd ed. Philadelphia: WB Saunders,1998.

MISCELLANEOUS

PATIENT TEACHING
The patient must be educated as to the particular risks and limitations of his or her type of congenital heart disease.

Activity
- The degree of exercise that is safe for an individual patient depends on the nature of the underlying congenital lesion. Lesions that are at least moderate risk for strenuous exercise:
  - Cardiomyopathy
  - Aberrant coronary artery that crosses between the aorta and the right ventricular outflow tract
  - Greater than moderate coarctation of the aorta, Marfan syndrome, or bicuspid aortic valve with significant aortic root dilation (patients should especially avoid isotonic exercise)
  - Moderate to severe aortic stenosis
  - Cyanotic heart disease
  - History of serious arrhythmia

Prevention
- Adequate prenatal care
- Fetal echocardiography for early diagnosis/treatment
- Genetic counseling in those with a family history of congenital heart disease

COR PULMONALE

Rajat Deo

 BASICS

DESCRIPTION

Right ventricular dilatation and hypertrophy due to pulmonary hypertension that results from an underlying pulmonary parenchymal or vascular disorder

- Symptoms are predominantly related to right ventricular failure.
- Chronic cor pulmonale is most frequently due to chronic obstructive pulmonary disease (COPD).
- Acute cor pulmonale is associated with pulmonary thromboembolism.

System(s) affected: Cardiopulmonary

EPIDEMIOLOGY

Predominant Age: Increases with advancing age

Pediatric Considerations
Unusual

Geriatric Considerations
Common

Prevalence
The true prevalence of cor pulmonale is difficult to estimate.

- However, because it is associated with common forms of pulmonary disease, it is encountered regularly in both the outpatient and inpatient settings.
- After age 50, cor pulmonale is the third most frequent form of cardiac disease after coronary artery atherosclerosis and hypertensive heart disease.
- It may play a role in up to 10–30% of hospital admissions for heart failure.

PATHOPHYSIOLOGY

- In the setting of lung disease, pulmonary hypertension develops primarily as a result of increased pulmonary vascular resistance. This alteration in vascular tone results from endothelial cell proliferation, thickening in arterioles, inhibition of endothelium derived nitric oxide (NO) and loss of the total cross-sectional area of the pulmonary circulation.
- Hypoxia resulting from pulmonary disease leads to muscularization of pulmonary arteries and arterioles in all three layers of the vessel.
- Hypoxia also leads to the inhibition of NO synthesis, which results in vasoconstriction.
- Reduction in the cross-sectional area of the pulmonary vascular bed may occur due to capillary destruction (emphysema), vascular obstruction (pulmonary embolism), or intimal thickening (primary pulmonary hypertension).
- Acidosis and hyperviscosity have a relatively small effect on the increase in pulmonary artery pressure.

ETIOLOGY

- Essentially any disease of the lung parenchyma or vasculature, if severe enough, can cause pulmonary hypertension and eventually right ventricular failure.
- The most common cause is COPD.
- Other causes include:
  - Pulmonary embolism
  - Cystic fibrosis
  - Infiltrative diseases (sarcoidosis, idiopathic pulmonary fibrosis)
  - Processes affecting thoracic cage movement (sleep apnea, kyphoscoliosis, neuromuscular disease)
  - Pulmonary tuberculosis
  - Drug-related lung diseases

ASSOCIATED CONDITIONS

- COPD
- Pulmonary embolus
- Primary pulmonary hypertension
- Restrictive lung disease
- Infiltrative lung disease
- Thoracic cage dysfunction
- Drug-related lung diseases

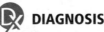 **DIAGNOSIS**

SIGNS AND SYMPTOMS

- The presence of underlying pulmonary disease is usually clinically evident. Therefore, many patients complain of cough, sputum production, and dyspnea.
- Patients with acute cor pulmonale due to pulmonary embolism also may complain of chest pain, which is usually pleuritic in nature.
- Symptoms related to right ventricular failure include:
  - Fatigue due to low cardiac output
  - Poor exercise capacity due to rapid increases in pulmonary artery pressures and right ventricular dysfunction.
  - Dependent edema
  - Abdominal pain (right upper quadrant) due to liver engorgement
  - Anorexia and bloating
  - Exertional syncope

Physical Exam
- Cyanosis/hypoxemia
- Distended neck veins with prominent *a* and *v* waves.
- Right ventricular (parasternal) heave
- Right ventricular third heart sound (S3)
- Holosystolic murmur at left lower sternal border that increases with inspiration (tricuspid regurgitation)
- Loud pulmonary component of the second heart sound (S2)
- Ascites
- Pitting edema

TESTS

- Electrocardiographic findings differ with respect to the acute and chronic forms of cor pulmonale and depending on whether obstructive airway disease is present.
- Electrocardiogram (ECG) is relatively insensitive for the detection of right ventricular hypertrophy.
- In general, the ECG should be examined for the following:
  - Right atrial enlargement (P waves >2.5 mm in leads II, III, and aVF or >1.5 mm in leads V_1 or V_2)
  - Right axis deviation >110 degrees (without right bundle branch block)
  - Incomplete right bundle branch block
  - R in V_1 = 7 mm in absence of right bundle branch block
  - R in V_1 = 15 mm with right bundle branch block
  - R or R′ > S in V_1
  - R in V_1 = S in V_5 or V_6 = 10 mm
  - RSR; sp; or qR pattern in lead V_1
  - S1, Q3, T3 pattern
  - ST segment depression with or without T-wave inversion in the right precordial leads (V_1–V_3)
  - R/S ratio in V_6 of <1
  - Low-voltage QRS
- Chest X-ray
  - Hyperinflation/diaphragmatic flattening
  - Enlarged central pulmonary arteries
  - Peripheral oligemia
  - Loss of the retrosternal airspace secondary to right heart enlargement

Lab
- Patients with advanced lung disease may manifest hypoxemia and hypercapnia on arterial blood gas (ABG) testing.
- In acute cor pulmonale due to pulmonary embolism, a widened alveolar to arterial (A–a) oxygen gradient may be present on the ABG.

Imaging
- Echocardiography
  - The echocardiogram can provide detailed structural and physiologic information.
  - The size and systolic function of the right ventricle can be assessed, as can regurgitation of the tricuspid and pulmonic valves.
  - If tricuspid regurgitation is present, its velocity can be used in the modified Bernoulli equation to obtain an estimate of right ventricular systolic pressure.
  - This can then be added to an estimate of mean right atrial pressure (based on the size of the inferior vena cava and its response to respiration) to obtain an estimate of the pulmonary artery systolic pressure.
  - An additional important function of the echocardiogram is to rule out significant left ventricular dysfunction, left-sided valvular disease, or congenital heart disease as potential causes of pulmonary hypertension.

Diagnostic Procedures/Surgery
- Cardiac catheterization
  - Right heart catheterization provides a direct measure of pulmonary artery pressure.
  - The diagnosis of cor pulmonale is supported by the finding of significant pulmonary hypertension with a normal pulmonary capillary wedge pressure.
  - The diagnosis of cor pulmonale can usually be made on the basis of the clinical picture, and electrocardiographic and echocardiographic findings.
  - Occasionally right heart catheterization is helpful, especially when the echocardiographic images are suboptimal.

Pathologic Findings
- Right ventricular hypertrophy
- Pulmonary vascular disease

DIFFERENTIAL DIAGNOSIS
- All of the previously noted symptoms and findings may be present in patients with biventricular failure of any cause.
- The presence of left-sided cardiac disease must be excluded before making the diagnosis of cor pulmonale.
- Shares some features with constrictive pericarditis, restrictive cardiomyopathy, and mitral stenosis
- Presence of advanced lung disease in a patient with symptoms and physical findings of right ventricular dysfunction makes the diagnosis of cor pulmonale most likely

 TREATMENT

GENERAL MEASURES
- Hospitalization if hemodynamically unstable or hypoxic
- The main thrust of therapy for cor pulmonale should be directed at improving the status of the underlying pulmonary disorder.
  - Superimposed infections should be aggressively treated.
  - Continuous oxygen therapy to correct hypoxia has been proved to improve survival.
  - Oxygen therapy results in a decrease in pulmonary artery pressure and pulmonary vascular resistance.
  - The progression of pulmonary hypertension may be halted or slowed.
  - In studies that compared duration of therapy, the greatest reduction in mortality was seen when oxygen was administered 24 hours per day.
- Supplemental oxygen should be prescribed for patients with a Pa_{O2} of <55 mmHg.
- Other measures
  - Periodic phlebotomy to maintain a hematocrit of <55% reduces blood viscosity and improves pulmonary blood flow.

 MEDICATION (DRUGS)

First Line
- Bronchodilators
  - By relieving bronchoconstriction, gas exchange is improved, which has a beneficial effect on hypoxia-mediated vasoconstriction.
- Warfarin
  - For patients with a thromboembolic etiology
  - Recurrent thromboembolism while on anticoagulation may call for placement of an inferior vena cava filter.
- Diuretics
  - Relieve fluid retention but have no documented positive effect on pulmonary hemodynamics in the absence of left ventricular failure.
  - Should be used with caution as they may reduce right ventricular end-diastolic volume and hence cardiac output.
- Contraindications
  - Refer to manufacturer's profile on each drug.
- Precautions
  - Refer to manufacturer's profile on each drug.
- Significant possible interactions
  - Refer to manufacturer's profile on each drug.

SURGERY
Markedly symptomatic patients with chronic cor pulmonale due to recurrent episodes of pulmonary thromboembolism may benefit from pulmonary thromboendarterectomy. This is a high-risk procedure that has limited clinical application.

 FOLLOW-UP

Close follow-up is recommended.

DISPOSITION
Patients may require additional assistance at home depending on their baseline functional status.

Admission Criteria
Patients who are profoundly hypoxic or hemodynamically unstable should be admitted.

Discharge Criteria
- Improvement in symptoms
- Evaluate whether patient will benefit from supplemental oxygen therapy.
  - Determine etiology for cor pulmonale.

Issues for Referral
- If etiology of underlying pulmonary disease is unclear, refer to pulmonary medicine for further work-up.
  - Cardiology evaluation is recommended prior to right heart catheterization.

PROGNOSIS
- The prognosis is closely related to the etiology and severity of the underlying lung disease and the degree of pulmonary hypertension.
- Patients with COPD who develop cor pulmonale have a 50% chance of surviving for 2–3 years, although this may be improved with oxygen therapy.

COMPLICATIONS
- Atrial arrhythmias are the most common nonpulmonary complication.
- Recurrences of atrial fibrillation and difficulty restoring sinus rhythm are found in patients with significant right atrial dilatation.

PATIENT MONITORING
- Arterial oxygen saturation should be monitored periodically.
- International normalized ratio (INR) needs to be periodically assessed in patients on warfarin.
- Renal function should be periodically assessed in patients on diuretics.

REFERENCES
1. Budev MM, Arroliga AC, Wiedemann HP, et al. Cor pulmonale: An overview. *Semin Respir Crit Care Med*. 2003;24:233–244.
2. Humbert M, Sitbon O, Simonneau G. Treatment of pulmonary arterial hypertension. *N Engl J Med*. 2004;351:1425–1436.

CODES
ICD9-CM
- 415.0 Acute cor pulmonale
- 416.9 Chronic cor pulmonale

PATIENT TEACHING
Diet
Low-sodium if right heart failure or hypoxia is present

Activity
Restricted if right heart failure or hypoxia is present

Prevention
Smoking is the most important modifiable risk factor.

FAQ
Q: What is the definition of cor pulmonale?
A: Cor pulmonale is an alteration in the structure and function of the right ventricle caused by an underlying pulmonary or vascular disorder.

Q: What therapies are available to treat patients with this disease?
A: Treat the underlying respiratory or vascular disorder.
- Oxygen therapy if warranted
- Bronchodilators
- Warfarin if thromboembolic etiology is detected
- Diuretics may be used for symptom relief.

COR TRIATRIATUM

Stéphanie Levasseur
Welton M. Gersony

 BASICS

DESCRIPTION

In this congenital anomaly, a fibromuscular membrane separates the left atrium (LA) into a posterior chamber (common pulmonary vein) receiving the pulmonary veins and an anterior chamber (true LA) communicating with the mitral valve and LA appendage. The presence of the atrial appendage in the anterior chamber is the feature distinguishing cor triatriatum from a supramitral ring. In the classic form, pulmonary venous chamber flow enters the mitral inflow chamber through a small communication. This results in restriction of the pulmonary venous return with secondary pulmonary hypertension. Presentation depends on the severity of obstruction between the common pulmonary vein and LA. An atrial septal defect is seen in 70–80% of cases; the communication is almost always at the level of the lower left atrial chamber. The "classical" form of cor triatriatum has no associated defects.

EPIDEMIOLOGY

Prevalence

Cor triatriatum is a rare cardiac anomaly. This diagnosis was made in 0.01–0.22% of patients in different surveys of children with congenital heart disease. The prospective Bohemian study reported a prevalence of 0.006 per 1,000 live births.

RISK FACTORS

No known risk factors

Genetics

No known genetic transmission

PATHOPHYSIOLOGY

Failure of complete incorporation of the common pulmonary vein into the LA or stenosis of the common pulmonary vein is the most accepted embryologic basis for cor triatriatum.

ETIOLOGY

No known etiology

ASSOCIATED CONDITIONS

Very rare reports of associated noncardiac lesions

 DIAGNOSIS

SIGNS AND SYMPTOMS

Signs and symptoms are almost invariably dependant on the severity of pulmonary venous obstruction and secondary increased pulmonary pressure.

History

- Some patients with minimal obstruction are asymptomatic or may have mild pulmonary symptoms.
- The great majority of patients present during early childhood with significant pulmonary venous obstruction.
- Presentations in infants and younger children:
  - Frequent respiratory infections, wheezing
  - Feeding difficulties, failure to thrive
  - Congestive heart failure with dyspnea, tachypnea, diaphoresis, lethargy
  - Hepatomegaly
  - Low cardiac output with pallor, decreased peripheral pulses
- Presentations in older children and adults:
  - Similar to mitral stenosis
  - Frequent respiratory infections
  - Dyspnea, orthopnea, paroxysmal nocturnal dyspnea
  - Symptomatology can be precipitated by failure to increase flow through the obstruction during exercise, pregnancy, infection, emotional stress
  - Atrial fibrillation
  - Hemoptysis
  - Symptomatology associated with right heart failure secondary to pulmonary hypertension: Edema, ascites, lethargy

Physical Exam

- In severe cases, pulmonary venous flow across the obstruction rarely causes more than a faint diastolic murmur. In mild cases, a louder diastolic murmur may be audible.
- Presence of an atrial septal defect (ASD) with left to right flow can cause a systolic outflow murmur.
- Pulmonary rales
- Evidence of pulmonary hypertension
  - Right ventricular heave
  - Loud pulmonary component of the second heart sound
- Evidence of right heart failure
  - Increased jugular venous pressure
  - Hepatomegaly
  - Ascites and edema
- Evidence of low cardiac output may be present.

TESTS

Lab

ECG

- Findings consistent with pulmonary hypertension
  - Right ventricular hypertrophy
  - Tall, peaked P-waves for right atrial hypertrophy
  - Broad, notched P-waves sometimes seen as a sign of dilation of the posterior chamber

Imaging

- Chest radiograph
  - Evidence of pulmonary venous congestion with interstitial edema and possible Kerley B lines
  - Possible evidence of pulmonary hypertension with an enlarged main pulmonary artery and right ventricular dilatation
  - Possible evidence of "LA" enlargement secondary to dilated posterior chamber
- Echocardiography:
  - Echocardiography is the specific modality for the diagnosis of cor triatriatum.
  - The membrane is seen as a linear echodensity in the LA. The severity of obstruction can be readily studied by Doppler evaluation. Secondary signs of pulmonary hypertension, the presence of an atrial septal communication and/or other anomalies are also readily evaluated by 2D and Doppler imaging.
  - 3-dimensional echocardiography also has been used to delineate the anatomy of this malformation.
- Magnetic resonance imaging:
  - MRI can be used to complement the echocardiogram in cases where echocardiographic images are more limited. It can help delineate associated anomalies and help refine the ventricular functional assessment.
- Computed tomography (CT)
  - CT also has been used to diagnose the intraatrial membrane of cor triatriatum.

Diagnostic Procedures/Surgery

Cardiac catheterization:

- Diagnostic catheterization is no longer routinely performed.
- Hemodynamic findings include pulmonary hypertension with an increased pulmonary arterial wedge pressure and normal LA anterior chamber pressure. A left to right shunt can be ruled out by oximetry. The intraatrial membrane can be identified by angiography. Other associated defects can be delineated.

Pathological Findings

The malformation consists of a fibromuscular membrane.

DIFFERENTIAL DIAGNOSIS

- Causes of pulmonary hypertension with pulmonary venous congestion:
  - Stenosis of the pulmonary veins
  - Small left-sided structures, including congenital mitral stenosis, with a restrictive atrial septum
  - Mitral valve stenosis
  - Left atrial thrombus
  - Left atrial myxoma
- Other causes of pulmonary hypertension:
  - Large left to right shunt from a ventricular septal defect (VSD), ASD, patent ductus arteriosus (PDA)
  - Complex congenital heart disease
  - Pulmonary disease
  - Primary pulmonary hypertension

 TREATMENT

GENERAL MEASURES

Supportive measures are necessary in the gravely ill patient. These include oxygen and ventilatory support if needed.

 MEDICATION (DRUGS)

- Medical treatment is aimed at relieving symptomatology before surgical correction and is only supportive in nature.
- In severely symptomatic patients, surgery should not be delayed.
- Postoperative treatment may require vigorous measures to reduce reactive pulmonary hypertension.

SURGERY

- Treatment of cor triatriatum is surgical and includes complete resection of the membrane on cardiopulmonary bypass. It is a relatively simple intervention with low operative mortality.
- Although balloon dilatation of the membrane has been reported, operative intervention remains the preferred treatment.

 FOLLOW-UP

PROGNOSIS

- Untreated patients presenting in the 1st year after birth have a mortality rate of 75% or more depending on severity of obstruction.
- Prognosis after surgical repair depends on patient status at the time of diagnosis. Postoperative risk is predominantly pulmonary hypertensive crises. For patients in good condition with the classical form, prognosis is excellent and late complications rare.

Pregnancy Considerations

Pregnancy is well tolerated after successful repair of cor triatriatum.

COMPLICATIONS

- Pulmonary infections
- Pulmonary hypertension
- Hemoptysis
- Right heart failure
- Atrial arrhythmias
- Systemic thromboembolic events
- Low cardiac output

PATIENT MONITORING

- Rarely, asymptomatic patients with unrestrictive membranes have been followed closely without intervention. No clear consensus exists as to the right course of action in these patients; some propose intervention in very active individuals and women who may become pregnant.
- After surgery, monitoring is easily done using serial echocardiography.

REFERENCES

1. Allen HD, et al., eds. *Moss and Adams' heart disease in infants, children, and adolescents: including the fetus and young adult,* 6th ed. Philadelphia: Lippincott Williams & Wilkins, 2001.
2. Alphonso N, Norgaard MA, Newcomb A, et al. Cor triatriatum: Presentation, diagnosis and long-term surgical results. *Ann Thorac Surg.* 2005;80: 1666–1671.
3. Bonow RO, Carabello B, de Leon AC Jr., et al. ACC/AHA guidelines for the management of patients with valvular heart disease. A report of the American College of Cardiology/American Heart Association. Task Force on Practice Guidelines (Committee on Management of Patients with Valvular Heart Disease). *J Am Coll Cardiol.* 1998;32:1486–1588.
4. Freedom RM, et al., eds. *The natural and modified history of congenital heart disease.* Elmsford, NY: Blackwell Pub./Futura, 2004.
5. Herlong JR, Jaggers JJ, Ungerleider RM. Congenital Heart Surgery Nomenclature and Database Project: pulmonary venous anomalies. *Ann Thorac Surg.* 2000;69(4 Suppl):S56–69.

 MISCELLANEOUS

CODES

ICD9-CM
746.82

PATIENT TEACHING

Diet
No dietary restrictions

Activity
No restriction of physical activities after the surgical repair.

CORONARY HEART DISEASE RISK FACTORS

Randal J. Thomas
Matthew E. Wiisanen

 BASICS

DESCRIPTION

- Risk factors are modifiable and nonmodifiable features that increase risk of atherosclerotic coronary artery disease (CAD).
- Long-term exposure to CAD risk factors is associated with clinical manifestations of CAD by interacting with the processes of atherosclerosis and thromboembolism.
- Clinical manifestations of CAD include angina pectoris, myocardial infarction (MI), and sudden cardiac death.

GENERAL PREVENTION

- Therapeutic lifestyle change including
  - Healthy dietary and exercise habits
  - Smoking cessation
- Medical therapy targeting control of hypertension (HTN), hyperlipidemia (HL), and diabetes (DM)

EPIDEMIOLOGY

- Over 250 identified risk factors, but majority of risk of CAD events is explained by DM, smoking, HTN, and HL.
- Risk factors contribute to the worldwide epidemic of cardiovascular disease (CVD)
- CVD is the leading cause of death in men >35 years and women >45 years.

Incidence

- DM: Approximately 1.4 million new cases between ages of 18–79 in 2004. Incidence has increased 54% from 1997.
- Smoking: More than 1.8 million Americans became daily smokers in 1996, with 66% under the age of 18.
- HTN: 7-year incidence of HTN is approximately 25% in U.S. adults.
- Majority of risk factors begin prior to adulthood.

Prevalence

- Generally, prevalence of CHD risk factors increases with age.
- Diabetes: Present in 8% of adults above 20 years of age; 18% of adults over 60. People aged 65 years or older account for almost 40% of the population with diabetes.
- Obesity, strongly correlated with DM, HTN, and HL, is increasing at alarming rates. 60% of adults are overweight or obese.
- Smoking rates have decreased over the past 3 decades. 44.5 million American adults (20%) now smoke.
- HTN is present in approximately 20% of adults.
- HL is present in approximately 20% of adults.
- Overall 58% prevalence of atherosclerosis in one autopsy study done in Olmsted County, MN.
- Atherosclerosis significantly higher in men than in women and in diabetic patients compared to nondiabetic controls.

RISK FACTORS

- Major modifiable risk factors:
  - Smoking
  - Hypertension (>140/90)
  - Elevated low-density lipoprotein (LDL) cholesterol (>13)
  - Low high-density lipoprotein (HDL) cholesterol (<40 mg/dL)
  - Physical inactivity
  - Diabetes (considered CHD equivalent by ATP III guidelines)
- Other risk factors:
  - Age: Males >50, females >60
  - Family history of early CHD (first-degree male relative <55 years, and first-degree female relative <65)
  - Male gender
  - Low socioeconomic status (SES)
  - Obesity
  - Family history of any vascular disease
  - Diet high in saturated fat
  - Estrogen deficiency
  - Left ventricular hypertrophy (LVH)
  - Psychosocial factors (positive and negative)
  - Hypertriglyceridemia
  - Elevated lipoprotein (a)
  - Hyperhomocysteinemia
  - Metabolic syndrome
- Other potential risk indicators:
  - Inflammatory markers (hs-CRP, others)
  - Thrombotic factors (fibrinogen, others)
  - Impaired endothelial function
  - Subclinical cardiovascular disease (coronary calcium score, ankle-brachial index (ABI), carotid intimal medial thickness (IMI))
- Risk factors can be used to estimate a person's risk of future CAD events (see references section).

Genetics

- A number of genetic links to CAD risk factors and to CAD have been suggested. Currently evaluated factors include:
  - Family history of heart disease
  - Familial hyperlipidemia syndromes
  - Elevated lipoprotein (a)
  - Homocysteine
- Future areas of study include gene–lifestyle and gene–drug interactions.

PATHOPHYSIOLOGY

- Risk factors are associated with a cycle of endothelial injury and repair, which leads to the development of subclinical CAD (an atherosclerotic plaque or atheroma).
- Continued exposure to risk factors leads to a disruption of atheroma, thrombosis, and clinical manifestations of CAD.

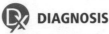 **DIAGNOSIS**

SIGNS AND SYMPTOMS

- HTN: Blood pressure (BP) >140/90; largely asymptomatic
- DM: Fasting glucose >125, two or more occasions; symptoms include polydipsia, polyuria, and polyphagia
- HL: LDL >130, HDL <40, triglycerides >150; largely asymptomatic

History

- Dietary and exercise habits
- Tobacco exposure
- Family history of CAD
- Past history of HTN, diabetes, previous CVD

Physical Exam

- BP, both arms
- Body composition (body mass index [BMI], waist and hip circumference, body fat percentage)
- Skin and eye exam looking for stigmata of hyperlipidemia (xanthomas, xanthelasma, arcus senilis)
- Funduscopic exam for stigmata of hypertensive eye disease (A-V nicking, copper wiring, flame-shaped hemorrhages) and diabetic retinopathy

TESTS

Lab

- Cholesterol profile
- Emerging lipid measurements (ApoB, LDL particle number)
- Fasting blood glucose
- Genetic markers (lipoprotein [a], homocysteine)
- Inflammatory markers (hs-CRP, others)

Imaging

- Coronary calcification CT scan
- Carotid ultrasound (IMT)
- Echocardiography to look for LVH

Diagnostic Procedures/Surgery

- Ambulatory BP monitor if HTN suspected
- Ankle-brachial index (ABI)

DIFFERENTIAL DIAGNOSIS

- Assess secondary causes of HTN.
  - Renovascular disease
  - Endocrine disorders
  - Sleep apnea
- Assess secondary causes of HL.
  - Hypothyroidism
  - Liver disease
  - Renal disease

TREATMENT

GENERAL MEASURES

- Therapeutic lifestyle change
  - Physical activity, including 30 min of brisk activity, at least 5 days a week. Strength training, at least 30 min/ week also is recommended, along with daily stretching/balance activities.
  - Healthy nutrition habits, including 5 or more servings of fruits and vegetables, whole grains high in fiber, healthy sources of protein that are low saturated fats, and a modest amount of healthy fats (unsaturated fats).
- Smoking cessation
- Management of diabetes
- Control of hypertension
- Control lipid abnormalities
- Maintaining ideal body weight (BMI 20–25 kg/m^2)

 MEDICATION (DRUGS)

- Elevated LDL cholesterol
  - First line
    - Statins (HMG Co-A reductase inhibitors)
    - Nicotinic acid
  - Second line
    - Ezetimibe
  - Bile acid resins
- Elevated triglyceride level
  - First line
    - Fibrates
    - Nicotinic acid
  - Second line
    - Ω-3 Fatty acids
- DM
  - First line
    - Metformin
    - Thiazolidinediones
    - α-Glucosidase inhibitors
  - Second line
    - Insulin secretogogues: Sulfonylureas, meglitinides
    - Insulin (first-line for Type 1 DM)
- HTN
  - First line
    - β-Blockers
    - Angiotensin-converting enzyme (ACE) inhibitors
    - Angiotensin receptor blockers
    - Thiazide diuretics
  - Second line
    - Calcium channel blockers
- Other treatments
  - LDL apheresis (consider for extreme elevation in LDL cholesterol not controlled with drug therapy)

 FOLLOW-UP

DISPOSITION
Issues for Referral
Consider referral to specialized center for patients with complex HTN, HL, or DM conditions.

PROGNOSIS
Long-term risk of future CAD events can be estimated by various models, including the Framingham Risk Score and risk estimates (see References section).

PATIENT MONITORING
- Monitor adherence and response to therapy.
- Monitor for potential side effects of medications.
- Assess attainment of goals for HTN, HL, and DM.
- HL: Monitor liver enzymes if patient is on a statin.
- DM: Monitor hemoglobin A1C to assess control of DM, assess urine microalbumin to assess renal status, undergo yearly eye evaluation.

REFERENCES

1. Hopkins PH, Williams RR. A survey of 246 suggested coronary risk factors. *Atherosclerosis*. 1981;40(1):1–52.
2. Kuller LH. Prevention of cardiovascular disease and the future of cardiovascular disease epidemiology. *Intern J Epidemiol*. 2001;20 Suppl:S66–S72.
3. Berenson GS, Smivasah SR. Cardiovascular risk factors in youth with implications for aging: The Bogalusa Heart Study. *Neurobiol Aging*. 2005;26(3):303–307.
4. Incidence of Initiation of cigarette smoking. United States, 1965–1996. *MMWR*. 1998;47(39):837–840.
5. He J, Klag MS, Appel LJ, et al. Seven-year incidence of hypertension in a cohort of middle-aged African Americans and whites. *Hypertension*. 1998;31(5):1130–1135.
6. Kullo IJ, Ballantyne CM. Conditional risk factors for atherosclerosis. *Mayo Clin Proc*. 2005;80(2):219–230.
7. Framingham Risk Calculator: http://hp2010.nhlbihin.net/atpiii/calculator.asp
8. http://www.cdc.gov
9. http://www.nhlbi.nih.gov/guidelines/cholesterol
10. http://www.americanheart.org
11. Roger VL, Weston SA, Killian JM, et al. Time trends in the prevalence of atherosclerosis: A population-based autopsy study. *Am J Med*. 2001 Mar:110(4):267–273.

ADDITIONAL READING
Preventive Cardiology: How can we do better? Proceedings of the 33rd Bethesda Conference. *J Am Coll Cardiol*. 2002;40(4):580–651.

CODES
ICD9-CM
- 401.0 Hypertension
- 272.0 Hypercholesterolemia
- 250.0 Diabetes
- 305.1 Tobacco abuse
- 278.0 Obesity

PATIENT TEACHING
Interactive, patient-centered action plans to help patients change lifestyle behaviors and follow recommendations for medical therapies.

Diet
Nutrition counseling indicated in patients with suboptimal dietary habits; consider counseling with registered dietitian.

Activity
Physical-activity counseling indicated in patients with suboptimal physical activity habits; consider formal exercise evaluation or fitness program with trained exercise personnel.

Prevention
Self-management training is indicated to help patients understand that much of CAD prevention depends on their individual lifestyle habits and adherence to preventive medications.

COUNTERPULSATION (AORTIC)

Gerald Cioce
Robert Hogan*
Gerard P. Aurigemma

 BASICS

DESCRIPTION

- Aortic counterpulsation is a means of assisting the failing heart by automatically removing arterial blood just before and during ventricular ejection and returning it to the circulation during diastole.
- Extracorporeal counterpulsation was first introduced in 1961.
- Intraaortic balloon pump (IABP) insertion via sheath/dilator was described in 1980.
- IABP is a standard in circulatory assistance (100,000 placed in the U.S. in 1993).
- Counterpulsation improves the myocardial oxygen supply–demand balance. Inflation of the IABP during diastole displaces a volume of blood, increasing diastolic blood pressure. Rapid balloon deflation just prior to systolic ejection reduces afterload and myocardial work.
- Hemodynamic effects:
  - Decrease in systolic arterial pressure
  - Increase in diastolic arterial pressure
  - No change in mean arterial pressure
  - Decrease in pulmonary capillary wedge pressure
  - Increase in cardiac output
  - Increase or no change in coronary blood flow
  - Increase in urine output
- Recently, enhanced external counterpulsation (sequential inflation of three cuffs from ankle to thigh on each leg during diastole) has been associated with fewer anginal episodes and with longer exercise duration without ECG evidence of ischemia.

 TREATMENT

- Indications for IABP
  - Acute coronary syndrome with:
    - Cardiogenic shock
    - Recurrent ischemic discomfort and signs of hemodynamic instability, poor LV function, or large area of myocardium at risk
    - Refractory ventricular tachycardia
    - Refractory pulmonary congestion
    - Mechanical complications of acute myocardial infarction (MI) (mitral regurgitation [MR] or ventricular septal defect [VSD])
  - Percutaneous coronary intervention in patients with:
    - Hemodynamic instability
    - High risk or complicated coronary intervention
  - Cardiac Surgery in patients with:
    - Severe left ventricular dysfunction
    - Severe left main coronary artery stenosis
    - Repeat coronary artery bypass surgery (CABG)
    - Critical aortic stenosis
    - Postcardiotomy cardiogenic shock
  - Hemodynamic support while awaiting transplant
- Absolute contraindications:
  - Significant aortic insufficiency
  - Aortic dissection
- Relative contraindications to femoral placement:
  - Abdominal aortic aneurysm
  - Severe calcific aortoiliac or femoral arterial disease
  - Recent groin incision at proposed site
  - Surgeons may place via intrathoracic route if femoral route not possible

GENERAL MEASURES

- IABP insertion:
  - Balloon catheter is introduced over wire via common femoral artery.
  - Balloon diameter should be no more than 80–90% of aortic diameter; the 40-mL balloon is adequate for most adults (30–34 mL if small, 50 mL if very large patient).
  - Tip of catheter is placed in descending aorta, just distal to left subclavian artery.
  - Balloon is inflated at dicrotic notch and deflated during isovolumic contraction (pressure monitored via central lumen in IABP catheter).
  - If ECG is used to control balloon, inflation occurs on T-wave, deflation on R-wave. Note: If patient is in atrial fibrillation, deflation on the R-wave is the preferred timing method to prevent ventricular contraction against an inflated balloon during a short R-R cycle.
  - IABP timing should be adjusted while assisting every other beat (1:2) so that assisted-beat waveforms can be compared with normal beats.
  - IABP catheter is attached to bedside control/monitoring console.
  - Helium gas (30–50 mL) is used to inflate balloon, due to its low viscosity (rapid shuttling needed in tachyarrhythmias).
- Management of IABP:
  - Heparin anticoagulation with partial thromboplastin time 50–70 sec
  - Evaluation of the involved limb for ischemia every 2–6 hours
  - Daily evaluation for evidence of sepsis, thrombocytopenia, blood loss, hemolysis, vascular obstruction, thrombus, embolus, or dissection

- Thrombocytopenia is expected due to traumatic platelet destruction, but counts rarely fall below 50,000–100,000/mL unless some other problem exists (e.g., disseminated intravascular coagulation, heparin-induced thrombocytopenia).
- Monitoring for normal pressure waveform (normally rectangular appearance with brief overshoot and undershoot artifacts)
- If rounding of the waveform occurs, consider a kink in the balloon or connection tubing, an incompletely inflated balloon, or an oversized balloon.
- Patients are kept on bed rest, with restricted hip flexion and head of bed elevated no more than 30 degrees.
- Prophylactic antibiotics (e.g., cefazolin) are not given routinely, but should be given at time of insertion if any compromise occurs in sterile technique.
- Daily chest radiograph to evaluate for proper catheter tip position at the level of the carina

PROGNOSIS

- 75% of patients who develop cardiogenic shock refractory to medication post-MI will respond to IABP therapy (ultimate outcome determined by coronary pathology; patients with operable disease achieve early survival as high as 93%).
- For ventricular septal rupture post-MI, IABP reduces left-to-right shunt; combined with urgent surgery allows 73–80% survival.
- For papillary muscle rupture post-MI, IABP increases coronary perfusion and reduces ischemic load, MR, and pulmonary capillary wedge pressure; mortality is related to extent of cardiac dysfunction and approaches 55%.
- For postcardiotomy cardiogenic shock, IAPB allows survival in 52–66%.
- 1-year survival in patients who require IABP pre-transplantation is 72–77%.

COMPLICATIONS

- Risk factors:
  - Diabetes mellitus
  - Low cardiac index
  - Female gender
  - Peripheral vascular disease
  - Extended use (e.g., >5 days)
- Complication rates range from 6% to 46%.
- Balloon rupture is rare.
- Major complications in 4–17% (leg ischemia requiring thrombectomy or amputation, aortic dissection, aortoiliac laceration or perforation, and deep wound infection requiring debridement)
- Minor complications in 7–42% (bleeding at insertion site, superficial wound infection, asymptomatic loss of peripheral pulse, and lymphocele)
- Vascular complications are most common (6–24%). Most are due to insertion procedure.
- If leg ischemia develops, IABP should be removed; if ischemia persists, surgical exploration is indicated.

REFERENCES

1. Aguirre FV, et al. Intraaortic balloon pump support during high-risk coronary angioplasty. *Cardiology*. 1994;84:175–186.
2. Antman EM, et al. ACC/AHA guidelines for the management of patients with ST-elevation myocardial infarction: A report of the American College of Cardiology/American Heart Association Task Force on Practice Guidelines (Committee to Revise the 1999 Guidelines for the Management of Patients with Acute Myocardial Infarction). *Circulation*. 2004;110:282–292.
3. Arora RR, et al. The Multicenter Study of Enhanced External Counterpulsation (MUST-EECP): Effect of EECP on exercise-induced myocardial ischemia and anginal episodes. *J Am Coll Cardiol*. 1999;33:1833–1840.
4. Baim D, *Grossman's cardiac catheterization, angiography, and intervention,* 7th ed. Philadelphia: Lippincott, Williams & Wilkins, 2006.
5. Braunwald E. *Heart disease: A textbook of cardiovascular medicine,* 6th ed. Philadelphia: WB Saunders, 2001.
6. Opie L. *The heart*. Orlando: Grune & Stratton, 1984.
7. Patel JJ, et al. Prospective evaluation of complications associated with percutaneous intraaortic balloon counterpulsation. *Am J Cardiol*. 1995;76:1205–1207.
8. Scheidt S, et al. Intra-aortic balloon counterpulsation in cardiogenic shock. Report of a co-operative clinical trial. *N Engl J Med*. 1973;288:979–984.
9. *Stedman's medical dictionary*, 25th edition. Baltimore: Williams & Wilkins,1990.

CUSHING'S SYNDROME AND THE HEART

Harsimran S. Singh
Deborah L. Ekery

 BASICS

DESCRIPTION

A combination of clinical features and biochemical abnormalities that occur as a result of excessive tissue exposure to cortisol

GENERAL PREVENTION

Exogenous or iatrogenic administration of steroids is included under the umbrella of Cushing syndrome (CS) and causes all the manifestations and complications of endogenous disease. Exogenous steroid use should be avoided as medically appropriate.

EPIDEMIOLOGY

Incidence

- Rare disease: Cushing disease estimated incidence ~0.1–1 new case per 100,000. Exogenous CS from therapeutic use of glucocorticoids is even more common.
- Pituitary hyperproduction of adrenocorticotropic hormone (ACTH) accounts for ~70% of all cases of CS.

Prevalence

Predominant Age: Varies with the cause

- Pituitary (corticotroph) adenoma: 25–40 years.
- Ectopic ACTH secretion: >40 years.
- Adrenal carcinoma: Bimodal age distribution with peaks in childhood/adolescence and late in life.
- Adrenal adenoma: Around 35 years.

Predominant Sex: Varies with the cause

- Adrenal adenomas, adrenal carcinomas, and corticotropin adenomas are 4–6 times more common in women than in men.
- Ectopic ACTH secretion is more common in men than women (may change as more women develop lung cancer, the most common cause of ectopic ACTH secretion).
- Predominant Race: None

RISK FACTORS

Genetic

- Multiple promising genetic targets have been implicated in the pathogenesis of CS:
  - Mouse model studies implicate D2 receptor inhibition as preventing hyperexpression of ACTH. Also, 7B2, a neuroendocrine protein, has been suggested to be integral in preventing the hypersecretion of ACTH in neuroendocrine cells.
  - In adrenal tumors—p53, p57, and insulin-like growth factor II have all been implicated as tumor suppressor genes.

PATHOPHYSIOLOGY

Normal Hypothalamic → Pituitary → Adrenal (HPA) Axis:

- Corticotropin-releasing hormone (CRH) synthesized in the hypothalamus is primary positive activator of ACTH production in anterior pituitary.
- ACTH, the principle product from a large precursor pro-opiomelanocortin (POMC), induces cortisol production from adrenal fasciculata.
- Cortisol, the primary glucocorticoid of the human body, plays a prolific role in metabolism including:
  - Protein and fat catabolism
  - Hepatic gluconeogenesis
  - Immunosuppression and antiinflammatory
  - Stress response
- Cortisol exerts autonegative feedback on the HPA axis at both the level of the anterior pituitary and the hypothalamus.
- CS is caused by any disruption in this axis (endogenous or exogenous) that results in hyperproduction of cortisol:
  - Increased production of ACTH (most common cause in adults) by an adrenal tumor (Cushing disease) or by other ectopic paraneoplastic malignancy.
  - Increased production of cortisol, most commonly because of adrenal adenomas, carcinomas, or hyperplasia.
  - Increased production of CRH (rare because of double-pronged negative feedback loop of cortisol).
  - Exogenous glucocorticoid/corticotrophin
- The hyperproduction of cortisol leads to the pathologic signs and symptoms notable in CS

ETIOLOGY

Exogenous (iatrogenic or factitious)

- CS secondary to use of high-dose glucocorticoids (most common cause of CS)

Endogenous

- ACTH (corticotropin)–dependent: Adrenal activation (overall ~80%).
  - Pituitary corticotroph adenoma (80%) = Cushing disease (CD)
  - Ectopic ACTH secretion (20%): Most commonly associated with small cell lung carcinoma; less commonly with carcinoid or islet cell tumors, pheochromocytoma, neuroblastoma, ganglioma, paraganglioma, and medullary carcinoma of the thyroid.
  - Ectopic corticotropin-releasing hormone (CRH)/corticotroph hyperplasia, corticotroph carcinomas very rare.
  - ACTH-independent: Adrenal activation (overall ~20%).
  - Adrenal adenoma (40–50%)
  - Adrenal carcinoma (40%–50%)
  - Macronodular adrenal hyperplasia
  - Micronodular adrenal hyperplasia (including Carney complex)

ASSOCIATED CONDITIONS

- Affective disorders
- Opportunistic infections
- Perforated viscus
- Renal calculi
- Metabolic syndrome
- Increased atherosclerosis and cardiac risk

 DIAGNOSIS

SIGNS AND SYMPTOMS

- Clinical course is slow and progressive – initial manifestations may be subtle and/or similar to other endocrine abnormalities, making the diagnosis difficult.
- Untreated CS can lead to a picture similar to metabolic syndrome or diabetes.

History

- Weight gain
- Fatigue
- Decreased libido
- Impotence
- Menstrual changes/infertility
- Psychiatric: Mood changes, depression, psychosis
- Impaired concentration or memory
- Insomnia
- Easy bruising
- Poor wound healing
- Fractures
- Headache, backache, abdominal pain

Physical Exam

- Obesity: Increased fat deposition in abdomen (truncal obesity, 96%), face (moon facies, 82%), supraclavicular or temporal fossae, dorsocervical area ("buffalo hump").
- Hypertension: Present in 80–90% of patients. Consider the diagnosis in patients with hypertension who are <40 years of age, especially if blood pressure is difficult to control.
- Striae: Purple, >1 cm in diameter, usually over the abdomen
- Hirsutism
- Fragile and thin skin
- Ecchymoses after minimal trauma
- Edema
- Acne
- Proximal muscle wasting and weakness with preservation of distal strength
- Female balding
- Growth retardation (in children)
- Exophthalmos
- Lisch nodules

Pediatric Considerations
- Unlike adults, the majority of children with CS will present with ACTH-independent CS, typically secondary to adrenal tumors.
- Excess cortisol affects bone growth, so consider screening all children with higher than normal weight patterns and yet stunted linear growth.
- Overall difficult to apply adult screening tests and hormone cutoffs to young children. Refer to well-versed specialty center for treatment.

TESTS
Patient's with central obesity or other cutaneous features; metabolic syndrome; hypogonadotrophic and hypogonadism; and osteoporosis at age <65 years old.

Lab
- White blood cell count ≥11,000/mm³
- Hypokalemic metabolic alkalosis
- Glucose intolerance: Hyperglycemia with resultant glucosuria and polydipsia.
- Elevated triglycerides, low-density lipoprotein (LDL) or high-density lipoprotein (HDL) levels.
- Decreased thyroid-stimulating hormone, luteinizing hormone, follicle-stimulating hormone levels
- Electrocardiographic abnormalities
- Accelerated atherosclerosis
- Osteopenia/osteoporosis on X-ray
  I. Establish the diagnosis of high cortisol

First-Line Screening:
- Salivary Cortisol at bedtime (~11:00 p.m.) – sensitivity/specificity approaching 95%
  - Recently introduced test, but many experts consider this as optimal first-line screening when available.
- 24-hour urine for free cortisol; generally on 2–3 consecutive days; 50% sensitive (improves with successive days of testing) and ~100% specific
- Low-dose dexamethasone suppression test
  - 2-Day dexamethasone suppression test: Administer 0.5 mg dexamethasone every 6 hours for eight doses. Urine free cortisol (UFC) levels >10 μg (>28 μmol) per 24 hours or urinary 17-hydroxycorticosteroid values >2.5 mg (6.9 μmol) per 24 hours indicate the presence of CS.
  - Overnight dexamethasone suppression test: Administer 1 mg dexamethasone at 11 p.m. or midnight. Plasma cortisol levels at 8 a.m. are >5 μg/dL (>138nmol/L) suggest the diagnosis of CS.

Second-Line Screening:
- Midnight plasma cortisol: Evening nadir is preserved in patients with pseudo-CS but not in those with CS. Difficult to obtain in natural setting.
- Dexamethasone-CRH test: In pseudo-CS, plasma cortisol levels are low (<1.4 μg/dL) after administration of dexamethasone and remain low when CRH is given soon after. In patients with CS, levels are higher. Expensive test and should be reserved when other screening tests remain equivocal.

II. CS versus pseudo-CS
- Insulin tolerance test: Plasma cortisol levels increase in response to insulin-induced hypoglycemia in patients with pseudo-CS but not in patients with CS.
- Administration of naloxone releases less CRH (and therefore less ACTH and cortisol) in patients with CS than in those with pseudo-CS.

III. Distinguish sub-type of CS
- Determine if CS is ACTH-dependent or ACTH-independent:
- Measurement of ACTH by radioimmunoassay
  - Levels <5 to 10 pg/mL suggest ACTH-independent (i.e., primary adrenal) CS
  - Levels >15 to 20 pg/mL suggest ACTH-dependent CS
- If ACTH-dependent, determine the source of excess ACTH secretion:
  - High-dose dexamethasone suppression test
    - 2-Day: Administer 2 mg dexamethasone every 6 hours for eight doses with measurement of UFC or urine cortisol metabolites. Suppression of UFC by more than 90% of mean basal values or suppression of 17-hydroxysteroid excretion by more than 64% is suggestive of a pituitary source of excess ACTH secretion (CD)
    - Overnight: Dexamethasone, 8 mg, is administered at 11 p.m., and plasma cortisol is measured between 7 a.m. and 8 a.m. that morning and the next morning. A decrease in plasma cortisol by ≥50% is suggestive of CD.
    - Sensitivity approaching 70% and specificity ~100% for Cushing disease
  - Metyrapone stimulation test
    - Metyrapone blocks the conversion of 11-deoxycortisol to cortisol, leading to a decrease in plasma cortisol, increase in ACTH secretion by the pituitary, increase in plasma 11-deoxycortisol, and urinary 17-hydroxycorticosteroid concentrations.
  - CRH stimulation test
    - Corticotropin-secreting tumors retain sensitivity to CRH, whereas noncorticotroph tumors do not respond to CRH.

Imaging
- Not useful for making the diagnosis of CS and should be used only for localization of tumors.
  - If the patient has ACTH-independent CS, thin-section computed tomography (CT) or magnetic resonance imaging (MRI) of the adrenal glands should be performed.
  - If the patient has ACTH-dependent CS with ACTH secretion that cannot be suppressed with dexamethasone, chest CT or MRI should be performed.
  - If the patient has CD, high-resolution CT or MRI of the sella turcica should be performed to determine the location of the adenoma and to locate bony landmarks prior to transsphenoidal surgery.

Diagnostic Procedures/Surgery
- Bilateral inferior petrosal sinus sampling
  - Most precise and direct way of measuring ACTH levels from region proximal to pituitary—may be the most sensitive/specific test for Cushing disease.
  - Consider performing this test only if the results of two or more noninvasive tests are inconsistent, as the test is invasive and operator-dependent.

DIFFERENTIAL DIAGNOSIS
- Glucocorticoid resistance: Compensatory increases in ACTH and excessive glucocorticoid production
- Pseudo-CS: Mild glucocorticoid excess of unclear pathophysiology seen in affective disorders, renal failure, chronic alcoholism, withdrawal from alcohol, hypoglycemia, strenuous exercise (UFC threefold normal), and HIV (may be secondary to antiretroviral therapies).
  - Up to 80% of patients with major depression have abnormal regulation of cortisol.
  - In pseudo-CS evening plasma cortisol concentrations may be preserved and the degree of hypercortisolism is usually mild and transient—may consider insulin tolerance test and naloxone induction test if need further assistance in differential.
- Many signs/symptoms of CS are common in the general population (hypertension, obesity, mood changes, and menstrual irregularities). Also must consider metabolic syndrome/diabetes, polycystic ovarian syndrome, thyroid/parathyroid abnormalities, and hypogonadotrophic hypogonadism.

 TREATMENT

GENERAL MEASURES
- Generally not an acute illness—although long-term cardiovascular complications and risk of infections may mandate prompt stabilization and treatment.
- These patient's should be considered in a similar framework as metabolic syndrome patients or diabetics—cardiac risk factors and disease should be assessed and treated aggressively.
- Hypertension and cardiovascular disease should be assessed and treated prior to surgery.
- Impaired glucose tolerance should be treated with insulin.
- For iatrogenic CS, weaning and eventual discontinuation of glucocorticoid ingestion should be attempted. If this is not possible, a change in dose may improve symptoms of CS.
- Other therapy: Pituitary irradiation
  - As second line, if transsphenoid surgery not curative and if patient not suitable for second operation.
- Disorders of increased cortisol can be difficult to diagnose and have long-term implications.
- A thorough history and physical examination can help in raising clinical suspicion of the disease.
- An awareness of the complications of CS is crucial—the complications include hypertension, metabolic syndrome, increased cardiac mortality, opportunistic infections, and mood disorders.

MEDICATION (DRUGS)

- Medications should be considered second-line therapies for patients who cannot safely undergo surgery or for those with occult or metastatic tumors.
- Used in conjunction with radiation therapy for CD patients who are not candidates for surgery.
- Agents that modulate CRH or ACTH release at HPA level (rarely effective alone):
  - Serotonin antagonists: Cyproheptadine, ritanserin, miterngoline, ketanserin
  - Dopamine agonists: Bromocriptine, lisuride
  - γ-Aminobutyric acid (GABA) reuptake inhibitors: Valproic acid
  - Somatostatin analog: Octreotide
- Agents that inhibit steroidogenesis at adrenal level—most effective category of the drugs—generally work via cytochrome P450:
  - Mitotane* most commonly used
  - Trilostane
  - Metyrapone
  - Aminoglutethamide
  - Ketoconazole
  - Etomidate
- Agents that bind competitively to the glucocorticoid receptor and inhibit the action of the endogenous ligand.
  - RU 486 (Mifepristone)***

SURGERY

Directed toward resection of abnormal tissue (ACTH- or cortisol-producing).

In Cushing disease:

- Trans-sphenoidal Selective Adenomectomy
  - Most widely accepted treatment modality
  - Total remission rates of ~80–90% (success criteria is undetectable post-operative plasma cortisol level).
  - Patients require exogenous glucocorticoid until HPA recovery (~4–12 months).

In Primary Adrenal Hypersecretion:

- Bilateral adrenalectomy
  - 100 % cure rate—with life long glucocorticoid and mineralocorticoid replacement (hydrocortisone 20–30 mg daily and fludrocortisones 50–100 ug daily).
  - Also viable option in Cushing's disease patients who fail trans-sphenoidal surgery and radiotherapy.
  - Carcinomas generally continue progression.
  - Risk of developing Nelson syndrome with dark pigmentation, high ACTH levels, and radiographic pituitary adenoma.

 FOLLOW-UP

PROGNOSIS

- The life expectancy of patients with nonmalignant causes of CS has improved significantly with effective surgical and medical treatments, antibiotics, antihypertensive agents, lipid-lowering agents, and glucocorticoids.
- Prognosis is affected by age, clinical severity, presence of major depression, high urine free cortisol levels, and post-treatment ACTH levels.
- The life expectancy of patients with malignant causes of CS varies depending on the type of tumor.
- Survival analysis suggests that up to 99% of Cushing's disease patients remain in remission after successful pituitary surgery after 2 years and ~75% after 10 years.
- Recurrence of CS after surgical resection varies depending on the cause. It is common with adrenal carcinoma, rare with adrenal adenoma, and relatively uncommon with pituitary adenoma.
- Surgical skill and experience is paramount in achieving surgical outcomes.

COMPLICATIONS

Given hypercoaguable state of CS patients – all should be treated with heparin prophylaxis while in hospital to prevent thrombosis complications.

ALERT
Pregnancy
- Up to 75% of CS patients have ovulatory disturbances secondary to high cortisol levels.
- Difficult to make the diagnosis of CS during pregnancy because of physical and biochemical changes that are common in both conditions (hypertension, glucose intolerance, weight gain, fatigue, striae).
- Potential complications of pregnancy are maternal diabetes, hypertension, preeclampsia, and heart failure and in the fetus, spontaneous abortion and premature delivery.
- Some evidence of improved pregnancy options with treatment.
- Use of ketoconazole, aminogluthemide, or mitotane is contraindicated in pregnancy.
- Cardiac Disease/Metabolic Syndrome
  – Untreated CS patients go on to develop a clinical picture and risk profile similar to Metabolic Syndrome.
    • Metabolic syndrome shares many of the common clinical features as CS—both lead to decreased insulin sensitivity, increased abdominal girth (waist-to-hip ratio), dyslipidemia, and hypertension.
    • Leads to greater risk of cardiac events.
  – Cortisol also directly leads to progression of atherosclerosis through vascular remodeling.
  – Limited evidence on the cardiac risk of surgically treated CS patients, but ~20%–50% of patients remain obese, hypertensive, dyslipidemic, etc., despite treatment.
    • While cardiac risk improves with treatment of CS, it does not appear to return to that of the baseline population.

PATIENT MONITORING
- Most patients have underlying suppression of the hypothalamic–pituitary–adrenal axis that is unmasked after surgical correction of CS.
- Once routine postoperative supraphysiologic doses of glucocorticoids have been tapered off, patients should have morning serum cortisol and daily urine free cortisol measured for 3 days.
- If these levels are persistently low, physiologic replacement doses of hydrocortisone should be initiated and continued until recovery of the adrenal axis.
- Recovery of the adrenal axis can be assessed by evaluation of the patient's signs and symptoms and by the cortisol response to synthetic ACTH; initial testing should be done at 6–9 months postoperatively.
- After pituitary surgery, patients should have serum osmolality, serum sodium, and urine output monitored, because diabetes insipidus is a potential complication.
- After bilateral adrenalectomy, patients will need lifelong glucocorticoid and mineralocorticoid replacement.

REFERENCES
1. Arnaldi G, Angeli A, Atkinson B, et al. Diagnosis & complications of Cushing's syndrome: A consensus statement. *J Endocrinol Metab.* 2005;88:5593–5602.
2. Bornstein SR, Stratakis CA, Chrousos GP. Adrenocortical tumors: Recent advances in basic concepts and clinical management. *Ann Int Med.* 1999;130:759–771.
3. Boscaro M, Barzon L, Fallo F, et al. Cushing's syndrome. *Lancet.* 2001;357:783–791.
4. Jacobson L. Hypothalamic-pituitary-adrenocortical axis regulation. *Endocrinol Metabol Clin.* 2005;34:271–292.
5. Kaplan NM. Systemic hypertension: Mechanisms and diagnosis. In: Braunwald E, ed. *Heart Disease,* 5th ed. Philadelphia: WB Saunders,1997;829.
6. Lindsay JR, Nieman LK. Differential Diagnosis and Imaging in Cushing's Syndrome. *Endocrinol Metabol Clin.* 2005;34:403–421.
7. Nieman L, Cutler GB. Cushing's syndrome. In: Degroot LJ, ed. *Endocrinology,* 3rd ed. Philadelphia: WB Saunders, 1995;1741–1769.
8. Orth DN. Cushing's Syndrome. *N Engl J Med.* 1995;332:791–803.
9. Pivonello R, Faggiano A, Lombardi G, et al. The metabolic syndrome and cardiovascular risk in Cushing's syndrome. *Endocrinol Metabol Clin.* 2005;34:327–339.
10. Shomali ME, Hussain MA. Cushing's Syndrome: From patients to proteins. *Eur J Endocrinol.* 2000;143:313–315.
11. Williams GH, Lilly LS, Seely EW. The heart in endocrine and nutritional disorders. In: Braunwald E, ed. *Heart Disease,* 5th ed. Philadelphia: WB Saunders, 1997;1896.

MISCELLANEOUS
- National Adrenal Diseases Foundation (NADF), 505 Northern Boulevard, Great Neck, NY 11021; (516)487-4992. http://www.medhelp.org/nadf/
- Cushing's Support and Research Foundation, 65 East India Row, Suite 22-B, Boston, MA 02110 http://world.std.com/~csrf/

CODES
ICD9-CM
255.0

PATIENT TEACHING
- Patients should wear an identification bracelet that notes the requirement for glucocorticoids.
- Patients should be aware of the importance of compliance with the daily dose of glucocorticoids and the signs and symptoms of adrenal insufficiency.
- Patients should be aware of the need to increase the oral dose of glucocorticoids for fever, nausea, and diarrhea and of the need for parenteral administration of glucocorticoids and medical evaluation for emesis, trauma, or severe medical stress.

C

CYTOKINES AND THE HEART

Benjamin Prentiss
Stefano Perlini
Gerard P. Aurigemma

 BASICS

DESCRIPTION

Cytokines are locally acting polypeptide mediators, or autocoids, that act as autocrine (acting on the cell of origin), paracrine (acting on neighboring cells), or juxtacrine (acting on adjacent cells) agents. Beyond exerting a crucial role as mediators of inflammatory and immune responses, cytokines play an important role in the pathogenesis of atherosclerosis and in the cardiac dysfunction that accompanies systemic sepsis, viral myocarditis, cardiac allograft rejection, ischemic–reperfusion injury, and congestive heart failure syndromes.

Cytokines and the Heart

- Under different forms of stress (such as mechanical load, oxidative stress, ischemic–reperfusion, lipopolysaccharide exposure), the heart is able to produce different proinflammatory cytokines—namely tumor necrosis factor α (TNF-α), interleukin 1 (IL-1), IL-6, and interferon γ (IFN-γ)—that may play an important role in initiating and integrating short-term homeostatic responses within the heart.

  When chronically elevated, these stress-activated cytokines have the potential to induce cardiac dysfunction and modulate peripheral vascular resistance via nitric oxide–dependent and – independent mechanisms. These cytokines also appear to precipitate pulmonary edema, reduce peripheral organ perfusion, induce ventricular remodeling, activate the fetal gene program and the apoptotic process, and induce cachexia, resulting in further skeletal muscle dysfunction.

- Stress-activated cytokines have been involved in the induction of programmed cell death (apoptosis) of cardiomyocytes and of endothelial cells.
- Antinflammatory cytokines such as IL-10, IL-4, and IL-13, secreted by T-helper lymphocytes and other cells, inhibit the production of proinflammatory cytokines.

TNF-α Receptors

- The widespread biologic effects of TNF-α are modulated by two specific receptors: TNF-R1 and TNF-R2. Both receptors are present in equal proportions in normal myocardium, and have a similar affinity for TNF-α.
- The negative inotropic effects of TNF-α are mediated by its interaction with TNF-R1 and not with TNF-R2.
- Compared with the nonfailing myocardium, the expression of myocardial TNF-α receptors is decreased in the failing myocardium, whereas the circulating levels of the soluble forms of TNF-R1 and TNF-R2 (namely the soluble TNF-α receptors) are elevated in patients with moderate-to-severe heart failure.

PATHOPHYSIOLOGY

Cytokines and Atherosclerosis

- Cardiovascular disease is now commonly accepted as having a significant inflammatory component. In fact, the well-known risk factors for cardiovascular disease may likely be the cause of chronic inflammation in vascular tissues.
- Cytokines, appear to influence the chronic development of atherosclerosis through their inflammatory signaling pathways.
- The unstable plaque, characterized by its thin fibrous cap covering a voluminous lipid core, is known to be a culprit lesion in the majority of acute coronary syndromes. These plaques exhibit an accumulation of proinflammatory cytokines including TNF-α and IL-1.
- Cytokines have been implicated in the overgrowth of smooth muscle cells, a second key component of the atherogenic process. IL-1 and TGF-β have been shown to induce autocrine platelet-derived growth factor (PDGF) loops in smooth muscle cells. By this mechanism a transient secretion of cytokines from activated leukocytes may give rise to prolonged activation of smooth muscle cell proliferation.

Cytokines and Hypertension

- Altered profiles of pro- and antiinflammatory cytokines have been demonstrated in patients with essential hypertension. These findings are consistent with peripheral monocyte activation in the circulation. The clinical significance and implications of these findings is yet to be elucidated.
- Both preeclampsia and pregnancy-induced hypertension have also been associated with altered pro- and antiinflammatory cytokine profiles when compared to normal pregnant subjects.

Cytokines and Heart Failure

- The role of stress-induced cytokines in heart failure relates to the observation that many of the untoward pathophysiologic responses of the failing circulation might be explained by these compounds.
- It has been shown that several inflammatory cytokines (particularly TNF-α and IL-1) induce reversible contractile dysfunction *in vitro* and *in vivo*.
- Injection of TNF-α into the circulation of animal models causes a marked decrease in left ventricular ejection fraction and end-systolic and -diastolic volume. The depressed left ventricular (LV) function has been shown to be independent of the cytokine-induced loading changes.
- TNF-α overexpression has been shown to lead to cardiomegaly. This cytokine is present in the normal myocardium and is elevated in patients with heart failure, particularly in advanced stages of the disease. This suggests that TNF-α overproduction plays a role in the development of cardiac remodeling and eventual organ failure.

- Patients with AIDS-associated cardiomyopathy have also been demonstrated to have increased plasma levels of TNF-α. This is secondary to overproduction by peripheral monocytes in patients with AIDS and is believed to play a key role in the development of AIDS-associated cardiomyopathies.
- Treatment with TNF-α antagonists in patients with advanced heart failure for up to 3 months resulted in a significant dose-dependent improvement in LV structure and function and a trend toward improvement in patient functional status.
- Treatment of patients with long-term TNF-α receptor antagonists for myriad inflammatory conditions has led to many case reports documenting the development of new heart failure while patients are treated with these cytokine blockers.
- Thus, the elaboration of cytokines, similar to the upregulation of neurohormones, may represent a biochemical mechanism that is responsible for producing symptoms in heart failure patients.

Cytokines and Cardiac Cachexia

- TNF-α levels are elevated in patients with chronic heart failure, particularly in patients with cardiac cachexia, a multifactorial neuroendocrine and immunologic disorder characterized by generalized body wasting.
- It has been shown that cardiac cachexia is predictive of poor survival independent of age, functional class, ejection fraction, and exercise capacity.
- In patients with advanced heart failure, the increased levels of TNF-α may be responsible for the induction of body wasting and cachexia.

Cytokines and Sepsis

- The possibility that the sera of patients and experimental animals with systemic sepsis (or other forms of systemic inflammatory response) contained a myocardial depressant factor was suggested more than 25 years ago.
- The systemic inflammatory response syndrome (SIRS) is characterized by hypotension, tachypnea, hypo- or hyperthermia, and leukocytosis, as well as other clinical signs and symptoms, including a depression in myocardial contractile function.
- SIRS is a major determinant of survival in patients with advanced viral or bacterial infection, or following severe trauma or burns complicated by multiorgan failure.
- Although the cause of cardiac contractile dysfunction in this syndrome is still largely unknown, cytokines may contribute to the pathogenesis of heart failure in this syndrome.

Cytokines and Myocarditis

- Most cases of myocarditis (in regions where Chagas disease and diphtheria are not endemic) are likely the result of viral infection. The secondary immune response to viral infection likely plays a greater role in disease pathogenesis than the primary infection itself. This is evident in the autoimmune phase of viral myocarditis where T cells seek out virus-infected cells and destroy them by cytokine production and cytolysis. Although the immune response is intended to be protective, continued autoimmune activation in this fashion is ultimately detrimental to the host, because both cytokine-mediated and direct T-cell–mediated myocyte damage reduce the number of contractile units.
- Patients with myocarditis have been shown to have marked plasma elevation of cytokines including TNF-α, IL-1, and IL-6.
- The recovery of some patients with severe LV dysfunction with viral myocarditis is probably secondary to short-term exposure to the autoimmune response and subsequent cytokine toxicity. In fact, patients with acute fulminant myocarditis have better survival compared to patients with more chronic myocarditis likely as a result of the limited exposure to the overproduced inflammatory cytokines.

Cytokines and Ischemic Heart Disease

- Recent evidence has implicated proinflammatory mediators such as TNF-α in the pathophysiology of ischemia–reperfusion injury.
- Clinically, serum levels of TNF-α are increased after myocardial infarction and after cardiopulmonary bypass. Both of these represent clinically relevant instances of cardiac ischemia-reperfusion injury.
- Moreover, cytokines may induce cardiac depression and are important in regulating the reparative process, which is activated following myocardial ischemic damage.
- The intense inflammatory reaction following reperfusion of the infarcted myocardium has been implicated as a factor in extension of injury.

REFERENCES

1. Bozkurt B, et al. Results of targeted anti-tumor necrosis factor therapy with etanercept (ENBREL) in patients with advanced heart failure. *Circulation*. 2001;103:1044.
2. Kwan HJ, et al. Case reports of heart failure after therapy with a tumor necrosis factor antagonist. *Ann Intern Med*. 2003;138:10:807–811.
3. Liu PP, Mason JW. Advances in the understanding of myocarditis. *Circulation*. 2001;104:1076.
4. Thompson E. *The Cytokine Handbook*, 3rd ed. San Diego: Academic Press, 1998.
5. Wilczynski JR, Tchorzewski H, et al. Cytokine secretion by decidual lymphocytes in transient hypertension of pregnancy and preeclampsia. *Mediators Inflamm*. 2003;11:105–111.
6. Willerson JT, Cohn JN, eds. *Cardiovascular Medicine*, 2nd ed. Philadelphia: Churchill Livingstone, 2000.
7. Young JL, Libby P, Shonbeck U. Cytokines in the Pathogenesis of Atherosclerosis. *Thromb Haemost*. 2002;88:554–567.

MISCELLANEOUS

CURRENT PERSPECTIVES

- Clarifying the role and the regulation of cytokine production and cellular signaling is an area of active research.
- This may aid the development of drugs that reduce cytokine-mediated cardiac contractile depression, that modulate myocardial damage following ischemic-reperfusion injury, and that prevent progressive cardiomyocyte loss, particularly by inhibiting cytokine-induced apoptosis.
- More broadly, modulation of "stress activated" cytokines may represent a new frontier in the management of heart failure.

C

TRANSPOSITION OF THE GREAT ARTERIES

Ismee A. Williams
Welton M. Gersony

 BASICS

DESCRIPTION

Transposition of the great arteries (TGA) is a form of cyanotic congenital heart disease.

- In complete transposition (D-TGA) there is:
  - Atrioventricular concordance
  - Ventriculoarterial discordance
  - The aorta arises anterior from the right ventricle.
  - The pulmonary artery (PA) arises posterior to the left ventricle.
  - The systemic and pulmonary circulations are separated, and unless communications exist between the two circulations, the baby will not survive.
  - In classic D-TGA, the aorta is to the right of the PA.
- In corrected transposition (L-TGA) there is:
  - Atrioventricular discordance
  - Ventriculoarterial discordance
  - Physiologic correction of the circulation
  - The aorta arises to the left of the PA

GENERAL PREVENTION

Not applicable

EPIDEMIOLOGY

Males > Females (3:1)

Incidence

Occurs in 20.5–30.1/100,000 live births

Prevalence

TGA accounts for 5%–7% of all congenital heart disease (CHD)

RISK FACTORS

- Prenatal factors associated with increased risk of CHD in general include:
  - Maternal diabetes
  - Alcohol exposure
  - Viral illnesses including rubella
  - Advanced maternal age
- It is unclear if any of these factors lead to TGA specifically.

Genetics

TGA is rarely associated with genetic syndromes, although recurrence in families has been reported.

PATHOPHYSIOLOGY

- Pulmonary and systemic circulations operate in parallel to each other instead of in series.
- Oxygenated blood from the lungs cannot pass to the body organs.
- Deoxygenated blood from the body cannot pass to the lungs.
- Unless sufficient communications between the 2 circulations exist, the baby will die.
- A small patent foramen ovale (PFO) will allow some degree of mixing in the newborn period.

ETIOLOGY

Most often multifactorial

ASSOCIATED CONDITIONS

- <10% have associated extracardiac lesions
- 50% of TGA have only PFO or patent ductus arteriosus (PDA)
- 40–45% have ventricular septal defect (VSD)
  - Pulmonary Stenosis (PS) will accompany 30% of TGA/VSD cases.
  - Taussig-Bing variant of DORV is seen with anterior malalignment type of VSD, causing subaortic stenosis and aortic arch anomalies.
- 25% have left ventricular outflow tract obstruction (LVOTO)/Pulmonary Stenosis (PS)
  - Measured gradients of PS usually overestimate the true obstruction due to high pulmonary blood flow
  - Stenosis is more severe in TGA with VSD than with intact ventricular septum (IVS)
  - Causes of LVOTO include:
  - Dynamic subpulmonary obstruction due to leftward bowing of the ventricular septum in the setting of high right ventricular (RV) pressure (20% of cases of TGA/PS/IVS)
  - Subpulmonary membrane
  - Fibromuscular tunnel
  - Abnormal mitral valve attachments
  - Pulmonary valve stenosis is less common
- 10% have VSD/PS
- 5% have a true secundum atrial septal defect (ASD)
- 5% have aortic coarctation or interrupted arch
- Pulmonary atresia
- 2–5% leftward juxtaposition of the atrial appendages
- Variations in coronary artery anatomy and alignment of the cusps of the pulmonary and the aortic valve
  - Intramural coronaries
  - Multiple ostia
  - Absence of one of the coronary branches
  - Unusual epicardial course

DIAGNOSIS

SIGNS AND SYMPTOMS

Any infant in the nursery with evidence of cyanosis and suspected CHD should undergo prompt echocardiography to ascertain a diagnosis. This is especially true in the setting of TGA as the clinical exam, electrocardiogram (ECG), and chest x-ray (CXR) may all appear normal.

- With intact ventricular septum, severe cyanosis is noted shortly after birth.
- In patients with large VSD or PDA, congestive heart failure will develop with respiratory distress and feeding difficulties.

History

- Cyanosis from birth
- CHF may manifest during infancy with VSD

Physical Exam

- Moderate to severe cyanosis
- Tachypnea
- Tachycardia
- Palpable liver edge
- Hepatomegaly with TGA/VSD
- Normal to prominent pulses
- Single loud second heart sound (S_2) due to anterior position of the aortic valve
- With TGA and intact ventricular septum, usually there is no murmur
  - In TGA/VSD, a loud pansystolic murmur, gallop and mid-diastolic rumble may develop within 2–6 weeks

TESTS

Hyperoxia Test

- Room air arterial blood gas (ABG) shows PaO_2 <30 mmHg
- Despite 100% oxygen, PaO_2 <45 mmHg

Differential cyanosis

- Pre-ductal O_2 saturations (arms) < post-ductal O_2 saturation (legs)
- Indicates there is a large PDA with shunting from PA to Ao
- May indicate an aortic arch anomaly

ECG

- Usually normal for age in the first days after birth
- Persistence of right axis deviation (+90 to +200 degrees) and right ventricular hypertrophy is noted in the older infant with upright T waves in the right precordial leads and prominent RV forces
- Signs of left ventricular hypertrophy may also develop in the setting of a large VSD, PDA, or LVOTO
- 60–80% of TGA/VSD demonstrate combined ventricular hypertrophy and 70% have a Q wave in V_6
- Sinus rhythm is the norm

Lab

- Arterial hypoxemia is marked and does not improve significantly with the administration of inhaled oxygen.
- Acidosis, hypoglycemia, and hypocalcemia may be present.

Imaging

Chest x-ray

- May be normal in the newborn
- Classic findings include:
  - Mild cardiomegaly
  - Increased pulmonary vascular markings
  - "Egg on a string" shape of the heart due to a narrow superior mediastinum with the great vessels arising in parallel
- Right aortic arch is seen in 4% of TGA/IVS and 11% of TGA/VSD cases
- Cardiomegaly and pulmonary vascular markings are more prominent in the setting of a large VSD

Echocardiography

- Usually provides all the necessary information for diagnosis and management
- Must look for important associated defects: VSD, LVOTO, AVV attachments, and coronary artery anatomy
- Great vessels exit parallel to each other
- Great vessel arising from the LV bifurcates
- Great vessel arising from the RV gives off coronary arteries and head vessels
- Evaluation of the atrial septum, the ventricular septum, and the PDA is necessary to determine if mixing is adequate
- Evaluate LVOT, RVOT, pulmonary valve, aortic arch, and coronary artery anatomy to determine surgical options
- If VSD is present, must evaluate size and location along with AVV attachments

Diagnostic Procedures/Surgery

Cardiac Catheterization

- Usually to perform a balloon atrial septostomy (Rashkind procedure)
- Rarely indicated for diagnosis alone
- In complex cases of TGA, cardiac catheterization may assist in the identification of associated VSDs, coronary artery anatomy, assessment of LVOTO, and measurement of pulmonary artery pressures and vascular resistance

Oxygen Saturations:

- In TGA/IVS:
  - IVC saturations are usually 40%
  - Systemic arterial, RV, and RA saturations are usually only 5–10% higher than the IVC
  - Pulmonary venous saturations are usually normal
  - LA and LV saturations may be 4–8% lower than pulmonary venous saturations
  - Classic finding is higher saturations in the PA than in the aorta
- In TGA/VSD:
  - IVC saturations may be reduced modestly
  - RA saturations increase by 5–10%
  - RV and systemic arterial saturations rise to 70–85%
  - Pulmonary venous, LA and LV saturations may be decreased if significant congestive heart failure (CHF) is present
  - PA saturations may be decreased due to preferential streaming from the RV across the VSD
  - PA saturations and aortic saturations may be similar if there is significant intracardiac mixing

Pressures:

- LA pressures may be elevated up to 20 mm Hg, saturation and a prominent V wave may be seen if the interatrial communication is not adequate
- In the setting of TGA/large VSD, LV and RV systolic and end-diastolic, and aorta and pulmonary systolic pressures are equal
- Pulmonary end diastolic and mean pressures should be lower than those of the aorta unless pulmonary vascular resistance is high
- Entering the pulmonary artery to measure pressure may be difficult

Angiography:

- Allows identification and description of VSDs, LVOTO, AVV, and coronary artery anatomy
- In the lateral view, the anterior position of the aorta relative to the pulmonary artery is readily seen
- The aortic valve is located higher than normal due to the presence of subaortic conal tissue

D

Interventional Catheterization/Balloon Atrial Septostomy
- Access can be obtained using either the umbilical or the femoral vein
- A deflated balloon-tipped catheter is advanced across the PFO into the LA
- Catheter position in the LA is confirmed by either fluoroscopy or echocardiography prior to balloon inflation
- Balloon is inflated with contrast material to a diameter of 12–15 mm and is rapidly and firmly withdrawn into the RA/IVC junction in order to rupture the septum primum flap of the fossa ovalis
  - Slow pulling of the balloon from the LA to the RA can lead to stretching instead of tearing of the septum and may be disadvantageous
- Procedure is repeated multiple times with the balloon inflated to greater volumes
- Complications may include:
  - Damage to or perforation of the LA, pulmonary vein, IVC, or AVV
  - Balloon rupture and air embolism if strict caution is not taken to avoid the entry of air into the balloon during inflation
  - Leftward juxtaposition of the atrial appendages may lead to false placement of the catheter in the right atrial appendage instead of the LA
- In older infants, a blade atrial septostomy or the Brockenbrough technique using a transseptal needle may be necessary due to a thickened atrial septum

DIFFERENTIAL DIAGNOSIS

Other forms of cyanotic heart disease including tricuspid atresia with severe pulmonary stenosis and tetralogy of Fallot with pulmonary atresia

 TREATMENT

GENERAL MEASURES
- Obtain arterial blood gas (ABG) and perform a Hyperoxia Test to confirm the presence of cyanotic CHD
- Administer oxygen, correct acidosis, and electrolyte imbalances

 MEDICATION (DRUGS)

- Used to stabilize the infant prior to surgery or to treat complications following surgery
- Surgical repair is the first line of treatment without which the infant will die

First Line
- Prostaglandin E_2 infusion to maintain ductal patency until surgical repair is undertaken
- Complications of PGE include fever, decreased systemic vascular resistance, apnea, and rash

Second Line
- Inotropes and diuretics may be of benefit in the setting of significantly increased pulmonary blood flow
- Balloon atrial septostomy if mixing is inadequate

SURGERY
- Arterial Switch Operation (ASO) or the Jatene operation consists of transecting the aorta and the PA directly above the levels of the valves and reimplanting them above the correct ventricle
  - Coronary arteries are transferred from the native to the new aorta
  - Includes the Lecompte maneuver: The aorta is brought posterior to the branch pulmonary arteries
  - Benefits include anatomic and physiologic correction of the defect and avoidance of many of the long-term complications seen with the atrial switch
  - Necessary components of a successful ASO include:
    - LV capable of pumping against systemic arterial pressures
    - Favorable coronary artery patterns
    - No LVOTO and normal pulmonary valve
  - Usually performed within 2 weeks after birth
  - 2–5% surgical mortality
  - 82% overall 5-year survival rate
  - Complications include:
    - Supravalvar pulmonary stenosis (5–30%)
    - Neoaortic stenosis (5–10%)
    - Aortic root dilatation and aortic regurgitation (20%)
    - Complete heart block (5–10%)
    - Coronary artery injuries
  - Long-term effects on coronary artery function remain to be seen
  - Benefits of the ASO over the atrial switch include:
    - Preservation of systemic LV function
    - Avoidance of dysrhythmias
- Atrial switch (Senning or Mustard procedure) consists of baffling systemic venous return to the LV and the PA and allowing pulmonary venous return to flow into the RV and out the aorta. The atrial switch is not currently used for simple D-TGA

  - Complications include:
    - Systemic RV failure (10%)
    - Tricuspid regurgitation (1–2% with TGV/IVS and 5–10% with TGV/VSD)
    - Sick sinus syndrome and/or atrial arrhythmias related to surgical scars and atrial dilation (>50%)
    - Sudden death (2–10%)
    - Obstruction of pulmonary venous return (<5%)
    - Obstruction of systemic venous return (<5%)
    - Residual intraatrial baffle shunt (<20%)
    - Pulmonary vascular disease
    - Preferential blood flow to the right lung due to the orientation of the LVOT
    - Poor exercise performance
  - Pharmacologic control of arrhythmias may be difficult as tachyarrhythmias and bradyarrhythmias may coexist
  - Survivors of the atrial switch with failing RV may undergo LV retraining and an arterial switch
  - Most common application is in the setting of "corrected" transposition (L-TGA)
  - May be offered to poor ASO candidates due to unfavorable coronary artery anatomy
  - Atrial switch is most commonly done between 3 and 9 months of age
- Rastelli Operation
  - Indication: TGA/VSD and PS not amenable to surgical resection
  - VSD is closed with tunneling of LV outflow to the aorta
  - RV to PA continuity is accomplished using a valved conduit
  - Anterior enlargement of the VSD may be necessary to prevent development of LVOTO
  - Typically performed after 1 year of age to allow placement of a large RV to PA conduit
  - Infants with severe PS may receive a BTS or may undergo an early Rastelli
  - Surgical mortality is <5%
- REV Procedure: Alternative to the Rastelli for patients with TGA/VSD/PS
  - High, anterior RV is opened and the outlet septum is excised
  - The aorta is connected to the LV with a short tunnel
  - The native pulmonary valve is closed and the main PA is transected and directly attached to the RVOT
  - Benefits over the Rastelli:
    - Perform at a younger age
    - Avoid a prosthetic conduit
    - Avoid LVOTO
  - Impact of long-term free PI on RV has yet to be seen
- Fontan or single ventricle palliation is offered to infants with TGA/VSD and straddling AVV or infants with TGA and multiple VSDs not amenable to closure

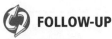

FOLLOW-UP

DISPOSITION

Pregnancy

- The first patients who underwent an ASO are just now reaching child-bearing age; it is anticipated that pregnancy will be well tolerated.
- Patients who underwent an atrial switch are at high risk for complications such as arrhythmia and RV failure, and pregnancy is not recommended for this group. However, there have been reports of successful pregnancies in asymptomatic patients with good repairs.

Issues for Referral

- Patients who underwent an atrial switch may develop arrhythmias requiring referral to an electrophysiologist.
- Failing systemic ventricular function should prompt referral for heart transplantation evaluation

PROGNOSIS

- Long-term prognosis for the infant with TGA is good.
- 5-year survival following the ASO is reported to be 82%.
- Recent improvements have led to a decrease in early mortality rates to <2%.
- In the absence of treatment, 30% of infants will die within the 1st week after birth, 70% will die before the age of 6 months, and 90% will die by 1 year of age.

COMPLICATIONS

- Specific to surgical procedure performed
- After the atrial switch, patients may develop arrhythmias, RV failure, TR, and exercise intolerance.
- The risk of coronary artery obstruction following the ASO is under current investigation.

PATIENT MONITORING

- After the atrial switch, follow-up occurs every 6 to 12 months in order to monitor for atrial arrhythmias, systemic or pulmonary venous obstruction, TR, poor exercise tolerance, and RV failure.
- After the ASO, regular follow-up is necessary to assess for: LVOTO, pulmonary stenosis, coronary artery obstruction, ventricular dysfunction, arrhythmias, aortic root dilation, and aortic and pulmonary regurgitation.

REFERENCES

1. Allen HD, et al. *Moss and Adams' Heart Disease in Infants, Children, and Adolescents: Including the Fetus and Young Adult*, 6th ed. Philadelphia: Lippincott Williams and Wilkins, 2001.
2. Freedom RM, et al. *The Natural and Modified History of Congenital Heart Disease*. Elmsford, NY: Blackwell Pub. 2004.
3. Park MK. *Pediatric Cardiology for Practitioners*. Chicago: Year Book Medical Publishers, 1984.
4. Schwartz ML, Gauvreau K, del Nido P, et al. Long-term predictors of aortic root dilatation and aortic regurgitation after arterial switch operation. *Circulation*. 2004;110[suppl II]:II128–II132.

ADDITIONAL MATERIAL

- http://www.americanheart.org/presenter.jhtml?identifier=1682
- http://www.pediheart.org/parents/defects/TGA.htm
- http://www.nlm.nih.gov/medlineplus/ency/article/001568.htm

MISCELLANEOUS

- Fetal diagnosis of TGA is easily obtained and is readily available at most tertiary care centers.
- Neurodevelopmental outcomes studies have demonstrated that infants with TGA are at risk for developmental delay.

CODES

ICD9-CM

745.1

PATIENT TEACHING

Diet

Regular diet

Activity

- For ASO: Regular activity, self-limited
- For atrial switch with poor RV systemic ventricular function: May benefit from exercise restriction

Prevention

- Close follow-up with pediatric cardiologist and eventually an adult congenital specialist is necessary for surveillance of complications following surgical repair.
- Endocarditis prophylaxis is recommended.

FAQ

- TGA is a severe form of cyanotic congenital heart disease that is almost uniformly fatal within the first year of life without surgical correction.
- TGA may be associated with a variety of additional lesions that impact prognosis and choice of surgical repair.
- Prognosis is favorable with access to modern medical and surgical techniques.
- Lifelong follow-up care is needed.

DERMATOMYOSITIS AND THE HEART

James A. Kong

 BASICS

DESCRIPTION

Dermatomyositis (DM) is an inflammatory muscle disease similar to polymyositis. Both are characterized by symmetric muscle weakness, but specific cutaneous manifestations or rash also accompany DM. Potential cardiovascular manifestations include myocarditis; pericarditis; conduction abnormalities, including bundle branch blocks and complete heart block (CHB); congestive heart failure (CHF); coronary artery vasculitis (rare); and mitral valve prolapse.

- Most cardiovascular conditions are secondary to inflammatory injury of cardiac myocytes with subsequent fibrosis.
- Specifically, the pericardium, myocardium, and conduction system may be involved. For example, CHF results from left ventricular (LV) diastolic dysfunction imparted by myocardial fibrosis and pericardial constriction.
- Electrical conduction abnormalities are due largely to fibrosis of the myocardial conduction system.
- The incidence and significance of these lesions in terms of prognosis has not been well studied.

Systems Affected
- Cardiovascular, skeletal muscle, skin

EPIDEMIOLOGY

- Predominant Age: DM is bimodal (child and adulthood). Cardiac manifestations are more common in older patients or those with a longer duration of DM.
- Predominant Sex: Female
- Predominant Race: Black

Prevalence

- Prevalence in the hospitalized population in the United States is 5/1,000,000.
- Electrocardiographic abnormalities are detected in 72%, myocarditis in 30%, and pericardial effusion in 5–25%.

ETIOLOGY

Inflammatory injury of cardiac myocytes and the conduction system

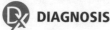 **DIAGNOSIS**

SIGNS AND SYMPTOMS

Patients typically are asymptomatic from a cardiovascular perspective.

- Cardiovascular manifestations usually are encountered in the setting of active skeletal muscle involvement.
- Patients may present with conduction abnormalities or arrhythmias and their attendant signs, symptoms, and complications.
- They also may present with myocarditis and pain mimicking angina.
- CHF is a possible presenting syndrome.
- LV dysfunction may be present, but the degree of dysfunction may or may not correlate with the degree of DM activity.

TESTS

- Electrocardiogram (ECG)
  - No findings specific to DM have been described.
  - Some electrocardiographic abnormalities may be observed in up to 53% of patients with DM, including nonspecific ST- and T-wave abnormalities, ECG evidence for LV hypertrophy (with or without a history of hypertension), and conduction abnormalities.
- Ambulatory ECG
  - Most common abnormalities are premature ventricular contractions.

Lab

- Creatinine kinase and myocardial band fraction (CK-MB)
  - Serum levels of CK are almost always elevated in DM patients with active myopathy, sometimes accompanied by elevations in serum aldolase.
  - CK-MB also may be elevated due to significant skeletal myopathy, with no cardiac involvement.
  - Myocarditis should be considered if CK-MB is >3%.

Imaging

- Echocardiography
  - LV diastolic dysfunction
  - Hyperdynamic LV (ejection fraction >75%)
  - Focal wall-motion abnormalities
  - Mitral valve prolapse (MVP)
  - Septal/endocardial fibrosis
  - Pericardial effusion
- Nuclear perfusion scan
  - Thallium scintigraphy may reveal areas of hypoperfusion that correlate with regions of myocarditis and not ischemia.
  - These perfusion defects may resolve with steroid therapy.

Diagnostic Procedures/Surgery

- Cardiac catheterization: Coronary angiography is usually normal. Rarely is vasculitis seen.
- Myocardial biopsy: See subsequent text.

Pathologic Findings

- Myocardial biopsy reveals myocardial necrosis, loss of cross-striations, and conduction system fibrosis.
- Postmortem examination: Fibrinous pericarditis has been rarely reported as an incidental finding at autopsy.

DIFFERENTIAL DIAGNOSIS

Patients with DM may present with various syndromes of cardiovascular dysfunction as described in the preceding text.

- More common causes of these conditions, for example, coronary artery disease (CAD) and myocardial ischemia leading to CHF or CHB, must be excluded.
- Diagnosis can be difficult because a patient with DM can present with symptoms similar to those of a patient with CAD, with ECG changes, with focal wall-motion abnormalities on echocardiogram, and with elevated cardiac enzymes.
- Myocarditis may be associated with other connective tissue diseases, including systemic lupus erythematosus or scleroderma.

TREATMENT

GENERAL MEASURES
- Routine cardiac evaluation in patients with DM has been advocated by some, although this is controversial.
- At the least noninvasive measures should be considered, including ECG and echocardiography.
- Cardiac catheterization should be performed if CAD is suspected or cannot be safely excluded. At that time, myocardial biopsy may be considered.

 ## MEDICATION (DRUGS)

First Line
- Corticosteroids and other immunosuppressants such as methotrexate, azathioprine, and cytoxan
  - Steroid therapy can lead to resolution of electrocardiographic changes, perfusion defects by thallium scintigraphy, and regional wall-motion abnormalities.
  - Usual dosing is prednisone 60–80 mg daily for 6–8 weeks.
  - Further immunosuppressive therapy should be directed by a rheumatologist experienced with the other agents listed previously; however, these other medications have not been shown to be effective when prednisone has failed.
  - Precautions
    - Complications associated with long-term steroid use include osteopenia, hyperglycemia, immunosuppression, adrenal suppression, weight gain, truncal obesity, myopathy, fluid retention, avascular necrosis, gastrointestinal complaints, and skin changes.
  - Significant possible interactions
    - Variable

Second Line
- Methotrexate
- Azathioprine
- Cytoxan

 ## FOLLOW-UP

PROGNOSIS
- The presence of cardiac manifestations is the most important factor associated with a poor prognosis in DM.
- CHF is considered the greatest negative outcome predictor of the various cardiovascular manifestations.
- Degree of CK-MB elevation also may correlate directly with poor outcomes; the highest levels of CK-MB are seen in CHF.

PATIENT MONITORING
- No specific guidelines
- Serial noninvasive monitoring may be warranted, including CK-MB and echocardiography, especially for patients with known cardiovascular involvement.

REFERENCES
1. Askari AD. The heart in polymyositis and dermatomyositis. *Mount Sinai J Med*. 1988;55:479–482.
2. Dalakas M, Bohan A, eds. Polymyositis and Dermatomyositis. Boston: Butterworth, 1988;26, 177.
3. Gonzalez-Lopez L, et al. Cardiac manifestations in dermato-polymyositis. *Clin Exp Rheumatol*. 1996;14:373–379.
4. Hochberg ML, et al. Adult onset polymyositis/dermatomyositis: An analysis of clinical and laboratory features and survival in 76 patients with a review of the literature. *Semin Arthritis Rheum*. 1986;15:168–178.
5. Tami LF, Bhasin S. Polymorphisms of the cardiac manifestations in dermatomyositis. *Clin Cardiol*. 1993;16:260–264.

 ## MISCELLANEOUS

SEE ALSO: CONGESTIVE HEART FAILURE, COMPLETE HEART BLOCKCODES
ICD9-CM
710.3 Dermatomyositis (acute) (chronic)

PATIENT TEACHING
Organizations
- Muscular Dystrophy Association, USA National Headquarters, 3300 E. Sunrise Drive, Tucson, AZ 85718; (800)572-1717; http://www.mdausa.org/home.html
- Myositis Association of America, 755 Cantrell Ave, Suite C, Harrisonburg, VA 22801; (540)433-7686; http://www.myositis.org/
- National Institute of Arthritis & Musculoskeletal & Skin Diseases, Building 31, Room 4C05, Bethesda, MD 20892-2350; (301)496-8188; http://www.nih.gov/niams/
- National Organization for Rare Disorders (NORD), P.O. Box 8923, New Fairfield, CT 06812-1783; (800)999-6673

D

DIASTOLIC VENTRICULAR FUNCTION

Gerard P. Aurigemma

 BASICS

DESCRIPTION

Diastolic mechanisms contribute importantly to many, if not most, of the instances of heart failure seen in the United States in view of the following considerations:

- Hypertension is an underlying risk factor in most patients with congestive heart failure.
- The prevalence of hypertension increases substantially with age.
- Roughly 1/3 to 1/2 of patients hospitalized with congestive failure have normal systolic ejection fraction at the time of hospitalization or thereafter.
- The proportion of heart failure patients with normal ejection fraction parallels the age of the study population. The older the mean age of the heart failure population being studied, the higher the proportion of patients with normal ejection fraction. Most patients with heart failure and normal ejection fraction have demonstrable abnormalities in diastolic function and an elevated left ventricular (LV) end-diastolic pressure.

PATHOPHYSIOLOGY

LV diastolic filling occurs in two phases: Passive filling followed by atrial systole. Normal diastolic filling may be characterized as the ability of the ventricle to fill optimally at normal pressures. This capability is influenced by both the active (energy requiring) and passive (compliance) properties of the left ventricle.

- Underlying mechanisms
  - Filling occurs as the left ventricle relaxes and pressure decays; this filling takes place during isovolumic relaxation (time between the aortic second sound and mitral valve opening) and during the early part of diastole, during which rapid filling takes place.
  - The rapid pressure decay in the left ventricle, in association with untwisting and elastic recoil of the left ventricle, promotes a pressure gradient (diastolic suction).
  - Because the ventricular myocardium is relaxed and distensible during diastole, pressures are low in what is effectively the common chamber, comprising the left ventricle, left atrium, and pulmonary veins. Therefore, filling in the normal ventricle is associated with a low or normal pulmonary capillary wedge pressure.
  - Atrial systole, an active process whereby blood is pumped into the left ventricle, assumes greater importance as aging or myocardial disease renders the LV myocardium less distensible (increasing stiffness, decreasing compliance).
  - Major influences on the compliance of the LV myocardium include the extent of fibrosis (scar from prior infarction, unrelieved pressure and/ or volume overload) and whether hypertrophy is present.

- LV and therefore left atrial, pulmonary vein, and pulmonary capillary pressures are also influenced by LV volume. Because even the normal LV does not have infinite compliance, a much larger than normal LV volume will result in abnormal elevation in LV diastolic pressures.
- As implied by the preceding discussion, the two major pathophysiologic problems comprise abnormalities in relaxation and abnormalities in LV compliance.
- Some of the more common underlying abnormalities include:
  - Myocardial hypertrophy (generally associated with long-standing hypertension)
  - Interstitial fibrosis
  - Ischemia contributes directly and indirectly to diastolic dysfunction, the latter acting by decreasing the ability of the myocardium to relax and compromising the normal decay in diastolic pressure. Ischemia also increases LV chamber stiffness and thereby alters the normal pressure volume relationship. Thus, in the ischemic LV, the ability of the heart to fill at normal pressure is compromised.
- Diastolic dysfunction generally comprises one or both pathophysiologic mechanisms:
  - Abnormalities in myocardial relaxation are generally associated with a diminution in the E wave and a prolongation in the time from peak E to zero velocity (diastasis). There is often an accompanying increase in A velocity as the atrial contraction increases in force. This may correspond to the fourth heart sound (S4) on physical examination.
  - Compliance abnormalities generally reflect more advanced disease, reflective of myocardial fibrosis. The Doppler pattern associated with compliance abnormalities includes a decrease in the time from peak E to diastasis (deceleration time <140 msec) and a diminution in the A velocity, reflecting increased atrial afterload. Thus, the E to A ratio may increase and approach that seen in normal, healthy adults. In this regard the deceleration time of the E wave will distinguish a pseudonorrmal E/A ratio from the left ventricle with severe compliance abnormalities.

TESTS

In the heart failure patient, bedside clinical assessment may not completely distinguish the heart failure patient with normal systolic function from the patient with systolic dysfunction. In both, individual signs of increased central venous and pulmonary venous volume may be present. Therefore, additional testing is necessary. Echocardiography is generally the test of choice in the assessment of the patient with heart failure and is the most common clinical test ordered to assess LV diastolic function.

Imaging

- The presence of a normal ejection fraction greatly increases the likelihood that diastolic dysfunction contributes importantly to the heart failure syndrome.
- Doppler echocardiography is used in everyday practice to assess LV filling and to determine the mechanism of congestive heart failure.
- The Doppler inflow pattern consists of two velocity profiles:
  - Early (E) wave, which corresponds to passive filling
  - Late (A) wave, which corresponds to atrial systole
  - In normal subjects the ratio of early to late filling is ≥1 because the atrial contraction tends not to be particularly forceful.
  - With advancing age, the ratio of peak E velocity to peak A velocity approaches 1 in normal individuals at around age 70.

TREATMENT

GENERAL MEASURES

- Proper patient management is obviously predicated on making the proper diagnosis. An assessment of systolic function, presence of valvular heart disease, extent of hypertrophy, and LV filling is essential. Echocardiography generally provides these data noninvasively. Regional wall-motion abnormalities present on the resting echocardiogram imply that coronary heart disease may be a contributing mechanism.
- Once the diagnosis is established, the following measures are in order:
  - Manage presenting symptoms generally including hypertension and coronary artery disease.
  - Maintenance of normal sinus rhythm and the avoidance of tachycardia have beneficial results.
  - Reduce congested state: Diuretics, salt restriction, angiotensin inhibitors (or angiotensin II receptor blockers)
  - Avoid tachycardia and promote bradycardia; this is usually accomplished with β-blockers and rate-lowering calcium channel blockers.
- Treat ischemia.

REFERENCES

1. Aurigemma GP, Gaasch WH. Diastolic heart failure. *N Engl J Med*. 2004;
2. Gaasch WH. Diagnois and treatment of heart failure based on left ventricular diastolic function. *JAMA*. 1994;271:1276–1282.
3. Gandhi SK, Powers JC, Nomeir AM, et al. The pathogenesis of acute pulmonary edema associated with hypertension. *N Engl J Med*. 2001;344:17–22.
4. Garcia MJ, Thomas JD, Klein AL. New Doppler echocardiographic applications for the study of diastolic function. *J Am Coll Cardiol*. 1998;32:865–875.
5. Levy D, Larson MG, Vasan RS, et al. The progression from hypertension to congestive heart failure. *JAMA*. 1996;275:1557–1562.
6. Nagueh SF, Middleton KJ, Kopelen HA, et al. Doppler tissue imaging: A noninvasive technique for evaluation of left ventricular relaxation and estimation of filling pressures. *J Am Coll Cardiol*. 1997;30:1527–1533.
7. Nishimura RA, Tajik AJ. Evaluation of diastolic filling of left ventricle in health and disease: Doppler echocardiography is the clinician's Rosetta Stone. *J Am Coll Cardiol*. 1997;30:8–18.
8. Rakowski H, Appleton C, Chan KL, et al. Canadian consensus recommendations for the measurement and reporting of diastolic dysfunction by echocardiography: From the Investigators of Consensus on Diastolic Dysfunction by Echocardiography. *J Am Soc Echocardiogr*. 1996;9:736–760.
9. Redfield MM, Jacobsen SJ, Burnett JC Jr, et al. Burden of systolic and diastolic ventricular dysfunction in the community: Appreciating the scope of the heart failure epidemic. *JAMA*. 2003;289:194–202.
10. Vasan RS, Levy D. Defining diastolic heart failure: A call for standardized diagnostic criteria. *Circulation*. 2000;101:2118–2121.
11. Vasan RS, Levy D. The role of hypertension in the pathogenesis of heart failure. A clinical mechanistic overview. *Arch Intern Med*. 1996;156:1789–1796.
12. Zile MR, Brutsaert DL. New concepts in diastolic dysfunction and diastolic heart failure: Part I: diagnosis, prognosis, and measurements of diastolic function. *Circulation*. 2002;105:1387–1393.
13. Zile MR, Brutsaert DL. New concepts in diastolic dysfunction and diastolic heart failure, II: Causal mechanisms and treatment. *Circulation*. 2002;105:1503–1508.
14. Zile MR, Gaasch WH, Carroll JD, et al. Heart failure with a normal ejection fraction: Is measurement of diastolic function necessary to make the diagnosis of diastolic heart failure? *Circulation*. 2001;104:779–782.

D

DIGITALIS TOXICITY

Lisa D. Wilsbacher
Jarvis W. Lambert

 BASICS

DESCRIPTION
Although the role of the cardiac glycoside therapy has been the subject of debate, the drug is generally accepted as effective treatment for heart failure due to systolic dysfunction and rate control in atrial fibrillation. A common complication of digoxin therapy is toxicity, which in its mildest form may go unrecognized and in its severest form can be fatal.

Pregnancy Considerations
- Digoxin crosses the placenta, and fetal umbilical cord venous blood levels of the drug are similar to maternal blood levels.
- Digoxin is a Pregnancy Category C drug, and thus should only be given to a pregnant woman if absolutely needed.

EPIDEMIOLOGY
The incidence and severity of digoxin intoxication decreased significantly with the introduction of digoxin assays in 1969.
- Occurs in 4–15% of patients at some point during therapy
- Mortality with current day treatment of digoxin intoxication is 5–24%.

RISK FACTORS
A number of risk factors influence an individual's sensitivity to cardiac glycosides.
- Advanced age: Diminished glomerular filtration rate; comorbid cardiac conditions
- Renal failure: Prolongs the drug half-life; increases serum concentrations; reduces volume of distribution
- Thyroid status: Hypothyroidism prolongs the half-life of digoxin.
- Pulmonary disease: Hypoxemia and respiratory failure increase arrhythmogenesis.
- Underlying heart disease
  - Preexisting conduction and automaticity abnormalities
  - Cardiac amyloid and ischemic cardiomyopathy increase sensitivity to digoxin.
  - Heart failure reduces volume of distribution.

- Hypochlorhydria (gastric pH >7 in older patients and those on H_2 blockers): Reduces gastric metabolism and nonrenal clearance of digoxin
- Electrolyte abnormalities
  - Hypokalemia: Increases binding of digoxin to the sodium pump, causing sensitization of the myocardium to the effects of digoxin and exacerbation of arrhythmias.
  - Hyperkalemia: Further depolarization of myocardial conduction tissue potentiates conduction abnormalities.
  - Hypomagnesemia: Causes hypokalemia
  - Hypercalcemia: Increases ventricular automaticity, exacerbation of arrhythmias
- Pharmacokinetic interactions (see the Appendix for the table on Effect on Digoxin Concentration).

PATHOPHYSIOLOGY
Toxic levels of digoxin lead to increased automaticity and arrhythmias.
- Digoxin blocks $Na^+K^+ATPase$ (the "sodium pump")
- Increased intracellular Na^+ leads to increased intracellular Ca^{2+}
  - Myocardial effect: Increased arrhythmogenic after-depolarizations

ETIOLOGY
Digoxin toxicity is frequently seen in the clinical setting of advancing age, renal insufficiency, drug interaction, diuretic use, or accidental/deliberate overdose.

ASSOCIATED CONDITIONS
See Risk Factors

 DIAGNOSIS

SIGNS AND SYMPTOMS
The features of digoxin toxicity are nonspecific and can be divided into cardiac and noncardiac.
- Cardiac
  - Digitalis is known to induce every known arrhythmia. Although there is no single electrocardiographic abnormality that is pathognomonic of digitalis excess, the combination of enhanced automaticity and impaired conduction is the hallmark of toxicity.
  - Most common: Premature ventricular contractions (PVCs), atrial tachycardias with block, and nonparoxysmal junctional tachycardia
  - Enhanced automaticity: Ectopic rhythms, nonparoxysmal junctional tachycardia, PVCs, ventricular tachycardia (VT), ventricular fibrillation (VF), accelerated escape, and atrioventricular (AV) dissociation
  - Abnormal conduction: Sinoatrial (SA) nodal arrest, SA block, AV block, exit block
  - Combination (rare but highly suggestive): Fascicular tachycardia, bidirectional VT, and alternating right- and left-axis deviation
- Noncardiac
  - Electrocardiographic signs of toxicity may be preceded by noncardiac manifestations such as:
    - Gastrointestinal: Anorexia, nausea, vomiting
    - Neurologic: Confusion, agitation, anxiety, lethargy, headaches, and nightmares
    - Ophthalmologic: Visual disturbances, usually described as halos around bright objects
    - Renal: Renal dysfunction

TESTS
Lab
Digoxin plasma level concentration has limited clinical value and may be useful only to confirm clinical signs of toxicity.
- Digoxin is rapidly absorbed with a peak serum concentration within 1.5–6 hours after ingestion.
- The therapeutic range of serum digoxin is considered 0.8–2.0 ng/mL.
- Overt digitalis toxicity tends to emerge at two- to threefold higher serum concentration than the target, but it must always be remembered that a substantial overlap of serum levels exists among patients who exhibit signs and symptoms of intoxication.
- Patients can manifest toxic symptoms at a level below the therapeutic range.
- Hyperkalemia is often seen in massive overdoses and results from extracellular redistribution of potassium because of inhibition of the $Na^+K^+ATPase$ pump.

DIFFERENTIAL DIAGNOSIS
Arrhythmias identical to those of digoxin intoxication also can be caused by primary heart disease, drugs other than digoxin, and a variety of extracardiac factors.

TREATMENT

The key to successful treatment of digoxin toxicity is early recognition that an arrhythmia or other signs and symptoms may be related to intoxication. Life-threatening arrhythmias require immediate, aggressive treatment.

- Electrical cardioversion
  - Great caution should be used in treating atrial and ventricular arrhythmias with direct current cardioversion due to the increased sensitivity of the digoxin-toxic myocardium, and the propensity to develop further arrhythmias.

GENERAL MEASURES

- Supportive care
  - Minor electrocardiographic changes (first-degree AV block, accelerated AV junctional pacemaker, atrial fibrillation with slow ventricular response, ectopy) can be treated by temporary discontinuation of the drug, monitoring, and future dose adjustment.
  - Conduction abnormalities (sinus bradycardia, sinus arrest, exit block, and second- and third-degree AV block) may respond to atropine or require temporary cardiac pacing.
  - Treat conditions that increase the likelihood of digitalis intoxication: Myocardial ischemia, hypovolemia, hypoxemia, acidosis, renal impairment.
  - Activated charcoal within 4 hours of overdose may be very effective.
- Electrolyte management
  - Hypokalemia: Potassium levels should be kept >4 mM/L. Potassium supplementation even in the setting of normal serum potassium is useful for atrial and AV junctional or ectopic rhythms. Parenteral potassium may be beneficial for severe arrhythmias such as VT but should be given only under close monitoring.
  - Hyperkalemia: Associated with a worse prognosis and can precipitate complete heart block; may be an indication for digoxin-specific Fab antibody fragments.
  - Hypocalcemia: Calcium supplementation should be avoided because it may increase automaticity and predispose to life-threatening ventricular arrhythmias.
  - Antiarrhythmics
  - Lidocaine or phenytoin may be beneficial for suppressing life-threatening arrhythmias. Both have little or no adverse effect on cardiac conduction.
  - Quinidine and procainamide should be avoided due to their suppression of AV conduction and proarrhythmic effects.
  - Amiodarone increases the steady-state concentration of digoxin.
- Hemodialysis is ineffective in the treatment of digoxin toxicity.

MEDICATION (DRUGS)

Digoxin-Specific Fab Antibody Fragments
- Most effective treatment available
- High affinity and specificity for cardiac glycosides; have been shown to reverse digoxin toxicity and reduce the risk of death.
- 80% will have complete resolution, 10% will improve, and 10% may not respond
- Indications:
  - Ventricular tachyarrhythmias
  - Symptomatic bradycardia, second- or third-degree AV block
  - Progressive hyperkalemia
  - Serum level >10 ng/mL
  - Total ingestion >10 mg
- Dosage: Each 40-mg vial of Fab fragment neutralizes 0.6 mg of digoxin. Determine "drug load" of digoxin using either plasma concentration or amount ingested.
  - Drug load = [serum level (ng/mL) × volume of distribution (5.6 L/kg) × weight (kg)]/1,000 or
  - Drug load = amount ingested (mg) × digoxin bioavailability (0.8)
  - Fab dose (mg) = drug load (mg) × 64 (based on equimolar dose of Fab [molecular weight (MW) = 50 daltons] to digoxin [MW = 781 daltons]
- Dose should be infused over 15–30 minutes.
- Improvement in signs and symptoms occur within 40 minutes.
- Digoxin–Fab fragment complexes are cleared from the system via renal excretion.
- Total serum digoxin levels are no longer meaningful following administration of Fab fragments, but free digoxin levels may be obtained and can be helpful.
- Common adverse side effects include hypokalemia and exacerbation of CHF.
- Anaphylaxis, serum sickness, and febrile reactions are potential complications, especially with repeated administrations.

FOLLOW-UP

DISPOSITION
Admission Criteria
- Most patients with clinical signs or symptoms of digoxin intoxication should be admitted to the hospital.
- They should be monitored closely for arrhythmia until the symptoms of toxicity have resolved and serum digoxin concentrations are in the therapeutic range.

PROGNOSIS
Several factors have been associated with a worse prognosis and higher overall mortality.
- Elderly
- Male
- Underlying heart disease
- Hyperkalemia

PATIENT MONITORING
- Cardiac monitoring should be considered and intensive care may be required in all patients with signs and symptoms of digoxin intoxication or in suspected overdose cases.
- In cases where cardiac toxicity is limited to ectopic beats or first-degree AV block, temporary drug withdrawal may be all that is needed.

REFERENCES
1. Borron SW, Bismuth C, Muszynski J. Advances in the management of digoxin toxicity in the older patient. *Drugs Aging.* 1997;10:18–33.
2. Hauptman PJ, Kelly RA. Digitalis. *Circulation.* 1999;99:1265–1270.
3. Kelly RA, Smith TW. Recognition and management of digitalis toxicity. *Am J Cardiol.* 1992;69:1086–1196.

CODES
ICD9-CM
972.1 Digitalis toxicity

PATIENT TEACHING
Diet prevention of digoxin toxicity is enhanced by taking the following measures:
- Discuss and emphasize the importance of proper dosing with patients.
- Awareness of drug–drug interactions
- Avoid use of drug in high-risk patients.
- Consider digitoxin, which is metabolized by the liver, in patients with renal disease.

D

DYSLIPIDEMIA
Luis Eng-Ceceña
Jorge F. Trejo

 BASICS

DESCRIPTION
Dyslipidemia is defined as the plasma lipid concentration that is associated with risk for disease, primarily atherosclerotic vascular disorders. Therefore, it is no longer defined according to the "normal" distribution levels of Western societies, which is shifted toward pathologic values.

GENERAL PREVENTION
Therapeutic lifestyle changes (TLC, see first-line therapy)

EPIDEMIOLOGY
- ~50% of U.S. adults have elevated total cholesterol level
- Elevated cholesterol and cardiovascular disease risk association is firmly established
- Most patients with atherosclerotic vascular disease have some form of dyslipidemia
- 35–40% of all cases of coronary heart disease (CHD) occur in patients with total cholesterol <200 mg/dL
- For each 1% decrease in low-density lipoprotein (LDL) cholesterol (LDL-C) and for each 1% increase in high-density lipoprotein (HDL) cholesterol (HDL-C), the risk of cardiovascular events is reduced by 2% and 3%, respectively
- Benefits extends to LDL-C levels of 50–70 mg/dL

RISK FACTORS
See secondary causes under Etiology.

Genetics
- If total cholesterol >300 mg/dL or a genetic disorder is discovered, a family history and measurement of cholesterol in other family members are needed
- Primary (genetic) dyslipidemia include (U.S. prevalence in parenthesis)
- Heterozygous familiar hypercholesterolemia (1/500); LDL-C 190–350 mg/dL
- Homozygous familiar hypercholesterolemia (1/1,000,000); LDL-C 400–1,000 mg/dL
- Polygenic hypercholesterolemia (~1/20); LDL-C ≥190 mg/dL
- Familial combined hyperlipidemia (FCH); total cholesterol 200–350 mg/dL, triglycerides (TGs) 150–500 mg/dL, or both
- Type III hyperlipidemia (familial dysbetalipoproteinemia); total cholesterol 300–600 mg/dL, TGs 400–800, but may be higher
- Familial hypertriglyceridemia (FH); TGs 200–500 mg/dL in type IV phenotype >1,000 mg/dL in type V phenotype; Total cholesterol only moderately elevated; LDL/HDL reduced
- Familial low HDL cholesterol (hypoalphalipoproteinemia); HDL may be <35 mg/dL

PATHOPHYSIOLOGY
Hypertriglyceridemia results from a combination of increased very-low-density lipoprotein (VLDL) production (as in FCH) and clearance defects (i.e., type 2 diabetes). Severe hypercholesterolemia (>300 mg/dL) usually results from defects in LDL receptor function (i.e., hypothyroidism or FH). Mixed hyperlipidemia is due to clearance abnormalities of VLDL, intermediate-density lipoprotein (IDL) or remnant particles.

ETIOLOGY
The most frequent primary hyperlipidemias are FCH (4–8%) and polygenic hypercholesterolemia. The most frequent secondary causes are: High-fat diets, type 2 diabetes, hypothyroidism, metabolic syndrome, and several drugs (excessive alcohol, isotretinoin, thiazide diuretics, β-blockers, estrogens, testosterone, glucocorticoids, cyclosporine, mycophenolate mofetil, protease inhibitors)

ASSOCIATED CONDITIONS
See secondary causes under Etiology

ALERT
- Many physicians initiate statin therapy at a low dose and fail to titrate upward to a dose needed to achieve LDL targets recommended by National Cholesterol Education Program Adult Treatment Panel III (NCEP-ATP III).
  When indicated, statins should be dosed to reduce LDL cholesterol levels by at least 30–40%.
- Although rare, the physician must remember the possibility of statin-associated myopathy, especially in the following risk states:
  – Age >80 years
  – Small body frame and frailty
  – Multisystem disease (e.g., renal failure)
  – Perioperative periods
- Multiple medications
  – Specific concomitant medications such as: Fibrates, nicotinic acid, cyclosporine, azole antifungals, macrolide antibiotics, protease inhibitors, nefazodone, verapamil, amiodarone, large quantities of grapefruit (>1 quart/day), alcohol abuse (independently predisposes to myopathy)

Geriatric Considerations
- Advanced age (>65 years) by itself should not preclude diet and drug therapy for dyslipidemia, especially in patients with established coronary artery disease or other manifestations of atherosclerosis.
- There is insufficient evidence in the management of individuals ≥80 years of age with dyslipidemia. Preliminary data suggest that greater benefit of LDL cholesterol reduction is observed in presence of low HDL cholesterol (<40 mg/dL).

Pediatric Considerations
- Pediatric age may be the best time to teach healthy behaviors that have impact on the development of dyslipidemia
- If a genetic dyslipidemia is discovered, a family history and lipid measurements are needed in other family members.

Pregnancy Considerations
- All statins are contraindicated in pregnancy and should not be used during breast feeding
- The use of fibrates requires individual risk–benefit assessment, and breast feeding is not recommended
- Bile-acid–binding resins and nicotinic acid use requires individual risk–benefit assessment. Breast feeding is not contraindicated.

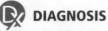 **DIAGNOSIS**

SIGNS AND SYMPTOMS
- Angina/myocardial infarction
- Transient ischemic attack/stroke
- Claudication
- Arterial bruits
- Xanthelasmas/xanthomas
- Lipemia retinalis
- Premature arcus senilis

History
- Investigate family history
- Exclude secondary causes of dyslipidemia

TESTS
Lab
- Fasting (9–12 hours) lipoprotein analysis (total cholesterol, LDL-C, HDL-C, and TG) for all adults ≥20 years old in a steady state (absence of active weight loss, acute illness, recent trauma or surgery, pregnancy, or recent change in diet), repeated at least once every 5 years
- The measurement of the following is still under validation: Lipoprotein (a); apolipoproteins B and A1; small and dense LDL; oxidized LDL; HDL subspecies; lipoprotein-associated phospholipase A_2; lipoprotein remnant particles

Pathologic Findings
Atheroma

 TREATMENT

GENERAL MEASURES
- LDL-C lowering is the primary goal of therapy for dyslipidemia.
- LDL-C goals vary inversely with CHD risk. Persons at highest risk have the lowest targets
- If TG ≥200 mg/dL, non–HDL-C (LDL + VLDL cholesterol, calculated by substracting HDL-C from total cholesterol) is a secondary goal of therapy
- Metabolic syndrome increases the risk of coronary events at any level of LDL-C. Specific therapy has benefit beyond LDL-C lowering

Therapeutic Goals
- High risk (CHD or CHD risk equivalents; 10-year risk of CHD >20%): LDL-C <100 mg/dL (optional <70 mg/dL); non–HDL-C <130 mg/dL (optional <100 mg/dL)
- Moderately high risk (≥2 risk factors; 10-year risk of CHD 10%–20%): LDL-C <130 mg/dL (optional <100 mg/dL); non–HDL-C <160 mg/dL (optional <130 mg/dL)
- Moderate risk (≥2 risk factors; 10-year risk of CHD <10%): LDL-C <130 mg/dL; non–HDL-C <160 mg/dL
- Lower risk (0–1 risk factors): LDL-C <160 mg/dL; non–HDL-C <190 mg/dL
- If acute coronary ischemic syndromes or revascularization, start therapy in the hospital

TREATMENT
- Beneficial effects of lipid therapy are due more to plaque stabilization than to changes in stenosis severity, which are generally modest and disproportionate to the 25–50% reduction in major cardiovascular events

- Control comorbidity, especially diabetes and hypertension.

First-Line Therapy

- TLC: Diet modification, increased physical activity, weight control, smoking cessation (<10% total cholesterol lowering)
- Food composition in ATP III diet is: Total fat 25–35% of total calories (saturated fat <7%; polyunsaturated fat, up to 10%; monosaturated fat, up to 20%; trans fats should be kept to a minimum); carbohydrates 50–60% of total calories (more than half as complex carbohydrates from whole grains, fruit, vegetables); fiber 20–30 g/day; protein ~15% of total calories; cholesterol <200 g/day; total calories, sufficient to achieve/maintain desirable body weight
- Basic components of a Mediterranean diet include: Omega-3 rich fish 1–2 times per week or omega-3 supplements; monounsaturated cooking oils (olive, flaxseed, or canola); wide variety of fresh fruit and vegetables (5–10 servings per day); vegetable protein from nuts and beans 1–2 times per week; limit saturated fats to <10–20 g/day; avoid trans fats; increase dietary fiber to 20–30 g/day; at least one source of high-quality protein with every meal

Second-Line Therapy (Drug)

- HMG-CoA inhibitors (statins): Lovastatin t = (Mevacor) 20–80 mg/day, simvastatin (Zocor) 20–80 mg/day, pravastatin (Pravachol) 20–80 mg/day, fluvastatin (Lescol) 40–80 mg/day, atorvastatin (Lipitor) 10/80 mg/day, rosuvastatin (Crestor) 10–40 mg/day
  - Expected benefit: LDL-C ↓ 18–55%, HDL-C ↑ 5–10%, TG ↓7–30%
  - Drugs of choice for most patients with LDL-C elevation
  - Absolute contraindications: Active or chronic liver disease, pregnancy, lactation
  - Relative contraindications: Concomitant use of cyclosporine, macrolide antibiotics, various antifungal drugs, cytochrome P450 inhibitors, previous intolerance to statins due to myalgias, elevated liver transaminases, other side effects
  - Side effects: Myopathy, reversible elevation in liver transaminases
- Cholesterol absorption inhibitors: Ezetimibe (Zetia) 10 mg/day
  - Expected benefit: LDL-C ↓ 18–25%, HDL-C ↑ 1%, TG ↓ 8%
  - Safe and effective adjunct to statins when further LDL-C lowering is required
  - Contraindications: Combination with statin in patients with active liver disease or unexplained persistent transaminase elevations
  - Side effects: Gastrointestinal (GI) complaints
- Nicotinic acid (niacin): Immediate-release form 50 mg to 4.5 g/day, sustained-release form and extended-release form (Niaspan, Slo-Niacin) 500 mg –2 g/day
  - Expected benefit: LDL-C ↓ 5–25%, HDL-C ↑ 15–35% , TG ↓ 20–50%
  - Useful in nearly all dyslipidemias. Uniquely effective in atherogenic dyslipidemia. Also useful for elevated Lp(a) levels and as an adjunctive therapy for mixed dyslipidemia
  - Absolute contraindications: Chronic liver disease, severe gout
  - Relative contraindications: Hyperuricemia, high doses (>3 g/day) in type 2 diabetes; caution in active liver or peptic ulcer disease, hyperuricemia, gout

- Side effects: Flushing, hyperglycemia, hyperuricemia/gout, upper gastrointestinal distress, hepatotoxicity (especially sustained-release form)
- Bile-acid sequestrants: Colesevelam (WelChol) 3.8–4.4 g/day, cholestyramine (Questran) 4–24 (4–16) g/day, colestipol (Colestid) 5–30 (5–20) g/day
  - Expected benefit: LDL-C ↓15–30%, HDL-C ↑ 3–5% , TG usually not affected (may ↑)
  - Major use: Moderate hypercholesterolemia; younger patients with ↑ LDL-C, especially women who are considering pregnancy; useful as adjunctive therapy with statins
  - Absolute contraindications: Familial dysbetalipoproteinemia, TG >400 mg/dL
  - Relative contraindications: TG >200 mg/dL
  - Side effects: GI complaints common; decreased absorption of warfarin, thiazides, thyroxine, digitalis, phenobarbital, tetracycline
- Fibric acid derivatives: Gemfibrozil 600 mg b.i.d. (Lopid), fenofibrate (Tricor, Triglide) 160 mg/day
  - Expected benefit: LDL-C ↓ 5–20% (may increase LDL-C with baseline elevation of TG), HDL-C ↑10–35%, TG ↓ 20–50%
  - Major use: Hypertriglyceridemia, atherogenic dyslipidemia (especially in type 2 diabetes)
  - Absolute contraindications: Severe hepatic or renal dysfunction, primary biliary cirrhosis, gallbladder disease
  - Relative contraindications: Combined therapy with statins (occasional occurrence of severe myopathy or rhabdomyolysis; less with fenofibrate); caution when combining with warfarin or cyclosporine
  - Adverse effects: Dyspepsia, upper gastrointestinal complaints, cholesterol gallstones, myopathy
- Omega-3 acid fatty acids: 3–4 g/day of docosahexaenoic (DHA) + eicosapentaenoic (EPA) acids. (Omacor: Each tablet approx. 840 mg of DHA+EPA)
  - Expected benefit: ↓ TG 45%, ↑ LDL-C 44%, ↑HDL- C 9%, ↓ non HDL-C 14%
  - Major use: Hypertriglyceridemia (TG > 500 mg/dL) that has not responded to TLC, fibrates or nicotinic acid
  - Contraindications: Hypersensitivity to any component of medication
  - Adverse effects: Rash, burping, dyspepsia, dysgeusia, back pain
- Current research focuses upon drugs that increase HDL-C protective effect (Apo A-1 Milano, Cholesteryl ester transfer protein inhibition). Emphasis is placed in combined treatment to decrease LDL-C plus drugs to increase HDL-C

SURGERY

Gastrointestinal surgery (gastric restriction or bypass) should be reserved for motivated patients with extreme obesity (BMI ≥40 kg/m² or ≥35 kg/m² with comorbidity) despite nonsurgical intervention

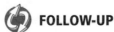 FOLLOW-UP

Issues for Referral

In general, patients with severe refractory lipid disorders should be referred

PROGNOSIS

See Epidemiology

COMPLICATIONS

See Signs and Symptoms

PATIENT MONITORING

- Check lipid panel 4–6 weeks after institution or change of therapy. If desirable lipid profiles on stable therapy, monitor yearly
- Liver function tests after 2 weeks with HMG-CoA reductase inhibitors and niacin

REFERENCES

1. Grundy SM, Cleeman JI, Bairey Mertz CN, et al. Implications of recent clinical trials for the National Cholesterol Education Program Adult Treatment Panel III Guidelines. *Circulation.* 2004;110:227–239.
2. Third Report of the National Cholesterol Education Program (NCEP) expert panel on detection, evaluation, and treatment of high blood cholesterol in adults (Adult Treatment Panel III) final report. *Circulation.* 2002;106:3143–3421.

 MISCELLANEOUS

- Internet sites:
  - American Heart Association: www.americanheart.org
  - American College of Cardiology: www.acc.org and www.cardiosource.com
  - National Cholesterol Education Program: rover.nhlbi.nih.gob./chd

CODES

ICD9-CM

- 272.0 Pure hypercholesterolemia
- 272.1 Pure hypertriglyceridemia
- 272.2 Mixed hiperlipidemia

PATIENT TEACHING

Diet

- Suggested diets are those recommended in the ATP III guidelines or a Mediterranean style diet. Emphasis in low saturated and *trans* fats, low in simple sugars, rich in vegetables and fruits, and high content of soluble fiber.
- Patients should learn how to read and apply information in food labels to their eating habits.

Activity

Regular aerobic exercise (30–60 minutes daily) increases HDL cholesterol, lowers triglycerides and blood glucose, and can help to achieve a healthier weight

Prevention

Pediatric age may be the best time to teach healthy behaviors that have an impact on the development of dyslipidemia

FAQ

- What is the optimal target to lower LDL-C for secondary prevention of CHD? Probably <70 mg/dL, suggested as optional in the guidelines
- How safe is the long-term treatment with statins? Statins are very well tolerated, with infrequent and reversible adverse events. In large placebo-controlled studies the frequency of adverse effects was similar to placebo. There has been no evidence of cancer associated with long-term use.

EBSTEIN'S DISEASE AND UHL'S ANOMALY

Beth Feller Printz
Welton M. Gersony

 BASICS

DESCRIPTION

- Ebstein anomaly (EA) is a congenital abnormality of the tricuspid valve with inferior displacement of the septal and/or posterior tricuspid leaflets from the atrioventricular ring, leading to partitioning of the right ventricle (RV) into "atrialized" and functional components.
- Tricuspid leaflets typically dysplastic and tethered to the right ventricular endocardium. The anterior leaflet may be normal or enlarged and "sail-like."
- Tricuspid regurgitation (TR), right atrial enlargement, and right-to-left shunting through an interatrial communication are characteristic, with impaired RV compliance and systemic cyanosis. Pulmonary stenosis may be present. Tricuspid stenosis occurs rarely.
- Atrial arrhythmias are common, due to associated Wolff-P-White (WPW) syndrome and/or right atrial enlargement.
- Clinical presentation of Ebstein anomaly is variable: (i) Severe malformations presenting prenatally with intrauterine death; (ii) severe cyanosis in infancy; (iii) exercise intolerance, cyanosis, arrhythmias and/or congestive heart failure presenting during childhood; (iv) cardiac arrhythmias in adults; or (v) mild TR in virtually asymptomatic adults.

EPIDEMIOLOGY

Rare congenital heart lesion, occurs equally in male and female patients.

Incidence

5/100,000 live births

Prevalence

Approximately 0.5% of all cases of congenital heart disease

RISK FACTORS

- Association with maternal lithium therapy:
  - Among women who receiving lithium during the first trimester of pregnancy: Low (0.05–0.1%), but 5 to 1 relative risk of EA compared with those women who did not receive lithium.

Genetics

- Most cases occur sporadically.
- Incidence of congenital heart disease in the offspring of women with EA reported as 6%. Risk of a fetus having EA less than 1%.
- No genetic basis elucidated to date.

PATHOPHYSIOLOGY

Large RA with atrialized RV inflow and tricuspid insufficiency most often is associated with right to left shunting across a ***PFO or ASD, and decreased RV filling. The small and sometimes dysfunctional RV with or without PS also contributes to symptoms of low cardiac output.

ETIOLOGY

The etiology has not been established.

ASSOCIATED CONDITIONS

- Inter-atrial communication (secundum atrial septal defect or patent foramen ovale (PFO)) present in approximately 90% of cases.
- Pulmonary stenosis and pulmonary atresia can be seen. May be due to decreased antegrade flow through the RV during early fetal development. With low RV cardiac output and PDA "pseudopulmonary atresia" may be noted (no forward blood flow over normal pulmonary valve). VSD occurs rarely.
- Diastolic and/or systolic RV dysfunction. A decrease in the absolute number of RV muscle fibers has been observed.
- Left ventricular (LV) systolic and diastolic dysfunction may occur. In part, may be related to diastolic bowing of the interventricular septum. LV hypertrophy, fibrosis, and dysplasia have been reported.
- Wolff-Parkinson-White (WPW) syndrome in approximately 20% of patients. AV nodal re-entrant tachycardia and atrial flutter/fibrillation can also be seen.
- Ebstein's-like anomaly of the left-sided tricuspid valve may occur in association with congenitally corrected transposition (l-transposition) of the great arteries transposition.

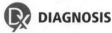 **DIAGNOSIS**

SIGNS AND SYMPTOMS

- Extreme variability in tricuspid valve morphology influences the clinical presentation.
- Presentation of Ebstein's anomaly also affected by the degree of TR, the presence of an inter-atrial communication, the degree of RV or LV dysfunction, and the presence of arrhythmias.
- May be dissociation between the severity of valve dysplasia, the degree of TR, and the severity of symptoms.

History

- **Fetal:** Fetal diagnosis can almost always be made by fetal echocardiography when significant TR is present.
  - Right atrial enlargement, often massive with severe TR
  - Lungs may be hypoplastic due to massive cardiomegaly
  - Congestive heart failure with pericardial effusion, ascites, and hydrops fetalis may occur, with high rate of intrauterine demise in these severe cases
  - Uncommonly, a fetus with Ebstein's anomaly may be diagnosed after an arrhythmia is noted (usually atrial flutter or supraventricular tachycardia in the presence of WPW)
- **Neonatal:** Cases diagnosed in the neonatal period most often are associated with severe TR and right-to-left shunting across an inter-atrial communication, leading to significant systemic cyanosis and heart failure. RV outflow obstruction may or may not be present.
- **Older Children and Adults:** Present with increasing cyanosis, dyspnea or exercise intolerance, and/or arrhythmias. Asymptomatic patients may also be diagnosed solely by an abnormal cardiac examination leading to a chest x-ray and echocardiogram.

Physical Exam

- Neonatal:
  - Murmur may or may not be audible
  - Evidence of RV dysfunction: Elevated venous pressure, hepatomegaly, and ascites.
  - Elevated pulmonary vascular resistance (PVR) during the immediate postnatal period can accentuate the severity of cyanosis, with increased right-to-left inter-atrial shunting and decreased antegrade flow through the RV to the pulmonary artery.
  - Low volume of antegrade flow may make it extremely difficult to differentiate functional pulmonary atresia from true valvar pulmonary atresia. Inhaled nitric oxide has been used to differentiate these conditions.
  - If supported through the first few days of life as PVR falls, the degree of cyanosis typically improves in the patient and may remain clinically stable for months to years. However, if true pulmonary atresia is present, the patient's condition will continue to deteriorate.
  - Less symptomatic infants: Mild cyanosis, heart murmur, and/or atrial arrhythmias
- Older children and adults:
  - Mild to moderate cyanosis with clubbing common.
  - Hepatomegaly or a pulsatile liver from increased right atrial and systemic venous pressure may be noted in patients with only small inter-atrial communications.
  - Peripheral edema
  - Cardiac examination:
    - Quiet precordium with a prominent RV impulse.
    - Characteristic "gallop" rhythm with multiple extra heart sounds (due to widely split first and second heart sounds, as well as S3 and/or S4 from abnormal ventricular filling).
    - A "scratchy" systolic murmur is audible at the left mid to upper sternal border, and a low intensity systolic regurgitant murmur (TR) may be heard along the left lower sternal border. A short, soft diastolic murmur may also be present (tricuspid inflow).
  - Many previously undiagnosed adolescent and adult patients present with arrhythmias. These patients may be virtually acyanotic with relatively mild tricuspid abnormalities.
  - Atrial arrhythmias common, a result of right atrial enlargement and/or accessory conduction pathways (WPW syndrome).
  - Ventricular arrhythmias occur less frequently.

TESTS

Lab

- **Hemoglobin concentration:** Increased proportionate to the degree of cyanosis. Serial analysis demonstrating increasing hemoglobin is consistent with increasing cyanosis.
- **Electrocardiographic abnormalities:**
  - First degree AV block common (1/4 to 1/3 of patients)
  - The P-wave usually enlarged (right atrial enlargement)
  - Right bundle branch block with low voltage R' pattern typical.
  - Short PR interval and a delta wave in patients with WPW syndrome. The accessory pathway is usually right-sided or in the interventricular septum.

Imaging

- Chest x-ray shows cardiomegaly (may be massive) with increased right atrial size. There may be decreased pulmonary vascularity when there is marked right-to-left inter-atrial shunting.
- Echocardiography: Imaging modality of choice (2-D, 3-D, and/or TEE)
  - Inferior displacement of the effective tricuspid valve annulus and dysplasia of the tricuspid leaflets
  - Color Doppler imaging will demonstrate TR originating from the effective valve annulus within the right ventricle. An inter-atrial communication with right-to-left inter-atrial shunting can be visualized.
  - Cardiac chamber enlargement, ventricular dysfunction, and associated lesions can be identified.

Diagnostic Procedures/Surgery

- Cardiac catheterization is not necessary solely for diagnosis, and is associated with increased risk.
  - Historic: Simultaneous demonstration of atrial pressure with ventricular electrogram within atrialized portion of RV
  - Generally reserved for assessment of associated lesions or preoperative evaluation of adult patients
  - Can be combined with electrophysiologic testing to evaluate accessory pathways

DIFFERENTIAL DIAGNOSIS

- Depends on the severity of the defect and degree of cyanosis.
- Must be differentiated from other cyanotic lesions, including tricuspid atresia and pulmonary atresia, as well as persistent pulmonary hypertension of the newborn (PPHN).
- Rarely, patients may present with isolated TR and a dysplastic tricuspid valve in the absence of Ebstein's anomaly.
- Mildly cyanotic patients with RV dysfunction must be differentiated from other causes of right-sided heart failure (including primary pulmonary hypertension).
- **Uhl's anomaly** ('parchment right ventricle') should also be differentiated from Ebstein's anomaly. Uhl's anomaly is an extremely rare malformation in which the right ventricle myocardium is absent and replaced by fibroelastic tissue. There is usually right heart failure with peripheral edema and ascites. Arrhythmias may occur. Most patients do not survive childhood.

 TREATMENT

GENERAL MEASURES

- Symptomatic cyanotic neonates without anatomic pulmonary obstruction: Often improve spontaneously as pulmonary vascular resistance (PVR) falls. Persistently critically ill patients may need urgent intervention to expedite the physiologic fall in PVR in order to increase antegrade flow through the RV:
  - Intubation with hyperventilation, sedation, Alkalinization
  - Inhaled nitric oxide may improve oxygenation in those severely symptomatic neonates without anatomic pulmonary obstruction
  - For most extreme cases, neonatal surgery may be attempted. Extra-corporeal membrane oxygenation (ECMO) or cardiac transplantation may be considered as rescue therapy. Prognosis is grave.
  - Neonates with significant anatomic pulmonary stenosis: Prostaglandin infusion to maintain ductal patency, followed by surgical intervention.
  - Symptomatic patients beyond the perinatal period with continued moderate or severe cyanosis: Surgical intervention
  - Patients with mild (or no) symptoms can be followed serially without surgical intervention.
  - Endocarditis prophylaxis recommended for all patients

E

MEDICATION (DRUGS)

First Line
- Anticongestive treatment for symptomatic heart failure
- Antiarrhythmic therapy in cases of WPW syndrome or atrial arrhythmias due to atrial enlargement

SURGERY
- Goal: Decrease TR and eliminate right-to-left inter-atrial shunting
- Indications for surgical intervention not clearly established
  - In recent years, results of non-neonatal surgical repair of Ebstein's anomaly have improved significantly, with low operative morbidity and mortality and good early and medium-term results.
  - Improved results have led most to conclude that any patient who has deteriorated to NYHA class III or IV despite medical management should undergo surgery.
  - Technique: Reconstruction or replacement of dysplastic tricuspid valve, atrial plication, and closure of inter-atrial communication to eliminate right-to-left shunting. May include tricuspid annuloplasty with valve ring placement. Reported methods for tricuspid valve reconstruction vary. Tricuspid valve replacement using a porcine bioprosthetic valve is performed as an alternative to repair in certain surgical centers, particularly in adult populations.

- Surgical repair of the tricuspid valve has not been shown to alter the risk of sudden death from arrhythmias.
- Tricuspid valve repair or replacement can be combined with intra-operative cryoablation, radiofrequency ablation, or Maze procedure in those patients with atrial tachyarrhythmias.
- Neonates with severe EA who are critically ill despite measures aimed at decreasing PVR have a poor prognosis with standard surgical repair.
  - Can attempt surgical palliation by closure of tricuspid valve and shunt placement, with later staged single ventricle-type surgery (bidirectional Glenn and Fontan)
- Radiofrequency catheter ablation or intra-operative cryoablation or Maze procedure may be considered in patients with atrial arrhythmias

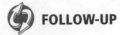 ## FOLLOW-UP

PROGNOSIS
- Quite variable, ranging from Ebstein's anomaly diagnosed as an incidental finding in an older adult, to high risk of fetal demise in severely symptomatic fetuses.
- Severity of tricuspid regurgitation, size of functional RV, and the function of RV and LV can influence prognosis of EA.
- Neonates with severe cyanosis and heart failure have high mortality despite attempts at intervention (medical or surgical)
- Survivors of neonatal period may have improvement in cyanosis and remain clinically stable for months or years; later may develop progressive TR leading to clinical de-compensation
- Some children with only mild cyanosis may develop arrhythmias with hemodynamic deterioration during adolescence or adulthood
- Less severe malformations of the tricuspid valve and RV are usually associated with a more benign prognosis. Some patients may remain asymptomatic into old age; a heart murmur may be present.
- Sudden death does occur rarely, and may not be predicted by the presence of symptoms, prior arrhythmias or pre-excitation syndrome.

PATIENT MONITORING

- Serial evaluation by physical examination, EKG, echocardiography and exercise testing with pulse oximetry: To evaluate for increasing cyanosis, exercise intolerance, or significant deterioration of tricuspid valve or ventricular function.
- Holter monitor or event recorder if there is evidence of palpitations or tachyarrhythmia.
- Electrophysiologic testing has been suggested for those Ebstein's anomaly patients with tachyarrhythmias in whom tricuspid valve surgery is planned

Pregnancy Considerations

Pregnancy in women with Ebstein's anomaly is generally well tolerated. Risk of fetal miscarriage, premature delivery, and low birth weight are increased with maternal cyanosis.

REFERENCES

1. Atz AM, Munoz RA, Adatia I, Wessel DL. Diagnostic and therapeutic uses of inhaled nitric oxide in neonatal Ebstein's anomaly. *American Journal of Cardiology*. 2003;91:906–908.
2. Celermajer DS, Bull C, Till JA, et al. Ebstein's anomaly: Presentation and outcome from fetus to adult. *JACC*. 1994;23:170–176.
3. Chen JM, Mosca RS, Altmann K, et al. Early and medium-term results for repair of Ebstein anomaly. *JTCVS*. 2004;127:990–999.
4. Cohen LS, Friedman JM, Jefferson SW, et al. A reevaluation of risk of in utero exposure to lithium. *JAMA*. 1994;271:146–150.
5. Correa-Villasenor A, Ferencz C, Neill C, et al. Ebstein's malformation of the tricuspid valve: Genetic and environmental factors. *Teratology*. 1994;50:137–147.
6. Khositseth A, Danielson GK, Dearani JA, et al. Supraventricular tachyarrhythmias in Ebstein anomaly: Management and outcome. *JTCVS*. 2004;128:826–833.
7. MacLellan-Tobert SG, Porter CJ. Ebstein's Anomaly of the Tricuspid Valve. In: Garson A, et al. *The Science and Practice of Pediatric Cardiology*. Baltimore, MD: Williams & Wilkins; 1998.
8. Mair DD. Ebstein's anomaly: Natural history and management. *JACC*. 1992;19:1047–1048.
9. Wald RM, Adatia I, Van Arsdell GS, et al. Relation of limiting ductal patency to survival in neonatal Ebstein's anomaly. *Am J Cardiol*. 2005;96:851–856.

CODES
ICD9-CM
746.2

PATIENT TEACHING
Diet
No restrictions

Activity

- Patients should be restricted from rough competitive sports with other restrictions dependent on the severity of their condition.
- Usually no other restrictions for patients in NYHA class I and II. They can participate in physical activities as tolerated; some may develop marked cyanosis with mild exertion.

Prevention
See above regarding maternal Lithium exposure and risk of Ebstein's anomaly.

E

EHLERS DANLOS SYNDROME AND THE HEART

James A. Kong

 BASICS

DESCRIPTION

Ehlers Danlos syndrome (EDS) is a heterogeneous group of heritable connective tissue disorders characterized by varying degrees of skin elasticity, joint hyperextensibility, and cutaneous fragility classified as types I–X.

- Cardiovascular (CV) manifestations (based mainly on case reports of types I–IV, with little prospective survey data):
  - Aortic dilation (more common in Marfan syndrome)
  - Bicuspid aortic valve
  - Pulmonic root dilation
  - Pulmonic stenosis
  - Mitral valve prolapse (MVP)
  - Tricuspid valve prolapse
  - Ventricular or atrial septal defects
  - Sinus of Valsalva ectasia or aneurysm
  - Myocardial infarction due to coronary artery dissection (rare)
  - Type I and especially type IV: Spontaneous rupture of large-/medium-sized arteries and viscera (e.g., gravid uterus)
- Cardiac manifestations are less common and peripheral vascular effects are more common in type IV EDS, presumably due to the paucity of type III collagen in the heart.
- CV effects may be present in the absence of obvious external manifestations of EDS.

Systems Affected

- Cardiovascular (including peripheral vasculature), skin, visceral organs

EPIDEMIOLOGY

Predominant Age: Congenital to adult

Incidence

- EDS occurs in 1/5,000 births; types I–III are most common (90%).
- In one series, the presence of congenital CV manifestations in a hospitalized population was as high as 47%.

Prevalence

Prevalence in the general population is unknown.

RISK FACTORS

Pregnancy Considerations

Women with Ehlers-Danlos type IV are of increased risk of vascular rupture and, therefore, pregnancy may be hazardous. Careful consideration and counseling are warranted.

Genetics

The most common EDS types are autosomal dominant/recessive; few, rare types are sex-linked. The pattern of CV effects is unknown.

ETIOLOGY

EDS type IV is due to a defect of type III collagen. Underlying biochemical defects of other types are unknown.

 DIAGNOSIS

SIGNS AND SYMPTOMS

- Asymptomatic to acute CV decompensation from structural heart disease or arterial/visceral rupture
- Severe cases may have hemorrhage leading to death.
- The most common presentations are referable to underlying valvulopathy or shunt, with chest pain, dyspnea, and/or congestive heart failure.
- Severe valvulopathy (e.g., mitral regurgitation, aortic insufficiency) and aortic dissection have been reported.

TESTS

- No pathognomonic findings for electrocardiography are described.
- Conduction delays, chamber hypertrophy, among others, secondary to cardiac structural defects have been described.

Lab

Molecular techniques may identify collagen defects, although these tests are not routinely available. In general, diagnostic biochemical tests are unavailable.

Imaging

- Echocardiography may reveal findings characteristic of the lesions mentioned previously, including valvular abnormalities.
- Structural and functional chamber abnormalities associated with these particular valvulopathies also may be seen.
- Progression of disease may be followed by echocardiography or nuclear cardiography.

Diagnostic Procedures/Surgery

- Cardiac catheterization may be indicated for evaluating valvular disease or for preoperative or medical management.
- Peripheral vascular lesions may require angiography in some cases (e.g., for preoperative management).

Pathologic Findings

As for the particular lesions noted in the preceding text

DIFFERENTIAL DIAGNOSIS

Similar aortic vessel and aortic valve disease may be observed in Marfan syndrome. In cases of congenital heart disease or great vessel dilation, consider EDS.

 TREATMENT

GENERAL MEASURES

- Screening echocardiography for patients with EDS, particularly types I and II
- Appropriate antibiotic prophylaxis for valvular disease (e.g., MVP)
- Especially in patients with EDS types I and IV, who are at risk for spontaneous rupture of blood vessels and viscera
  - Avoid contact sports and heavy physical activity.
  - Handle invasive procedures with care due to the risk of scar formation, bleeding, dissection, and arterial rupture.
  - Administer anticoagulants (including antiplatelet agents) cautiously.
  - Avoid intramuscular and intravenous therapies if possible.
  - Control hypertension.

 MEDICATION (DRUGS)

Vitamin C, despite its importance in collagen synthesis, has little efficacy in the treatment of EDS.

- Precautions
  - Antiplatelet therapy as noted in the preceding text

SURGERY

- Often met with unsatisfying results; surgical therapy is directed toward valvular replacement or repair of arterial dissection or rupture
- Although successful aortic valve replacements have been reported, surgery is complicated by variable wound healing and widened scars, wound dehiscence, and failure of tissue–graft unions.
- Bleeding may be excessive.

FOLLOW-UP

DISPOSITION
Admission Criteria
- Asymptomatic or mildly symptomatic CV abnormalities may be evaluated on an outpatient basis.
- Hemodynamic instability should be evaluated and treated emergently.

PROGNOSIS
- Variable
- Those with EDS type IV have a shorter life expectancy, usually surviving to only the fourth decade, due to the catastrophic nature of their CV abnormalities.

PATIENT MONITORING
- Objective evaluation of cardiac function, either with echocardiography or nuclear cardiography
- Referring a patient for surgery should follow conventional guidelines for treatment of valvular abnormalities, while considering the patient's clinical status and symptoms.
- Potential for progression of CV abnormalities, especially in cases of congenital abnormalities, is an important factor, weighed against the risks of surgery in EDS.

REFERENCES
1. Ades L C, et al. Myocardial infarction resulting from coronary artery dissection in an adolescent with Ehlers-Danlos syndrome type IV due to a type III collagen mutation. *Br Heart J.* 1995;74:112–116.
2. Antani J, Srinivas HV. Ehlers-Danlos syndrome and cardiovascular abnormalities. *Chest.* 1973;63:214–272.
3. Dolan AL, et al. Clinical and echocardiographic survey of the Ehlers-Danlos syndrome. *Br J Rheumatol.* 1997;36:459–462.
4. Leier CV, et al. The spectrum of cardiac defects in the Ehlers-Danlos syndrome, types I and III. *Ann Intern Med.* 1980;92:171–178.
5. Pyeritz RE. Cardiovascular manifestations of the heritable disorders of connective tissue. *Prog Med Genet.* 1983;5:191–301.
6. Shohet I, et al. Cardiovascular complications in the Ehlers-Danlos syndrome with minimal external findings. *Clin Genet.* 1987;3:148–152.
7. Steinmann B, et al. *Connective Tissue and its Heritable Disorders.* New York: Wiley-Liss, 1993;351–407.

 MISCELLANEOUS

See also: Marfan's syndrome

CODES
ICD9-CM
756.83 Ehlers-Danlos syndrome

PATIENT TEACHING
Organizations
- Ehlers Danlos National Foundation, 6399 Wilshire Blvd., Suite 510, Los Angeles, CA 90048; (323)651-3038; http://www.ednf.org/ The Foundation publishes a quarterly newsletter, *Loose Connections.*
- National Institute of Arthritis & Musculoskeletal & Skin Diseases, Building 31, Room 4C05, Bethesda, MD 20892-2350; (301)496-8188; http://www.nih.gov/niams/

Activity
Some patients with EDS should avoid strenuous activity or contact sports.

E

EISENMENGER'S SYNDROME

Robyn J. Barst
Welton M. Gersony

BASICS

DESCRIPTION AND PATHOBIOLOGY
- Pulmonary vascular obstructive disease related to congenital heart disease (i.e., Eisenmenger syndrome) develops after a period of left-to-right shunting with increased pulmonary flow and elevated pulmonary artery pressure.
- Shear stress on pulmonary arterioles creates medical and intimal proliferation and increasing pulmonary vascular obstruction.
- System(s) affected: Cardiovascular

EPIDEMIOLOGY
Predominant Sex: More females than males
Incidence
In the United States:
- Maximal estimate of incidence of pulmonary vascular obstructive disease in uncorrected congenital heart disease is 32%.
- The incidence is approximately equal in males and females for posttricuspid defects. When the disease occurs in adults, there appears to be an increased incidence among female patients, with Eisenmenger syndrome associated with an atrial septal defect (similar to the increased incidence in females with idiopathic pulmonary arterial hypertension, previously termed primary pulmonary hypertension).
- Although pulmonary vascular obstructive disease has been reported in children younger than 2 years of age with posttricuspid (interventricular or great artery) defects, it is uncommon except with Down syndrome and certain cyanotic heart diseases associated with pulmonary arterial hypertension (e.g., truncus arteriosus, transposition of the great vessels, ventricular septal defect).

RISK FACTORS AND ASSOCIATED CONDITIONS
- High altitude
- Complicated neonatal history (e.g., spontaneous pneumothorax) may trigger maintenance of high pulmonary vascular resistance after birth.
- Family history of pulmonary arterial hypertension (i.e., pulmonary vascular obstructive disease)
- Autoimmune abnormalities
- Down syndrome
- Sleep disorders
- Genetic mutations

Pregnancy Considerations
- Pregnancy is associated with significant risk to fetus and mother. Spontaneous abortion occurs in 20–40%, premature delivery in 50%, and term delivery in only 25%. At least 30% of infants have intrauterine growth retardation; 8–28% die perinatally. The maternal mortality rate is 45%.
- Pregnant patients with the Eisenmenger syndrome should be advised to have an elective abortion without delay.

Genetics
- The same genetic mutations reported in idiopathic pulmonary arterial hypertension (e.g., bone morphogenetic protein receptor 2 mutations), also occur in some patients with Eisenmenger syndrome.
- The Eisenmenger physiology begins in infancy in patients with posttricuspid defects: Ventricular septal defects of all types, single ventricles, and aortopulmonary communications (patent ductus arteriosus, aortopulmonary windows, and large surgical shunts).
- It is uncommon in patients with pretricuspid defects (e.g., atrial septal defects of all types, sinus venosus defects, common atrium), but when it occurs, it does so most often during adult life.

DIAGNOSIS

SIGNS AND SYMPTOMS
- Natural history
  - Many patients have a history of failure to thrive and congestive heart failure during infancy (due to large left-to-right shunt), which improves spontaneously as pulmonary vascular resistance increases.
- Most common signs and symptoms
  - Exercise intolerance
  - Syncope
  - Chest pain
  - Hemoptysis
  - Congestive heart failure
  - Squatting
  - Central cyanosis
  - Digital clubbing
- Other signs and symptoms
  - Normal jugular venous pressure
  - Normal or narrow peripheral arterial pulse pressure
  - Right ventricular lift
  - Increased pulmonary closure with variable splitting of the second heart sound
  - Pulmonary ejection click
  - Pulmonary ejection murmur or left sternal border systolic murmur
  - High-pitched protodiastolic murmur of pulmonary valve insufficiency at the left sternal border
  - Pansystolic murmur of tricuspid regurgitation at the left sternal border
  - Third heart sound

TESTS
Lab
Hemoglobin normal to markedly increased

Imaging; Diagnosis
- Electrocardiogram (ECG)
  - Right axis deviation
  - Right ventricular hypertrophy with or without strain
- Chest x-ray
  - Right ventricular enlargement on lateral projection
  - Enlarged central pulmonary arteries
  - Normal to decreased pulmonary vascular markings peripherally.

- Echocardiography (2D)
  - Normal to decreased right ventricular function
  - Dilated right heart
  - Right ventricular hypertrophy
  - Flattened to posterior bowing of the interventricular and interatrial septa
  - Bidirectional shunting or right-to-left shunting via defects
- Cardiac catheterization
  - Increased pulmonary vascular resistance
  - Pulmonary arterial hypertension
  - Bidirectional shunt or right-to-left shunt via the pretricuspid or posttricuspid defects

Pathologic Findings
- Progressive pulmonary vascular changes (Heath-Edwards classification grade I–VI)
  - Medial hypertrophy
  - Intimal proliferation
  - Intimal fibrosis
  - Plexiform lesions
  - Dilatation lesions
  - Necrotizing arteritis

DIFFERENTIAL DIAGNOSIS
- Pulmonary arterial hypertension (including idiopathic pulmonary arterial hypertension, familial pulmonary arterial hypertension, portal hypertension, HIV infection, connective tissue disease, and toxin/drug exposure)
- Lung disease
- Chronic thromboembolic disease
- Pulmonary venous hypertension
  - Cor triatriatum
  - Mitral stenosis
  - Left ventricular dysfunction

TREATMENT

GENERAL MEASURES
- Aggressive antibiotic therapy for significant upper respiratory tract infections
- Antipyretic therapy for febrile illnesses
- Dietary and/or medical therapy for constipation to prevent Valsalva maneuvers from precipitating abrupt decreases in cardiac output
- Yearly flu vaccine and pneumonia vaccine as indicated
- Supplemental oxygen with airplane flying to prevent alveolar hypoxia from exacerbating the underlying pulmonary vascular disease by hypoxic pulmonary vasoconstriction
Precautions
- Avoidance of circumstances or substances that may aggravate the pulmonary vascular disease, for example, oral contraceptives, anorectic agents, smoking; exercise should be guided by symptoms (avoid isometric exercise) and exposure to high altitude may worsen pulmonary arterial hypertension by producing hypoxic-induced pulmonary vasoconstriction due to alveolar hypoxia.
- Dehydration (e.g., from physical activity, environmental effects, diarrhea) can precipitate a significant decrease in cardiac output and should be prevented or treated if it occurs.

- Although airplane travel is generally safe, supplemental oxygen therapy may be advisable. Pregnancy, oral contraceptives, and appetite suppressants should be avoided. Avoid high altitude.
- Patients with Eisenmenger syndrome who become pregnant are at increased risk of sudden death both within the course of delivery and immediately postpartum.
- In patients with symptomatic hyperviscosity, phlebotomy with replacement of fluid (e.g., plasma or albumin) is helpful in cyanotic congenital heart disease in which severe hypoxemia has evoked a large increase in red blood cell mass. Caution is required to avoid depletion of iron stores and to avoid reduction of the circulating blood volume. Routine phlebotomy compromises oxygen tissue delivery and thus increases the risk of stroke.
- Special anesthesia management
- Special care with angiography and noncardiac surgery

Special Problems
- Increased uric acid (less commonly gout)
- Renal dysfunction
- Cholelithiasis
- Scoliosis
- Arthropathy (osteochondrosis)
- Acne
- Risk of systemic infection
  - Brain abscess (focal neurologic symptoms not to be confused for hyperviscosity symptoms)
- Hemoptysis
- Menorrhagia
- Arrhythmias (atrial and ventricular)
- Syncope
- Right heart failure (late, ominous sign)

MEDICATION (DRUGS)

- Oxygen/digitalis/diuretics
  - Supplemental oxygen with sleep may slow the progression of polycythemia; ambulatory supplemental oxygen may improve exercise capacity.
  - Digitalis and diuretics may be beneficial for patients with severe right ventricular failure, although excessive diuresis can lead to a decrease in cardiac output in patients who are highly preload dependent.
- Anticoagulation
  - Anticoagulation has been demonstrated to improve survival in patients with idiopathic pulmonary arterial hypertension, although its usefulness in patients with Eisenmenger syndrome is unknown.
- Vasodilator/antiproliferative therapy
  - Chronic vasodilator therapy, for example, prostacyclins, endothelin receptor antagonists or phosphodiesterase type 5 (PDE5) inhibitors have been shown to improve quality of life, hemodynamics, exercise capacity, and survival in patients with idiopathic pulmonary arterial hypertension; limited data also suggest efficacy with Eisenmenger patients, although long-term data are limited.

SURGERY
- Prevention: Early correction in infancy of unrestrictive ventricular septal defect(s) or other posttricuspid communications
- "Corrective cardiac surgery" in older children and adults if pulmonary vasoreactivity is demonstrated with acute vasodilator drug testing, for example, inhaled citric oxide, intravenous prostacyclins, inhaled prostacyclins, intravenous (IV) adenosine
  - If a patient with elevated pulmonary vascular resistance is considered for surgery, with the increased risk of perioperative pulmonary hypertensive crises, short-term pulmonary vasodilator therapy (e.g., inhaled nitric oxide, prostacyclin or PDE5 inhibitor) in the perioperative period may be needed to treat acute pulmonary hypertensive crises.
  - Consideration of creating a "palliative atrial septal defect" during corrective cardiac surgery also may be indicated.
- Palliative atrial septostomy may be helpful in select patients with advanced pulmonary vascular obstructive disease, intractable right heart failure, and/or recurrent syncope who have previously undergone surgical repair of their congenital heart defects.
- Transplantation
  - Heart/lung, single lung, bilateral lung, and living-related lung transplantation have all been performed successfully for patients with pulmonary vascular disease, although the long-term outlook remains unknown with 1-, 3-, 5-, and 10-year survival rates with lung transplantation for pulmonary vascular disease currently 65%, 54%, 45% and 20%, respectively (United Network of Organ Sharing 2004).

FOLLOW-UP

Admission Criteria
- Hemoptysis
- Systemic infection
- Dehydration
- Right heart failure
- Pneumonia

PROGNOSIS
- The natural history of Eisenmenger syndrome demonstrates a wide spectrum of variability, although the overall survival is significantly better than with idiopathic pulmonary arterial hypertension.
- This wide variability suggests that the immunogenetic predisposition demonstrated in idiopathic pulmonary arterial hypertension also may play a significant role in the development of Eisenmenger syndrome.
- Overall 80% 5-year and 40% 20-year survival rates have been reported with Eisenmenger syndrome versus a 2- to 3-year mean survival after diagnosis in idiopathic pulmonary arterial hypertension.
- This underscores the need to individualize therapeutic options for patients based on risk–benefit considerations of the various therapeutic modalities currently available.

PATIENT MONITORING
Close regular visits for assessment of signs/symptoms to serially optimize chronic medical/surgical therapeutic regimen

REFERENCES
1. Barst RJ, Miller WM. Pulmonary arterial hypertension in infants and children. *Prog Pediatr Cardiol.* 2001;12:219–340.
2. O'Fallon WM, Weidman WH, eds. Long-term follow-up of congenital aortic stenosis, pulmonary stenosis and ventricular septal defect—report from the Second Joint Study on the Natural History of Congenital Heart Defects. *Circulation.* 1993;87[Suppl]:1–126.
3. Rosenzweig EB, Barst RJ. Treatment options for children with pulmonary arterial hypertension. In: *Tracleer CHD-International Scientific Advisory Board (INSAB).* New York, New York: Marcel Dekker, 2006.
4. Rosenzweig EB, Gersony WM, Barst RJ. Eisenmenger syndrome in ventricular septal defect patients. *Prog Pediatr Cardiol.* 2001;14:175–180.
5. Rosenzweig EB, Barst RJ. Clinical management of patients with pulmonary hypertension. In: Allen HD, Gutgesell HP, Clark EB, et al., eds. *Moss and Adams' Heart Disease in Infants, Children and Adolescents,* 7th ed. Baltimore: Lippincott Williams & Wilkins, 2006.
6. Wood P. The Eisenmenger syndrome or pulmonary hypertension with reversed central shunt. *Br Med J.* 1958;2:701–709, 755–762.
7. Young D, Mark H. Fate of the patient with Eisenmenger syndrome. *Am J Cardiol.* 1971;28:658–669.

CODES
ICD9-CM
- 416.0 Pulmonary hypertension, primary
- 416.8 Pulmonary hypertension, secondary

PATIENT TEACHING
Organization
Pulmonary Hypertension Association
  801 Roeder Road, Suite 400,
    Silver Spring, MD 20910
    Phone: 1-800-748-7274
    www.phassociation.org
    Publication: Pulmonary Hypertension, a Patient's Survival Guide, 3rd Edition

ENDOCARDIAL CUSHION DEFECTS

Howard D. Apfel
Welton M. Gersony

 BASICS

DESCRIPTION

Atrioventricular (AV) canal defects include a spectrum of anomalies caused by maldevelopment of the endocardial cushions.

- Three major potential hemodynamic disturbances contribute to the pathophysiology, natural history, and medical and surgical management of these lesions.
- The relative effects of interatrial shunting, interventricular shunting, and AV valve function will determine the general course of patients with uncomplicated AV canal defects.
- The term *complete atrioventricular canal defect* refers to a heart with both significant ventricular and atrial components, whereas *partial atrioventricular canal defect* refers to a predominant primum atrial defect, cleft mitral valve, or restrictive or no ventricular shunting.
- *Unbalanced canal defect* refers to hearts with a right or left dominant ventricle.
- These are often associated with hypoplasia or atresia of one side of the common AV valve.

EPIDEMIOLOGY

- AV canal defects occur in 4–5% of patients diagnosed with congenital heart disease.
- Among patients with Down syndrome, 40–50% will have congenital heart disease, and, among those, approximately 40% will have AV canal defects.

Pregnancy Considerations

- Fetal diagnosis of AV canal defects is readily made on the four-chamber view of the fetal heart alone.
- Identifying features include absence of primum atrial septum, loss of the offsetting of the mitral valve above the tricuspid valve at the crux of the heart, and an inlet ventricular septal defect.
- The relative size of the atrial and ventricular septal defects, the size of the left and right ventricles, and the degree of AV valve insufficiency, if any, should be specifically evaluated.
- Currently, no specific *in utero* management other than prenatal counseling is available for this diagnosis.

Genetics

- Complex AV canal defects with hypoplasia of one ventricle and/or variable degrees of pulmonic stenosis are associated with heterotaxy syndromes.
- Families in which several members had AV canal defects not associated with trisomy 21 have been described.

ASSOCIATED CONDITIONS

Associated cardiac anomalies include straddling, stenosis, or atresia of part of the AV valve, often associated with hypoplasia of a ventricular chamber. Occasionally, complete AV canal defects are seen in combination with tetralogy of Fallot.

 DIAGNOSIS

SIGNS AND SYMPTOMS

- Patients with mainly atrial shunting are generally recognized following detection of a cardiac murmur on routine pediatric evaluation.
- The examination is similar to that noted in patients with isolated secundum atrial septal defects [systolic pulmonic flow murmur with fixed wide splitting of second heart sound (S2)], often with the additional finding of an apical blowing systolic murmur of mitral regurgitation.
- A low-pitched diastolic rumble may be appreciated at the mitral area. Patients with complete AV canal defects are usually symptomatic by 4–6 weeks of life.
- Those noted to have earlier signs of congestive heart failure in the first or second week often have significant AV valve regurgitation.
- This occurs in up to 20% of patients. Failure-to-thrive tachypnea, tachycardia, and poor feeding are common presenting symptoms.
- Physical examination also may reveal a pulmonary flow murmur, fixed splitting of the S2, a blowing systolic murmur of AV valve regurgitation, and often a mid-diastolic low-pitched rumble.
- When the ventricular septal defect is unrestrictive, it often does not generate a prominent separate systolic murmur.

TESTS

Generally, cardiac catheterization is unnecessary in uncomplicated cases, unless pulmonary vascular disease or associated cardiac lesions such as tetralogy of Fallot are suspected.

Lab

The electrocardiogram (ECG) usually shows a right ventricular conduction delay pattern, and PR interval prolongation may be present. A left superior QRS axis is almost always noted.

Imaging

- The diagnosis of all variants is readily confirmed on two-dimensional (2D) echocardiography.
- Occasionally, a dilated coronary sinus secondary to a left superior vena cava can be identified incorrectly as a primum atrial septal defect.
- Careful visualization of the intact primum septum (anterior to the coronary sinus) and tracing of the course of the left superior vena caval connection help differentiate this possibility.
- Color flow Doppler is helpful in estimating the degree of mitral regurgitation.
- Searching for evidence of increased right ventricular pressure (ventricular hypertrophy, septal orientation, and Doppler estimation of pressure on the basis of tricuspid regurgitation) is important in the echocardiographic assessment of these defects.
- In complete AV canal defects, attention should be directed to the morphology and attachments of the AV valve leaflets and estimating the sizes of the right and left ventricles.
- These observations are important in determining the type of surgical management.

DIFFERENTIAL DIAGNOSIS

- Patients with mainly atrial shunting may present similarly to patients with isolated secundum atrial septal defects.
- If a restrictive ventricular septal defect is present, a left sternal border pansystolic murmur may be dominant, suggesting an isolated ventricular septal defect.
- Complete AV canal defects may present similarly to moderate to large ventricular septal defects.

 TREATMENT

GENERAL MEASURES

- Medical intervention in the form of inotropes, afterload reduction, or diuretics are usually not indicated in the group of asymptomatic patients with partial AV canal defects.
- Endocarditis prophylaxis is required in the presence of AV valve regurgitation.
- Most patients with complete AV canal defects require inotropic and diuretic therapy in the first weeks to months of life to control symptoms of congestive heart failure and improve feeding intake and weight gain.
- Often it is difficult to determine the primary cause of poor feeding in the setting of patients with Down syndrome who may be feeding poorly because of noncardiac issues despite optimal medical management.

MEDICATION (DRUGS)

Early management involves close observation until signs of congestive heart failure appear, when digoxin and diuretic therapy will most likely be necessary to control symptoms.

SURGERY
- Surgical repair in partial AV canal patients is indicated when there is a clearcut defect identified and clinical or echocardiographic evidence of cardiac chamber dilation.
- The timing of repair is elective and similar to that for closure of isolated secundum atrial septal defects.
- The majority of defects should be closed by 2–5 years of age.
- Patients with trivial defects can be followed medically.
- Surgical repair in complete AV canal patients is indicated in the setting of severe symptoms resistant to medical therapy or failure to thrive.
- Patients whose conditions are well controlled with adequate weight gain on medical therapy nevertheless should undergo complete repair prior to 4–5 months of age to avoid irreversible pulmonary vascular disease.
- Relatively early repair is particularly important in the large subgroup of patients with Down syndrome.
- This group has been shown to have a greater degree of elevation of pulmonary vascular resistance in the first year of life and may have more rapid progression to fixed pulmonary obstructive disease than children with normal chromosomes.

PROGNOSIS
- Results of surgical repair of primum atrial septal defects and partial AV canal defects have been excellent, with a mortality rate of <1% and a reoperation rate of <3%.
- Late death after surgery is rare, reported in 0–4% of patients.
- The overall long-term survival of patients with primum atrial septal defect following repair was found to match that of the general population.
- Residual interatrial communication rarely occurs.
- Left AV valve regurgitation is the major cause of late morbidity in all forms of AV canal defects.
- In partial canal repair follow-up studies, the incidence of significant regurgitation requiring reoperation ranges from 7–10% of patients.
- Subaortic stenosis is noted in less than 5% of postoperative patients.
- The early postoperative mortality rate following repair of complete AV canal defects has been reduced from approximately 20–25% in the past to 3–4% in the current era.
- Strong risk factors for early death included postoperative pulmonary hypertensive crisis, immediate postoperative severe left AV regurgitation, and double-orifice left AV valve.
- Improved surgical skills, postoperative care of small infants, and management of perioperative pulmonary hypertension are undoubtedly responsible for the notable decline in early mortality.
- Intraoperative transesophageal echocardiography has been noted to favorably alter surgical treatment in some patients by detecting inadequate repair in the operating room.
- Heart block, residual ventricular septal defect, left ventricular outflow tract obstruction, and mitral valve dysfunction are potential long-term complications that must be considered in patients following repair of complete AV canal defects.
- Although heart block and residual ventricular septal defect are uncommon in the current era, left ventricular outflow tract obstruction and mitral insufficiency continue to be significant long-term issues.
- Persistent elevation of pulmonary vascular resistance may be an issue in some patients, especially if surgical correction was delayed, or pulmonary vascular resistance was marginal at the time of surgery.
- Reoperation for residual mitral regurgitation, recently has been reported at rates varying from 2–10%.

PATIENT MONITORING
Close regular visits for assessment of adequacy of weight gain and or signs of congestive heart failure

REFERENCES
1. Castaneda AR, Jonas RA, Mayer JE, et al. Atrioventricular canal defects. In: *Cardiac Surgery of the Neonate and Infant.* Philadelphia: WB Saunders; 1994;167–186.
2. Feldt RH, Porter CJ, Edwards WD, et al. Atrioventricular septal defects. In: Adams FH, Emanouilides GC, Riemenschneider TA, et al. *Heart Disease in Infants,* Children and Adolescents. Baltimore: Williams & Wilkins; 1989;704–723.
3. Kirklin JW, Barrat-Boyes BG. Atrioventricular canal defect. In: *Cardiac Surgery.* New York: Churchill Livingstone 1993;693–749.
4. Laks H, Pearl JM. Primum atrial septal defect. *Semin Thorac Cardiovasc Surg.* 1997;9:2–7.
5. Pearl JM, Laks H. Intermediate and complete forms of atrioventricular canal. *Semin Thorac Cardiovasc Surg.* 1997;9:8–20.
6. Permut LC, Mehta V. Later results and reoperation after repair of complete and partial atrioventricular canal defect. *Semin Thorac Cardiovasc Surg.* 1997;9:44–54.

E

ENDOCARDITIS
Chandan Devireddy

 BASICS

DESCRIPTION
Endocarditis is a disease caused by a microbial infection of the endothelial lining of the heart. Vegetations are characteristic, with involvement of heart valves and possibly endocardium. Endocarditis is classified by several definitions:
- Acute bacterial endocarditis (ABE): Aggressive course usually caused by highly virulent organisms such as *Staphylococcus aureus* with diagnosis usually made in less than 2 weeks; often affects normal heart valves
- Subacute bacterial endocarditis (SBE): Indolent course over weeks to months caused by low virulence organisms such as viridans streptococci; usually develops on previously abnormal valves
- Early prosthetic valve endocarditis (PVE): Infection of an artificial heart valve within the first 2 months after surgery
- Late prosthetic valve endocarditis: Infection 2 months after valve implantation
- Nonbacterial thrombotic endocarditis (NBTE): Any endocardial sterile vegetation (wide spectrum of presentations)

EPIDEMIOLOGY
Incidence
Incidence is estimated at 1.6–6.0 cases/100,000 person-years in developed countries. In intravenous (IV) drug users alone, the incidence is estimated at 11.6/100,000 person-years.

RISK FACTORS
Conditions predisposing to development of endocarditis:
- High risk: Prosthetic heart valves, previous endocarditis, cyanotic congenital heart disease, preexisting rheumatic heart disease, acquired valvular disease, aortic valve disease, mitral regurgitation with or without stenosis, ventricular septal defect, patent ductus arteriosus, coarctation of aorta
- Intermediate risk: Mitral valve prolapse with regurgitation, pure mitral stenosis, tricuspid disease, pulmonary valve disease, asymmetric septal hypertrophy, degenerative valve disease, intracardiac prosthetic implants (nonvalvular), intracardiac catheters
- Other factors: IV drug abuse, arteriovenous shunt for hemodialysis, creation of persistent portals of entry (wounds, catheters), perinatal infective complications

ETIOLOGY
Most patients who develop infective endocarditis have a preexisting cardiac condition.
- NBTE: Endothelial damage leads to platelet aggregation and deposition with fibrin deposition and development of sterile thrombotic vegetations.
- ABE/SBE: Microbes probably colonize preexisting NBTE or even directly invade endothelium in the case of ABE. Microbial adherence is a crucial factor for selection of organisms that colonize the endocardium.
- Valves normally involved (downstream side of high/low-pressure valves): Mitral > aortic > tricuspid > pulmonary
- Valves involved in IV drug abusers: Tricuspid > mitral = aortic > pulmonary
- Patients secondarily develop embolic phenomena from friability of vegetation and immune complex damage secondary to humoral reaction to bacterial proliferation in vegetation.

Causative Agents
- ABE: *S. aureus, Haemophilus influenzae, Neisseria gonorrhoeae, Streptococcus pneumoniae, Enterococcus* species
- SBE: Alpha-hemolytic streptococci (viridans), *Streptococcus bovis* (group D strep), enterococcal species, HACEK group (*Haemophilus aphrophilus, Actinobacillus actinomycetemcomitans, Cardiobacterium hominis, Eikenella corrodens, Kingella kingae*), *S. aureus*
- Early PVE: *S. aureus, Staphylococcus epidermidis,* gram-negative rods, *Aspergillus* species
- Late PVE: Alpha-hemolytic streptococci (viridans), enterococcal species, *S. epidermidis, Aspergillus* species
- Intravenous drug abusers: *S. aureus, Pseudomonas aeruginosa,* other gram-negative rods, enterococcal species, *Candida* species

 DIAGNOSIS

SIGNS AND SYMPTOMS
- Fever (low-grade or severe if acute)
- Chills, rigors, night sweats
- Pallor, malaise, anorexia, weight loss
- New or prominent murmur (also may be absent)
- Myalgias, arthralgias, back pain
- Focal neurologic signs (embolic phenomenon or meningeal reaction)
- Delirium or headache
- Chest pain, dyspnea, cough, hemoptysis
- Flank pain, hematuria, left upper quadrant pain (evidence of distal emboli or immune complex glomerulonephritis)
- Cold painful extremity
- Splenomegaly
- Petechiae (Roth spots if retinal)
- Osler nodes (tender erythematous extremity nodules)
- Janeway lesions (flat nontender red spots)
- Splinter hemorrhages (linear, subungual)
- Clubbing of digits
- Rales, gallops

TESTS
Duke Endocarditis Service Criteria for diagnosis of infective endocarditis: Two major criteria, or one major and three minor criteria, or five minor criteria
- Major Criteria
  – Typical microorganism for infective endocarditis from two separate blood cultures (viridans strep, strep bovis, HACEK group, community-acquired *S. aureus*, or enterococci in absence of primary focus), or persistently positive blood culture, defined as recovery of a microorganism consistent with infective endocarditis from blood cultures drawn more than 12 hours apart, or all or a majority of four positive with first and last drawn 1 hour apart
  – Positive echocardiogram for infective endocarditis
    • Oscillating intracardiac mass, on valve or supporting structures, or in the path of regurgitant jet or on implanted material, in the absence of an alternative anatomic explanation, or abscess, or new partial dehiscence or prosthetic valve, or new valvular regurgitation (increase or change in preexisting murmur not sufficient)
- Minor Criteria
  – Predisposing heart conditions or IV drug use
  – Fever (>38°C)
  – Vascular phenomena: Major arterial emboli, septic pulmonary infarcts, mycotic aneurysm, intracranial hemorrhage, conjunctival hemorrhages, Janeway lesions
  – Immunologic phenomena: Glomerulonephritis, Osler nodes, Roth spots, rheumatoid factor
  – Microbiologic evidence: Positive blood culture but not meeting major criterion as previously defined or serologic evidence of active infection with organism consistent with infective endocarditis
  – Echocardiogram: Consistent with infective endocarditis but not meeting major criteria as previously defined

Lab

- Blood cultures (draw three separate samples first day)
- Complete blood count (anemia and leukocytosis possible)
- Elevated erythrocyte sedimentation rate in 90%
- Elevated C-reactive protein
- Urinalysis (microscopic hematuria in 50%)
- Rheumatoid factor positive in 35–50% of SBE
- Special serology tests (*Coxiella*, *Bartonella*)

Imaging

- Echocardiography crucial for diagnosis
- Transthoracic echo with color flow Doppler sensitivity for detection of vegetation is 60–75%.
- Transesophageal echo more sensitive (>95%), especially with mitral involvement, abscesses, valve perforation, rupture of sinus of Valsalva; echo also helpful with ventricular function
- Cardiac catheterization: Depending on age of patient, catheterization may be necessary for coronaries when surgery of valve is considered.
- Radionuclide studies: No technique justified for detection of vegetations
- Chest x-ray: Evaluate for signs of congestive heart failure (CHF), septic emboli, widening of aorta (mycotic aneurysm)

Diagnostic Procedures/Surgery

ECG: Disturbance of conduction may suggest extension of infection into myocardium from abscess formation. It also may reveal embolic phenomena causing myocardial ischemia.

DIFFERENTIAL DIAGNOSIS

Pneumonia, pleurisy, meningitis, brain abscess, stroke, malaria, acute pericarditis, vasculitis, disseminated intravascular coagulation, rheumatic fever, osteomyelitis, tuberculosis, intraabdominal infection, glomerulonephritis, salmonellosis, brucellosis, myocardial infarction, atrial myxoma, occult malignancies, septic pulmonary infarction, fever of unknown origin

TREATMENT

GENERAL MEASURES

- Eliminate offending organism as soon as possible.
- Determine if surgical intervention is necessary and when is the best time to perform.
- Treat symptoms (CHF, embolic phenomena, immune complex phenomena).
- Adjust length of treatment to patient's presentation and offending organism (usually 4–6 weeks).

MEDICATION (DRUGS)

First Line

Antibiotics

- Bactericidal antibiotics are drugs of choice secondary to inadequate host defense within vegetation.
- Be suspicious for emerging drug-resistant organisms.
- Penicillin-sensitive streptococci (viridans): Penicillin G 4 million units every 6 hours IV.
- Penicillin-resistant streptococci: Penicillin G 4 million units IV every 4 hours plus gentamycin 1.0 mg/kg every 12 hours IV, or vancomycin 15 mg/kg IV every 12 hours
- Enterococci: Penicillin G 18–30 million units/day IV plus gentamycin 1 mg/kg IV every 8 hours, or ampicillin 12 g/day IV plus gentamycin 1 mg/kg IV every 8 hours, or vancomycin 15 mg/kg IV plus gentamycin 1 mg/kg IV every 8 hours
- Staphylococci (no prosthetic material): Nafcillin 2 g IV every 4 hours, or vancomycin 15 mg/kg IV every 12 hours if methicillin resistant
- Staphylococci (prosthetic material): Nafcillin 2 g IV every 4 hours and gentamycin 1.0 mg/kg IV every 8 hours, or vancomycin 15 mg/kg IV every 12 hours plus gentamycin 1 mg/kg IV every 8 hours and rifampin 300 mg orally every 8 hours if methicillin resistant
- HACEK group: Ceftriaxone 2 g IV once daily
- *P. aeruginosa*: Extended-spectrum penicillin or third-generation cephalosporin or imipenem plus aminoglycoside

SURGERY

Major Indications

- Moderate or severe heart failure not responding to medical treatment, valvular obstruction, periannular or myocardial abscess, prosthetic valve dehiscence, persistent bacteremia despite appropriate antibiotics, fungal infection

Relative Indications

- Recurrent emboli, staphylococcal and gram-negative infections, persistent fever despite treatment, vegetations enlarging despite treatment

FOLLOW-UP

DISPOSITION

Admission Criteria

Patients with suspected endocarditis should be hospitalized for IV antibiotics with option for home parenteral treatment in selected cases for remainder of duration.

PROGNOSIS

- Fatal unless treated; median time from onset of symptoms to death in untreated SBE is 6 months.
- Median time from onset of symptoms to death in untreated ABE is <4 weeks. Adverse prognostic factors include central nervous system complications, CHF, renal failure, culture-negative disease, gram-negative or fungal infection, prosthetic valve infection, and abscesses of myocardium or valve ring.
- Favorable prognostic factors include youth, early diagnosis and treatment, mitral valve prolapse infection, and penicillin-sensitive SBE infection. Rates of cure depend on classification of endocarditis and microbiologic diagnosis, from 98% cure in native valve viridans strep SBE to <1% cure in fungal infection of prosthetic valves.

PATIENT MONITORING

Inpatient monitoring and diligent observation if treated as outpatient

REFERENCES

1. Alexander RW, et al., eds. *Hurst's the Heart*, 9th ed. New York: McGraw-Hill; 1998.
2. Dajani AS, et al. Prevention of bacterial endocarditis: Recommendations by the American Heart Association. *Circulation*. 1997;96:358–366.
3. Fauci AS, et al., eds. *Harrison's Principles of Internal Medicine*, 14th ed. New York: McGraw-Hill; 1998.

CODES

ICD9-CM

- 421.0 Acute and subacute bacterial endocarditis
- 421.9 Acute endocarditis, unspecified
- 424.9 Endocarditis, valve unspecified, unspecified cause

PATIENT TEACHING

- Prophylaxis: Most cases of endocarditis are not attributable to an invasive procedure. Determine the risk posed by the preexisting cardiac lesion and inherent risk posed by the procedure itself.
- High risk: Prosthetic heart valves, previous history endocarditis, complex cyanotic congenital heart disease, surgically constructed systemic pulmonary shunts or conduits
- Moderate risk: Most other congenital cardiac malformations, acquired valvar dysfunction, hypertrophic cardiomyopathy, mitral valve prolapse with valvar regurgitation and/or thickened leaflets
- Procedures for which prophylaxis is recommended: Dental procedures with significant bleeding from hard or soft tissues, and surgical procedures involving respiratory, intestinal, or genitourinary mucosa
- Standard general prophylaxis: Amoxicillin 2.0 g orally 1 hour before procedure only

E

ENDOTHELIN

Rishi R. Vohora
Helge U. Simon*
Gerard P. Aurigemma

 BASICS

DESCRIPTION

Endothelin is a 21 amino-acid peptide released by endothelium, which acts locally (paracrine activity) to produce vasoconstriction. Four structurally similar isopeptides of endothelin have been sequenced: endothelin-1, endothelin-2, endothelin-3, and endothelin-4

- Endothelin-1 is the main isoform, and is present in human vasculature. In fact, endothelin-1 is the most powerful vasoconstrictor yet discovered.
- Endothelin-2 is present in the kidney and intestine.
- The physiologic roles of endothelin-3 and endothelin-4 are unclear, but they also have vasoconstrictive properties.
- Messenger RNA (mRNA) coding for endothelin-1 is induced by shear stress, ischemia, and hypoxia.
- Endothelin-1 has a plasma half-life of 4–7 minutes, and 80% is eliminated during its first passage through the lung.
- Plasma endothelin-1 levels may correlate with the severity of heart failure, may give prognostic information, and may be assayed.
- There are two main endothelin receptors: Endothelin-A and endothelin-B.
  - Both endothelin-A and endothelin-B receptors have been shown to mediate vasoconstriction, indicating that a dual receptor antagonist, such as bosentan or tezosentan, may be necessary to fully inhibit the vasoconstrictor effects of endothelin-1.
  - Activation of endothelin-B receptors on vascular endothelial cells also has been shown to causes vasodilation via release of nitric oxide and prostaglandins.

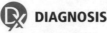 **DIAGNOSIS**

Pathologic Findings
Cardiovascular Pathology
Elevated endothelin levels appear to be an epiphenomenon of endothelial damage and are observed in the following disorders.

- Heart Failure
  - Endothelin plays the role of vasoconstrictor, prodysrhythmic potentiator of other neurohormones, and mediator of increased vascular permeability.
  - Endothelin-1 increases angiotensin I to angiotensin II conversion and aldosterone production.
  - Angiotensin itself increases endothelin 1 production.
  - Circulating endothelin-1 may contribute to dyspnea caused by direct bronchoconstriction mediated by endothelin receptors.
  - Plasma concentration in heart failure is closely related to disease severity, and among the strongest predictors of dysrhythmia and death.

- Ischemia
  - Atherosclerosis is generally associated with endothelial dysfunction, both a reduction in nitric oxide and increased endothelin effects.
  - Acute injury: in animal models, high endothelin levels are observed downstream from endothelial injury. Antiendothelin antibody reduces myocardial injury by 40–45%.
  - Nitric oxide, prostacyclin, and arterial natriuretic peptide inhibit endothelin-1 production.
  - Reperfusion injury appears to be related to endothelin release.
  - Endothelin appears to play a role in restenosis: Neointima formation after balloon angioplasty in rats may be linked to mitogenic properties of endothelin and prevented by blocking of the endothelin receptor.
  - The mortality rate 1 year after myocardial infarction (MI) correlates with endothelin-1 levels on day 3 following MI.
- Hypertension
  - Administration of bosentan, a dual receptor antagonist, has been shown to decrease blood pressure in patients with mild-to-moderate essential hypertension, suggesting that elevated levels of endothelin-1 contribute to hypertension in these patients.
- Pulmonary Hypertension
  - High local endothelin-1 concentrations are found in primary pulmonary hypertension and asthma.

TREATMENT

GENERAL MEASURES

- Measurements of serum levels are technically difficult (cross-reactivity with the prehormone, big endothelin, and endothelin-2 and -3, adherence of the protein to glassware and plastic). This, in combination with other simpler diagnostic tools to detect acute ischemia or heart failure greatly limits the usefulness of endothelin-1 as a diagnostic tool.
- Furthermore, overlap in conditions associated with endothelin release and plasma levels may underestimate local ET levels and action.

PROGNOSIS

Therapeutic Roles in Heart Failure

- The therapeutic effects of both selective and dual receptor antagonists in heart failure are still being evaluated, but trials thus far have been discouraging.
- Tezosentan, a nonselective endothelin receptor antagonist, has been shown to improve cardiac index and decrease PCWP in acute and chronic heart failure NYHA Class III–IV, but had significant dose-related side effects including hypotension, renal failure, and dizziness.

Therapeutic Roles in Pulmonary Hypertension

- Bosentan, a dual selective antagonist, improves cardiac hemodynamics and exercise capacity in patients, with primary pulmonary hypertension or pulmonary hypertension associated with scleroderma.

REFERENCES

1. Benigni A, Remuzzi G. Endothelin antagonists. *Lancet*. 1999;353:133–138.
2. Cowburn PJ, Cleland JG, McArthur JP, et al. Endothelin-B receptors are functionally important in mediating vasoconstriction in the systemic circulation in patients with left ventricular systolic dysfunction. *J Am Coll Cardiol*. 1999;33:932–938.
3. Homcy CJ. Signaling hypertrophy: How many switches, how many wires. *Circulation*. 1998;97:1890–1892.
4. Kaddoura S and Poole-Wilson P. Endothelin-1 in heart failure: A new therapeutic target?; *Lancet*. 348:418–419.
5. Krum H, et al. The effect of an endothelin-receptor antagonist, bosentan, on blood pressure in patients with essential hypertension. *N Engl J Med*. 338:784–791.
6. Rubin LJ, et al. Bosentan therapy for pulmonary arterial hypertension. *N Engl J Med*. 346:896–903.
7. Schrier RW, Abraham WT. Hormones and hemo-dynamics in heart failure. *N Engl J Med*. 1999;341:577–585.
8. Teerlink JR. Overview of randomized clinical trials in acute heart failure syndromes. *Am J Cardiol*. 2005;96:59–67.
9. Torre-Amione G, Young JB, Colucci WS, et al. Hemodynamic and clinical effects of tezosentan, an intravenous dual endothelin receptor antagonist, in patients hospitalized for acute decompensated heart failure. *J Am Coll Cardiol*. 2003;42:140–147.

E

EOSINOPHILIC HEART DISEASE

Gary S. Francis
Deepak L. Bhatt
Apur R. Kamdar

 BASICS

DESCRIPTION

Patients are occasionally seen with striking eosinophilia and cardiomyopathy.

- The eosinophilia can persist for many years before the cardiomyopathy appears.
- The major cause of death and disability is progressive, restrictive heart disease.
- The contents of the eosinophil can be toxic to many organs, including the heart, but it is not clear if this is the mechanism of cardiac fibrosis.
- In 1936, Löffler recognized the association of eosinophilia, constrictive cardiomyopathy, a thickened endomyocardium, and intraventricular mural thrombus.
  - This disorder is now considered part of a continuum of disease that has been termed *hypereosinophilic syndrome* (HES).
  - More than 75% of patients with HES have severe heart failure.

EPIDEMIOLOGY

- HES tends to occur between the ages of 20 and 50 years.
- Occasionally it occurs in children.
- Multiple organs may be involved.
- Men tend to have more myocardial involvement.

Incidence

The incidence is unknown, but hypereosinophilic heart disease is relatively uncommon.

RISK FACTORS

None known

ETIOLOGY

- The mechanism of HES and subsequent organ involvement (including heart) is unknown.
- HES patients develop multiorgan damage.
- The eosinophils may have decreased granules and abnormal cytoplasmic inclusions.
- Eosinophils are attracted to a region of the heart (i.e., the endocardium), apparently in response to foreign antigenic stimulus.
- It is not clear if the eosinophilic contents are actually toxic to the myocardium.
- It appears that the tropical form (Davies endomyocardial fibrosis) may differ significantly in pathophysiology and etiology from the temperate form (Loeffler fibroplastic endocarditis).
- Clinical picture and underlying pathology differ from acute eosinophilic necrotizing myocarditis and drug-related hypersensitivity myocarditis.
- Extent of organ infiltration does not appear to explain the amount of organ dysfunction.

ASSOCIATED CONDITIONS

Major organ involvement includes the heart, lungs, gastrointestinal tract, liver, urinary bladder, central and peripheral nervous system, skin, spleen, lymph nodes, and vasculature.

 DIAGNOSIS

SIGNS AND SYMPTOMS

- Elevated venous pressure
- Heart is not dilated.
- Mitral and tricuspid regurgitation
- Systemic embolization
- Hepatosplenomegaly
- Dyspnea
- Cough
- Fatigue
- Ascites
- Peripheral edema

TESTS

- Electron microscopy of eosinophils is sometimes performed.
  - Eosinophils have large, round, and homogeneously electron-dense cytoplasmic inclusions.
  - The inclusions are usually larger than normal, mature granules.

Lab

- Eosinophils may have decreased number of granules and vacuolation of the cytoplasm.
- Anemia and thrombocytopenia may be present.
- Myelodysplastic features such as increased vitamin B_{12} levels, abnormal leukocyte alkaline phosphatase, and cytogenic abnormalities are sometimes present.

Imaging

- An echocardiogram should be performed and will show restricted diastolic filling.
- It will usually demonstrate marked thickening of the walls of both ventricles, a pattern suggestive of infiltrative cardiomyopathy and mural thrombus.

Pathologic Findings

- Acute inflammatory eosinophilic myocarditis
- Thrombosis, fibrinoid change, and inflammation of intramural coronary vessels
- Mural thrombus containing eosinophils
- Fibrotic thickening

DIFFERENTIAL DIAGNOSIS

- Patient must have sustained blood eosinophilia >1,500/mm³ present for longer than 6 months.
- The amount of eosinophilia may vary from 20–90%.
- Other etiologies for eosinophilia must be absent, including parasitic infections and allergic disease.
- Other restrictive or infiltrative cardiomyopathies such as amyloidosis and sarcoidosis should be excluded.

TREATMENT

GENERAL MEASURES

- Eosinophilic heart disease may be reactive, although some cases of HES are believed to be leukoproliferative.
- Prognosis is poor, with a mean survival from diagnosis of about 9 months.
- Occasionally there is prolonged survival for decades.
- When there is organ involvement such as cardiac disease, a short course of prednisone may sometimes suppress the eosinophilia.
- 38% of patients respond well to prednisone and 31% respond partially to prednisone.
- Patients unresponsive to prednisone may respond to hydroxyurea.
- Vincristine has helped an occasional patient, as has interferon α and cyclosporine.
- Pheresis does not seem to help.
- Supportive therapy for heart failure including diuretics may be helpful.
- Both anticoagulation and antiplatelet agents have been administered to reduce thromboembolic events.

MEDICATION (DRUGS)

As for restrictive cardiomyopathy of any cause

SURGERY

- Mitral and tricuspid valve replacement or repair have been performed with benefit in occasional patients.
- Patients receiving mechanical valves have experienced thrombosis of the valves.
- If valve replacement is contemplated, a bioprosthesis should be used.
- Rarely, mitral and tricuspid stenosis can occur, and valve replacement may be helpful.

FOLLOW-UP

PROGNOSIS

Prognosis for restrictive cardiomyopathy is very poor.

PATIENT MONITORING

Patients need careful, regular follow-up by the cardiologist and hematologist, especially if chemotherapy is used.

REFERENCES

1. Parillo JE. Heart disease and the eosinophil. *N Engl J Med*. 1990;323:1560–1561.
2. Solley GO, Maldonado JE, Gleich GJ, et al. Cardiomyopathy with eosinophilia. *Mayo Clin Proc*. 1976;51:697–708.
3. Weller PF, Bubley GJ. The idiopathic hypereosinophilic syndrome. *Blood*. 1994;83:2759–2779.
4. Zipes DP. *Braunwald's Heart Disease: A Textbook of Cardiovascular Medicine*, 7th ed., 2005.

CODES

ICD9-CM

428.0 Failure, heart, congestive

PATIENT TEACHING

As for restrictive cardiomyopathy of any cause

E

FABRY'S DISEASE AND THE HEART

Apur R. Kamdar
Deepak L. Bhatt
Gary S. Francis

 BASICS

DESCRIPTION

Glycosphingolipid metabolism is disordered due to deficiency of the lysosomal enzyme α-galactosidase A.

- This deficiency leads to intracellular accumulation of the glycolipid ceramide trihexoside.
- Angiokeratoma corporis diffusum universale is another name for this disease.

EPIDEMIOLOGY

Occurs in 1/40,000 births

RISK FACTORS

Pregnancy Considerations

Prenatal diagnosis is possible.

PATHOPHYSIOLOGY
ETIOLOGY

- X-linked, with full expression in males and only partial expression in females
- Several possible mutations in the *Gal* gene at Xq22; some atypical forms, due to partial gene deletions and point mutations, lead to isolated myocardial disease that presents later in life
- Women typically have either no symptoms or mild disease; skin lesions and corneal deposits may be present.

ASSOCIATED CONDITIONS

- Kidney failure and proteinuria
- Hypertension (due to renal involvement)

 DIAGNOSIS

SIGNS AND SYMPTOMS

- Fever
- Purple skin lesions (angiokeratoses)
- Corneal opacities
- Paresthesias
- Edema
- Mitral valve prolapse
- Cardiomegaly
- Hypertension
- Vasospastic angina, myocardial infarction, mitral regurgitation
- Renal failure

TESTS

- Cardiac catheterization typically reveals normal coronary arteries.
- Endomyocardial biopsy can make the diagnosis.

Lab

- Decreased α-galactosidase A activity in leukocytes
- The *Gal* mutation should be looked for to detect heterozygous women.
- On electrocardiogram (ECG), left ventricular hypertrophy (LVH), atrial fibrillation, conduction abnormalities, and ventricular ectopy are seen. Short PR interval may be seen.

Imaging

- Chest x-ray
  - Shows cardiomegaly, aortic root dilation
- Echocardiography
  - Shows massive LVH and LV dilation
  - Mitral valve prolapse and aortic root dilation also may occur.
- Doppler reveals diastolic dysfunction.

Pathologic Findings

Glycolipid substrate accumulation in lysosomes of cardiac tissues.

DIFFERENTIAL DIAGNOSIS

Other causes of cardiomegaly such as amyloidosis and hypertrophic obstructive cardiomyopathy

 TREATMENT

GENERAL MEASURES

- Enzyme replacement with recombinant human α-galactosidase A.
- May reduce hypertrophy and improve cardiac function.
- Dialysis
- Antiplatelet agents, anticoagulants
- Analgesics

MEDICATION (DRUGS)

As for heart failure of any etiology

SURGERY
Renal transplantation

 ## FOLLOW-UP

PROGNOSIS
- Cardiac and renal failure in the third and fourth decades of life
- Increased risk of stroke

PATIENT MONITORING
As for heart failure of any etiology

REFERENCES
1. Bleiden LC, Moller JH. Cardiac involvement in inherited disorders of metabolism. *Prog Cardiovasc Dis*. 1974;26:615–631.
2. Desnick RJ. Fabry disease, an under-recognized multisystemic disorder: Expert recommendations for diagnosis, management, and enzyme replacement therapy. *Ann Intern Med*. 2003;138:338–346.
3. Eng CM, Guffon N, Wilcox WR, et al. Safety and efficacy of recombinant human alphagalactosidase A—Replacement therapy in Fabry's disease. *N Engl J Med*. 2001;345:9.
4. Masson C, et. al. Fabry disease: A review. *Joint Bone Spine*. 2004;71:381–383.
5. Topol EJ, ed. *Textbook of Cardiovascular Medicine*. Philadelphia: Lippincott Williams & Wilkins, 2002.
6. Zipes DP. *Braunwald's Heart Disease: A Textbook of Cardiovascular Medicine*, 7th ed., 2005.

CODES
ICD9-CM
- 272.7 Fabry's disease (angiokeratoma corporis diffusum)
- 428.0 Failure, heart, congestive

PATIENT TEACHING
As for heart failure of any etiology

F

FORAMEN OVALE

Adhar Seth
Christopher Abadi*
Gerard P. Aurigemma

BASICS

DESCRIPTION

The foramen ovale is an opening in the midportion of the interatrial septum, in the developing fetus, at the junction of the septum primum and septum secundum.

- A flaplike membranous portion of the septum primum covers this opening. *In utero*, the high right atrial pressure allows right-to-left shunting of blood and delivery of oxygenated blood to the unborn fetus.
- Normal changes in the intracardiac pressures with elevation of the left atrial pressure after delivery of the infant results in the flaplike membrane closing the foramen ovale such that no shunting of blood can occur.
- Fusion of the membrane with permanent closure of the foramen normally occurs in the majority of people. Patency of the foramen ovale does occur and has been associated with unexplained stroke.
- Systems affected: Cardiovascular, Cerebrovascular

EPIDEMIOLOGY

Incidence

A patent foramen ovale (PFO) is present in 10–20% of the general population by autopsy series. Patency may be related to conditions where there are abnormal intracardiac pressures.

- Specifically, congenital heart disease or other conditions associated with high right atrial pressure may predispose people to maintenance of patency of the foramen ovale and may result in right-to-left shunting.
- Patients with unexplained stroke have a higher incidence of PFO (up to 50%). This may be due to paradoxical embolus—a venous embolus passing through the PFO and causing an arterial embolic event—but there may be other mechanisms as well.

DIAGNOSIS

SIGNS AND SYMPTOMS

- No specific signs or symptoms are associated with an isolated PFO with no shunting of blood.
- Unexplained stroke should lead to an evaluation of a cardiac source of embolus, including PFO.
- In conditions where the right atrial pressure is high and significant right-to-left shunting of blood occurs through a PFO, symptoms of dyspnea and fatigue with associated hypoxia may be present.
- Clubbing, cyanosis, and erythrocytosis may occur in severe hypoxia.
- Findings seen with an atrial septal defect (ASD), such as wide, fixed splitting of the second heart sound and right ventricular conduction delay, have not been clearly associated with a PFO.
- Electrocardiogram (ECG) with an isolated PFO is generally normal.
- Migraine and vascular headache may be related to PFO. The mechanism is not yet clearly understood. Several studies have documented either complete resolution or marked reduction in frequency of migraines in patients undergoing transcatheter PFO closure.

Imaging

- Echocardiography is the diagnostic test of choice for identifying a PFO.
- PFO may be found, incidentally, during an echocardiogram obtained for other reasons.
- Transesophageal echocardiography (TEE) is superior to transthoracic echo (TTE) and transcranial doppler (TCD) in identification of PFO and differentiation of ASD or atrial septal aneurysm (ASA) from a PFO. Both 2D and color flow Doppler are used for PFO evaluation. Injection of agitated saline with both TEE and TTE improves the sensitivity for the diagnosis of PFO.

- Having a patient cough or perform a Valsalva maneuver during agitated saline contrast injection also increases the sensitivity for identification of PFO.
- Patients with unexplained stroke should undergo echocardiography as part of the work-up, with the ordering physician specifically requesting a saline contrast study with and without Valsalva maneuver.
- If a TTE is nondiagnostic, TEE should be considered.
- Specific Echocardiographic Findings of Patent Foramen Ovale
  - Thinning of the interatrial septum
  - Atrial septal aneurysm or Chiari network may be present in association with PFO.
  - Color flow Doppler demonstration of interatrial shunting
  - Pulsed Doppler through the interatrial septum may demonstrate shunting.
  - Calculation of a shunt ratio can be performed when significant shunting is present.
  - Right atrial and/or left atrial enlargement may occur with significant shunting.
  - Saline contrast study with the presence of microbubbles in the left heart within three to five cardiac cycles is consistent with intracardiac shunting.
  - Work-up for a deep venous thrombosis should be performed in patients with a PFO and a cerebral ischemic event. Further testing of patients with unexplained stroke and a PFO also may include cardiac catheterization to determine the shunt size, as well as intracardiac pressures.

DIFFERENTIAL DIAGNOSIS

- For patients with interatrial shunting, the differential would include an ASD or ASA.
- Echocardiography should be able to differentiate a PFO from an ASD or an associated ASA.
- For patients with unexplained stroke and no interatrial shunting, mitral valve prolapse, mitral annular calcification, valvular vegetations, aortic atherosclerotic plaque, atrial and ventricular thrombus, and left atrial myxoma have been associated.

TREATMENT

GENERAL MEASURES

- In asymptomatic patients with the incidental finding of a PFO, no specific treatment is indicated.
- In patients with unexplained stroke and the finding of a PFO, treatment options include antiplatelet therapy, anticoagulation therapy, transcatheter closure, and surgical closure.
- Currently there is no consensus as to which treatment is most effective.

MEDICATION (DRUGS)

- In patients with an unexplained stroke and PFO, antiplatelet therapy with aspirin has been associated with a higher recurrence rate of stroke or transient ischemic attack than in patients treated with anticoagulant therapy with coumadin, but other studies have shown no statistical difference.
- The consideration of potential bleeding risk on coumadin needs to be considered when deciding on treatment. Overall, the available data suggest that the recurrence rate of cerebral ischemic events is relatively low (0–4%) in individuals treated medically with antiplatelet therapy alone or in combination with short-term anticoagulant therapy.
- If a deep venous thrombus is present, anticoagulant therapy would be indicated.

SURGERY

- In patients with an unexplained stroke and PFO, surgical closure has been performed with a low incidence of complications and recent studies reporting no serious complications.
- Residual shunting and recurrent stroke or transient ischemic attack has been reported after surgical closure, with one study reporting a 35% incidence of recurrent events in a group of patients over the age of 45 and zero recurrent events in patients under the age of 45.
- Catheter-based closure devices have been deployed with low complication rates, but the experience with this is relatively new. Efficacy ranges from 86–100%.
- Among 1,355 patients undergoing percutaneous closure, the rate of recurrent stroke or transient ischemic attack was 0–4.9% at 1 year. These values compare favorably to 1-year recurrence rates among 895 patients receiving medical therapy (3.8–12.0%); however, the differences in the study design and clinical characteristics do not allow for meaningful comparison.

REFERENCES

1. Bogousslavsky J, Devuyst G, Nendaz M, et al. Prevention of stroke recurrence with presumed paradoxical embolus. *J Neurol*. 1997;244:71–75.
2. Gin FG, Huckel VF, Pollick C, et al. Femoral vein delivery of contrast medium enhances transthoracic echocardiography detection of patent foramen ovale. *J Am Coll Cardiol*. 1993;22:1994–2000.
3. Hara H, Virmani R, Ladich E, et al. Patent foramen ovale: Current pathology, pathophysiology, and clinical status. *J Am Coll Cardiol*. 2005;46:1768–1776.
4. Haussmann D, Mugge A, Becht I, et al. Diagnosis of patent foramen ovale by transesophageal echocardiography and association with cerebral and peripheral embolic events. *Am J Cardiol*. 1992;70:668–672.
5. Homma S, Di Tullio MR, Sacco RR, et al. Surgical closure of patent foramen ovale in cryptogenic stroke patients. *Stroke*. 1997;28:2376–2381.
6. Kizer JR, Devereux RB. Patent foramen ovale in young adults with unexplained stroke *N Engl J Med*. 2005;353:2361–2372.
7. Lechat PH, Mas JL, Lascault G, et al. Prevalence of patent foramen ovale in patients with stroke. *N Engl J Med*. 1988;318:1148–1152.
8. Mas JL, Zuber M. Recurrent cerebrovascular events in patients with patent foramen ovale, atrial septal aneurysm, or both and cryptogenic stroke or transient ischemic attack. *Am Heart J*. 1995;30:1083–1088.
9. Siostrzonek P, Zangeneh M, Gossinger H, et al. Comparison of transesophageal and transthoracic echocardiography for the detection of patent foramen ovale. *Am J Cardiol*. 1991;68:1247–1249.

CODES
ICD9-CM
745.60

F

HEART FAILURE (DIAGNOSIS AND MANAGEMENT)

Gary S. Francis
Apur R. Kamdar
Deepak L. Bhatt

 BASICS

DESCRIPTION

Heart failure is a clinical syndrome characterized by signs and symptoms of exertional dyspnea due to structural and/or functional heart failure.

- Virtually any form of heart disease can lead to heart failure.
- There are many secondary manifestations: fatigue, circulatory congestion, edema, muscle wasting, etc.

GENERAL PREVENTION

- Treat risk factors for developing CHF: [American Hearth Association/American College of Cardiologists AHA/ACC) Stage A]—asymptomatic patients
  - Hypertension, atherosclerotic disease, diabetes, obesity, metabolic syndrome, patients on cardiotoxic drugs, and with family history of cardiomyopathy

EPIDEMIOLOGY

- An estimated 5 million people in the United States have heart failure, and it is believed to be present in 10% of patients older than the age of 65 years.
- >550,000 patients are newly diagnosed with heart failure yearly.
- Heart failure is the most common Medicare DRG and carries the highest Medicare financial cost.
- Coronary disease is present in about 60–65% of patients with heart failure.

RISK FACTORS
Pregnancy Considerations

- Pregnancy can sometimes be accompanied by heart failure.
- Stress of delivery can precipitate acute heart failure in patients who are predisposed to have heart failure (i.e., mitral stenosis, congenital heart disease).
- In general, pregnancy is contraindicated or is to be strongly discouraged in patients with heart failure or who are at risk to develop heart failure.

ETIOLOGY

- There are as many etiologies of heart failure as there are types of heart disease.
- The most common etiologies of heart failure in the United States are coronary artery disease and hypertension.
- Valvular heart disease, dilated cardiomyopathy, left ventricular hypertrophy, and abnormal diastolic function are common etiologic factors.

ASSOCIATED CONDITIONS

Numerous associated conditions occur with heart failure, including renal insufficiency, peripheral vascular disease, cerebral vascular disease, arrhythmias, pneumonia, uncontrolled diabetes mellitus, hyperthyroidism, and volume overload, among others.

 DIAGNOSIS

SIGNS AND SYMPTOMS

- Exertional dyspnea
- Fatigue
- Cough
- Edema
- S3 (third heart sound)
- Rales
- Elevated jugular venous pressure

TESTS

- Occasionally, patients undergo metabolic exercise testing with measurement of total body oxygen consumption.
- Although myocardial biopsy is not routinely performed, it is useful in selected patients in whom infiltrative cardiomyopathy or inflammatory myocarditis is being considered.

Lab

- Electrocardiogram (ECG)
- Chest x-ray
- Complete blood count (CBC)
- Blood urea nitrogen
- Serum creatinine
- Urinalysis
- Fasting glucose
- Thyroid function tests, in some cases
- Liver function tests
- Ferritin

Imaging

- Imaging studies are critical to the diagnosis of heart failure because they help to distinguish systolic dysfunction from diastolic dysfunction.
- Echocardiography with Doppler should be performed in virtually every new patient with the diagnosis of heart failure.
- The ECG provides information regarding cardiac size and function, and valuable information regarding valvular stenosis and incompetence.

Diagnostic Procedures/Surgery

- Coronary arteriography should be considered in all patients presenting with heart failure.

DIFFERENTIAL DIAGNOSIS

- Any cause of breathlessness, such as chronic obstructive lung disease or asthma
- It is sometimes difficult to distinguish the cause of shortness of breath in patients who have chronic obstructive lung disease and heart failure.

 TREATMENT

GENERAL MEASURES

- Sodium restriction, continued physical activity (including modest or recreational dynamic exercise), avoidance of isometric exercise, and careful and frequent follow-up by a physician knowledgeable about heart failure
- Fluid restriction is rarely necessary unless there is concomitant hyponatremia, provided that salt restriction is strictly maintained.
- Most patients are advised to follow a 2 g per day low-sodium diet.

 MEDICATION (DRUGS)

First Line

- Cornerstones of therapy are the angiotensin-converting enzyme (ACE) inhibitors and the β-blockers.
- ARBs are indicated if patient is intolerant of ACE inhibitor or previously on this medication.
- Patients with evidence of fluid retention may require a loop diuretic.
- For patients with moderately severe to severe heart failure and no associated renal insufficiency, spironolactone 12.5–25 mg daily is sometimes prescribed.
- Hydralazine and nitrates may be considered as add-on therapy, especially in African Americans patients.
- Non-steroidal antiinflammatory drugs (NSAIDs), most antiarrhythmics, and most calcium channel blockers should be avoided if possible.

Second Line

- Digoxin may be considered to decrease incidence of hospitalization.

SURGERY

- Implantable cardioverter–defibrillator is recommended for primary prevention of sudden cardiac death in patients with left ventricular ejection fraction (LVEF) less than 30%.
- Cardiac resynchronization therapy is indicated in patients with LVEF less than 35%, New York Heart Association (NYHA) Class III symptoms, and QRS >120 msec.
- A patient with advanced heart failure may sometimes benefit from left ventricular assist devices or volume reduction surgery, such as the Dor procedure.
- In some cases, coronary artery bypass surgery has improved left ventricular performance remarkably.
- Heart transplantation is the ultimate palliative therapy.

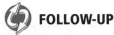

FOLLOW-UP

DISPOSITION
Admission Criteria
• Patients should be admitted to the hospital for:
  – Respiratory distress
  – Acute pulmonary edema
  – Desaturated blood that is not due to underlying lung disease
  – Concomitant medical illnesses that are poorly controlled or need treatment, such as diabetes mellitus, rapid atrial fibrillation, pneumonia, syncope, or demonstrate refractoriness to standard therapy
• Patients with anasarca who are unable to comply with medical therapy should be considered for hospitalization.
• The average hospital stay for heart failure is 5–7 days.
• Patients can usually be safely discharged when there is obvious clinical improvement, reduction in weight, and the ability to ambulate in the hospital without obvious difficulty.

PROGNOSIS
• The course of heart failure may wax and wane, with some patients demonstrating prolonged stability and others requiring frequent hospitalization.
• The prognosis generally is poor, with an annual mortality rate that varies from 9–12%.

PATIENT MONITORING
• Follow-up for patients with heart failure is extremely important.
Patients discharged from the hospital should be seen in 1–2 weeks and every 1–3 months thereafter.
• Heart failure care may increasingly be delivered by multidisciplinary disease management programs.

REFERENCES
1. Francis GS. Congestive heart failure. In: *Stein's Internal Medicine*, 5th ed. St. Louis: CV Mosby, 1998:156–175.
2. Francis GS. Congestive heart failure. In: Rake RE, ed. *Conn's Current Therapy*. Philadelphia: WB Saunders, 1998:292–296.
3. Francis GS. Pathophysiology of the heart failure syndrome. In: Topol EJ, ed. *Textbook of Cardiovascular Medicine*. Philadelphia: Lippincott Williams & Wilkins, 1998:2179–2303.
4. Hunt, SA et. al. Diagnosis and Management of Chronic Heart Failure in the Adult. ACC/AHA Guideline *(Based on 2005 Guideline Update)*, August 2005.

CODES
ICD9-CM
428.0 Failure, heart, congestive

PATIENT TEACHING
• Patient education is critical.
• Patients should be informed about the natural history of their disease, the prognosis, and should have ample information regarding their medications and how to use them.

H

HEART RATE VARIABILITY

John Respass
Theofanie Mela

 BASICS

DESCRIPTION

- Heart rate variability (HRV) is a measure of the variable periodicity of the heart rate due to interactions between ongoing perturbations to the cardiovascular system and the response of control mechanisms, which serve to regulate cardiovascular function.
- The perturbations may be exogenous or endogenous (e.g., changes in posture, the mechanical effects of respiratory variation in intrathoracic pressure on the filling and emptying of cardiovascular structures, autoregulatory adjustments in local vascular resistance in different tissue beds that lead to fluctuations in total vascular resistance). Responses to these stimuli are mediated primarily by variable inputs from the sympathetic and parasympathetic systems.
- Analysis of HRV using nonlinear dynamics has demonstrated that variability is nonrandom and demonstrates fractal properties. Similar variations are demonstrated over a wide range of time scales. The loss of these properties represents increased randomness of HR behavior and is associated with increased mortality, including sudden cardiac death.

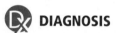 **DIAGNOSIS**

- HRV can be used as a quantitative tool to investigate autonomic function:
- Independent risk factor of mortality after myocardial infarction (MI)
- Marked derangement of HRV in patients with severe congestive heart failure (CHF)
- Decreased HRV a predictor of death in patients with CHF

TESTS

- Time-domain techniques
  - The most simple and straightforward technique involves the detection of each QRS complex in a continuous electrocardiogram (ECG) recording and the determination of normal-to-normal (NN) intervals or the instantaneous heart rate. Ectopic or nonconducted beats are not included.
  - Statistical methods: The simplest variable to calculate is the standard deviation of the NN intervals (SDNN), that is, the square root of variance.
  - Geometric methods: The series of NN intervals also can be converted to a geometric pattern; a simple formula is then used that judges the variability on the basis of the geometric and/or graphic properties of the resulting pattern.
  - Frequency-Domain Techniques: The use of spectral analysis implies that the event series can be represented by a sum of sinusoidal components of different amplitude, frequency, and phase values, using the Fast Fourier transform algorithm (FFT) or on an autoregressive (AR) methodology. The main spectrum calculated from short-term recordings of 2–5 minutes includes very low frequency power (VLFP), low-frequency power (LFP), and high-frequency power (HFP) components. The distribution of the power and the central frequency of LFP and HFP vary in relation to changes in autonomic modulations of heart period. When the spectrum is calculated from the entire 24-hour period, the result also includes an ultra low frequency power (ULFP) component.
  - Results of the frequency–domain analysis are generally equivalent to those of the time-domain analysis, which is easier to perform.

- Nonlinear dynamics (Chaos Theory and Fractals)
  - Based on chaos theory: Apparently erratic behavior can be generated by a nonlinear deterministic structure
  - Quantified in various ways, the most powerful of which is the short-term fractal scaling exponent (alpha), a measure of short-term correlation of fluctuations in the R-R interval.
- Physiologic correlates of HRV
  - The HRV reflects modulations of heart rate related to fluctuations in autonomic activity but not mean levels of autonomic tone.
  - The efferent vagal activity is a major contributor to the HFP component. The determinants of the LFP component is less clear but likely includes both sympathetic and vagal influences.
  - There is a circadian pattern, with higher values of LFP in the daytime and of HFP at night. Maneuvers such as 90-degree tilt, standing, mental stress, and moderate exercise in healthy subjects increase LFP as does moderate hypotension, physical activity, or occlusion of a coronary artery or common carotid arteries in conscious dogs. Conversely, an increase in HFP is induced by controlled respiration, cold stimulation of the face, and rotational stimuli.
- Changes of HRV related to specific pathologies and clinical use of HRV: Myocardial infarction
  - HRV is decreased early after acute MI and begins to recover within a few weeks; it is maximally but not fully recovered by 6–12 months after MI. HRV measured late (1 year) after acute MI also predicts further mortality.
  - To date, the most practical clinical utility of HRV is its prognostic power after MI, which is independent of other factors established for risk stratification.

- SDNN <50 msec measured 11 days post-MI conferred a relative risk (RR) of mortality of 2.8 over 2–4 years of follow-up
- In ATRAMI (autonomic tone and reflexes after myocardial infarction—1988) SDNN again an independent predictor of mortality with an RR of 5.9 in patients with low SDNN and LVEF (left ventricular ejection fraction) <35%
- Sub-study of DIAMOND compared time domain, frequency domain, and fractal indices of HRV: found alpha (short-term fractal scaling coefficient) most sensitive and specific for mortality (all-cause, arrhythmic and nonarrhythmic) within 2 years after an MI resulting in LVEF <35%.
- La Rovere et al. assessed a multivariate survival model to predict sudden death in patients with heart failure, identifying FLP <12 msec^2 and >83 PVCs (premature ventricular contractions) per hour as independent risk factors for mortality. More importantly, the absence of both factors (in a surprising 62% of a population with a mean LVEF <30%) conferred sudden cardiac death risk of only 3% over 3 years. This finding suggests the presence of a population of patients with reduced LVEF who may not benefit from prophylactic implantable cardioverter–defibrillator (ICD) implantation.

- Myocardial Dysfunction
  - Although there is poor correlation between HRV and asymptomatic LV dysfunction, reduced HRV has been observed consistently in patients with congestive heart failure. The circadian pattern also reveals an absence of the usual diurnal variation in day–night HRV.
- Cardiac transplantation
  - A very reduced HRV with no definite spectral components was reported in patients with a recent heart transplant, likely representing the denervated state of the donor heart.
- Diabetic neuropathy
  - A reduction in time–domain parameters of HRV seems not only to carry negative prognostic value but also to precede the clinical expression of diabetic neuropathy.

TREATMENT

MEDICATION (DRUGS)

- Flecainide and propafenone but not amiodarone decrease time–domain measures of HRV in patients with chronic ventricular arrhythmia.
- β-Blockade induces a significant increase in HRV parameters.
- Captopril increases both time and frequency domain indices of variability.

REFERENCES

1. Frenneaux MP. Autonomic changes in patients with heart failure and in post-myocardial infarction patients. *Heart.* 2004;90:1248–1255.
2. Huikuri H, Makikallio T, et al. Fractal correlation properties of r-r interval dynamics and mortality in patients with depressed left ventricular function after an acute myocardial infarction. *Circulation.* 2000;101:47–53.
3. La Rovere MT, et al. Short-term heart rate variability strongly predicts sudden cardiac death in chronic heart failure patients. *Circulation.* 2003;107:565–570.
4. Lombardi F. Chaos theory, heart rate variability, and arrhythmic mortality. *Circulation.* 2000;101:8–10.
5. Kleiger RE, Miller JP, Bigger JT, et al. and the Multicenter Post-infarction Research Group. Decreased heart rate variability and its association with increased mortality after acute myocardial infarction. *Am J Cardiol.* 1987;59:256–262.
6. Nolan J, Batin PD, Andrews R, et al. and the United Kingdom Heart Failure Evaluation and Assessment of Risk Trial. Prospective study of heart rate variability and mortality in chronic heart failure. *Circulation.* 1998;98:1510–1516.
7. Reed MJ, Robertson CE, Addison PS. Heart rate variability measurements and the prediction of ventricular arrhythmias. *Q J Med.* 2005;98:87–95.
8. Task force of the European Society of Cardiology and the North American Society of Pacing and Electrophysiology. Heart rate variability: Standards of measurement, physiological interpretation and clinical use. *Circulation.* 1996;93:1043–1065.

MISCELLANEOUS

- Measurements of HRV offer a simple, noninvasive, and reliable approach to the clinical assessment of the cardiac autonomic modulation in healthy and diseased hearts.
- So far, the clinical utility of HRV resides mainly in the ability to risk-stratify post-MI patients with respect to outcome events.
- For clinically meaningful ranges of sensitivity, the predictive value of HRV alone is modest and should be combined with other factors.
- HRV has promise to aid in further selection of ICD candidates within the MADIT II population.

H

HEART TRANSPLANTATION

Apur R. Kamdar
Deepak L. Bhatt
Gary S. Francis

 BASICS

DESCRIPTION

Heart transplantation entails the surgical implantation of a recently explanted heart from a brain-dead human, for severely symptomatic or end-stage heart failure.

- In the absence of significant symptoms, transplantation should not be performed, even if ventricular function is markedly impaired.
- There are many contraindications, and due to donor shortage, patients must be rigorously screened.

EPIDEMIOLOGY

- More than 4,000 patients are currently on the waiting list for heart transplantation in the United States.
- More than 2,200 heart transplantations are performed per year in the United States and more than 3,500 worldwide at >200 medical centers.
- The mortality of patients on the waiting list is about 10% per year.
- Organ shortage continues to be a major problem despite liberalization of criteria for organ donation.

RISK FACTORS

- Absolute indications (in appropriate patients) include refractory cardiogenic shock, dependence on intravenous (IV) inotropic support, peak Vo_2 <10 mL/kg, severe ischemia that is not revascularizable, refractory ventricular arrhythmias.
- Absolute contraindications to heart transplantation include severe, fixed pulmonary hypertension, active infection, and active malignancy.
- Although transplantations are increasingly being performed for older patients, advanced age is a relative contraindication for the procedure.
- Other relative contraindications include severe, longstanding diabetes with end-organ damage, severe peripheral vascular disease, obesity, and the presence of alloantibodies.
- Social support and psychological stability are requisite.

Pregnancy Considerations

Has been successful in patients who have undergone heart transplantation

ETIOLOGY

- Heart transplantation is used for end-stage heart failure of almost any cause.
- Ischemic cardiomyopathy and dilated cardiomyopathy are the most frequent indications.
- Reversible etiologies, such as alcoholic cardiomyopathy, should be sought.
- Furthermore, spontaneous improvement may occur in the first 6 months after initial presentation with many cardiomyopathies.

ASSOCIATED CONDITIONS

- Immunosuppressive therapy predisposes to infections (including unusual ones) and skin cancers.
- Hypertension, renal insufficiency
- Hyperlipidemia
- Coronary artery disease (i.e., allograft vasculopathy)

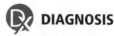 **DIAGNOSIS**

SIGNS AND SYMPTOMS

- Fever, even low grade, can signify infection or rejection.
  - Rejection
  - Fatigue
  - Dyspnea
  - Pericardial rub
  - Supraventricular arrhythmias

TESTS

- Cardiopulmonary stress testing is useful to decide upon the need for transplantation in outpatient: peak Vo_2 measurements.
- Endomyocardial biopsy is mandatory if rejection is suspected.
  - Allows grading of the degree of rejection
  - Helps guide immunosuppressive therapy

Lab

- Electrocardiogram (ECG) may show dual sinus node activity (from donor and recipient atria).
- Typical ECG shows an incomplete right bundle branch block.
- Blood cultures, sputum Gram stain, and culture if infection is suspected

Imaging

With rejection, echocardiography may show pericardial effusion, left ventricular systolic dysfunction, and myocardial edema reflected as increased ventricular wall thickness.

 TREATMENT

MEDICATION (DRUGS)

- Immunosuppressants
  - Cyclosporine, azathioprine, prednisone, tacrolimus (FK506), mycophenolate mofetil, ATG, OKT3, and rapamycin/everolimus.
  - Monoclonal antibodies such as daclizumab appear promising.
- Antihypertensives are usually necessary due to the hypertensive effects of cyclosporine.
- Cholesterol-lowering medications
  - Pravastatin is the preferred statin
  - Increased risk of rhabdomyolysis with concomitant cyclosporine
- Atropine and digoxin may not be effective, due to denervation of the transplanted heart.
- Trimethoprim/sulfamethoxazole for *Pneumocystis carinii* prophylaxis
  - Monthly inhaled pentamidine is a less effective alternative for patients who are allergic to sulfa drugs.

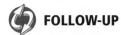

FOLLOW-UP

DISPOSITION

Admission Criteria
Suspicion of rejection or infection is usually an indication for admission.

Issues for Referral
- All reasonable options should be considered prior to transplantation including optimal medication regimen and/or biventricular pacing/defibrillator.
- Left ventricular assist devices (LVADs) are increasingly being used as a "bridge" to transplantation and as destination therapy in place of transplantation.

PROGNOSIS
- 1-Month survival rate is 93%.
- 1-Year survival rate is 85%.
- 3-Year survival rate is 76%.
- Primary graft rejection and infection are the most common causes of early mortality.
- Infection with bacteria, viruses, fungi, or protozoa
- Human papilloma virus infection can lead to cutaneous warts or to cervical cancer.
- Rejection most commonly occurs in the first 3 months posttransplantation.
- Transplant vasculopathy can be problematic because there is no established therapy.
  - Many cardiologists increase the level of immunosuppression when vasculopathy is detected.
  - Angina is often absent due to denervation of the transplanted heart, even in the presence of significant arterial obstruction.
  - The coronary vasculopathy is diffuse and not typically amenable to angioplasty.
  - Vasculopathy can progress rapidly and is a cause of sudden death.
  - Transplant vasculopathy has an incidence of 20% over 5 years and remains the major cause of late mortality.
  - Rapamycin and its synthetic derivative, everolimus, can limit disease progression.
  - Retransplantation has been performed successfully, but has a much higher associated mortality.
- Skin cancers (squamous cell carcinoma, basal cell carcinoma, and keratoacanthomas) are common.
- Lymphoma (posttransplant lymphoproliferative disorder, PTLD)
- Osteoporosis (secondary to steroids)

PATIENT MONITORING
- Yearly endomyocardial biopsies to monitor for rejection
- Yearly coronary angiography, potentially accompanied by intravascular ultrasonography, is recommended to monitor for transplant vasculopathy.
- Dobutamine stress echocardiography also appears to have powerful prognostic ability and may be a means to noninvasively assess the presence of vasculopathy.
- Female patients should have routine 6-month Pap smears to monitor for human papilloma virus–induced cervical dysplasia.

REFERENCES
1. Johnson FL. Heart transplantation: An update and review. *Minerva Cardioangiol*. 2003;51:245–255.
2. Poston RS, Griffith BP. Heart transplantation. *J Intensive Care Med*. 2004;19:3–12.
3. Shumway SJ, Shumway NE. *Thoracic Transplantation*. Cambridge, MA: Blackwell, 1995.
4. Smith JA, McCarthy PM, Sarris GE, et al. *The Stanford Manual of Cardiopulmonary Transplantation*. Armonk, NY: Futura, 1996.
5. Spes CH, Klauss V, Mudra H, et al. Diagnostic and prognostic value of serial dobutamine stress echocardiography for noninvasive assessment of cardiac allograft vasculopathy: A comparison with coronary angiography and intravascular ultrasound. *Circulation*. 1999;100:509–515.

CODES

ICD9-CM
- 428.0 Failure, heart, congestive
- 996.83 Transplanted heart: failure, infection, rejection

PATIENT TEACHING
- Regular skin self-examinations
- Use sunscreen (minimum SPF of 15).
- Report fevers.
- Organizations
  - United Network for Organ Sharing: www.unos.org

H

HIGH OUTPUT HEART FAILURE

Deepak L. Bhatt
Gary S. Francis
Apur R. Kamdar

 BASICS

DESCRIPTION
The symptoms of high-output heart failure are associated with an increased cardiac output as opposed to the typical decreased cardiac output.

EPIDEMIOLOGY
Extremely rare, especially in the United States

RISK FACTORS
Depends on the etiology

Pregnancy Considerations
- Pregnancy not advisable until the underlying condition has been corrected
- Pregnancy itself can be associated with a high-output state, rarely leading to failure.

ETIOLOGY
- Chronic anemia
- Arteriovenous fistulas
- Osler-Weber-Rendu disease (hereditary hemorrhagic telangiectasia)
- Hyperthyroidism
- Paget disease
- Thiamine deficiency (beriberi)
- Multiple myeloma
- Pregnancy
- Albright syndrome (fibrous dysplasia)
- Obesity
- Glomerulonephritis
- Cor pulmonale
- Polycythemia vera
- Carcinoid syndrome

ASSOCIATED CONDITIONS
Peripheral neuropathy with beriberi

 DIAGNOSIS

SIGNS AND SYMPTOMS
- Wide pulse pressure
- Tachycardia
- Brisk carotid upstroke
- Third heart sound (S_3)
- Fourth heart sound (S_4)
- Branham sign (reduction in heart rate during manual compression of an arteriovenous fistula)
- Edema

Physical Exam
Varies according to etiology

TESTS
- Right heart catheterization reveals elevated cardiac output and low systemic vascular resistance.
- Oxygen extraction is increased and the arterial-mixed venous o_2 difference is decreased.

Lab
- Hemoglobin, thyroid function tests, thiamine levels
- Elevated alkaline phosphatase in Paget disease

Imaging
Echocardiography can help assess left ventricular function.

DIFFERENTIAL DIAGNOSIS
An elevated cardiac output secondary to conditions such as fever must be distinguished from true high-output heart failure.

 ## TREATMENT

GENERAL MEASURES
Correction of underlying cause if possible

 ## MEDICATION (DRUGS)

First Line
- In cases of beriberi, thiamine replacement is critical.
- Diuretics and digoxin also may be useful.
- β-Blockers may be used judiciously in hyperthyroidism.

 ## FOLLOW-UP

DISPOSITION
Admission Criteria
As for heart failure of any etiology

PROGNOSIS
The underlying condition must be treated before any improvement in symptoms.

PATIENT MONITORING
As for heart failure of any etiology

REFERENCE
1. Zipes DP. *Braunwald's Heart Disease: A Textbook of Cardiovascular Medicine,* 7th ed., 2005.

CODES
ICD9-CM
- 428.0 Failure, heart, congestive
- 265.0 [425.7] Cardiomyopathy, beriberi
- 242.9 [425.7] Cardiomyopathy, thyrotoxic

PATIENT TEACHING
As for heart failure of any etiology

H

HURLER'S SYNDROME AND THE HEART

Jeff Ciaramita,
Steven C. Herrmann
Bernard R. Chaitman

 BASICS

DESCRIPTION
Hurler syndrome is one of the mucopolysaccharidosis diseases in which a deficiency occurs of lysosomal enzymes involved in degrading glycosaminoglycans.
• Synonym(s): Mucopolysaccharidoses, MPS IH

Pregnancy Considerations
Screening is not routinely performed in pregnancy.

EPIDEMIOLOGY
Usually diagnosed in infancy

Incidence
Approximate incidence is 1/100,000.

RISK FACTORS
Genetics
Autosomal recessive, caused by mutations in IDUA gene, localized on chromosome 4p16.3

ETIOLOGY
• Afflicted individuals appear normal at birth, and are typically diagnosed at 6 months to 2 years of age.
• Caused by a deficiency of α-L-iduronidase

 DIAGNOSIS

SIGNS AND SYMPTOMS
• Infants with Hurler syndrome usually present in the first 2 years after birth with severe mental retardation, hepatosplenomegaly, skeletal deformities, and corneal clouding.
• Patients usually die of obstructive airway symptoms and respiratory infection.
• Cardiac involvement usually presents before age 5 and includes premature coronary artery disease and myocardial infarction, pulmonary hypertension with hypoxemia, valvular involvement including mitral and aortic insufficiency, pseudohypertrophic cardiomyopathy, and endocardial fibroelastosis.

TESTS
Confirmation of the diagnosis is obtained by leukocyte DNA analysis and demonstration of lack of α-l-iduronidase in white cells.

Lab
High concentrations of both heparin and dermatan sulfate in the urine suggest evidence of biochemical defect.

Imaging
A radiographic skeletal survey is recommended and will demonstrate a characteristic MPS pattern known as *dysostosis multiplex*.

Pathologic Findings
• Deficiency of α-L-iduronidase results in the increase of both heparin and dermatan sulfate in the interstitium.
• The increase in undegraded glycosaminoglycans results in abnormal tissue function.

DIFFERENTIAL DIAGNOSIS
• Scheie syndrome
• Hunter syndrome
• Hurler-Scheie syndrome
• Sanfilippo A-D syndromes
• Morquio syndrome
• Maroteaux-Lamy syndrome
• Sly syndrome
• Hyaluronidase syndrome

TREATMENT

GENERAL MEASURES
- Hematopoietic stem-cell and cord-blood transplantation have been shown to be effective treatments, increasing life span, preventing cardiac disease progression, and reducing hepatosplenomegaly.
- Enzyme replacement therapy with recombinant (α)-L-iduronidase also has been FDA approved.

 MEDICATION (DRUGS)

None

PROGNOSIS
Most patients die before age 10.

PATIENT MONITORING
Annual cardiac evaluations using echocardiography are recommended to assess for valvular disease, heart failure, cor pulmonale, and cardiomyopathy.

REFERENCES
1. Braunwald E, ed. *Heart disease: A textbook of cardiovascular medicine*, 7th ed. Philadelphia: WB Saunders, 2005.
2. Mueuzer J, et al. Advances in the treatment of mucopolysaccharidosis type 1. *N Engl J Med*. 2004;350(19):1932–1934.
3. Wappner RS, ed. *Oski's pediatrics: Principles and practice*, 3rd ed. Philadelphia: Lippincott, 1999.

 MISCELLANEOUS

See also: Scheie Syndrome; Hunter Syndrome; Hurler-Scheie Syndrome; Sanfilippo Syndrome; Morquio Syndrome; Sly Syndrome

CODES
ICD9-CM
277.5

PATIENT TEACHING
Diet
No restrictions
Activity
Limited

H

HYPERTROPHIC CARDIOMYOPATHY

Brian Ristow

 ## BASICS

DESCRIPTION

Cardiac manifestations are among the earliest as well as the most consistent features of hyperthyroidism. All-cause and cardiovascular mortality are increased by hyperthyroidism.

- T_3 (triiodothyronine) is the active thyroid hormone and is converted from T_4 (thyroxine) by 5'-deiodinase in the liver and kidney.
- T_3 binds to nuclear receptors and regulates gene expression. Direct myocardial effects include:
  - Increased heart rate
  - Increased contractility
  - Increased diastolic relaxation
  - Increased cardiac output
- Systemic effects of thyroid hormone include:
  - Increased blood volume (increased sodium retention)
  - Decreased systemic vascular resistance (SVR) by direct effect on smooth muscle
  - Increased systolic BP and increased pulse pressure
  - Increased tissue thermogenesis and oxygen consumption
- Myocardial ischemia (with or without coronary artery disease) can occur secondary to increased oxygen consumption or coronary vasospasm.
- Tachycardia can lead to reversible hyperthyroid cardiomyopathy (5% of cases occur in absence of cardiac disease).
- Hyperthyroidism can cause decompensation of underlying heart disease leading to congestive heart failure (CHF).
- The risk of atrial fibrillation is increased in both hyperthyroidism and subclinical hyperthyroidism (the clinical entity of low thyrotropin [TSH] and normal T_3 or T_4).
- System(s) affected: Cardiovascular; Endocrine

GENERAL PREVENTION

Monitor TSH and free thyroxine levels when hyperthyroidism is suspected.

EPIDEMIOLOGY

- Predominant age: Young adults and the elderly
- Predominant sex: Female > Males

Incidence

- Thyroid disease becomes more common with advancing age.
- Graves disease is especially common in the 3rd and 4th decades of age and affects 0.02–0.4% of the U.S. population.
- Graves disease is more frequent in women (4:1 to 10:1).

Geriatric Considerations

- Apathetic thyrotoxicosis may present with weakness and depression rather than classic symptoms of hyperthyroidism.
- Atrial fibrillation is a common presentation.

Pediatric Considerations

Rare

Prevalence

Women 2%; men 0.2%

RISK FACTORS

Autoimmune diseases (type 1 diabetes, vitiligo, pernicious anemia, and myasthenia gravis) are associated with Graves disease.

Genetics

Genetics play an important role in Graves disease.

- Increased frequency of haplotypes HLA-B8 and -DRw3 in white patients
- Increased frequency of haplotype HLA-Bw36 in Japanese patients
- Increased frequency of haplotype HLA-Bw46 in Chinese patients

PATHOPHYSIOLOGY

Graves disease is caused by thyroid-stimulating antibodies.

ETIOLOGY

- The most common cause of hyperthyroidism in the U.S. is Graves disease (60–80%).
- Other causes are toxic multinodular goiter, toxic adenoma, thyroiditis (lymphocytic, postpartum, or subacute), and rarely tumors (thyroid, ovarian, or pituitary).
- Excess exogenous thyroid hormone:
  - Overtreatment of hypothyroidism
  - Treatment to reduce thyrotropin levels in thyroid cancer
- Amiodarone-induced hyperthyroidism:
  - Type 1: Iodine excess (increased radioiodine uptake)
  - Type 2: Inflammatory (low radioiodine uptake)

ASSOCIATED CONDITIONS

- Atrial fibrillation
- CHF
- Hypertension
- Myocardial ischemia

 ## DIAGNOSIS

SIGNS AND SYMPTOMS

Cardiovascular findings

- Sinus tachycardia
- Atrial arrhythmias (especially atrial fibrillation)
- Wide pulse pressure
- Hypertension
- Mid-systolic ejection murmur (left sternal boarder)
- Active apical impulse
- Loud S1, loud P2, and occasional S3
- Means-Lerman scratch (rare systolic scratch heard in the second left intercostal space during expiration)
- Increased stroke volume, cardiac output, and cardiac work with decreased peripheral resistance

Pregnancy Considerations

- Metabolic demands of pregnancy will exacerbate symptoms.
- Radioiodine and methimazole are contraindicated in pregnancy; propylthiouracil (PTU) can be used.
- Careful management with an obstetrician and endocrinologist is desirable.

History

- Nervousness, insomnia, tremors
- Palpitations
- Diarrhea
- Heat intolerance
- Weight loss despite preserved or increased appetite
- Increased perspiration
- Weakness and fatigue
- Oligomenorrhea or amenorrhea
- Stare, lid lag
- Exertional dyspnea

Physical Exam

- Elevated systolic blood pressure, tachycardia, weight loss
- Dry skin, thin hair, brittle nails
- Exophthalmos (Graves disease) or lid lag
- Goiter or thyroid nodule
- Tremor, hyperreflexia

TESTS

- ECG (common but nonspecific)
  - Sinus tachycardia (40% of patients)
  - Atrial fibrillation (15–25% of patients)
  - Shortening of atrio-ventricular conduction time along with functional refractory period transmits rapid atrial impulses.
  - Intraatrial conduction disturbance causes prolongation or notched P-wave and prolongation of the P-R interval (5–15% of patients).
  - Interventricular conduction disturbances (right bundle branch block most common)
  - 2nd- or 3rd-degree heart block (rare)

Lab

- Suppressed TSH and increased free thyroxine index (FTI), a measurement of free T_4
- Subclinical hyperthyroidism is defined by low TSH and normal FTI
- Serum T_3 only rarely needed (i.e., cases of T_3 toxicosis when both FTI and TSH are low)
- High FTI and high TSH indicate a TSH-producing tumor or peripheral hormone resistance.
- Thyroid-stimulating immunoglobulin assay if diagnosis is unclear
- Hypokalemia is common in hyperthyroidism.
- Drugs that may alter laboratory results: Amiodarone is an iodine-rich benzofuran derivative that causes both hyperthyroidism and hypothyroidism. It also may affect thyroid function tests in the absence of clinical disease.

Imaging

- Echocardiography
  - Measurement of cardiac chamber sizes, wall thickness, diastolic function, and ejection fraction
  - Evaluation for associated mitral valve prolapse in Graves disease
- Chest radiograph (nonspecific)
  - Prominent left ventricle, aorta, and pulmonary artery
  - Generalized cardiac enlargement
  - Pulmonary edema (late)

Diagnostic Procedures/Surgery

Radioactive iodine uptake can be used in the differential diagnosis of hyperthyroidism with diffuse goiter, and in the diagnosis of ectopic struma ovarii, thyroiditis, and thyrotoxicosis factitia.

Pathologic Findings
Multinodular goiter, thyroiditis, ophthalmopathy, dermopathy; no specific cardiovascular pathology

DIFFERENTIAL DIAGNOSIS
- Emotional anxiety
- Pheochromocytoma
- Metastatic carcinoid
- Sprue
- Hyperparathyroidism

TREATMENT

GENERAL MEASURES
- Minor symptoms can be controlled medically as an outpatient.
- Unstable symptoms (i.e., thyroid storm or decompensated heart failure) require aggressive management and hospitalization.
- Prompt treatment of the hyperthyroid state is essential to the reduction of cardiovascular symptoms.
- Cardiovascular manifestations (CHF, atrial fibrillation) attributed solely to hyperthyroidism are reversible with treatment.

MEDICATION (DRUGS)

First Line
- β-Adrenergic blockade (e.g., propranolol 40–120 mg/day or atenolol 100 mg/day) reduces symptoms.
- β-Blockade reduces heart rate, but direct inotropic effects of T_3 persist.
- β-Blockers, verapamil, and diltiazem can rapidly rate-control superventricular arrhythmias and reduce the hyperdynamic state (see Supraventricular Tachycardia chapter for dosing).
- Digitalis glycosides can control ventricular rate in atrial fibrillation and are especially helpful in patients with heart failure. Higher doses may be required due to metabolic clearance. Target ventricular rate should be approximately 120 beats/min to avoid drug toxicity in the acute setting.
- Thyroid-suppressive drugs such as PTU (100 mg q2h during thyrotoxic crisis) or methimazole (20 mg/day) are the preferred drugs when heart failure complicates severe hyperthyroidism. Each blocks thyroid hormone and thyroid-stimulating immunoglobulin production. PTU also inhibits extrathyroidal conversion of T_4 to T_3.
- Radioiodine (^{131}I) ablation of thyroid tissue can provide definitive treatment of most causes of hyperthyroidism, such as Graves disease.
- Diuretics reduce volume overload and pulmonary vascular congestion (see Congestive Heart Disease chapter for dosing).
- Warfarin therapy in atrial fibrillation for embolic prophylaxis except in young patients with no other cardiovascular disease
- β-Blockers, calcium channel blockers, and nitrates for angina pectoris (see Angina chapter for dosing)

SURGERY
Thyroidectomy may be required in patients with a large, toxic, nodular goiter after medical stabilization or in medical therapeutic failures.

FOLLOW-UP
Check TSH and T_4 regularly to guide therapy for adequate thyroid replacement.

DISPOSITION
Ensure adequate treatment and follow-up for treatment of both hyperthyroidism and cardiac manifestations.

Admission Criteria
- Congestive heart failure, arrhythmia, or unstable vital signs
- Medical, radioactive, or surgical treatment of hyperthyroidism often requires admission.

Discharge Criteria
- Stable cardiac rhythm, blood pressure, and symptoms
- Adequate follow-up

Issues for Referral
Consultation with an endocrinologist generally is recommended.

PROGNOSIS
- Overall symptomatic improvement in 1–2 weeks with euthyroidism by 2 months
- Cardiac manifestations usually take longer to resolve. Cardiovascular mortality and the risk of stroke remain increased for at least 12 months after treatment.
- Recurrence of hyperthyroidism is possible (up to 50%), depending on treatment modality used.

COMPLICATIONS
- Agranulocytosis, vasculitis, hepatitis, and aplastic anemia are seen infrequently with suppressive therapy using PTU and methimazole.
- Hypothyroidism with ^{131}I
- Hypothyroidism or hypoparathyroidism after subtotal thyroidectomy

PATIENT MONITORING
- Depends on frequency and severity of symptoms
- In Graves disease, treat with PTU or methimazole for 6–12 months and follow-up for recurrence
- Treatment of arrhythmias and heart failure can be weaned as symptoms resolve.
- Repeat thyroid levels to access for euthyroidism
- CBC and liver functions to evaluate for complications of suppressive therapy (see Complications above)

REFERENCES
1. Braverman LE, Utiger RD. *The thyroid: A fundamental and clinical text*, 6th ed. Philadelphia: JB Lippincott, 1991.
2. Klein I, Ojamaa K. Mechanisms of disease: Thyroid hormone and the cardiovascular system. *N Engl J Med*. 2001;344:501–509.

ADDITIONAL READING
Boelaert K, Franklyn JA. Thyroid hormone in health and disease. *J Endocrinol*. 2005;187:1–15.

MISCELLANEOUS

CODES
ICD9-CM
242.9 + 425.7 Hyperthyroid heart disease

PATIENT TEACHING
American Heart Association, 7320 Greenville Ave., Dallas TX 75231; (214) 373-6300

Diet
Low-sodium and low-fat (if underlying coronary artery disease)

Activity
As tolerated, after consulting with a physician

Prevention
Check TSH when hyperthyroidism suspected to prevent heart failure, arrhythmias, or other complications

FAQ
- Should patients with thyrotoxicosis and atrial fibrillation receive anticoagulation?
  - Anticoagulation with warfarin is recommended except for young individuals with no other risk factors for thromboembolism.
- Does subclinical hyperthyroidism increase the risk for atrial fibrillation?
  - The risk of atrial fibrillation is increased 6-fold compared with the general population among individuals with subclinical hypothyroidism, especially in the elderly.

H

HYPOPLASTIC LEFT HEART SYNDROME

Jeffrey H. Kern
Welton M. Gersony

 BASICS

DESCRIPTION
Hypoplastic left heart syndrome (HLHS) is described as underdevelopment of the left-sided cardiac structures, including the mitral valve, left ventricle, aortic valve, and aortic arch. Aortic and mitral valves may be either atretic or stenotic.

EPIDEMIOLOGY
Slight male predominance

Incidence
- Incidence is 0.016–0.036% of live births.
- 1.5% of infants with congenital heart disease

Genetics
Recurrence risk for sibling of 0.05%; not associated with single specific chromosomal abnormality

ASSOCIATED CONDITIONS
- Noncardiac
  - Associated with many different syndromes, including Turner, Noonan, and Holt-Oram; 28% of HLHS patients have a genetic disorder or extracardiac anomalies, including brain malformations.
- Cardiac
  - Associated with ventricular septal defects, small foramen ovale, anomalous pulmonary venous return
  - HLHS may occur in the context of a double-outlet right ventricle or unbalanced atrioventricular canal defect.

 DIAGNOSIS

SIGNS AND SYMPTOMS
- Many infants are prenatally diagnosed through fetal echocardiography
- Postnatally, typically presents in first week of life with signs of poor cardiac output.

Physical Exam
- Signs of low cardiac output, pallor, poor respiratory effort, decreased responsiveness, poor feeding, seizures, and oliguria.
- Physical findings include mild cyanosis, poorly palpable femoral pulses, and an active precordium with a single second heart sound (S_2).
- There may be a nonspecific grade II/VI systolic murmur heard along the left sternal border.
- The murmur may be holosystolic and of a harsher quality in the presence of tricuspid regurgitation.
- The liver may be enlarged.

TESTS
Electrocardiogram (ECG) findings include the following:
- Right superior axis deviation
- Right ventricular hypertrophy
- Right atrial enlargement
- Diminished R waves in leads V_5 and V_6

Lab
- Arterial blood gas reveals low pCO_2, slightly low pO_2.
- Following ductal closure, the infant develops a profound metabolic acidosis with elevation of liver enzymes and serum creatinine.

Imaging
- Chest x-ray findings are nonspecific and include:
  - Cardiomegaly with a globular appearance
  - Increased pulmonary vascular markings
- Echocardiography is the primary diagnostic study to be performed, and findings include the following:
  - Mitral and aortic atresia or stenosis
  - Markedly diminished left ventricular size, sometimes too small to be visualized
  - Hypoplasia of the ascending aorta and transverse arch
  - The ductus arteriosus is seen with flow from the pulmonary artery to the aorta.
  - Retrograde flow from the site of ductal entry up to the proximal aortic arch and coronary arteries
  - Flow across the foramen ovale from the left atrium to the right atrium
- Echocardiographers must evaluate for tricuspid regurgitation, restriction to flow across the foramen ovale, pulmonary venous anatomy, right ventricular outflow tract obstruction, and right ventricular function.

Diagnostic Procedures/Surgery
- Cardiac catheterization is not necessary for the diagnosis of HLHS.
  - See below for surgical procedures.

DIFFERENTIAL DIAGNOSIS
- Prior to ductal closure: persistent pulmonary hypertension of the newborn [PPHN, or persistence of the fetal circulation (PFC) syndrome].
- Sepsis, critical coarctation of the aorta, interrupted aortic arch

TREATMENT

GENERAL MEASURES

- Continuous positive airway pressure (CPAP) or intubation and mechanical ventilation may be required.
- Limitation of pulmonary blood flow may be achieved through hypoventilation and avoidance of supplemental oxygen.
- Balloon atrial septostomy may be required urgently if the atrial communication is restrictive.

MEDICATION (DRUGS)

- Continuous intravenous (IV) infusion of prostaglandin E_1 at 0.05–0.2 μg/kg/minute is necessary to maintain ductal patency and systemic output.
- Diuresis and inotropic support are frequently required, especially for patients with a prolonged preoperative period.

SURGERY

- Surgical repair may be delayed until liver, brain, and renal function recover.
- Surgical approach usually consists of the staged Norwood procedure.
- Surgical management of HLHS consists of three stages:
  - Stage 1: performed in the neonatal period. The right ventricle is used as the systemic ventricle. The proximal pulmonary artery is reconstructed to form the ascending aorta and is anastomosed to the descending aorta. Controlled pulmonary blood flow is supplied via either (i) a Blalock-Taussig shunt between the innominate artery and the pulmonary artery (Norwood operation) or (ii) via a conduit between the right ventricle and pulmonary artery (Sano procedure). The atrial septum is resected to allow unobstructed flow from the left atrium to the right atrium. The aortic coarctation is repaired.
  - Stage 2: The bidirectional Glenn procedure usually is performed at 4–8 months of age. Cardiac catheterization is required prior to stages 2 and 3 to assess the hemodynamics and pulmonary artery anatomy. The shunt is taken down and the superior cava is connected directly into the pulmonary artery.
  - Stage 3: The Fontan procedure, in which the inferior vena caval flow is also directed into the pulmonary artery, usually is completed at approximately 18–36 months of age. Cyanosis is relieved, although some desaturation may persist, especially if the Fontan is "fenestrated" (right atrium to left atrium (RA/LA) connection to maintain cardiac output in early postoperative period).
- Combined approach entails planned transplantation with crossover to Norwood procedure if no donors are available. Cardiac transplantation may follow any stage in the face of unfavorable hemodynamics and severe symptoms.
- No intervention: This approach is occasionally used, but less commonly in recent years.

PROGNOSIS

- 100% mortality without surgical intervention
- Norwood procedure
  - Greatest mortality in the immediately postoperative stage 1 period
  - Additional deaths may occur between stages 1 and 2.
  - Low mortality following stages 2 and 3
  - Morbidity due to recurrent coarctation of the aorta, restriction to flow across the atrial septum.
  - Morbidity following stage 3 is similar to that in other Fontan patients, including pleural effusions, protein-losing enteropathy, poor cardiac output, and ventricular failure.
- Cardiac transplantation
  - Significant mortality awaiting transplantation due to shortage of neonatal donors
  - If transplantation is performed, survival is approximately 85%.
  - Significant morbidity present due to chronic immunosuppression and risks of infection and graft rejection
- 5-year survival is approximately 65–70% in both groups when also considering deaths of infants awaiting transplantation.

PATIENT MONITORING

- Frequent visits required
- Echocardiography, oxygen saturation, and hemoglobin measurements periodically obtained

REFERENCES

1. Chang RKR, Chen AY, Klitzner TS. Clinical management of infants with hypoplastic left heart syndrome in the United States, 1988–1997. *Pediatrics*. 2002;110:292–308.
2. Garson A, et al., eds. *The Science and Practice of Pediatric Cardiology*, 2nd ed. Baltimore: Lippincott Williams & Wilkins; 1998.
3. Iannettoni MD, Bove EL, Crowley DC, et al. Improving results with first-stage palliation for hypoplastic left heart syndrome. *J Thorac Cardiovasc Surg*. 1994;107:934–940.
4. Norwood WI, Kirklin JK, Sanders SP. Hypoplastic left heart syndrome: Experience with palliative surgery. *Am J Cardiol*. 1980;45:87–91.
5. Sano S, Kawada M, Yoshida H, et al. Norwood procedure to hypoplastic left heart syndrome. *Jpn J Thorac Cardiovasc Surg*. 1998;46:1311–1316.

PATIENT TEACHING

Parents of affected infants should be careful regarding maintaining adequate hydration after the Norwood operation, because clotting of the shunt is a life-threatening event. Antibiotic prophylaxis against bacterial endocarditis is required prior to selected procedures.

H

HYPOTHYROID HEART DISEASE

Rajni K. Rao

 BASICS

DESCRIPTION

Cardiovascular manifestations of hypothyroidism include heart failure, pericardial effusion, arrhythmias, and premature atherosclerosis. Heart failure in hypothyroid patients usually occurs secondary to exacerbation of preexisting cardiac disease by the hemodynamic effects of hypothyroidism. Occasionally, hypothyroidism alone may cause a cardiomyopathy with associated heart failure.

EPIDEMIOLOGY

- Predominant Age
  - Peak incidence between the ages of 30 and 60 years.
- Predominant Sex
  - Female

Incidence

- Congenital hypothyroidism rare. Hypothyroidism occurs in 2% of adult women and 0.1–0.2% of adult men in North America.
- Incidence at least 3–10% with chronic amiodarone use.

Geriatric Considerations

- Overt and subclinical hypothyroidism common
- Subclinical hypothyroidism with TSH >7 mU/L associated with a 2–3 fold increase in heart failure events among the elderly.

Pediatric Considerations

- Rare

Pregnancy Considerations

- Heart disease due to hypothyroidism is unusual.

RISK FACTORS

- Preexisting heart disease increases the likelihood of cardiac involvement.
- Even subclinical hypothyroidism may increase the risk of coronary heart disease

PATHOPHYSIOLOGY

- Decreased contractility
  - Thyroid hormone regulates sarcomeric calcium fluxes (e.g., phospholamban)
- Increased peripheral vascular resistance
  - Thyroid hormone causes vasodilation through nitric oxide release
- Reduced LDL receptor expression
  - Accelerated atherosclerosis, often without angina
- Reduced oxygen consumption

ETIOLOGY

Decreased secretion of both thyroxine (T_4) and triiodothyronine (T_3), either due to thyroid gland destruction or due to pituitary or hypothalamic pathology.

ASSOCIATED CONDITIONS

- Hypopituitarism
- Addison's disease
- Amiodarone use

 DIAGNOSIS

SIGNS AND SYMPTOMS

- Symptoms
  - Exertional dyspnea
  - Fatigability, muscle weakness, lethargy
  - Erectile dysfunction, menstrual irregularities
  - Rarely syncope
  - Angina during hormone replacement
- Signs
  - Bradycardia
  - Weak arterial pulses
  - Distant heart sounds
  - Non-pitting edema
  - Hypertension, usually diastolic hypertension
  - Hypotension in severe myxedema
  - Rarely cardiac tamponade

TESTS

- ECG
  - Sinus bradycardia
  - Decreased P-wave amplitude
  - Reduced QRS voltage
  - T wave flattening/inversion
  - Prolonged QTc interval of 450–519 msec in 14%–21% of hypothyroid patients
  - Rarely QTc interval $\geq$520 msec (increased risk of malignant ventricular arrhythmias)
  - Atrioventricular and intraventricular conduction disturbances; incomplete or complete right bundle branch block

Lab

- Thyroid-stimulating hormone (TSH) ↑ in most cases, but rarely may be normal or undetectable in pituitary or hypothalamic hypothyroidism
- ↓Serum T_4 and free thyroxine index (FTI) are common to all types of hypothyroidism.
- Serum T_3 in thyroid hypothyroidism may be reduced to a lesser degree than serum T_4.
- Increased LDL and total cholesterol.
- CK ↑ common – usually the CK-MM type
  - CK-MB occasionally ↑ but troponin normal
- ↑ Total cholesterol, LDL, +/− triglycerides

Imaging

- Chest x-ray
  - Cardiac enlargement due to chamber enlargement and/or pericardial effusion
  - Small heart with pituitary hypothyroidism and adrenal insufficiency

Diagnostic Procedures/Surgery

- Potential echocardiographic findings:
  - Pericardial effusion in approximately 1/3 of patients with myxedema
  - Rarely cardiac tamponade
  - Left ventricular dilatation
  - Systolic dysfunction at rest or with exertion
  - Isolated diastolic dysfunction
- Coronary angiography in hypothyroid patients with angina often reveals severe coronary artery disease.

Pathologic Findings

- Heart often pale, flabby, and grossly dilated in frank myxedema
- Microscopic examination in myxedema reveals myofibrillar swelling, loss of striations, and interstitial fibrosis.

DIFFERENTIAL DIAGNOSIS

- The nephrotic syndrome may resemble myxedema (facial puffiness, pallor, anemia, and hypercholesterolemia).
- Myxedematous heart failure differs from other causes of heart failure because:
  - There is usually a normal chronotropic response to exercise
  - Pulmonary edema is rare
  - Pleural/pericardial effusions have a higher protein content

 TREATMENT

GENERAL MEASURES

- Usually a normal metabolic state should be restored gradually in patients with heart disease. In adults, levothyroxine may be initiated at 25 μg/day and increased by 12.5- to 25-μg increments every 4–6 weeks until a euthyroid state is achieved.
- In known or suspected pituitary and hypothalamic hypothyroidism, treatment with hydrocortisone should precede thyroid replacement to avoid unmasking adrenal insufficiency. Also, hydrocortisone should be given during rapid thyroid hormone treatment.
- Pericardiocentesis for rare cardiac tamponade

MEDICATION (DRUGS)

- Unless contraindicated, beta-blocking drugs can be added if thyroid hormone therapy exacerbates myocardial ischemia.
- Digitalis glycosides may be beneficial.
- When severe heart failure or cardiogenic shock results from hypothyroidism, intravenous T_3 is recommended.
- Subclinical hypothyroidism
  – L-T_4 25 μg/day decreases lipoprotein (a) levels
- Hypothyroidism
  – Titration to daily L-T_4 doses of 150 μg or higher prevents atherosclerosis progression.
- Severe angina pectoris
  – Surgical or percutaneous revascularization may be performed with low-dose thyroid replacement, followed by postoperative or post-procedural full thyroid replacement.
  – Beta-blockers may be tried cautiously if no contraindication. Beware of severe bradycardia.
- Hypothyroidism due to amiodarone use:
  – Amiodarone discontinuation may restore euthyroid state within 2–4 months if no anti-thyroid antibodies present.
  – Thyroid hormone replacement usually added while amiodarone continued. Higher dose of thyroxine replacement may be needed.

 FOLLOW-UP

Admission Criteria
- Moderate to severe heart failure
- QTc $\geq$520 msec, syncope, or ventricular tachycardia (monitored bed)
- Evidence of cardiac tamponade
- Severe angina or acute coronary syndrome

Discharge Criteria
- Stabilization/treatment of heart failure, acute coronary syndrome, or tamponade.

PROGNOSIS
- Full recovery of arrhythmias, hypertension, edema, hyperlipidemia is expected. Coronary artery disease is not reversible. Cardiomyopathy may be reversible with thyroid and heart failure treatment.

COMPLICATIONS
- Unstable angina, heart failure, and pericardial tamponade

PATIENT MONITORING
- Thyroid tests (T_4, T_3, and TSH) should be measured every 4–6 weeks until a euthyroid state is attained. Optimum L-T_4 dose should be based on TSH and serum T_3.
- After patient becomes euthyroid on appropriate L-T_4 dose, measure TSH annually.
- With concurrent amiodarone use
  – Transient (<3 mo), mild, benign TSH and T4 ↑ may occur early with amiodarone use (TSH usually <20mU/L though); repeat TSH needs to be followed closely, and if TSH normalizes, thyroid replacement therapy unnecessary
  – In all patients: Check TSH prior to starting drug, then every 3–6 months for up to 1 year after discontinuation of amiodarone

REFERENCES
1. Walsh JP, et al. Subclinical thyroid dysfunction as a risk factor for cardiovascular disease. *Arch Intern Med*. 2005;165:2467–2472.
2. Rodondi N, et al. Subclinical hypothyroidism and the risk of heart failure, other cardiovascular events, and death. *Arch Intern Med*. 2005;165:2460–2466.
3. Vorperian VR, Havighurst TC, Miller S, et al. Adverse effects of low dose amiodarone: A meta-analysis. *J Am Coll Cardiol*. 1997;30(3):791–798.
4. Tadei S, Caraccio N, Virdis A, et al. Impaired endothelium-dependent vasodilation in subclinical hypothyroidism: Beneficial effect of levothyroxine therapy. *J Clin Endocrinol Metab*. 2003;88(8):3731–3737.
5. Basaria S, Cooper DS. Amiodarone and the thyroid. *Am J Med*. 2005;118(7):706–714.

 MISCELLANEOUS

CODES
ICD9-CM
244.9 + 429.9 Hypothyroid heart disease

Diet
- No-added-salt diet
- Reduced saturated fat and cholesterol diet

Prevention
- Judicious monitoring of thyroid function in patients with known thyroid disease or with risk factors for thyroid disease (such as other autoimmune disease or amiodarone use).

FAQ
- In a patient with symptomatic CAD and hypothyroidism, when and how should thyroxine replacement be initiated?
  – Low dose replacement should be slowly titrated once the patient has been revascularized or medically optimized.
- How frequently do thyroid function tests need to be checked in patients taking amiodarone?
  – Every 3–6 months
- Does amiodarone have to be discontinued if a patient develops hypothyroidism?
  – Not usually. Thyroxine replacement may be added if amiodarone therapy is essential.

H

HYPOXIC HEART SYNDROME, AND HIGH-ALTITUDE PULMONARY EDEMA (HAPE)

Gerald A. Charlton

BASICS

DESCRIPTION
- High-altitude pulmonary edema (HAPE) is a form of noncardiogenic pulmonary edema that occurs after ascending to altitudes above 8,000 feet.
  - Usually occurs in young, healthy persons who have quickly ascended to altitude and then engaged in physical exertion before they have become acclimated
  - Can also occur in persons who reside at high altitude and return home after a few days at lower altitude
- Systems affected: Pulmonary
- Synonym(s): Noncardiogenic pulmonary edema

GENERAL PREVENTION
- Rate of ascent and altitude achieved are critical in development of HAPE
  - Slow rate of ascent
  - Average increase in sleeping altitude 1,000–1,200 ft/day above 8,000 feet
  - No ascent to higher altitude with symptoms of acute mountain sickness (AMS)
  - Descent when symptoms of AMS do not improve after a day of rest
- Limit activity for first 1–2 days.
  - Vigorous exercise should be avoided until acclimatized to altitude.
- Diet high in carbohydrates may be beneficial.
- Avoid alcohol.
- Drink plenty of fluids.

EPIDEMIOLOGY
- Predominant age: Young adults
- Predominant sex: Males > Females

Pediatric Considerations
- Children more susceptible
- Upper respiratory tract infection or bronchitis may be precipitating factors.

Geriatric Considerations
Recovery may be slower

Incidence
Incidence ranges from 1/10,000 Colorado skiers to 1/50 climbers on Mt. McKinley.

Prevalence
In the U.S., occurs in 0.2–15% of the population, depending on factors such as age, sex, and rate of ascent

RISK FACTORS
- Altitude achieved (increased incidence with higher altitude)
- Rate of ascent (increased incidence associated with more rapid ascents)
- Cold exposure
- Upper respiratory infection may increase risk
- Prior history of HAPE

Pregnancy Considerations
- Women with low-risk pregnancies should experience no difficulties up to approximately 10,000 feet.
- Women with high-risk or late-term pregnancies should avoid high altitudes.

Genetics
Unknown

PATHOPHYSIOLOGY
- Pronounced hypoxia-induced patchy pulmonary vasoconstriction may lead to overperfusion of the less obstructed portions of the vascular bed, leading to endothelial injury and pulmonary edema.
- Pulmonary edema is thought to be secondary to increased capillary permeability and increased pulmonary artery pressure without increased pulmonary capillary wedge pressure.

ETIOLOGY
Hypoxia (decreased inspired PO_2) plays a central role.

ASSOCIATED CONDITIONS
- Hypothermia
- Acute mountain sickness
- High-altitude cerebral edema

DIAGNOSIS

SIGNS AND SYMPTOMS
- Symptoms begin within 2–5 days of a rapid ascent.
- Most cases are preceded by symptoms of AMS.

History
- Early symptoms
  - Dyspnea
  - Fatigue
  - Decreased exercise tolerance
  - Weakness
  - Dry cough
- Late symptoms
  - Confusion

Physical Exam
- Tachycardia
- Tachypnea
- Rales
- Pink-tinged frothy sputum
- Cyanosis
- Fever (usually <38.5°C)

TESTS
- No diagnostic tests; diagnosis is made on clinical grounds.
- ECG
  - Usually shows sinus tachycardia and may demonstrate right ventricular strain, right-axis deviation, right bundle branch block, and P-wave abnormalities.

Lab
- No characteristic findings in common laboratory tests
- CBC: Frequent leukocytosis
- Arterial blood gas: Respiratory alkalosis and low oxygen saturation

Imaging
- Chest radiograph
  - Normal cardiac size
  - Diffuse, peripheral patchy infiltrates, may be unilateral or bilateral
  - Becomes more homogeneous in advanced cases and during recovery

Pathologic Findings
Lung edema

DIFFERENTIAL DIAGNOSIS
- Viral or bacterial upper respiratory infection
- Pneumonia
- Congestive heart failure
- Asthma
- Hyperventilation syndrome
- Mucus plugging
- Myocardial infarction
- Pulmonary embolus

TREATMENT

GENERAL MEASURES
- Immediate improvement in oxygenation is the treatment of choice:
  - Descent is critical, at least 3,000 feet as soon as possible
  - Supplemental oxygen at 2–6 L/min to keep oxygen saturation above 90%
  - If descent not feasible, use a hyperbaric bag to simulate descent
  - May benefit from continuous positive airway pressure mask if available

 ## MEDICATION (DRUGS)

First Line
- High-flow oxygen to maintain oxygen saturation above 90%
- Nifedipine SR 30 mg every 12–24 hours, only necessary when supplemental oxygen is unavailable and descent is impossible
  - Contraindications: Refer to manufacturer's literature.
  - Precautions: Refer to manufacturer's literature.

 ## FOLLOW-UP

DISPOSITION
- If patient can maintain oxygen saturation above 90%, discharge on home oxygen with next day follow-up.
- Must have reliable person with them to observe for worsening condition

Admission Criteria
- Required for patients unable to maintain saturations above 90% with supplemental oxygen
- Patients with concomitant high-altitude cerebral edema also should be hospitalized.

Discharge Criteria
When clinically improved and maintaining oxygenation

PROGNOSIS
- Mild cases show improvement in symptoms within hours and complete recovery within 2–3 days.
- Untreated and unable to descend, mortality rate >50%
- Severe, advanced cases may require prolonged hospital course.

COMPLICATIONS
Death, arrhythmias, cardiac arrest

PATIENT MONITORING
Pulse oximetry to monitor arterial oxygen saturation

REFERENCES
1. Auerbach P. *Wilderness medicine*, 3rd ed. St. Louis: CV Mosby, 1995.
2. Bartsch P. High altitude pulmonary edema. *Med Sci Sports Exerc*. 1999;31(Suppl):23–27.
3. Hackett PH, Roach RC. High-altitude illness. *N Engl J Med*. 2001;345:107–114.
4. Hultgren HN. High-altitude pulmonary edema: Current concepts. *Annu Rev Med*. 1996; 47:267–284.
5. West JB. The physiologic basis of high-altitude diseases. *Ann Intern Med*. 2004;789–800.
6. Zafren K, Honigman B. High-altitude medicine. *Emerg Med Clin North Am*. 1997;15:191–221.

 ## MISCELLANEOUS

CODES
ICD9-CM
518.4 Acute edema of lung

PATIENT TEACHING
Persons with history of HAPE are at increased risk of recurrence.

Activity
As tolerated during recovery

Prevention
- Nifedipine 20 mg every 8 hours or 30 mg of sustained release every 12–24 hours in patients with history of HAPE
- Rate of ascent and altitude achieved are critical in development of HAPE
  - Slow rate of ascent
  - Average increase in sleeping altitude 1,000–1,200 ft/day above 8,000 feet
  - No ascent to higher altitude with symptoms of acute mountain sickness (AMS)
  - Descent when symptoms of AMS do not improve after a day of rest
- Limit activity for first 1–2 days
  - Vigorous exercise should be avoided until acclimatized to altitude

FAQ
Q: Who is at risk of developing HAPE?
A: Persons who ascend quickly to altitudes above 8,000 feet, and participate in vigorous exercise before becoming acclimated. Other risk factors include a history of prior high-altitude illness and a concurrent upper respiratory tract infection. Physical fitness does not appear to be protective against high-altitude illness.

Q: Can HAPE be prevented?
A: The incidence of HAPE can be reduced by reducing the rate of ascent (limiting increases in sleeping altitude to 1,000–1.200 feet per day at altitudes above 8,000 feet) and limiting vigorous physical activity for 1–2 days post ascent.

Q: What is the treatment for HAPE?
A: The key to treating HAPE is in treating the hypoxia that causes the pulmonary vasoconstriction and pulmonary edema. This is best done with supplemental oxygen and/or descent to a lower altitude.

H

KAWASAKI'S DISEASE

Peter C. Grow
Nanette K. Wenger

 BASICS

DESCRIPTION

- Kawasaki disease (KD) (i.e., Kawasaki syndrome) is an acute, self-limited, generalized systemic vasculitis of infancy and childhood first described by Dr. Tomisaku Kawasaki in 1967 and initially designated as the mucocutaneous lymph node syndrome.
- KD is the leading cause of acquired, noncongenital heart disease in children in North America and Japan, surpassing acute rheumatic fever.
- The classic diagnosis of KD has been based on the presence of ≥5 days of fever and ≥4 of the 5 principal clinical features (see Signs and Symptoms). Patients with fever and <4 principal features can be diagnosed as having KD when coronary artery disease is detected by two-dimensional (2D) echocardiography or coronary angiography.
- Three described phases:
  - Acute febrile phase (days 1–11): high spiking (>39°C) and persistent fever unresponsive to antipyretics and antibiotics lasting a mean of 11 days but up to 3–4 weeks without appropriate therapy. Other clinical findings include irritability, bilateral conjunctival injection without exudate, polymorphous exantham, cervical lymphadenopathy (>1.5 cm in diameter), erythema and edema of the palms and soles, and changes in the lips and oral cavity including erythema, dryness, fissuring, cracking, and strawberry tongue.
    - Cardiovascular manifestations are prominent in the acute phase and are the leading cause of long-term morbidity and mortality. They include coronary artery ectasia and aneurysms (CAA), myocarditis, congestive heart failure, pericarditis, pericardial effusion, arrhythmia, and mitral/aortic regurgitation.
    - CAA occurs in approximately 15–25% of untreated patients during the acute phase and is pathognomonic of KD when identified in the setting of a compatible febrile illness. Aneurysms have been detected around 3 days of onset of illness but more commonly occur from 10 days to 4 weeks after onset of symptoms. They may also occur in the renal, iliac, and axillary arteries.
  - Subacute phase (days 12–21): resolution of the fever, persistent irritability and conjunctival injection, and exfoliative changes of the skin of the feet and hands around the nails
  - Convalescent phase (days 22–60): begins when all signs of illness have disappeared and continues until acute-phase reactants [erythrocyte sedimentationrate (ESR) and C reactive protein (CRP)] have resolved
    - The most significant clinical finding that persists is the presence of CAA.
- 10–45% of KD cases may have an incomplete or atypical course. Incomplete disease should be considered in all children with unexplained fever for ≥5 days associated with 2–3 of the principal clinical features. In atypical cases, lymph nodes are usually normal and there is no rash, whereas 90% have mucosal changes.

EPIDEMIOLOGY

- Considerable geographic, seasonal, and racial variability
  - Peak incidence between 6 months and 5 years of age (85% of cases <5 years old)
  - Recurrence rate of ~4%
  - Males > Females by ~1.5–1.7:1
  - More common in children in Japan and children of Japanese or Pacific Island ancestry
  - More common in winter and early spring months

Incidence

- Increasing globally
- Japan incidence ~120–150 cases per 100,000 children <5 years old
- In the United States, incidence highest in children of Asian and Pacific Island descent (32.5/100,000 <5 years old), intermediate in non-Hispanic African Americans (16.9/100,000 <5 years old) and Hispanics (11.1/100,000 <5 years old), and lowest in whites (9.1/100,000 <5 years old).

Prevalence

- Asians > blacks > whites

RISK FACTORS

- Reported possible linkage to exposure to freshly cleaned carpets, humidifier use, and residence near a body of water
- Antecedent respiratory illness and pre-existing eczema reported associated with KD
- Disease onset at <6 months at higher risk for coronary aneurysms

Genetics

- KD is associated with certain gene polymorphisms and major histocompatability alleles in different populations
- Proportion of cases with positive family history is ~1%
- Siblings have >10-fold risk of developing disease within 1 year after onset of first case in a family

PATHOPHYSIOLOGY

- Vasculitic lesions marked by endothelial cell edema, proliferation, necrosis, and adhesion of polymorphonuclear leukocytes
- Immune activation with increasing levels of circulating cytokines and CD4 and CD8 cells, polyclonal hypergammaglobulinemia, and circulating immunoglobulin G (IgG) and IgM immunocomplexes
- Matrix metalloproteinases (MMPs) and their endogenenous tissue inhibitors (TIMPs) may play a role

ETIOLOGY

- Unknown
- Infectious etiology suspected because of acute, self-limited course and periodic outbreaks
  - Another hypothesis is a bacterial superantigen stimulating the disease process

ASSOCIATED CONDITIONS

- HIV
  - KD rarely seen in adults. Among adult patients with KD that have been described, a disproportionate number are infected with HIV.

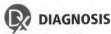 **DIAGNOSIS**

SIGNS AND SYMPTOMS

- Diagnosis of KD is based on the presence of ≥5 days of fever, ≥4 of the 5 principal clinical features in the following list, and by lack of another known disease process to explain the illness.
  - Bilateral conjunctival injection
  - Changes of the mucous membranes of the upper respiratory tract: injected pharynx; injected, fissured lips; strawberry tongue
  - Polymorphous rash
  - Changes of the extremities: peripheral edema, peripheral erythema, periungual desquamation
  - Nonpurulent cervical lymphadenopathy

History

- Irritable child
- Fever
- Gastrointestinal complaints in one third of patients
- Arthralgias

Physical Exam

- Cardiac auscultation may reveal hyperdynamic precordium, tachycardia, gallop rhythm, friction rub, innocent flow murmur, mitral regurgitation
- Mucosal membrane changes
- Skin rash, erythema, or edema
- Cervical lymphadenopathy

TESTS

- Electrocardiogram (ECG) may show arrhythmia, prolonged PR interval, decreased voltage, nonspecific ST- and T-wave changes, ST-segment changes consistent with myocardial injury
- Echocardiography may reveal CAA, pericardial effusion
- ECG-gated magnetic resonance imaging (MRI) and magnetic resonance angiography (MRA) are alternative methods of visualization of the coronary arteries (limited data exist)
- Ultrafast CT is an option for imaging coronary arteries (limited data exist)

Lab

- No specific laboratory test
  - In acute phase, positive inflammatory markers present: leukocytosis, elevated ESR, higher CRP
  - Other nonspecific lab abnormalities: hypochromic anemia, thrombocytosis, hypoalbuminemia, hyponatremia, albuminuria or sterile pyuria, elevated total bilirubin, SGOT/SGPT, lactate dehydrogenase (LDH), creatine phosphokinase (CPK), and troponin-I

Imaging

- Coronary angiography gold standard for diagnosing coronary artery aneurysms (CAAs)
- Screening echocardiography (ECHO) is the noninvasive study of choice to demonstrate CAA
- MRI/MRA may delineate CAA
- Spiral CT

Diagnostic Procedures/Surgery

- Cardiac stress testing for reversible ischemia indicated to assess existence and functional consequences of CAA
- Coronary angiography

Pathologic Findings

- Coronary artery ectasia or aneurysms
  - Thrombosed CAA may undergo recanalization, forming two or more new arteries that each possess a normal wall architecture, braided together within the original artery known as "arteriae in arteria"
- Vasculitis

DIFFERENTIAL DIAGNOSIS

- Viral infections (e.g., measles, adenovirus, enterovirus, Epstein-Barr virus)
- Scarlet fever
- Staphylococcal scalded skin syndrome
- Toxic shock syndrome
- Bacterial cervical lymphadenitis
- Drug hypersensitivity reactions
- Stevens-Johnson syndrome
- Juvenile rheumatoid arthritis
- Rocky Mountain spotted fever
- Leptospirosis
- Mercury hypersensitivity reaction (acrodynia)

 MEDICATION (DRUGS)

First Line

- Acute phase: Aspirin (ASA) 80–100 mg/kg/day in 4 doses with intravenous immunoglobulin (IVIG, see subsequent text)
- Reduce ASA dose to 3–5 mg/kg/day after child is afebrile for 48–72 hours, and maintain it until the patient shows no evidence of coronary changes by 6–8 weeks
- Continue ASA indefinitely in children who develop coronary abnormalities
  - Reye syndrome is a risk in patients who take salicylates while infected with active varicella or influenza, and has been reported in children with KD
  - Salicylates should be avoided for at least 6 weeks after the administration of a live virus vaccine
- IVIG, 2 g/kg in a single infusion together with ASA
  - ≥10% of patients with KD fail to defervesce with initial therapy, and a retreatment with IVIG, 2 g/kg is recommended
  - Measles and varicella immunizations should be deferred for 11 months after a child receives IVIG
- Thrombolytic therapy has been given to patients who develop an acute myocardial infarction or intraaneurysmal thrombus
- Patients with giant aneurysms (>8 mm in diameter) should receive low dose ASA + warfarin to prevent thrombosis

Second Line

- Corticosteroid use in KD is not well established
- Pentoxifylline treatment in KD is uncertain
- Plasma exchange has been reported to be effective in patients refractory to IVIG
- Limited data on use of percutaneous coronary interventions for coronary artery disease due to KD
- Abciximab plus standard therapy has been shown to cause a greater regression in maximum aneurysm diameter
- Cytotoxic agents, such as cyclophosphamide, have been reported to be useful in refractory cases

SURGERY

- Coronary artery bypass grafting (CABG) is generally indicated if there is severe obstruction of the left main coronary artery, or high-grade lesions in at least 2 of the 3 major coronary arteries
- Cardiac transplantation has been performed

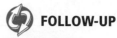 **FOLLOW-UP**

DISPOSITION

Admission Criteria

Patients with KD should be admitted to a pediatric cardiology service for aggressive therapy

Issues for Referral

- Pediatric cardiologist to follow CAA
- Serial ECHO to follow CAA
- Coronary MRI/MRA is an alternative noninvasive imaging technique for following CAA

PROGNOSIS

- Depends largely on the cardiac manifestations and size of CAA
  - Worst prognosis in children with giant CAA
- CAA regress in ~50–67% of vessels at 1–2 years

COMPLICATIONS

- Primary complications involve development and rupture of CAA
- Dehydration may result from fever or anorexia
- Joint inflammation in acute phase may limit mobility

PATIENT MONITORING

- Long-term monitoring and management depends on degree of coronary artery involvement
  - Practical guidelines have been published (see Newburger et al.)

REFERENCES

1. Burns JC, Glodé MP. Kawasaki syndrome. *Lancet*. 2004;364:533–544.
2. Newburger JW, Takahashi M, Gerber MA, et al. Diagnosis, treatment, and long-term management of Kawasaki disease: A statement for health professionals from the Committee on Rheumatic Fever, Endocarditis and Kawasaki Disease, Council on Cardiovascular Disease in the Young, American Heart Association. *Circulation*. 2004;110:2747–2771.
3. Wang CL, Wu YT, Liu CA, et al. Kawasaki disease: Infection, immunity and genetics. *Pediatr Infect Dis J*. 2005;24:998–1004.

CODES

ICD9-CM

446.1 Kawasaki disease

PATIENT TEACHING

- Internet resource
  - www.kdfoundation.org

K

L TRANSPOSITION OF THE GREAT ARTERIES

Leonardo Liberman
Welton M. Gersony

 BASICS

DESCRIPTION

Corrected transposition of the great arteries, ventricular inversion, or L transposition of the great arteries (L-TGA) is defined as a congenital cardiac malformation in which the systemic venous blood returns to an anatomic right atrium, which is connected to an anatomic left ventricle and then to the pulmonary artery. The pulmonary venous blood returns to an anatomic left atrium, which is connected to the anatomic right ventricle and then to the aorta. This combination of atrioventricular discordance and ventriculoarterial discordance results in a physiologically normal circulation.

EPIDEMIOLOGY

This is an uncommon cardiac defect that affects 0.6–0.9% of all patients with congenital heart defects. Only 1% of these patients have no other associated cardiac abnormalities. There is a higher incidence in males (63–76%).

ETIOLOGY

Unknown

ASSOCIATED CONDITIONS

L-TGA can be an isolated anatomic defect without major clinical manifestations. However, this lesion is usually associated with other cardiac malformations such as ventricular septal defect, pulmonary outflow tract obstruction, abnormalities of the systemic atrioventricular valve (Ebstein-type malformation), and conduction system defects. These patients have a fragile conduction system, and there can be a progressive incidence of developing complete heart block (1–2%/year). The presence of associated intracardiac malformations is so common that they should be considered as part of the disease.

 DIAGNOSIS

SIGNS AND SYMPTOMS

- The timing of presentation in cases of L-TGA is significantly influenced by the presence of associated malformations. The majority of the patients have signs or symptoms in the first few months of life, depending on the predominant associated lesion. The infant may present with signs or symptoms of congestive heart failure if the predominant associated lesion is a ventricular septal defect or systemic atrioventricular valve regurgitation, or with cyanosis if it is pulmonary outflow tract obstruction.
- Older patients can present with signs and symptoms of congestive heart failure secondary to poor systemic right ventricular function or progressive tricuspid (systemic) atrioventricular valve regurgitation. With balanced anomalies, patients can remain symptom free for years or even decades.
- Some patients are diagnosed during evaluation of a heart murmur or after seeing an abnormal chest x-ray obtained for other reasons.

Physical Exam

- The physical exam findings are determined by the presence of the associated lesions.
- Most patients are acyanotic unless severe pulmonary stenosis is present.
- A loud single second heart sound is characteristic in patients with L-TGA due to the anterior position of the aortic valve.
- The characteristics of the murmur depend on the predominant associated lesion (ventricular septal defect, pulmonary stenosis, or tricuspid regurgitation).

TESTS

- Electrocardiogram (ECG) usually shows reversed septal depolarization with Q waves that are present in the right precordial leads but absent over the left precordium (the initial ventricular septal activation is from right to left).
- Ambulatory 24-hour ECG recording (Holter) is periodically used to follow atrioventricular nodal function in this group of patients where progressive atrioventricular block is common.

Imaging

- Chest x-ray may show a leftward ascending aorta that can be seen in the left upper border of the cardiac silhouette. Like the other clinical findings, the radiographic findings depend on the position of the heart and the presence of associated lesions.
- Echocardiography is the optimal method for diagnosis and evaluation of L-TGA and associated lesions. The main finding is the presence of ventricular inversion. The anatomic right atrium connects through a mitral valve (with two papillary muscles) to a morphologic left ventricle with smooth wall located on the right side. The anatomic left atrium connects via a tricuspid valve to a morphologic left-sided right ventricle characterized by chordal attachments of the atrioventricular valve to the septum, coarse trabeculations, and the presence of a moderator band.
- Cardiac catheterization is not necessary to establish the diagnosis of L-TGA; however, it is needed to assess the hemodynamic status in certain cases before surgery. Special care should be taken to avoid catheter trauma to the delicate conduction system.
- Echocardiographic assessment of the function of a morphologic right ventricle is challenging because of the complex shape of this chamber. In recent years, cardiac magnetic resonance has evolved to be a good quantitative standard, especially for serial comparisons.

DIFFERENTIAL DIAGNOSIS

The differential diagnosis of L-TGA depends on the associated lesions.

- Patients with right ventricular outflow tract obstruction should be differentiated from patients with tetralogy of Fallot or ventricular septal defect with pulmonary stenosis.
- The differential diagnosis in patients with congestive heart failure includes ventricular septal defect, endocardial cushion defects, and patent ductus arteriosus.

 ## TREATMENT

GENERAL MEASURES

- Patients with L-TGA and no associated cardiac defects do not require intervention.
- The nature of the associated cardiac defect will determine the need for intervention. A neonate with severe cyanosis secondary to pulmonary outflow tract obstruction will need surgical palliation by placement of a systemic-to-pulmonary artery shunt. Conversely, an infant with congestive heart failure due to a large ventricular septal defect may need anticongestive therapy or even pulmonary banding or surgical closure of the defect.

 ## MEDICATION (DRUGS)

- In case of significant right ventricular outflow tract obstruction at birth, the newborn requires prostaglandin infusion to maintain ductal patency.
- Patients with large ventricular septal defects, right ventricular failure, or severe tricuspid valve regurgitation need anticongestive treatment and diuretics.
- Endocarditis prophylaxis

SURGERY

- A double switch operation has been considered an attractive surgical alternative for this cardiac defect. This can be accomplished by combining an atrial switch operation (Senning or Mustard operation) with either an arterial switch operation or, if pulmonary stenosis is present, the Rastelli procedure (tunneling the anatomic left ventricle to the aorta through a ventricular septal defect and placement of a right ventricle to pulmonary artery conduit). In this way, the morphologic left ventricle becomes the systemic ventricle and the morphologic right ventricle, the pulmonary ventricle.
- In case of complete heart block, permanent transvenous or epicardial pacemaker is implanted when the patient meets the criteria determined by the American Heart Association (AHA) and American College of Cardiology (ACC).

 ## FOLLOW-UP

PROGNOSIS

- The natural history of L-TGA is determined by the presence of associated cardiac defects and the onset of acquired changes. Although long life expectancy is possible, it is rare in this group of patients. There is a high incidence of systemic ventricular dysfunction and congestive heart failure, leading to high mortality rate, particularly in patients with tricuspid (systemic valve) regurgitation, heart block, or other associated cardiac defects.
- When the right ventricle fails as a systemic ventricle despite anticongestive therapy, cardiac transplantation is often needed.
- The results of pregnancy with L-TGA depend on the status of the ventricular function and the presence of associated lesions. Cardiac risks are increased in patients with cyanotic forms of this lesion.

PATIENT MONITORING

Frequent follow-up is necessary following the state of the tricuspid valve, ventricular function, and cardiac rhythm.

REFERENCES

1. Freedom RM. Discordant atrioventricular connections and congenitally corrected transposition. In: Anderson RH, Baker EJ, Macartney FJ, et al. *Pediatric Cardiology*. London: Churchill Livingstone, 2002:1321–1351.
2. Fyler DC. Corrected transposition of the great arteries. In: Fyler DC, ed. *Nadas' Pediatric Cardiology*. Philadelphia: Hanley and Belfus Inc; 1992:701–706.
3. Gregoratos G. Abrams J. Epstein AE, et al. ACC/AHA/NASPE 2002 guideline update for implantation of cardiac pacemakers and antiarrhythmia devices. *Circulation*. 2002;106:2145–2161.
4. Lundstrom U, Bull C, Wyse RKH, et al. The natural and "unnatural" history of congenitally corrected transposition. *Am J Cardiol*. 1990;65:1222–1229.
5. Prieto LR, Hordof AJ, Secir M, et al. Progressive tricuspid valve disease in patients with congenitally corrected transposition of the great arteries. *Circulation*. 1998;98:997–1005.
6. Rutledge JM, Nihill MR, Fraser CD, et al. Outcome of 121 patients with congenitally corrected transposition of the great arteries. *Pediatr Cardiol*. 2002;23:137–145.
7. Van Praagh R, Papagiannis J, Gründenfelder J, et al. Pathologic anatomy of corrected transposition of the great arteries: Medical and surgical implications. *Am Heart J*. 1998;135:772–785.

CODES
ICD9-CM
745.12

L

LEFT VENTRICULAR OUTFLOW OBSTRUCTIVE, NONVALVULAR

David A. Crowe
Welton M. Gersony

 BASICS

DESCRIPTION

Left ventricular outflow tract obstruction (LVOTO) may be valvar, subvalvar, or supravalvar. Combined lesions can occur. This chapter will discuss nonvalvular LVOTO.

- Subaortic obstructive defects include discrete fibromuscular ridges, hypertrophic cardiomyopathy idiopathic hypertrophic subaortic stenosis (HCM/IHSS) with systolic anterior motion of the mitral valve (SAM), accessory endocardial cushion tissue, and fibromuscular tunnel.
- Supravalvar aortic stenosis may occur as a discrete lesion immediately distal to the aortic valve, long segment narrowing of the transverse aortic arch, localized fibrous membrane, or discrete narrowing of the aorta, forming an aortic coarctation.

GENERAL PREVENTION

LVOTO obstruction is a congenital condition that may be progressive and requires serial follow-up as dictated by the cardiologist.

EPIDEMIOLOGY

- Subvalvar aortic stenosis constitutes 8–20% of left ventricular outflow tract obstruction. Supravalvar stenosis is the least common form.
- Discrete membranous subaortic obstruction: Male > female predominance (2:1)
- Obstruction in HCM/IHSS occurs in 30/100,000 population

RISK FACTORS

Pregnancy Considerations

- Potential poor tolerance of decreased systemic vascular resistance and increased blood volume, which accompanies pregnancy because of an inability to increase stroke volume; tachycardia may produce heart failure and myocardial ischemia
- HCM/IHSS may reduce outflow gradient related to increased blood volume.

Genetics

Supravalvar obstruction is associated with Williams syndrome in approximately 30–50% of cases; the remainder are non-Williams and are often familial.

PATHOPHYSIOLOGY

Obstruction to left-sided outflow can cause poor cardiac output; can be associated with poor exercise tolerance.

ETIOLOGY

- HCM/IHSS is related to autosomal dominance in 50%; may occur with Friedreich ataxia (autosomal recessive or dominant inheritance), LEOPARD syndrome, and Pompe disease (glycogen storage disorder).
- Supravalvar aortic obstruction can occur as an autosomal-dominant trait; an elastin gene abnormality (7q11) has been determined to cause Williams syndrome.
- No determined genetic etiology for other forms

ASSOCIATED CONDITIONS

- Subvalvar outflow obstruction is associated with valvar stenosis, aortic coarctation, ventricular septal defect, double outlet right ventricle, D-transposition of the great arteries, and endocardial cushion defects.
- Supravalvular outflow obstruction is associated with peripheral pulmonic stenosis, ventricular septal defect, patent ductus arteriosus, pulmonary valve stenosis, abnormalities of coronary arteries, and aortic coarctation. In Williams syndrome, both supravalvar aortic stenosis and peripheral pulmonic stenosis are most often present. In adult life, other arterial lesions may occur.

DIAGNOSIS

SIGNS AND SYMPTOMS

History

- Often asymptomatic; may be discovered only during referral for murmur evaluation
- Chest pain, dyspnea, and tachycardia are noted with severe HCM/IHSS, especially in adolescents and children. Chest pain is not anginal, although some studies have described evidence of ischemia.
- HCM/IHSS may present in infancy with congestive heart failure (CHF) with poor feeding/growth and respiratory distress.
- HCM/IHSS may be associated with supraventricular and ventricular arrhythmias; most common is nonsustained ventricular tachycardia.
- HCM is the most common cause of sudden death in the adolescent population; family history of sudden early death often can be confirmed.

Physical Exam

- Discrete subvalvar obstruction
  - Soft murmur at left medial/left lateral sternal border radiating to upper sternal border and suprasternal notch
  - No systolic ejection click
  - Early diastolic murmur of aortic insufficiency may be audible.
  - Pulses are usually symmetric.
- HCM/IHSS
  - Variable
  - Often healthy appearing, may have normal examination results
  - Often increased apical impulse
  - First heart sound (S_1) normal; second heart sound (S_2) may be paradoxically split with delayed closure of aortic valve
  - Systolic ejection murmur at left lower sternal border and apex; increases with decreased preload (i.e., Valsalva maneuver)
  - May be holosystolic murmur at apex and axilla with associated mitral regurgitation; often difficult to discern from outflow murmur

- Supravalvar obstruction
  - Features of Williams syndrome may be present, including elfin facies
  - Thrill often palpable at suprasternal notch and carotid vessels
  - No systolic click
  - Blood pressure differential between right and left arms may be present.
  - Systolic ejection murmur at base of heart radiating to neck
  - Murmur of aortic insufficiency may be present.
  - Coexistent murmur of peripheral pulmonic stenosis may be present.

TESTS

Lab

- Electrocardiogram (ECG)
  - LV hypertrophy in proportion to degree of obstruction: wide spectrum, may be minimal to severe
  - Prominent hypertrophy accompanied by ST- and T-wave changes
- Holter
  - Holter monitor and exercise study to screen for possible arrhythmias
  - Supraventricular arrhythmias and ventricular arrhythmias may be documented, especially runs of nonsustained ventricular tachycardia

Imaging

- Chest x-ray
  - Usually normal cardiac silhouette and pulmonary vascular markings, although a congestive heart may cause pulmonary vascular congestion
  - Cardiomegaly may be present late, and enlargement of the LV downward, leftward, and posterior gives the appearance of an elongated heart in the frontal view extending down to the left hemidiaphragm, whereas the lateral view reveals a convex and globular posterior shadow.
  - Aortic root is rarely severely dilated with fixed subaortic obstruction. May appear smaller with supravalvar stenosis.
  - Calcification generally is seen only with valvar stenosis.
- Echocardiogram
  - Excellent modality for diagnosis and examining 2D anatomy of obstruction
  - Allows for evaluation of degree/location of hypertrophy
  - Gradient across obstruction may be estimated by Doppler.
  - Visualization of supravalvar stenosis, degree of narrowing
  - Evaluation of LV size, and septal and free wall thickness
  - Differentiates discrete subaortic stenosis by a fibrous ridge from HCM with muscular obstruction. On occasion, both will be present.
  - Identifies associated lesions

- Cardiac catheterization/angiography
  - Mean left atrial pressure and left ventricular end-diastolic pressure may be elevated
  - Accurate measurement of gradient across obstruction
  - Ventriculogram shows location and dimensions of obstruction and quality of ventricular function
  - Identifies associated lesions, especially peripheral pulmonic stenosis
  - Often not required due to accuracy of noninvasive testing and imaging

Pathologic Findings
HCM/IHSS: Hypertrophy especially of interventricular septum with at times concentric hypertrophy. Myocyte disarray with varying hypertrophy/fibrosis. At times septal coronary vessels thickened with narrowed lumens.

DIFFERENTIAL DIAGNOSIS
Valvar aortic stenosis

TREATMENT

GENERAL MEASURES
- Dependent on nature/degree of obstruction
- Discrete membranous subaortic obstruction tends to be progressive; will usually be referred for surgical resection at time of identification if >30 mm Hg; some patients remain stable with mild gradients
- No vigorous physical activity (e.g., weight lifting, competitive sports)
- Dual-chamber pacing in HCM/IHSS may improve symptomatology and reduce outflow gradient.
- Increased degree of gradient in HCM/IHSS is not correlated directly to increased risk of sudden death.
- Gradient in HCM may be variable.

MEDICATION (DRUGS)

- Antiarrhythmic therapy not required in most cases
- Calcium channel blockers may improve diastolic function in HCM/IHSS
- Atrial fibrillation prominent in HCM/IHSS, especially following surgery
- High-dose β-adrenergic blockade may reduce gradient in HCM/IHSS; may be used for control of ventricular arrhythmias in HCM/IHSS
- Anticongestive measures for late LV dilation and CHF

SURGERY
- The fibromuscular ridge of discrete subvalvar membranous obstruction is resected surgically. Obstruction is generally removed circumferentially during cardiopulmonary bypass and accessed through the aortic valve; septal myotomy also may be performed. Recurrence rate is low with this approach.
- HCM/IHSS referred for myectomy; at times mitral valve repair, dependent on degree of obstruction
- Tunnel-type obstruction may have a history of repeated resections; use of Ross procedure (pulmonary autograft) is recommended.
- Removal of accessory endocardial cushion tissue to relieve LVOTO; may need mitral valve replacement.

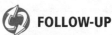

FOLLOW-UP

DISPOSITION
Dependent upon degree of residual obstruction following intervention

Admission Criteria
- Signs/symptoms of LV outflow compromise: Poor perfusion, hypotension, CHF, myocardial infarction, arrhythmia
- Progressive increase in degree of obstruction

Discharge Criteria
Resolution of above status after supportive care or surgical intervention

Issues for Referral
Increasing exercise intolerance, chest pain, palpitations, dizziness, syncope

PROGNOSIS
- Surgery for a discrete membranous obstruction usually yields a good result but can recur; gradient may persist despite surgical resection; reports vary on reoperation with range of 4–16%, subsequent surgery may be required for recurrence of obstruction; significant aortic insufficiency is rare
- HCM/IHSS courses are age dependent. Symptomatic infants have a poor prognosis, with high mortality. The usual course is slow progression of symptoms with risk of sudden death. Some patients remain stable for many years.
- Risk factors for death in HCM/IHSS include family history of sudden death, higher LV end-diastolic pressure, syncope, history of CHF.
- Supravalvar aortic stenosis within or outside the context of Williams syndrome may remain stable for years with mild obstruction. Surgical results are usually excellent. Peripheral pulmonary stenosis rarely leads to right ventricular dysfunction and may regress during childhood. Other arterial stenoses may emerge.

COMPLICATIONS
Subaortic membrane: Aortic insufficiency and heart block are potential complications of surgery.

PATIENT MONITORING
Dependent upon degree of obstruction, symptomatology, surgical history

REFERENCES
1. Berger S, Dhala A, Friedberg DZ. Sudden cardiac death in infants, children, and adolescents. *Pediatr Clin North Am*. 1999;46:221–234.
2. Bruce CJ, et al. Fixed left ventricular outflow tract obstruction presumed hypertrophic obstructive cardiomyopathy: Implications for therapy. *Ann Thorac Surg*. 1999;68:100–104.
3. Darcin OT. Discrete subaortic stenosis: Surgical outcomes and follow-up results. *Tex Heart Inst J*. 2003;30:286–292.
4. Emmanouildes GC, et al. *Moss & Adams*, 5th ed. 1995.
5. Erentug V. Surgical treatment of subaortic obstruction in adolescent and adults: long-term follow-up. *J Card Surg*. 2005;20:16–21.
6. Kim YM, et al. Natural course of supravalvar aortic stenosis and peripheral pulmonary arterial stenosis in William's syndrome. *Cardiol Young*. 1999;9:37–41.
7. Kitchiner D, et al. Prognosis of supravalve aortic stenosis in 81 patients in Liverpool (1960–1993). *Heart*. 1996;75:396–402.
8. Kizilbash AM, et al. Spontaneous variability of left ventricular outflow tract gradient in hypertrophic obstructive cardiomyopathy. *Circulation*. 1998;97:461–466.
9. Kuck KH. Arrhythmias in hypertrophic cardiomyopathy. *Pacing Clin Electrophysiol*. 1997;20(Part 2):2706–2713.
10. Morris CA. Genetic aspects of supravalvular aortic stenosis. *Curr Opin Cardiol*. 1998;13: 214–219.
11. Oakley CM. Pregnancy and congenital heart disease. *Heart*. 1997;78:12–14.
12. Ostman-Smith I, Wettrell G, Risenfeld T. A cohort study of childhood hypertrophic cardiomyopathy. *J Am Coll Cardiol*. 1999;34:1813–1822.
13. Rayburn ST, Netherland DE, Heath BJ. Discrete membranous subaortic stenosis: Improved results after resection and myectomy. *Ann Thorac Surg*. 1997;64:105–109.
14. Solomon NA, et al. Mild supravalvular aortic stenosis with left coronary obstruction in a neonate. *Ann Thorac Surg*. 2005;79:2153–2155.
15. Stassano P. Discrete subaortic stenosis: Long-term prognosis on the progression of the obstruction and of the aortic insufficiency. *Thorac Cardiovasc Surg*. 2005;53:23–27.
16. Takeuchi M, Abe H, Kuroiwa A. Effect of dual chamber pacing on coronary flow velocity in a patient with hypertrophic obstructive cardiomyopathy. *Pacing Clin Electrophysiol*.1996;19(Part 1):2153–2155.

CODES
ICD9-CM
- 425.4 HCM, nonobstructive
- 425.1 IHSS
- 746.81 Subvalvar aortic stenosis
- 745.9 Endocardial cushion defect
- 747.10 Aortic coarctation
- 747.22 Supravalvar aortic stenosis

PATIENT TEACHING
Diet
No specific dietary changes recommended

Activity
- No vigorous activity/competitive sports
- Higher incidence of sudden death with HCM/IHSS than general population, especially during or following exercise

Prevention
Endocarditis prophylaxis

L

LYME DISEASE AND THE HEART
Maria Cecilia Bahit

 BASICS

DESCRIPTION
Lyme disease is a multisystem infection caused by *Borrelia burgdorferi*, a spirochetal organism transmitted by the Ixodes tick (deer tick).
- Stage 1: Early localized (3–32 days after tick bite) erythema chronicum migrans (90%) and flulike illness
- Stage 2: Early disseminated (weeks to months) multiorgan involvement, most commonly neurologic (10%) and carditis (1–8%)
- Stage 3: Late disseminated (months to years) arthritis (up to 50%) and neurologic syndromes
  - Cardiac manifestations typically occur 1–2 months after onset of infection.
  - Conduction system disease: First-, second-, or third-degree atrioventricular (AV) block, bundle branch block, fascicular block
  - Tachyarrhythmias
    - Myocarditis and pericarditis
    - Cardiomyopathy and congestive heart failure rare in the United States

EPIDEMIOLOGY
- Lyme disease is the leading tick-borne disease in the United States.
- Between May and August
- Highest prevalence in northeastern coastal states, the upper Midwest, and northern California
- Can occur at any age, most common in children and young adults
- Males affected as often as females
- Myocarditis was reported in 8% of U.S. patients before widespread use of antibiotic for erythema migrans; most recent data <1%

Incidence
Overall incidence 4.4/100,000

RISK FACTORS
Exposure to tick-infested area

ETIOLOGY
- Causal microorganism *B. burgdorferi*, transmitted by the bite of Ixodes ticks
- Chronic arthritis related to HLA DR-4

 DIAGNOSIS

SIGNS AND SYMPTOMS
- Cardiac symptoms
  - Asymptomatic
  - Light-headedness
  - Dizziness
  - Syncope
  - Dyspnea
  - Palpitations
  - Chest pain

TESTS
- Electrocardiogram (ECG)
  - AV conduction system disease in up to 90% of patients with Lyme disease: First-, second-, or third-degree AV block, bundle branch block, fascicular block, tachyarrhythmias, nonspecific ST-segment or T-wave changes***

Lab
- Immunoglobulin G (IgG)–IgM burgdorferi antibodies [positive enzyme-linked immunosorbent assay (ELISA) or immunofluorescent assay result should be confirmed by Western blot]. Poor sensitivity early, as antibodies develop slowly: 30–40% seropositive patients early, 60–70% 2–4 weeks after infection
- Culture of skin lesions and polymerase chain reaction of skin biopsy and blood

Imaging
ECG***: Dilated cardiomyopathy is rare.

DIFFERENTIAL DIAGNOSIS
- Rheumatic myocarditis, viral myocarditis
- Juvenile rheumatoid arthritis
- Babesiosis, ehrlichiosis

 TREATMENT

GENERAL MEASURES
- Preventive measures when in grassy or wooded areas, including wearing light-colored clothing, long pants tucked into socks or boots, and long-sleeved shirts, and using tick repellent
- Prophylactic antibiotic therapy is not necessary.

 MEDICATION (DRUGS)

- Most manifestations of Lyme disease resolve spontaneously without treatment.
- Antibiotics may hasten resolution and prevent disease progression.
- Myocarditis
  - Oral treatment for first-degree heart block: doxycycline (100 mg b.i.d. for 14 days), amoxicillin (500 mg t.i.d. for 14 days), cefuroxime axetil 500 mg b.i.d. for 14 days
  - For advanced (second- or third-degree) heart block, no proof that intravenous (IV) treatment is more effective than oral treatment: Ceftriaxone (2 g IV daily for 14 days)
  - Vaccine LYMERIX: Recommended for individuals older than 15 years of age who live or work in grassy or wooded areas and whose exposure is frequent or prolonged

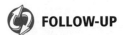

FOLLOW-UP

DISPOSITION
Admission Criteria
- Hospitalize patients with significant PR prolongation or second-degree or complete AV block until antibiotics have been initiated and the heart block has responded.
- Temporary pacing may be necessary.

PROGNOSIS
- Prognosis of cardiac manifestations of Lyme disease is usually good.
- Temporary pacemaker may be required in up to one third of cases.
- Complete recovery occurs in most (up to 90%).
- Late complications such as dilated cardiomyopathy occur rarely.

PATIENT MONITORING
Patients with severe Lyme disease should be monitored with ECG during weeks and months after tick bite to detect conduct abnormalities.

REFERENCES
1. Cox J, et al. Cardiovascular manifestations of Lyme disease. *Am Heart J.* 1991;122:1449–1455.
2. Nadelman RB, Wormser GP. Lyme borreliosis. *Lancet.* 1998;352:557–565.
3. Nagi K, et al. Cardiac manifestations of Lyme disease: A review. *Can J Cardiol.* 1996;12:503–506.
4. Sigal L. Early disseminated Lyme disease: cardiac manifestations. *Am J Med.* 1995;89[Suppl 4A]:25–29.

CODES
ICD9-CM
- 088-8 Other specific arthropod-borne disease
- 088-81 Lyme disease

PATIENT TEACHING
- Protection against tick exposure should be emphasized in endemic areas.
- American Lyme Disease Foundation, One Financial Plaza, Hartford, CT 66103; (860)525–2000; hotline (800)886–LYME; lymefnd@aol.com

L

MARFAN'S SYNDROME

Donna M. Timchak
Welton M. Gersony

 BASICS

DESCRIPTION

Marfan syndrome describes a clinical constellation reflecting connective tissue disease of varying severity.

- The clinical presentation ranges from severe congestive heart failure in the fetus/neonate, to the relatively asymptomatic adult.
- Genetic expression and penetrance determine the clinical manifestations.
- Mitral valve prolapse (MVP) with or without mitral regurgitation and aortic root dilation are the most common cardiac findings.
- The ultimate complication of the disease is aortic dissection with or without aortic valve insufficiency.
- The aim of management is to closely monitor or even retard aortic root growth and, if possible, replace the aorta prophylactically, before dissection occurs.
- Spontaneous pneumothorax, lens dislocation, and scoliosis/lordosis can all be among the presenting findings in Marfan syndrome.
- Patients may be unusually tall with long, slender fingers and toes.
- They may report being "double-jointed" (abnormal appendicular joint mobility).
- The trunk is short compared with leg length, and there can be anterior chest deformity (pectus excavatum or carinatum), giving the patient with Marfan syndrome a characteristic appearance.
- Hernias and lumbosacral spine widening of the neural canal (dural ectasia) also may be present.

EPIDEMIOLOGY

Marfan syndrome is relatively common.

- There is no predilection for race or sex.
- Age at presentation is usually dependent on the severity of the disease:
  - Mild scoliosis in a lanky child may result in a screening echocardiogram, which shows MVP and a dilated aortic root.
  - Ophthalmologic examination may result in the diagnosis of lens dislocation (50%).
  - In some cases, other members of the family with "familial tall stature" are then diagnosed with Marfan disease.
  - A hydropic fetus may have severe MVP/mitral regurgitation on fetal echocardiographic evaluation, and at birth be found to have long digits and heart failure syndrome.
  - Myriad presentations reflect Marfan as a multisystem disease with protean manifestations.

Prevalence

About 1/10,000 population in the United States

RISK FACTORS

The cardiovascular complications of Marfan syndrome are often more severe in young children (infantile type) with new mutations.

Pregnancy Considerations

- Many women with Marfan syndrome have had multiple successful pregnancies.
- Marfan syndrome patients with prominent cardiac manifestations are often discouraged from pursuing pregnancy because of increased risk of aortic dissection.

ETIOLOGY

- Marfan syndrome is autosomal dominant.
  - 25–30% are sporadic, new, dominant mutations; there is full penetrance, but considerable clinical variability.
  - Sporadic cases demonstrate a paternal age effect: In a small series, the fathers were older than fathers in the general population (37 years vs. 30 years).
  - Linkage to chromosome 15 has been established. The gene product, fibrillin, is abnormal in Marfan syndrome.
  - Linkage to chromosome 3, with resultant abnormal TGFβR2 (Transforming Growth Factor-β Receptor 2) is also reported.

ASSOCIATED CONDITIONS

- Marfan syndrome is a multisystem disease.
- In addition to the previously noted characteristics, dolichocephaly, high arched palate, arachnodactyly, striae atrophicae, hernias, and pes planus may all be seen.

DIAGNOSIS

SIGNS AND SYMPTOMS

- Near-sightedness (myopia) in a patient with subluxation of the lenses, should provoke concern for Marfan's syndrome.
- Acute chest pain or relentless "tearing" chest pain in an adolescent or adult with few risk factors for angina, should stimulate concern for ascending aortic or thoracoabdominal aortic dissection.
- Spontaneous pneumothorax in a person of tall stature, with prominent digits, and/or pes planus may be the first presentation of Marfan syndrome.
- Tall patients with scoliosis or lordosis should be evaluated carefully to see if any other criteria for Marfan syndrome are satisfied.
- Patients presenting with a new apical murmur, a mid-systolic click at the left lower sternal border, or a diastolic murmur at the left middle to right upper sternal border should be assessed for other Marfan criteria.

- The positive wrist sign indicates joint hyperextensibility in that the little finger covers the nail of the thumb when one hand is wrapped around the other, at the wrist.
- The positive thumb sign indicates joint hyperextensibility in that the thumb extends beyond the ulnar surface of the hand when the patient is asked to stretch the thumb across the palm.
- The upper-to-lower segment ratio averages 0.85 in patients with Marfan syndrome (normal ratio 0.93). The upper segment of height is the distance from the top of the head to the pubic bone; the lower segment is the length from the pubic bone to the bottom of the foot. This abnormally low ratio in patients with Marfan syndrome reflects their abnormally long limbs.
- The arm span is frequently longer than the height in patients with Marfan syndrome. In the general population, arm span is usually less than or equal to length.

TESTS

- Electrocardiogram (ECG) to evaluate left atrial and left ventricular enlargement complements echocardiography.
- Genetic sequencing may become routine in the future to identify and confirm the abnormality on chromosome 15, and the resultant deficit within fibrillin.

Lab

- Urine amino acid analysis in the absence of pyridoxine supplementation should be obtained to rule out homocystinuria.
- Blood can be obtained to search for deletions/alterations on genes 3 and 15 for research.

Imaging

- Transthoracic echocardiography looks for and quantifies aortic root dilation, compared with normal values for age and body surface area. MVP with or without regurgitation and aortic insufficiency as well as heart function are also assessed. In patients who image well, false lumina in the ascending aorta may be seen.
- CT angiography or magnetic resonance angiography delineates false lumina in patients presenting with possible aortic dissection.
- Arteriography is used to confirm aortic dissection.
- Lumbosacral magnetic resonance imaging (MRI) confirms the presence of dural ectasias.

DIFFERENTIAL DIAGNOSIS
- Homocystinuria
- Klinefelter syndrome
- Fragile-X syndrome
- Ehlers Danlos syndrome
- Erdheim cystic medial necrosis
- Congenital contractural arachnodactyly (Beals Syndrome)
- Stickler syndrome may present with similar connective tissue findings.
- Loeys-Dielz syndrome
- Diagnosis of Marfan's syndrome requires the presence of 2 major criteria plus several minor criteria in another system:
  - Positive family history fulfills 1 major criterion.
  - Other major criteria are ectopia lentis, dilation or dissection of the ascending aorta, and lumbosacral dural ectasias and 4 of 7 major skeletal manifestations:
  - At least 4 of the following should be present:
    - Pectus carinatum or pectus excavatum requiring surgery
    - Positive wrist sign and thumb sign
    - Reduced upper to lower segment ratio <0.86 or arm span to height ratio of >1.05
    - Scoliosis or spondylolisthesis
    - Protrusio acetabula
  - Spontaneous pneumothoraces, striae atrophicae, and recurrent hernias are also useful signs for diagnosis.
    - Pes Planus
    - Limited elbow extension (<170°)

TREATMENT

GENERAL MEASURES
- Adults and children are routinely followed by the cardiologist or pediatric cardiologist in addition to the primary caregiver. Depending on the level of aortic root dilation, and the rate of the dilation, follow-up intervals should be between 3 and 12 months.
- Because Marfan syndrome is the most common etiology of aortic dissection in youth, rough competitive sports are discouraged. Moderately strenuous or nonstrenuous recreational activities are permissible (e.g., badminton, curling, golf, table tennis, archery, bowling, and riflery).
- All patients with valvar involvement should receive endocarditis prophylaxis prior to dental work or invasive procedures.
- Chest pain, back pain, and abdominal pain in a Marfan syndrome patient should provoke a prompt evaluation for aortic dissection.

MEDICATION (DRUGS)

- Use of β-blockade or calcium channel blockers has been advocated in adults.
- Losartan, an angiotensin 2 receptor blocker, has been shown, in fibrillin—deficient mice, to normalize aortic root growth. It is clinical trials.
- Although wall stress is increased in the acute intravenous administration of these drugs in the catheterization laboratory, long-term use may decrease the rate of aortic root dilation.
- Advantages of long-term β-blockade have not been proven in growing children, whose aortic root size is predicated on their age and body surface area.
- Bacterial endocarditis prophylaxis for dental and invasive procedures

SURGERY
- Emergency surgery during dissection or rupture is mandatory.
- Prophylactic aortic root replacement should be performed when the aortic root diameter reaches or exceeds 5 cm, because the risk of dissection increases substantially at greater diameters.
- Mitral valve replacement may be necessary for severe regurgitation.

FOLLOW-UP

Admission Criteria
Management is on an outpatient basis, unless aortic dissection or elective aortic/mitral surgery is undertaken.

PROGNOSIS
Prognosis is predicated on which major manifestations of Marfan syndrome are present.
- Even with aggressive medical therapy and appropriate vigilance, aortic dissection and death have occurred.
- Replace the root prophylactically at 5–5.5 cm.
- Clinical course is dependent on the rate of aortic root dilation and on mitral valve status.
- Heart failure symptoms from mitral regurgitation can usually be medically managed.
- If accompanied by cardiomyopathy, the prognosis is more guarded; heart transplantation may be considered.
- Operative mortality rate for aortic root replacement is less than 2%, if myocardial function is good preoperatively.

PATIENT MONITORING
- Close regular visits for assessment of possible signs and symptoms.
- Serial echocardiography is mandatory, because aortic root dilation can occur without symptoms.

REFERENCES
1. Beighton P, et al., eds. *McKusick's Heritable Disorders of Connective Tissue*, 5th ed. St. Louis: Mosby–Year Book; 1993.
2. Gott VL, et al. Replacement of the aortic root in patients with Marfan's syndrome. *N Engl J Med*. 1999;340:1307–1313.
3. Haouzi A, et al. Heterogeneous aortic response to acute beta-adrenergic blockade in Marfan syndrome. *Am Heart J*. 1997;133:60–63.
4. Rios AS, et al. Effect of long-term beta-blockade on aortic root compliance in patients with Marfan syndrome. *Am Heart J*. 1999;137:1057–1061.

CODES
ICD9-CM
759.82 Marfan's syndrome

PATIENT TEACHING
The National Marfan Foundation of the United States can supply information and support, although treatment must be individualized by the cardiologist/pediatric cardiologist.

Diet
Diet should be the AHA diet for both children and adults.

Activity
Activities are limited, as discussed previously. Please see 36th Bethesda Conference recommendations: *JACC*. 45(8) p. 1342–1343, April 19, 2005.

M

MESENTERIC ISCHEMIA

Patrick Hu
Rosemary Mehl

 BASICS

DESCRIPTION

Primary mesenteric ischemia
- Interruption of abdominal vascular circulation by arterial embolus, arterial or venous thrombosis, atherosclerotic stenosis, or nonocclusive vasospasm
- Also known as mesenteric vasculopathy or mesenteric ischemic vasculopathy

Secondary mesenteric ischemia
- Compression of the vascular circulation from an extrinsic source

Pregnancy Considerations

Pregnancy increases the risk of arterial and venous thrombosis in patients with pre-existing hypercoagulable states.

EPIDEMIOLOGY

- Accounts for 1/1,000 hospital admissions.
- Mean age for acute arterial embolus is 68 years, for acute arterial thrombosis 77 years, and for acute venous thrombosis 47–60 years.
- Men and women are affected equally.
- Nonocclusive intestinal mesenteric ischemia accounts for 1/5,000 hospital admissions, 25–60% of all bowel infarctions.
- Chronic mesenteric ischemia may be present in 10–20% of elderly patients by autopsy series, probably underreported because of multisystem disease; predilection for women among symptomatic patients, with mean age of 60 years.

RISK FACTORS

- Embolus
  - Cardiac thrombi from atrial fibrillation, recent myocardial infarction, valvular heart disease, dilated left atrium, dilated ventricle with mural thrombus (risk significantly reduced in patients who are chronically anticoagulated)
- Arterial thrombosis and chronic mesenteric ischemia
  - Atherosclerosis with associated risk factors (age, smoking, diabetes, hypertension, hyperlipidemia); also vasculitis (Behçet, Buerger, Churg-Strauss, Kawasaki, polyarteritis nodosa, Takayasu, Wegener, rheumatoid arthritis, and lupus), hypercoagulable states (antiphospholipid antibodies; deficiency or mutations of protein C, protein S, and antithrombin III; sickle cell anemia; myeloproliferative disorders; oral contraceptives), trauma
- Venous thrombosis
  - Hypercoagulable states; also vasculitis, bowel obstruction, dehydration, pancreatitis, infections (appendicitis, diverticulitis), abdominal malignancy, abdominal trauma
- Nonocclusive intestinal mesenteric ischemia (NOMI)
  - Systemic hypotension (cardiogenic and cardiogenic shock), especially in elderly patients undergoing emergency cardiac or abdominal surgery; vasoconstricting drugs (e.g., cocaine, digoxin)

- Secondary mesenteric ischemia
  - Strangulated/ischemic bowel, abdominal malignancy, amyloidosis, neurofibromatosis, retroperitoneal fibrosis.

ASSOCIATED CONDITIONS

- Embolus
  - 20% have synchronous emboli to upper or lower extremities. Prior emboli (cerebral, renal, lower extremity) are common.
- Arterial thrombosis and chronic mesenteric ischemia
  - Typically, diffuse and extensive atherosclerotic disease (coronary, cerebrovascular, peripheral vascular)
  - Less commonly, systemic vasculitis
- Venous thrombosis: deep vein thromboses
- NOMI
  - Usually critically ill
  - With cardiogenic shock from aortic insufficiency
  - Myocardial infarction
  - Congestive heart failure
  - Renal failure (9–20% deaths among hemodialysis patients from NOMI)
  - Hypovolemic shock from dehydration
  - Pancreatitis
  - Burns
  - Diarrhea
- Secondary mesenteric ischemia
  - Intra-abdominal pathology (malignancy, infection, fibrosis, adhesions, trauma)

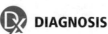 **DIAGNOSIS**

SIGNS AND SYMPTOMS

- Character, time-course, and predominance of symptoms vary, depending on the cause and on the anatomic site of the ischemia.
- Abdominal pain, usually out of proportion to findings at physical examination, often poorly localized, is precipitous with embolus, more insidious with thrombosis
- Urge to defecate (ischemic colitis)
- Classic triad (fear of eating, postprandial pain, weight loss) in chronic mesenteric ischemia
- Change in mental status (especially elderly patients)
- Abdominal distention (especially critically ill patients)
- Nausea and vomiting
- Diarrhea
- Lower gastrointestinal bleeding (common presenting sign in ischemic colitis)
- Fever
- Anorexia
- Upper gastrointestinal bleeding (in venous thrombosis, vague symptoms often delay diagnosis until esophageal variceal bleed)

- Physical signs minimal initially
- Later signs indicate bowel ischemia and necrosis
  - Fever
  - Tachycardia
  - Abdominal tympany
  - Peritoneal irritation
  - Abdominal distention from hypoperistalsis
  - Hypoactive bowel sounds from severe muscle ischemia
  - Fecal occult blood
  - In very late stages, hypotension, septicemia, and decreased mentation

TESTS

- Abdominal paracentesis not widely used, may reveal blood-tinged fluid with high leukocyte count and amylase level
- Endoscopy useful only in acute and chronic ischemic colitis; preferred over barium studies in these entities because it allows mucosal brushings to exclude other diagnoses

Lab

- Routine blood tests show nonspecific markers of bowel injury
  - Hemoconcentration
  - Leukocytosis with left shift
  - Metabolic acidosis
  - Hyperamylasemia
  - Elevated serum lactate
  - Elevated serum alkaline phosphatase
  - Azotemia
  - Bacteremia
  - Specialized coagulation studies should be performed in cases of mesenteric vein thrombosis (antiphospholipid antibody, assays for protein C, protein S, factor V Leiden, and antithrombin III).
  - Special labs such as assaying the alpha subunit of GST appear to be good predictors of acute mesenteric ischemia but are neither widely available nor widely used yet.

Imaging

- Plain films (chest and abdominal x-ray) are important to exclude other diagnoses.
- Selective mesenteric angiography and digital subtraction angiography should be performed immediately if acute mesenteric ischemia is suspected. They are the gold standard, are diagnostic, and can differentiate embolus from thrombus and allow for planning surgical revascularization, and may provide means of therapy (papaverine infusion).
- Computed tomography (CT) or magnetic resonance imaging (MRI) is diagnostic in 70–100% of mesenteric venous thrombosis, and helpful in extrinsic vascular compression; but is unhelpful in arterial ischemia and can delay diagnosis.
- Ultrasonography is not useful in acute ischemia, but excludes gallstones or appendicitis.
- Avoid barium studies if angiography is planned; utility is limited to acute ischemic colitis.

216

DIFFERENTIAL DIAGNOSIS
- Bowel obstruction
- Perforated viscus
- Adhesions
- Appendicitis
- Cholecystitis
- Infectious colitis
- Pancreatitis
- Abdominal aortic aneurysm
- Abdominal abscess
- Abdominal malignancy
- Toxic megacolon
- Crohn/ulcerative colitis
- Infectious colitis
- Pseudomembranous colitis

 TREATMENT

GENERAL MEASURES
- Aggressive fluid resuscitation to replace losses from ischemic bowel
- Supplemental oxygen
- Optimize cardiac function; treat failure and arrhythmia (Swan-Ganz and Foley catheter monitoring)
- Discontinue vasoconstricting drugs (e.g., digoxin, vasopressin)
- Correct electrolyte and acid–base imbalances
- Broad-spectrum antibiotics
- Nasogastric tube to decompress ischemic bowel
- Rectal tube for ischemic colitis

 MEDICATION (DRUGS)

- Heparin immediately if thromboembolism is suspected
- Warfarin long term to prevent recurrent embolus or thrombosis
- Papaverine via affected artery (never systemic) for NOMI and preoperative arterial embolus or thrombosis
- Thrombolytics considered experimental for poor surgical candidates

SURGERY
- Embolism
  - Immediate vascular surgery for embolectomy and resection of nonviable bowel; second operation at 24–48 hours to evaluate areas of questionable viability

- Arterial thrombosis
  - Revascularization (bypass grafting) with resection of nonviable bowel; second operation at 24–48 hours to evaluate areas of questionable viability
- Venous thrombosis
  - General surgery only to resect nonviable bowel
- NOMI: General surgery only to resect nonviable bowel
- Secondary mesenteric ischemia: General surgery to resect extravascular disease
- Acute ischemic colitis: 20% require bowel resection
- Chronic ischemic colitis: Only to relieve symptomatic stricture
- Chronic venous thrombosis: Portosystemic shunting for intractable variceal bleeding
- Chronic mesenteric ischemia: Arterial reconstruction for symptomatic patients
- Endovascular techniques are being tested versus traditional surgical techniques but have not been adopted mainstream

 FOLLOW-UP

DISPOSITION
Admission Criteria
Admit for any indication of bowel ischemia requiring angiographic or surgical intervention.

Discharge Criteria
Discharge when vascular supply sufficient to prevent bowel ischemia and necrosis.

PROGNOSIS
- Acute arterial ischemia
  - Overall mortality rate 50%
  - If diagnosed before peritoneal signs, survival rate is 90%.
  - If bowel necrosis at time of diagnosis, mortality rate is 70–90%.
  - Causes of death include extensive bowel necrosis, cardiopulmonary failure, hemorrhage, and recurrent emboli to other sites.
- Acute venous thrombosis
  - 25–30% mortality rate
  - Average hospital stay 26 days, with 55% incidence of major postoperative complications (infection, recurrent thrombosis)
- NOMI: very high mortality (70–100%) from underlying shock state and multiorgan failure

- Acute ischemic colitis
  - Most patients improve after 24 hours of expectant medical therapy (antibiotic, fluids, rectal tube).
  - 60% mortality rate in surgical cases
  - Recurrence unusual
  - 20% develop chronic colitis requiring elective surgery.
- Chronic arterial ischemia
  - 80–90% success following elective surgery
  - Myocardial disease and arterial reocclusion are important causes of death.

PATIENT MONITORING
- Life-long anticoagulation for most patients
- Monitor patients for extraintestinal emboli and thrombosis (coronary, cerebrovascular, peripheral vascular, deep vein thrombosis).

REFERENCES
1. Capell MS. Intestinal (mesenteric) vasculopathy, I: Acute superior mesenteric arteriopathy and venopathy. *Gastroenterol Clin North Am*. 1998;27:783–825.
2. Capell MS. Intestinal (mesenteric) vasculopathy, II: Ischemic colitis and chronic mesenteric ischemia. *Gastroenterol Clin North Am*. 1998;27:827–860.
3. Eldrup-Jorgenson J, Hawkins RE, Bredenberg CE. Abdominal vascular catastrophes. *Surg Clin North Am*. 1997;77:1305–1320.
4. Yasuhara, H. Acute mesenteric ischemia: The challenge of gastroenterology. *Surg Today*. 2005;35:185–195.

CODES
ICD9-CM
- 444.9 Embolism and thrombosis of unspecified artery or vein
- 557.9 Unspecified vascular insufficiency to intestine

PATIENT TEACHING
Because early intervention is key to survival, advise patients to seek immediate medical attention for symptoms of recurrent bowel ischemia.

M

METABOLIC SYNDROME

Carlos A. Aguilar-Salinas
Roopa Mehta

 BASICS

DESCRIPTION

- A cluster of metabolic risk factors associated with insulin resistance and/or abdominal obesity leading to increased cardiovascular morbidity and type 2 diabetes. These risk factors include dyslipidemia, arterial hypertension, hyperglycemia, and abdominal obesity.
  - Several diagnostic criteria exist. Some are based on the presence of insulin resistance (i.e., World Health Organization); others give a prominent role to abdominal obesity (i.e., International Diabetes Federation and the National Cholesterol Education Program's Adult Treatment Panel III (NCEP-ATPIII).
  - Regardless of which definition is used, the metabolic syndrome concept is a valuable tool; it provides an overview of the complex mechanisms by which the disease causes long-term complications.

GENERAL PREVENTION

- Healthy lifestyle
  - Regular physical activity
  - Avoidance of atherogenic diets

EPIDEMIOLOGY

- Prevalent disorder. More common among:
  - Certain ethnic groups (Asians, Native Americans, Hispanics). Disease expression varies among ethnic groups (e.g., low HDL cholesterol and diabetes are more common in Hispanics and Native Americans).
  - Urban, westernized societies
  - Age-dependent
  - HIV patients

Incidence

Has been rarely measured. Abdominal obesity, HDL cholesterol, and fasting glucose are the main determinants.

Prevalence

- The unadjusted prevalence (according to the original NCEP-ATPIII definition) increased from 23.1% in NHANES III (1988–1994) to 26.7 in NHANES 1999–2000. The age-adjusted prevalences were 24.1% and 27%, respectively. In nondiabetic cases the age-adjusted prevalences were 20.3% and 23.3%, respectively.
  - Prevalence is higher in women than in men (29 vs. 25.2%). The greatest increase in prevalence has been in women ages 20–39 (from 9.718% between surveys).
  - The highest prevalence is found in men >60 years (39.7%). This group had a 6.8% decrease in prevalence between surveys.
  - The contribution of the individual components are abdominal obesity 44%, hypertriglyceridemia 32.6%, low HDL cholesterol 39.9%, arterial hypertension 39.2%, fasting glucose >110 mg/dL 13.1%, fasting glucose >100 mg/dL 30.7%
  - Using the revised NCEP-ATPIII criteria (glycemia >100 mg/dL), the corresponding age-adjusted prevalences are 29.2% and 32.3% for the NHANES III and the NHANES 1999–2000 surveys, respectively.

- Prevalence varies in population-based surveys: Mexican-American (men 40.3%, women 44%), African American (men 24.5%, women 36.4%); Mexico 26.6%, Europe 21%, China 10.9%, Korea 28%

RISK FACTORS

- Genetic predisposition
  - Ethnicity
  - Family history of type 2 diabetes
- Environmental factors
  - Early life undernourishment
  - Childhood obesity
  - Sedentary lifestyle, stress
  - High fat/high carbohydrate diets
  - Cigarette smoking

Genetics

Loci on chromosomes 1p, 3,5,6q, 7,10p, 19q and genetic variants of several genes (e.g., adiponectin, Peroxisome proliferator-activator receptors [PPAR] gamma) have been linked to the disease.

PATHOPHYSIOLOGY

- Insulin resistance: Probably related to an overabundance of circulating fatty acids and/or abnormal lipid deposition in muscle, liver, and other tissues. May coexist with leptin resistance.
- Abdominal adiposity: Increased hepatic concentration of free fatty acids results in greater hepatic glucose and lipoprotein production. Hormones involved in inflammation [interleukin 6 (IL- 6)] and glucose/lipid metabolism (e.g., adiponectin, retinol binding protein 4, leptin) are also generated.
- Dyslipidemia: Hypertriglyceridemia and an increase in small dense low-density lipoproteins (LDLs) are caused by hepatic overproduction of lipoproteins, increased Cholesteryl Ester Transfer Protein (CETP) activity, and decreased clearance of triglyceride-rich particles. Low HDL cholesterol levels result from increased clearance of HDL particles.
- Arterial hypertension: Decreased insulin-mediated vasodilatation, increased sodium reabsorption, and higher concentrations of vasoconstrictors (endothelin-1, angiotensinogen) are among the putative mechanisms.
- Increased atherogenicity: In addition to the proatherogenic abnormalities discussed in the preceding text, the metabolic syndrome is associated with prothrombotic changes (increased fibrinogen, plasminogen activator inhibitor-1), decreased fibrinolysis, low-grade chronic inflammation, microalbuminuria, increased asymmetric dimethylarginine, and endothelial dysfunction).

ETIOLOGY

Interaction between genetic and environmental factors

ASSOCIATED CONDITIONS

- Nonalcoholic steatohepatitis
- Obstructive sleep apnea
- Polycystic ovary disease
- Hyperuricemia
- Primary hyperlipidemias (e.g., familial combined hyperlipidemia)

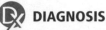 **DIAGNOSIS**

SIGNS AND SYMPTOMS

- According to the revised NCEP-ATPIII, ≥3 of the following criteria must be present:
  - Abdominal obesity (waist circumference >102 cm in men and >88 cm in women)
  - Arterial hypertension (≥130/85 mm Hg or on antihypertensive medication)
  - Hypertriglyceridemia (≥150 mg/dL)
  - Low-HDL cholesterol (<40 mg/dL for men and <50 mg/dL for women)
  - Fasting plasma glucose ≥100 mg/dL or type 2 diabetes
  - The requirement for 3 criteria is an arbitrary threshold. Diagnosis should be considered in the presence of any of the components. The risk for complications increases proportionally with the number of components, even in cases with only 1 or 2 criteria.
- The definition proposed by the International Diabetes Federation differs from the NCEP-ATPIII in the following manner:
  - Abdominal obesity is an obligate component; waist circumference thresholds vary among ethnic groups (white >94 cm in men and >80 cm in women); in other groups (except Japanese) >90 cm in men and >80 cm in women. Pharmacologic treatment for any of the components is synonymous with that for the metabolic syndrome.

History

Familial or personal history of type 2 diabetes, coronary heart disease, or any component of the metabolic syndrome

Physical Exam

- Waist circumference: Measured as the midpoint between the highest point of the iliac crest and the lowest part of the costal margin in the midaxillary line.
  - Acanthosis nigricans: Marker of insulin resistance

TESTS

- Cardiovascular risk stratification:
  - Individuals with atherosclerosis and/or type 2 diabetes are in the high-risk category.
  - In cases without atherosclerosis or diabetes, Framingham risk scoring is used to estimate 10-year risk for coronary heart disease (CHD). The performance of this score varies between ethnic groups.
  - Detecting the metabolic syndrome is only one part of overall cardiovascular risk assessment. *Per se* it is not an adequate tool to estimate 10-year risk for CHD. The metabolic syndrome is associated with a higher lifetime risk, but in the absence of diabetes, it is not necessarily associated with a high 10-year risk.
- Detection of diabetes, impaired glucose tolerance, or impaired fasting glucose
- The components of the metabolic syndrome should be investigated in first-degree relatives.

Lab

- Fasting lipid profile: Inclusion of apolipoprotein B is recommended.

- Oral glucose tolerance test: if fasting plasma glucose is 90–125 mg/dL
- Aspartate aminotransferase (AST), alanine aminotransferase (ALT), and Alkaline phosphatase (ALP) for the diagnosis of nonalcoholic steatohepatitis
- Uric acid
- C-reactive protein and microalbuminuria may help to estimate the risk for complications.

Imaging
Not required

Diagnostic Procedures/Surgery
Not required

Pathologic Findings
Increased fat deposition in liver and muscle

DIFFERENTIAL DIAGNOSIS
Not required

TREATMENT

GENERAL MEASURES
- The treatment goals are:
  - Reduce risk for clinical atherosclerotic disease
  - Prevent or treat diabetes
- Emphasis should be placed in achieving effective lifestyle changes and the management of each of the risk factors.
- Abdominal obesity: Reduce body weight by 7–10% by increasing physical activity, decreasing caloric intake, and use of behavior modification programs. Encourage maintenance of weight lost. Currently available weight-loss drugs have limited utility.
- Physical inactivity: 30 minutes of continuous or intermittent exercise at least 5 days a week
- Diet modification: Reduce intake of calories, saturated fat, trans fat, simple sugars, and cholesterol.
- Atherogenic dyslipidemia: The position statement (endorsed by the AHA/NHLBI) proposes LDL cholesterol as the primary target. Other important targets include non-HDL cholesterol, HDL-C, and triglycerides.
  - LDL goals are based on risk stratification:
    - High risk: LDL-C <100 mg/dL, <70 mg/dL optional
    - Moderately high risk: LDL-C <130 mg/dL, <100 mg/dL optional
    - Low risk: LDL-C <160 mg/dL
  - To obtain the non-HDL goals, add 30 mg/dL to the corresponding LDL-C goal.
  - Diet is critical for hypertriglyceridemia.
  - LDL-lowering drugs (statin ± ezetimibe) and fibrates are first-line drugs.
- Arterial hypertension: Reduce blood pressure to <140/90 mm Hg (or <130/80 if diabetes is present). If drug therapy is required, medication with positive or neutral effects on insulin sensitivity are preferred [i.e., angiotensin-converting enzyme (ACE) inhibitors].
- Hyperglycemia: For impaired glucose tolerance, encourage weight reduction and lifestyle modification. For diabetes, achieve and maintain HbA1c <7%.
- Prothrombotic state: Use low-dose aspirin in cases with high or moderately high risk.

MEDICATION (DRUGS)

Refer to: Treatment of arterial hypertension, dyslipidemia, obesity, and type 2 diabetes

SURGERY
Bariatric surgery is an option if the body mass index >35 kg/m^2.

FOLLOW-UP

DISPOSITION
Primary care physicians and internists manage the majority of cases.

Admission Criteria
Atherosclerosis- and diabetes-related complications

Issues for Referral
- Endocrinologist if diabetes, polycystic ovary syndrome, or obesity are present
- Lipid specialist if a severe primary hyperlipidemia exists
  - Gastroenterologist if nonalcoholic steatohepatitis is suspected

PROGNOSIS
The NCEP definition of the metabolic syndrome is associated with a relative risk of 1.27 (95% CI 0.90–1.78) for all-cause mortality, 1.65 (1.38–1.99) for cardiovascular disease, and 2.99 (1.96–4.57) for diabetes.

COMPLICATIONS
Type 2 diabetes and atherosclerosis

PATIENT MONITORING
- Body weight, waist circumference, and blood pressure
- Medical evaluation at least 3 times/year
  - Fasting glucose and lipid profile at least once a year (more often if abnormal)

REFERENCES
1. Aguilar-Salinas CA, Rojas R, Rios-Torres JM, et al. The metabolic syndrome: A concept hard to define. *Arch Med Res*. 2005;36:223–231.
2. Eckel R, Grundy SM, Zimmet P. The metabolic syndrome. *Lancet*. 2005;365:1415–1428.
3. Ford ES. Risk for all cause mortality, cardiovascular disease and diabetes associated with the metabolic syndrome. *Diabetes Care*. 2005;28:1769–1778.
4. Ford ES, Giles W, Mokdad A. Increasing prevalence of the metabolic syndrome among US adults. *Diabetes Care*. 2004;27:2444–2449.
5. Grundy SM, Cleeman J, Daniels S et al. Diagnosis and management of the metabolic syndrome. An America Heart Association/National Heart Lung and Blood Institute Scientific Statement. *Circulation*. 2005;112:2735–2752.

MISCELLANEOUS

Organizations
American Diabetes Association.
http://www.diabetes.org
American Heart Association.
http://www.americanheart.org
International Diabetes Federation. http://www.idf.org

CODES
ICD9-CM
277.7

PATIENT TEACHING
Lifestyle change is the cornerstone of treatment

Diet
Reduction in calories, saturated fat, trans fat, simple sugars, and cholesterol. Possible benefit from Mediterranean diet.

Activity
Regular exercise guided by physician

Prevention
- Primary prevention:
  - Adoption of healthy lifestyle early in life
- Secondary prevention:
  - Effective lifestyle change and management of each of the risk factors (hyperlipidemia, arterial hypertension, hyperglycemia, abdominal obesity)

FAQ
Q: What is the metabolic syndrome?
A: A cluster of metabolic risk factors including abdominal obesity, atherogenic dyslipidemia (high triglycerides, low HDL cholesterol, and high LDL cholesterol), arterial hypertension, insulin resistance, or glucose intolerance

Q: How many people have the metabolic syndrome?
A: Common worldwide with an estimated prevalence of 50 million in United States

Q: What are the complications of the metabolic syndrome?
A: Coronary heart disease and type 2 diabetes

M

MITRAL REGURGITATION, ADULT

Jeff Ciaramita
Steven C. Herrmann
Bernard R. Chaitman

 BASICS

DESCRIPTION

Mitral regurgitation (MR) is the backflow of blood from the left ventricle (LV) to the left atrium (LA) during systole.

Pregnancy Considerations

Patients with mitral regurgitation tolerate pregnancy well, but it might precipitate congestive heart failure in case of severe MR with LV systolic dysfunction.

ETIOLOGY

- Myxomatous degeneration (mitral valve prolapse, Marfan syndrome, Ehlers-Danlos syndrome) of the mitral valve is the most common cause of MR in U.S. It accounts for about 65% of causes of pure MR.
- Mitral annular calcification
- Rheumatic heart disease
- Congenital malformation
- Ruptured chordae tendineae
- Ruptured papillary muscle
- Infective endocarditis
- Marfan syndrome
- Ehlers-Danlos syndrome
- Pseudoxanthoma elasticum
- Systemic illness/drug effects (e.g., lupus vasculitis); fenfluramine
- Tumors (atrial myxoma)
- Functional
  - Ischemic
  - Dilated cardiomyopathy
  - Infiltrative/restrictive cardiomyopathy
  - Hypertrophic cardiomyopathy
  - Trauma

Prevalence

Estimates of disease prevalence are confounded by the observation that a small degree of physiologic MR can be detected on careful Doppler echocardiography in as many as 80% of normal healthy people. MR occurs in approximately 20% of post-MI patients.

PATHOPHYSIOLOGY

Pathology of the mitral valve apparatus (chordae tendineae, papillary muscles, mitral annulus) or leaflets may cause MR. Severe chronic MR is associated with LVH, LV dilation, increased LVEDP, and heart failure. Symptom onset is related to degree of LA compliance and underlying cause of the MR.

 DIAGNOSIS

SIGNS AND SYMPTOMS

- MR secondary to ischemic disease or dilated cardiomyopathy will have symptoms typical of the underlying disease. However, patients with MR secondary to leaflet disease may remain asymptomatic for many years.
- The typical initial presentation will be exercise intolerance in the form of exertional dyspnea. This is followed by symptoms of pulmonary congestion and congestive heart failure (CHF).
- The onset of symptoms may coincide with a period of increased hemodynamic burden (e.g., pregnancy, infection, etc.) or with the onset of atrial fibrillation.

History

Acute MR (e.g., ruptured chordae, endocarditis) may present with acute pulmonary edema, hypotension, and shock.

Physical Exam

- Brisk carotid upstroke with early peak and rapid decline secondary to backward flow into the LA instead of forward flow across the aortic valve. Stroke volume is increased early in the disease.
- Precordial palpation usually reveals a normal apical impulse early in the disease with a displaced diffuse apex late in the course of the disease due to LV dilatation.
- Left parasternal pulsations can be appreciated with the onset of right ventricular failure or with systolic expansion of the LA with anterior displacement of the right heart when severe MR is present.
- On cardiac auscultation, the patient with MR typically has a soft S1 with a holosystolic, soft-pitched, and blowing murmur that is loudest at the apex and radiates to the axilla. The intensity of the murmur correlates with the severity of MR of organic etiology, contrary to functional MR, when it is grade 4 or above or grade 2 or below.
- In patients with prolapse of the anterior mitral valve leaflet and a posteriorly directed regurgitation jet, the murmur may be auscultated by the spine.
- A widely split S2 is normal early in the disease, resulting from the shortening of left ventricular ejection. An accentuated pulmonary component of S2 can be appreciated with the onset of pulmonary hypertension. S3 can be heard over the apex, secondary to the increased rate and velocity of early diastolic filling.

TESTS

Imaging

- Electrocardiography
  - Findings in patients with MR are nonspecific and include LA enlargement, atrial fibrillation, and LV hypertrophy in patients with severe MR. About 15% of patients also exhibit right ventricular hypertrophy on ECG.
- Chest radiograph
  - Chest radiography may be normal early in the disease with LA enlargement later. During the decompensated stage, evidence of pulmonary edema becomes apparent.
  - Pulmonary hypertension is manifested as increased size of central pulmonary arteries with peripheral attenuation of pulmonary vessels.
- Transthoracic echocardiography
  - Echo Doppler study can estimate both LV and LA volumes/dimensions, LV ejection fraction (LVEF), and the severity of MR, and can help define the anatomic cause of MR.
  - Serial echocardiograms help in the decision regarding timing of surgery.
  - Echo should be performed after mitral valve surgery to establish the baseline hemodynamics of the repair of prosthesis.
- Transesophageal echocardiography
  - Useful for evaluation of patients in whom transthoracic echocardiography is inconclusive, and to establish the anatomic basis of MR and determine if MV repair is an option rather than MV replacement.
  - Cardiac catheterization can be performed to assess the severity of MR as well as to delineate coronary anatomy.

DIFFERENTIAL DIAGNOSIS

- The murmur of MR must be differentiated from aortic stenosis and hypertrophic cardiomyopathy.
- Dynamic auscultation is helpful in that situation; MR murmur increases with squatting and during the strain phase of Valsalva, but the murmur of aortic stenosis is diminished.
- Hand grip increases the murmur of MR due to increase in the afterload, with opposite effect on aortic stenosis and hypertrophic cardiomyopathy murmurs.

TREATMENT

GENERAL MEASURES

- Recommendations for invasive left ventriculography and hemodynamic measurement in MR:
  - When noninvasive tests are inconclusive regarding the severity of MR, LV function, or need for surgery
  - When discrepancy exists between clinical and noninvasive findings regarding severity of MR
- To determine coronary anatomy if MV surgery is necessary

 MEDICATION (DRUGS)

- Vasodilators
  - No long-term studies indicate benefit in asymptomatic patients with normal LV function and chronic MR.
  - Symptomatic patients and those with deteriorating LV function should be referred for surgery.
- Atrial fibrillation
- Rate control can be achieved using β-blockers, calcium channel blockers, digitalis, or, rarely, amiodarone if cardioversion is a consideration.
- Anticoagulation using warfarin is indicated in patients with MR and atrial fibrillation with a target INR of 2–3.
- Patients with symptoms of heart failure should be treated using standard drug therapy (diuretics, vasodilators, digoxin, etc.).
- Afterload reduction therapy is indicated for acute MR.

SURGERY

- Mitral valve replacement or repair
  - Acute symptomatic MR
  - Patients with severe MR and New York Heart Association (NYHA) class II–IV symptoms with EF >60% and end-systolic dimension <45 mm
  - Patients with severe MR with EF 50–60% and end-systolic dimension 45–50 mm regardless of the symptoms
  - Patients with severe MR with EF 30–50% and/or end-systolic dimension 50–55 mm regardless of the symptoms
  - Asymptomatic patients with severe MR and atrial fibrillation in the presence of preserved LV function
  - Asymptomatic patients with severe MR and severe pulmonary hypertension with preserved LV function

- Asymptomatic patients with severe MR with EF 50–60% or end-systolic dimension 45–50 mm
- Patients with severe LV dysfunction (EF <30% and/or end-systolic dimension >55 mm) in whom chordal preservation is likely
- Asymptomatic patients with severe MR and preserved LV function in whom mitral valve repair is highly likely
- Patients with mitral valve prolapse and severe MR in the presence of preserved LV function who have recurrent ventricular arrhythmias despite medical therapy
- Recommendations for coronary angiography in MR:
  - When mitral valve surgery is contemplated in patients with angina or history of MI
  - When mitral valve surgery is contemplated in patients with one or more risk factors for CAD
  - When ischemia is suspected as a causal factor in MR

 FOLLOW-UP

PROGNOSIS

- For patients with symptoms from severe MR, surgical intervention improves long-term outcome and quality of life.
- For patients with predominant MR and NYHA Class II–IV undergoing elective surgery, mortality rates are about 6%.
- Surgical treatment of MR secondary to LV dilation and systolic dysfunction, dilated cardiomyopathy, or ischemic heart disease remains controversial, with the possibility of worsening of LV function after surgery as a result of increased afterload.

COMPLICATIONS

- Atrial arrhythmias
- CHF
- Sudden cardiac death
- Pulmonary hypertension with right-sided heart failure
- Recurrent rheumatic fever
- Systemic embolization
- Prosthetic valve–related complications

PATIENT MONITORING

- Asymptomatic patients with normal LV function should be evaluated clinically on a yearly basis. For patients with normal or hyperdynamic LV function and good exercise tolerance, echocardiography is recommended every 6–12 months with severe MR.
- A baseline echocardiogram should be obtained and followed in patients postoperatively because some might worsen after surgery, and, in case of mitral valve replacement, they should be anticoagulated.

REFERENCES

1. Bonow RO, Carabello B, de Leon AC Jr., et al. ACC/AHA 2006 guidelines for the management of patients with valvular heart disease: A report of the American College of Cardiology/American Heart Association Task Force on Practice Guidelines (Writting Committee to Revise the 1998 Guidelins for the management of Patients With Valvular Heart Disease). American College of Cardiology Web Site. Available at: http://content.onlinejacc.org/cgi/reprint/48/3/e1
2. Botkin NF, Seth PS, Aurigemma GP. Asymptomatic valvular disease: Who benefits from surgery? Curr Cardiol Rep. 2005;7:87–93.
3. Bonow RO, Cheitlin MD, Crawford MH, et al. Task Force 3: valvular heart disease. J Am Coll Cardiol. 2005;45:1334–1340.
4. Enriquez-Sarano M, Avierinos JF, Messika-Zeitoun D, et al. Quantitative determinants of the outcome of asymptomatic mitral regurgitation. N Engl J Med. 2005;352:875–883.
5. Zoghbi WA, Enriquez-Sarano M, Foster E, et al. Recommendations for evaluation of the severity of native valvular regurgitation with two-dimensional and Doppler echocardiography. J Am Soc Echocardiogr. 2003;16:777–802.

CODES
ICD9-CM
424.0

PATIENT TEACHING

Asymptomatic patients should be educated to report any symptoms, which can be confirmed objectively using an exercise test or echocardiography.

Diet
Low-salt diet for CHF

Activity
- No limitation for asymptomatic patients with mild to moderate MR with normal LV function.
- No evidence suggests that vigorous exercise accelerates the progression of MR.

Prevention
Prophylaxis against infective endocarditis and recurrent rheumatic fever, if applicable, is indicated.

M

MITRAL REGURGITATION, PEDIATRIC

Erika Berman Rosenzweig
Welton M. Gersony

 BASICS

DESCRIPTION
Congenital abnormalities of the mitral valve result in incompetence during systole (ventricular contraction), causing regurgitation of blood into the left atrium (LA) with each left ventricular (LV) contraction.

RISK FACTORS
- Congenital mitral abnormality
- History of rheumatic fever
- Endocardial cushion defect
- Mitral valve prolapse
- Connective tissue disease

Genetics
Isolated congenital mitral insufficiency is a rare congenital anomaly in pediatric patients.

PATHOPHYSIOLOGY
Mitral regurgitation leads to volume loading in the LV because cardiac output must be maintained despite a regurgitant fraction returning to the LA through the incompetent mitral apparatus. Given the lower pressure in the LA, "unloading" of the LV occurs at low resistance. This may result in apparent normalization of LV function with ejection fractions that may not reflect true ventricular function.

ETIOLOGY
- Most often seen in association with other congenital heart defects, connective tissue disease, or metabolic/storage disease
- Secondary/acquired mitral regurgitation (MR) is seen following acute rheumatic fever, Kawasaki disease, cardiomyopathy, and endocarditis in children.

ASSOCIATED CONDITIONS
- Mitral insufficiency is a component of numerous congenital and acquired cardiac abnormalities. These include:
  - Endocardial cushion defects
  - Mitral valve prolapse
  - Cleft of the anterior leaflet
  - Rheumatic fever
  - Cardiomyopathy
  - Myocardial or papillary muscle infarction
  - Connective tissue disorders
  - Endocarditis
  - Kawasaki disease

 DIAGNOSIS

SIGNS AND SYMPTOMS
- General:
  - Symptoms usually depend on the severity and acuity of MR, although patients may be asymptomatic even with severe MR.
  - Chronic MR is usually well-tolerated in children.
- Most common signs and symptoms:
  - Shortness of breath
  - Tachypnea
  - Increased frequency of respiratory tract infections
  - Cough
  - Fatigue
  - Poor feeding
  - Exercise intolerance
- Other signs and symptoms:
  - Growth failure, if advanced

History
- Murmur
- Rheumatic fever
- Connective tissue disease
- Mitral valve prolapse
- Congenital cardiac abnormality

Physical Exam
- Increased precordial activity
- Right ventricular heave if associated with increased pulmonary arterial pressure
- Laterally displaced LV impulse
- Increased intensity of second heart sound if pulmonary arterial pressure is elevated
- S3 may be loud
- Murmur of MR is a high-frequency, blowing, pansystolic sound heard best at the apex, with radiation to the axilla (appreciated best when patient is supine and leaning leftward).
- If MR is moderate to severe, a low-frequency diastolic rumble may be appreciated at the apex, which represents increased diastolic flow across the mitral valve.

TESTS
- ECG:
  - May remain normal until MR is severe
  - LA enlargement (manifested by broad, notched P waves prominent in lead II)
  - Prominent LV forces
  - Right ventricular hypertrophy may eventually be present in severe cases with pulmonary hypertension.
  - If LA enlargement is severe, atrial arrhythmias may be observed.

Imaging
- Chest radiograph:
  - Cardiomegaly (enlarged LA and LV)
  - Pulmonary venous congestion
  - Pulmonary edema (if severe mitral regurgitation) with heart failure
- Echocardiography:
  - Detailed visualization of the mitral valve and valve apparatus
  - LV systolic function is normal to increased because the ventricle is unloaded. If "normal," it must be compared with previous echocardiogram to ensure that function has not deteriorated.
  - LA may appear dilated.
  - Color Doppler can be used to qualitatively assess MR.
  - If severe, pulmonary venous flow reversal may be observed (i.e., reflux into the pulmonary veins).
- MRI:
  - May use for LV volume assessment
  - Can be used to help quantify MR fraction
- Cardiac catheterization:
  - May be indicated if echocardiogram is not conclusive regarding the cause of MR, cardiac function, associated lesions, or degree of pulmonary hypertension
  - Mitral valve anatomy, cardiac output, pulmonary vascular resistance, and associated lesions should be assessed.
  - Pressure tracings demonstrate an elevated pulmonary capillary wedge pressure A-wave or an elevated left atrial A-wave if LA is entered.

DIFFERENTIAL DIAGNOSIS
- The main considerations for differential diagnosis of types of MR include:
- Acquired heart disease, such as acute rheumatic fever or chronic rheumatic heart disease
- Congenital mitral regurgitation alone or in association with endocardial cushion defects or mitral valve prolapse
- Connective tissue disease
- Acute trauma, infarcted papillary muscle:
  - On physical examination, the murmur should be distinguished from a ventricular septal defect murmur

TREATMENT

GENERAL MEASURES
- Outpatient. except for complications or surgery
- Treatment options are medical or surgical.
- For children, the size/age of the patient is an important factor in selecting a treatment plan because the smaller the patients are, the more likely they will need serial valve replacements as they outgrow an initial prosthetic valve.
- Manage medically, if possible. If medical therapy fails, consider valvuloplasty if technically feasible and use mitral valve replacement (MVR) as a final option.
- Timing of surgery is controversial; although recent literature indicates that in children, unlike adults, ventricular function appears to be preserved and improves postoperatively.

 MEDICATION (DRUGS)

- Mild to moderate chronic MR often can be managed medically with digoxin and diuretics.
- Angiotensin-converting enzyme inhibitors (ACE-Is) may be used for afterload reduction, although they usually are reserved for moderate to severe MR (long-term use in children has not been well studied).
- If MR is acute, patients are usually more symptomatic because the uncompensated LA has a sudden increase in volume overload. These patients usually require IV afterload reduction with nitroprusside or hydralazine, in addition to digoxin or IV inotrope and diuretics.
- If atrial arrhythmias are present, antiarrhythmic medications should be administered as needed.
- If MR is secondary to rheumatic fever, following initial treatment, long-term prophylaxis is necessary: 1.2 million units penicillin G benzathine IM every 4 weeks or penicillin V 250 mg orally twice daily.
- Bacterial endocarditis prophylaxis is necessary per AHA guidelines.
- For patients who undergo MVR, anticoagulation (heparin) should be started within 8–12 hours of surgery at a dose that achieves a partial thromboplastin time of 1.7–2.0 times normal. Oral anticoagulation also may be started once no active surgical issues are present, such as chest tubes or pacing wires requiring removal.
- Warfarin should be dosed to achieve an INR of 2.0–3.0. Discontinue heparin once warfarin is in the therapeutic range.
- Contraindications: Penicillin or other drug allergies
- Precautions: Refer to manufacturer's profile of each drug.

SURGERY
- Mitral valve repair and MVR are the surgical options and indicated if medical therapy fails.
- Mitral valve repair is preferred if technically feasible to avoid complications related to size and growth, as well as anticoagulation.
- The type of mitral valve repair depends on the type of mitral valve defect. For a regurgitant valve, annuloplasty or valvuloplasty is performed. In the larger child, the annulus may be supported by a DeVega or Carpentier ring (this will not grow with the child).
- Mitral valve leaflet cleft or chordae tendineae abnormalities usually can be repaired surgically.
- MVR is reserved for patients with moderate to severe MR who failed medical management and who are not candidates for valve repair.
- Most common type of prosthetic valve is the St. Jude bileaflet tilting disk valve for children.
- Current operative mortality rate is <5%.

 FOLLOW-UP

PROGNOSIS
- Preoperatively, most patients with mild to moderate mitral insufficiency can be medically managed; however, patients who demonstrate LV dysfunction or atrial arrhythmia may be at increased risk for surgery and for long-term postoperative arrhythmias.
- Although LV function may worsen in the immediate postoperative period, children generally appear to have recovery of LV function with time.
- After MVR in children, eventual re-replacement is required.

COMPLICATIONS
- Complications of anticoagulation may arise in patients with prosthetic mitral valves (i.e., bleeding or thrombosis).
- Recurrent rheumatic fever
- Bacterial endocarditis
- Pulmonary edema
- Atrial arrhythmias

PATIENT MONITORING
- Close, regular follow-up is essential to monitor for development or progression of symptoms or change in physical status.
- For all nonoperated and postsurgical patients, close attention should be directed to the echocardiographic appearance of the mitral apparatus at time intervals dependent on severity.
- Recommendations for unoperated patients regarding frequency of visits, serial echocardiograms, and ECGs depend on the severity of MR.
- Close monitoring of the INR during anticoagulation therapy following MVR
- Children are at particular risk for bleeding because of their activity level.
- Children have up to a 2% risk of thromboembolic events, even with appropriate anticoagulation.

Pregnancy Considerations
Pregnancy usually is well tolerated in women with mild to moderate mitral insufficiency.

REFERENCES
1. Bradley LM, et al. Anticoagulation therapy in children with mechanical prosthetic cardiac valves. *Am J Cardiol*. 1985;56:533–535.
2. Carpentier A, Branchini B, Cour C, et al. Congenital malformation of the mitral valve. Pathology and surgical treatment. *J Thorac Cardiovasc Surg*. 1976;7:854–857.
3. Emmanaulides GC, Allen HD, Riemenschneider TA, et al., eds. *Moss and Adams' heart disease in infants, children, and adolescents including the fetus and young adult*, 5th ed. New York: *Williams & Wilkins*, 1995.
4. Garson A Jr., Bricker JT, Fisher DJ, et al. *The science and practice of pediatric cardiology*, 2nd ed. New York: Williams & Wilkins, 1998.
5. Krishnan US, Gersony WM, Berman Rosenzweig E, et al. Late left ventricular function after surgery for children with chronic symptomatic mitral regurgitation. *Circulation*. 1997;96:4280–4285.
6. Skoularigis J, Sinovich V, Houbert G, et al. Evaluation of long-term results of mitral valve repair in 254 young patients with rheumatic mitral regurgitation. *Circulation*. 1994;90:167–174.

ADDITIONAL READING
- Khanna D, Miller AP, Nanda NC, et al. Transthoracic and transesophageal echocardiographic assessment of mitral regurgitation severity: Usefulness of qualitative and semiquantitative techniques. *Echocardiography*. 2005;22:748–769..
- Kon MW, Myerson SG, Moat NE, et al. Quantification of regurgitant fraction in mitral regurgitation by cardiovascular magnetic resonance: Comparison of techniques. *J Heart Valve Dis*. 2004;13:600–607.

CODES
ICD9-CM

PATIENT TEACHING
- Patients should be educated about signs of worsening symptoms or the presence of palpitations, which may indicate new onset of an atrial arrhythmia.
- Bacterial endocarditis prophylaxis as per AHA guidelines.
- Patients receiving anticoagulation with prolonged bleeding or easy bruisability should contact their physician. Children receiving anticoagulation must be restricted from rough physical activities.

Diet
No restrictions

Activity
- Adequate rest and reasonable physical activity
- Patients on oral anticoagulation are restricted from contact sports.

Prevention
- Bacterial endocarditis prophylaxis for dental and invasive procedures is continued for life.
- Rheumatic fever prophylaxis when indicated

M

MITRAL STENOSIS

Jennifer Lash
Steven C. Herrmann
Bernard R. Chaitman

 BASICS

DESCRIPTION
Mitral stenosis (MS) is caused by structural abnormalities in the mitral valve that prevent complete opening during diastole.

EPIDEMIOLOGY
Prevalence
- During the past 40 years, prevalence and incidence of rheumatic fever has decreased dramatically in Western countries.
- In 1960, MS accounted for 43% of all valve disease at European centers, compared with 9% in 1985.
- Rheumatic heart disease is still common in developing countries, with as many as 21 out of 1,000 school-age children affected in Asia.

RISK FACTORS
2/3 of all patients with rheumatic MS are women.

PATHOPHYSIOLOGY
Diastolic filling of the left ventricle (LV) is impaired by the stenotic mitral valve, leading to increased left atrial (LA) pressure (with orifice area $\sim<2$ cm^2). With critical MS (orifice area <1 cm^2), elevated LA pressure usually exceeds 25 mm Hg, causing symptoms of heart failure, particularly with tachycardia. LV diastolic pressure is usually normal in isolated MS.

ETIOLOGY
- Rheumatic heart disease is the most common cause of MS. 99% of valves removed for MS have rheumatic involvement.
  - Other rare causes of MS
  - Degenerative
    - Carcinoid syndrome
    - Fabry's disease
    - Mucopolysaccharidosis
    - Methysergide
    - Whipple's disease
    - Rheumatoid arthritis
    - Obstruction by large vegetation
  - Congenital mitral stenosis accounts for <1% of cases.

ASSOCIATED CONDITIONS
Lutembacher syndrome consists of MS and an atrial septal defect (ASD).

DIAGNOSIS

SIGNS AND SYMPTOMS
- Dyspnea is the most common complaint.
- Orthopnea, paroxysmal nocturnal dyspnea, lower extremity edema, and acute pulmonary edema
- Patients with mild MS usually are asymptomatic at rest and with mild exercise.
- Symptoms may be precipitated by factors that increase blood flow across the mitral valve or shorten the diastolic time, such as emotional or physical stress, infection, fever, pregnancy, or atrial fibrillation with rapid ventricular response.
- Mitral facies (malar flush), secondary to decreases in cardiac output in patients with severe MS, is rarely seen in the Western world.
- Atrial arrhythmias: About 30–40% of patients with MS develop atrial fibrillation.
- Hemoptysis is a rare manifestation of end-stage MS.
- Patients with MS are at increased risk for embolic events causing myocardial infarction (MI), stroke, or hypertension secondary to renal emboli.

Physical Exam
- Accentuated S1 in early MS while the valve leaflets are still flexible, because the prolonged mitral inflow prevents the leaflets from returning to the normal resting position before LV pressure increases abruptly at the onset of systole
- Accentuated pulmonary component of the second heart sound with the development of pulmonary hypertension, leading to a loss of physiologic split of S2 as pulmonary pressure increases
- Opening snap (OS) of mitral valve that moves closer to S2 as LA pressure increases. An S2–OS interval of 70 msec is seen in severe MS.
- Diastolic mid-diastolic rumbling murmur heard at the apex with presystolic accentuation coinciding with atrial contraction
- Findings of pulmonary hypertension and right-sided heart failure occur later in MS (i.e., elevated jugular venous pressure, hepatomegaly, ascites, lower extremity edema).

TESTS
Imaging
- ECG
  - Relatively insensitive technique for detection of MS
  - P mitrale, a sign of LA enlargement, is defined as a broad and bifid P-wave in lead II, >0.12 seconds, or broad and deep negative component of the biphasic P wave in lead V1, longer than 0.04 seconds and 1 mm in depth.
  - Atrial fibrillation or flutter may be seen.
  - Exercise testing may be useful in determining an objective measure of functional capacity in asymptomatic patients.
- Chest radiograph
  - The classic features are LA enlargement with normal LV contour and enlarged pulmonary artery.

  - Pulmonary congestion and interstitial edema (Kerley B-lines)
  - Other features may include hemosiderosis and mitral valve calcification.
- Echocardiography
  - 2-D and Doppler echocardiography is considered modality of choice for diagnosis and assessment of the severity of MS.
  - 2-D echo demonstrates thickening and calcification of the leaflets, with restricted mobility of the anterior leaflet with diastolic doming and a fixed posterior leaflet. Mitral valve area can be measured by direct visualization of the valve.
  - Doppler echo can be used to estimate the pressure gradient between the LA and LV and mitral valve area.
  - Echocardiography also is used to determine the appropriateness of the valve for balloon valvuloplasty.
- Cardiac catheterization
  - Invasive evaluation of valve stenosis when noninvasive studies are inadequate or if a discrepancy exists between clinical symptoms and noninvasive testing

Diagnostic Procedures/Surgery
- Percutaneous mitral balloon valvotomy
- Transesophageal echocardiography is usually performed before, or at the time of percutaneous mitral valvuloplasty to evaluate the suitability of the valve/and subvalvular structures for balloon valvuloplasty, the presence of mitral regurgitation (MR), and to evaluate the LA appendage for thrombus.

Pathologic Findings
- Most characteristic pathologic finding is fusion of the leaflet edges along the commissures between the anterior and posterior leaflets.
- Additional features include fusion, thickening, and shortening of the mitral valve chordae; fibrosis and thickening of the valve leaflets; and superimposed calcification.

DIFFERENTIAL DIAGNOSIS
- Causes of mid-diastolic murmur (MDM)
  - Austin-Flint: MDM over the mitral valve heard in patients with aortic insufficiency. The MDM results from reduced opening of mitral valve in diastole due to an eccentric jet of aortic regurgitation directly impinging on the anterior mitral valve leaflet or an increase in LV diastolic pressure causing partial mitral valve closure.
  - MDM with patent ductus arteriosus (PDA) and ventricular septal defect (VSD) occurs due to increased flow across the mitral valve.
- MDM in constrictive pericarditis secondary to constriction ring at the AV groove level
- Cor triatriatum
- Tricuspid stenosis: Its murmur increases during inspiration as well as during the release phase of Valsalva.
- Atrial septal defect (ASD): MDM over the tricuspid secondary to increased flow across the tricuspid valve

TREATMENT

GENERAL MEASURES

- Prophylaxis for recurrent rheumatic fever if indicated
- Endocarditis prophylaxis is recommended, because pure MS confers intermediate risk and MS with MR confers a relatively high risk.

 MEDICATION (DRUGS)

- MS is a mechanical limitation to diastolic filling. Medical therapy cannot be expected to cause regression or delay progression of disease but can improve symptoms by improving diastolic filling time.
- β-Blockers and calcium channel blockers can be used to manage exertional symptoms related to rapid heart rate.
- Intermittent diuretics can be used if evidence exists of pulmonary vascular congestion.
- Digitalis does not benefit patients with MS with normal sinus rhythm unless paroxysmal atrial fibrillation exists, with rapid ventricular response or ventricular dysfunction.
- Anticoagulation in patients with atrial fibrillation (either chronic or patients with prior embolic events), and patients with severe MS and a large left atrium (>-5.5 cm) on echocardiography

SURGERY

- Percutaneous mitral balloon valvotomy
  - Candidates for mitral valvotomy are evaluated on leaflet mobility, leaflet thickening, valvular calcification, and subvalvular thickening. Significant MR or LA appendage thrombus is a contraindication to valvotomy.
  - Patients with MS (mitral valve area <1.5 cm²) and New York Heart Association (NYHA) class II or more symptoms and valve morphology suitable for balloon valvotomy in the absence of atrial thrombus and moderate to severe MR
  - Patients with MS (mitral valve area <1.5 cm²) and pulmonary hypertension (pulmonary artery systolic pressure >50 mm Hg at rest and 60 mm Hg during exertion) and valve morphology suitable for balloon valvotomy in the absence of atrial thrombus and moderate to severe MR
  - Patients with MS (mitral valve area <1.5 cm²) and NYHA class III or more symptoms and a nonpliable calcified valve who are at high risk for surgery in the absence of atrial thrombus and moderate to severe MR
  - Patients with MS (mitral valve area <1.5 cm²) and valve morphology suitable for balloon valvotomy who have new-onset atrial fibrillation in the absence of atrial thrombus and moderate to severe MR
- Mitral valve replacement
  - Patients with MS (mitral valve area <1.5 cm²) and NYHA class II or more symptoms who are not candidates for balloon valvotomy and mitral valve repair
  - Asymptomatic patients with MS (mitral valve area <1.0 cm²) and severe pulmonary hypertension with NYHA class I–II symptoms who are not candidates for balloon valvotomy or mitral valve repair

 FOLLOW-UP

- Asymptomatic patients with moderate MS should be re-evaluated yearly.
- Strenuous exertion should be avoided in symptomatic patients.

PROGNOSIS

- In studies conducted before the surgical era, 10-year survival was related to symptoms present at diagnosis and varied from 80% with functional class I to 0% in functional class IV.
- In these historical studies, the incidence of heart failure was ~60%, and ~20% of the patients had embolic events.

COMPLICATIONS

- Atrial arrhythmias
- Pulmonary hypertension with right-sided heart failure
- Hemoptysis
- Recurrent rheumatic fever
- Systemic embolization may occur in 10–20% of patients with MS.

REFERENCES

1. Bonow RO, Carabello B, de Leon AC Jr., et al. ACC/AHA 2006 guidelines for the management of patients with valvular heart disease: A report of the American College of Cardiology/American Heart Association Task Force on Practice Guidelines (Writting Committee to Revise the 1998 Guidelines for the Management of Patients with Valvular Heart Disease). American College of Cardiology Web Site. Available at: http//content.onlinejacc.org/cgi/reprint/48/3/e1
2. Bonow RO, Cheitlin MD, Crawford MH, et al. Task Force 3: valvular heart disease. *J Am Coll Cardiol* 2005;45:1334–1340.
3. Guerios EE, Bueno R, Nercolini D, et al. Mitral stenosis and percutaneous mitral valvuloplasty (part 2). *J Invasive Cardiol.* 2005;17:440–444.
4. Vahanian A, Palacios IF. Percutaneous approaches to valvular disease. *Circulation.* 2004; 109P1572–1579.
5. Zipes DP, et al. *Braunwald's Heart Disease*, 7th ed. Philadelphia: Elsevier Saunders, 2005.

 MISCELLANEOUS

CODES
ICD9-CM
394.0

PATIENT TEACHING
Diet
Low-sodium diet with the development of congestive heart failure
Activity
Patients with mild MS have few physical limitations. Patients with moderate or severe limitations to diastolic filling should avoid vigorous physical activity and stress.
Prevention
Prophylaxis against infective endocarditis and rheumatic fever
Pregnancy Considerations
- Increased maternal morbidity, preterm delivery, intrauterine growth retardation with increasing severity of MS
- Consider percutaneous balloon valvuloplasty in nonpregnant women considering pregnancy with a mitral valve area of <1.0 cm².
- In pregnant women with MS, decrease heart rate and LA pressure with decreased activity and β-blockade.

M

MITRAL VALVE PROLAPSE, MYXOMATOUS DEGENERATION OF THE HEART

Steven Kuehn
Steven C. Herrmann
Bernard R. Chaitman

 BASICS

DESCRIPTION
- Mitral valve prolapse (MVP) is exaggerated billowing of the mitral valve leaflets into the left atrium (LA) during systole without valve coaptation, resulting in mitral regurgitation (MR).
  Synonym(s): Systolic click-murmur syndrome; Barlow's syndrome; Billowing mitral cusp syndrome; Myxomatous mitral valve; Floppy-valve syndrome; Redundant cusp syndrome

EPIDEMIOLOGY
- Age: MVP has been described in all groups, but is most common in young women.
- Sex: Female > Male (2:1)

Prevalence
One of the most prevalent cardiovascular abnormalities, affecting ~2% of the general population

RISK FACTORS
- MVP generally is a primary cardiovascular disorder. Several conditions may be associated with it (see below).
- MVP tends to be more common in patients with asthenic body habitus, straight backs, shallow chest wall, and pectus excavatum.

Genetics
MVP syndrome is thought to be at least partly heritable, with an autosomal-dominant mode of transmission with variable penetrance.

PATHOPHYSIOLOGY
Severe MVP is associated with MR. Severe MR may lead to heart failure symptoms.

ETIOLOGY
Myxomatous degeneration of the mitral valve apparatus; likely due to a connective tissue abnormality

ASSOCIATED CONDITIONS
- Hyperthyroidism
- Marfan's syndrome
- Ehlers-Danlos syndrome
- Pseudoxanthoma elasticum
- Periarteritis nodosa
- Osteogenesis imperfecta
- Myotonic dystrophy
- Von Willebrand's disease

DIAGNOSIS

SIGNS AND SYMPTOMS
- The majority of patients with MVP are asymptomatic.
- However, many patients have increased anxiety, fatigue, palpitations, orthostatic hypotension, and evidence of autonomic dysfunction, although it has not been confirmed that these symptoms occur more frequently than in the general population.
- Chest pain is a frequent complaint, although it is generally atypical with regard to angina.
- The chest pain with MVP usually occurs at rest and is sharp in character.
  – Thought to be due to abnormal tension on papillary muscles
  – Palpitations are common and can represent both benign atrial and malignant ventricular tachyarrhythmias. An increased associated of Wolf-Parkinson-White syndrome is noted in patients with MVP.

Physical Exam
- Auscultatory examination shows a systolic click at least 0.14 seconds after the first heart sound, occurring just after the carotid upstroke, which helps differentiate the click of MVP from an ejection click.
- The prolapse is a volume-dependent phenomenon; at low ventricular volumes more stress is placed on the abnormal mitral apparatus, and the valve may prolapse earlier or more so than in a volume-overloaded condition.
- The ejection click is best heard with the stethoscope diaphragm at the left sternal border and is followed by a mid to late crescendo systolic murmur lasting until the second heart sound.
- Occasionally, only the ejection click or the murmur alone is present.
- The duration of the murmur corresponds with the severity of MR.
- Arterial vasodilation, augmented contractility, and decreased venous return cause the click and murmur to move toward S1.
- Dynamic auscultation with amyl nitrate, early Valsalva, or upright posture causes the click and murmur to move toward S1.
- Squatting, leg raise, and isometric exercise delays the click and murmur toward S2.

TESTS
Cardiac catheterization can visualize the mitral valve leaflets prolapsing into the atrium as well as a scalloped appearance of the leaflets consistent with redundant tissue; should be considered in patients with chest pain and abnormal noninvasive ischemia test results.

Imaging
- The ECG is usually normal in asymptomatic patients. However, biphasic T-waves and nonspecific ST-segment abnormalities, perhaps secondary to papillary muscle ischemia, may be noted in leads II, III, and aVF.
- Paroxysmal supraventricular tachycardia is the most frequent arrhythmia noted with MVP, although premature atrial beats, ventricular beats, and sinus node dysfunction with bradyarrhythmias are also common.
- In patients with dizziness, syncope, or QT prolongation, consider 24-hr ECG monitoring if no clear explanation for these symptoms exists.
- M-mode echocardiography shows posterior movement of the mitral valve leaflets in mid-systole.
- On 2-D echocardiography, the valve leaflets are thickened and redundant and prolapse back into the atrium during systole.
- The parasternal view is the most specific for the diagnosis of MVP.
- Color-flow Doppler usually shows a mitral regurgitant jet.

Diagnostic Procedures/Surgery
- MVP was previously grossly overdiagnosed before more stringent clinical and echocardiographic criteria were accepted.
- For diagnosis, patients must have 1 of the following:
  – Mid to late systolic click with late murmur or whoop
  – Marked superior displacement of the mitral valve leaflets (≥2 mm) above the annulus
  – Mild to moderate superior displacement of the MV leaflets above the annulus, along with other supportive findings on echo or physical exam (classic click, murmur in a young patient, or whoop)

Pathologic Findings
- Myxomatous proliferation of the middle layer (spongiosa) of the valve, resulting in increased mucopolysaccharide deposition and myxomatous degeneration
- By electron microscopy, the collagen fibers in the valve leaflets are disorganized and fragmented.
- With increased stroma deposition, the valve leaflets enlarge and become redundant.
- The endothelium is usually noncontiguous and a frequent site for thrombus or infective vegetation.

DIFFERENTIAL DIAGNOSIS
- Mitral regurgitation
- Tricuspid regurgitation
- Tricuspid valve prolapse
- Papillary muscle dysfunction
- Hypertrophic cardiomyopathy

TREATMENT

GENERAL MEASURES
- Reassurance is necessary with the asymptomatic patient.
- Patients with a documented focal neurologic event should be considered for aspirin or anticoagulation therapy.
- Patients with significant MR should be treated with afterload reduction or considered for mitral valve repair or replacement.
- Patients with arrhythmias or long QT syndromes should have 24-hour ECG monitoring.
- Electrophysiologic studies may be considered in symptomatic patients because of the rare association of MVP and sudden cardiac death.
- Endocarditis prophylaxis is recommended for patients with systolic click and murmur of MR and in those with the systolic click and echo findings of prolapse. No prophylaxis is recommended for an isolated systolic click.

MEDICATION (DRUGS)

First Line
- β-Blockers are drug of choice for patients with MVP and palpitations.
- Chest pain syndromes are also best treated with β-blockers.
- Angiotensin-converting enzyme (ACE) inhibitors and angiotensin receptor blockers may be used to reduce blood pressure and regurgitation in the appropriate clinical setting, but should not be used in the presence of severe MR and left ventricular remodeling without consideration of mitral valve repair.

Second Line
Hydralazine and nitrates in combination for afterload reduction

SURGERY
Indications are the same as for MR.

PROGNOSIS
- For asymptomatic patients, prognosis is excellent.
- For patients with severe MR or reduced ejection fraction, the prognosis is similar to nonischemic MR.

COMPLICATIONS
- Sudden cardiac death (very rare)
- Chordae rupture with acute mitral insufficiency
- Endocarditis
- Fibrin emboli
- Heart failure with progressive MR

PATIENT MONITORING
- Asymptomatic patients should be followed with transthoracic echocardiogram every 3–5 years.
- Patients with more severe MR should be followed annually.

REFERENCES
1. Hayek E, Gring CN, Griffin BP. Mitral valve prolapse. *Lancet*. 2005;365:507–518.
2. Maron BJ, Ackerman MJ, Nishimura RA, et al. Task Force 4: HCM and other cardiomyopathies, mitral valve prolapse, myocarditis, and Marfan syndrome. *J Am Coll Cardiol*. 2005;45:1340–1345.
3. Wu WC, Aziz GF, Sadaniantz A. The use of stress echocardiography in the assessment of mitral valvular disease. *Echocardiography*. 2004;21:451–458.

MISCELLANEOUS

See also: Mitral Regurgitation

CODES
ICD9-CM
354.9

PATIENT TEACHING
Patient education on avoidance of alcohol, caffeine, stimulants, and nicotine may be sufficient to control symptoms in some instances.

Diet
Sodium and water restriction should be encouraged if the MR is severe enough to affect left ventricular function.

Activity
No limitations unless heart failure or anginal symptoms predominate

Prevention
- Endocarditis prophylaxis is recommended for patients with both the mid-systolic click and mitral regurgitant murmur, with click and echo findings, or with typical echo findings (see above).
- Women under the age of 45 with the systolic click only may not require prophylaxis unless undergoing upper respiratory or genitourinary procedures.

M

MUSCULAR DYSTROPHY AND THE HEART

Nezar Amir

 BASICS

DESCRIPTION

A diffuse group of heritable disorders of the skeletal muscles in which direct involvement of the cardiac muscle and/or the cardiac conducting system is present to a variable degree.

Manifestations

- Progressive skeletal muscle wasting and weakness involving specific groups of muscles
- Cardiac disease manifested as heart failure, arrhythmias, and sudden cardiac death due to:
  - Cardiomyopathy
  - Conduction system disease
- Other organ systems

Classification is based on the mode of inheritance, pattern, and distribution of skeletal muscle weakness.

- X-linked dystrophinopathies
  - Duchenne muscular dystrophy
  - Becker muscular dystrophy
- Myotonic muscular dystrophy
- Emery-Dreifuss and associated disorders
- Limb-girdle muscular dystrophy
- Fascioscapulohumeral muscular dystrophy

EPIDEMIOLOGY

- X-linked dystrophinopathies
  - Duchenne
    - Males, all ethnic groups
    - Onset in childhood, by 5 years all are involved
    - Death by 20–25 years from cardiac/respiratory failure
  - Becker
    - Males and females
    - Age of onset is variable (5–45 years)
    - Most survive to 40–50 years
- Myotonic muscular dystrophy
  - Most common neuromuscular disease in patients presenting in adulthood
  - Commoner in French Canadians
  - Age of onset is 20–25

- Emery-Dreifuss and associated disorders
  - Rare familial disease with prominent cardiac involvement
  - Male
- Limb-girdle muscular dystrophy
  - Usual age of onset is <30 years
- Fascioscapulohumeral muscular dystrophy
  - Cardiac involvement is rare in this disease and therefore will not be discussed any further

PEDIATRIC CONSIDERATIONS

Usual age of onset for X-linked dystrophinopathies

Incidence

- X-linked dystrophinopathies:
  - Duchenne: Incidence 1/3,300 male, live births (13–33/100,000)
  - Becker: Incidence 3–6/100,000 male births
- Myotonic muscular dystrophy
  - Global incidence is 1/8,000
- Emery-Dreifuss and associated disorders
  - Rare disease
- Limb-girdle muscular dystrophy
- Fascioscapulohumeral muscular dystrophy

Prevalence

- X-linked dystrophinopathies
  - Duchenne muscular dystrophy: 3/100,000
  - Becker muscular dystrophy: Hard to predict
- Myotonic muscular dystrophy
- Emery-Dreifuss and associated disorders
- Limb-girdle muscular dystrophy
- Fascioscapulohumeral muscular dystrophy

Pregnancy Considerations

- Female carriers could have serious conducting system disease
- Exacerbation and decompensation of left ventricular (LV) function during pregnancy
- Mild cases may require further genetic testing and counseling during pregnancy

RISK FACTORS

Family history

Genetics

- X-linked dystrophinopathies
  - X-linked recessive
  - Gene is located on the short arm of X chromosome
  - Gene product is dystrophin protein
  - 1/3 is sporadic
  - Females are affected in Becker
- Myotonic muscular dystrophy
  - Unstable trinucleotide repeat
  - Chromosome 19
  - Number of copies correlate with severity of muscular and cardiac disease
- Emery-Dreifuss
  - X-linked
  - Female carriers have cardiac conduction system disease
  - Gene product is emerin, Lamin A&C
- Limb-girdle muscular dystrophy
  - Autosomal recessive
  - Gene products are dystrophin-associated proteins and Lamin A&C

PATHOPHYSIOLOGY

- Absent or abnormal gene products predispose to cardiac dysfunction
- Absent dystrophin leads mainly to cardiomyopathy
- Absent Lamin leads to selective conduction system disease

ETIOLOGY

Hereditary

ASSOCIATED CONDITIONS

Respiratory insufficiency, Pneumonias, Mild retardation, Duchenne dystrophy, Myotonic dystrophy, Chronic bronchitis, Brochiectasis, Cataract, Baldness, Gonadal Atrophy, Megacolon megacolon (myotonic dystrophy)

DIAGNOSIS

History
- Positive family history
- Age of onset depends on the type
- Proximal muscle weakness, difficulty in standing from a chair, climbing stairs and in children delayed motor milestones
- Cardiac involvement
  - Shortness of breath, edema
  - Palpitations, presyncope, syncope, sudden cardiac death
- Noncardiac manifestations depending on the type: mild mental retardation, diabetes, recurrent chest infections

Physical Exam
- X-linked dystrophinopathies
  - More severe and earlier onset with Duchenne
  - Becker can present with minimal muscle disease but significant cardiac involvement
  - Muscular involvement
    - Clumsy, waddling gait, frequent falls, difficulties rising from floor; wheelchair bound
    - Pseudohypertrophy of calves, lumbar lordosis and kyphoscoliosis
    - Later respiratory muscle weakness leads to pneumonia and impaired cough
  - Cardiovascular
    - Sinus tachycardia, atrial flutter
    - Displaced and forceful apical impulse due to thoracic deformity, loud pulmonic component of the second heart sound (P_2), pan-systolic murmur (PSM) of mitral regurgitation due to posterior papillary muscle dysfunction
    - Impaired LV function as early as 5 years in Duchenne
    - Skeletal muscle involvement may underestimate the severity of cardiac involvement.

- Myotonic muscular dystrophy
  - Many subtypes, the commonest is type 1
  - Muscular involvement: mainly weakness of the fascial and neck muscles and distal muscles of the extremities that exhibit the typical myotonic delayed relaxation response
  - Cardiac involvement
    - Conduction system disease resulting in atrioventricular (AV) block, trial and ventricular tachycardia
    - Dilated cardiomyopathy is rare
  - Other features: Diabetes mellitus, frontal baldness, and mild mental retardation
- Emery-Dreifuss disease
  - Female carriers develop conduction system disease
  - Early contractures of the elbow, Achilles tendon, and posterior cervical muscles
  - Slowly progressive weakness
  - Cardiac involvement
    - Conduction system disease and arrhythmias in the form of complete heart block, atrial flutter, and ventricular tachycardia and sudden cardiac death is common <50
  - Dilated cardiomyopathy is rare
- Limb-girdle muscular dystrophy
  - Difficulty in walking due to pelvic girdle involvement
  - Slow progression of muscular disease
- Cardiac involvement is heterogeneous; cardiomyopathy is rarely reported; arrhythmias and conduction system disease are the most serious manifestation and may develop when Lamin A&C are defective; there is high risk of sudden cardiac death despite pacing and may point to implantable cardioverter defibrillator (ICD) as the ideal treatment option.

TESTS
Duchenne

Lab
- ECG
  - X-linked dystrophinopathies:
  - Characteristic features due to selective inferolateral fibrosis
  - Tall right precordial R waves and increased R/S amplitude, Deep Q waves on leads I, aVL, V_5–V_6. Abnormal terminal force of P waves, especially in V_1 with negative deflection >20 msec and 0.1 mV, or broad and notched P waves in V_2, short P-R interval, or in late stage prolonged P-R interval.
  - The other muscular dystrophies have no specific electrocardiographic changes
- Elevated creatinine kinase (CK) CK and MB fraction (CK-MB); not useful for diagnosis of cardiac involvement. The highest is seen in Duchenne and Becker and to a lesser extent in fascioscapulohumeral and Emery-Dreifuss.

Imaging
- X-linked dystrophinopathies
  - Duchenne
    - Chest x-ray includes thoracic deformity, high diaphragms, decreased anteroposterior (AP) dimensions, evidence of heart failure in the advanced stages
    - Echocardiography: Inferolateral and inferior basal-mid hypokinesis, impaired diastolic function, and, at later stages, impaired systolic function, mitral regurgitation due to inferolateral pap muscle dysfunction and prolapse
    - Thallium scintigraphy/single protein emission computed tomography (SPECT)

Regional perfusion defects (posterobasal and lateral LV wall) in metabolic abnormal but viable myocardium

M

Becker, Emery-Dreifuss, Myotonic dystrophy

- Chest x-ray
  - May show evidence of heart failure with enlarged heart and prominent pulmonary vasculature
- Echocardiogram
  - May show dilated cardiomyopathy
  - For myotonic dystrophy, normal systolic function is common, with evidence of diastolic dysfunction.

Diagnostic Procedures/Surgery

- Diagnosis of muscular dystrophy and its type
  - CK levels
  - Electromyogram (EMG) and nerve conduction studies
  - Skeletal muscle biopsy [hematoxylin and eosin (H&E) stains, histochemistry and E/M]
  - Analysis of the defective gene products (dystrophin levels, Lamin A&C, sarcoglycan levels)
  - Genetic testing: To detect the deletion(s) and trinucleotide repeats in myotonia
- Cardiac involvement: The diagnostic procedures are dictated by the type of the clinical presentation.
  - Heart failure: cardiac biopsy
  - Arrhythmias or high risk asymptomatic electrocardiographic abnormalities suggestive of conduction system disease: cardiac electrophysiologic study

Pathologic Findings

Duchenne:

- Predilection for specific regions of the myocardium: the inferolateral and inferior LV walls (fibrous replacement) with relative sparing of interventricular septum (IVS), right ventricle, and atria
- Often there is a small vessel coronary arteriopathy characterized by hypertrophy of media with luminal narrowing.

DIFFERENTIAL DIAGNOSIS

- Other causes of heart failure, especially with mild clinical involvement and in sporadic cases
- Arrhythmogenic right ventricular dysplasia (ARVD) in isolated right ventricle involvement in Becker
- Pulmonary hypertension in patients with Duchenne may be suspected based on the abnormal cardiac examination and the electrocardiogram (ECG); however, measurement of right ventricular pressures by echocardiogram is normal.
- Other major causes for arrhythmias and conduction system disease

TREATMENT

GENERAL MEASURES

- Hospitalization only for those with heart failure, arrhythmias, or other serious illness
- Supportive, prevention of contractures, bilevel positive airway pressure (BIPAP) at night (Duchenne)
- Symptomatic, treatment of heart failure and serious arrhythmias (sotalol used with variable success in limb-girdle type)
- Treatment follows guidelines used for cardiomyopathy and conduction abnormalities due to any cause.
- The American College of Cardiology (ACC)/American Heart Association (AHA) guidelines for pacing put this group of patients as a high risk.

MEDICATION (DRUGS)

Steroids are used for boys younger than 5 years with Duchenne and remain the mainstay of treatment.

- There are a number of medications that should be avoided in these patients:
  - Procainamide/phenytoin: May worsen muscle weakness.
  - Verapamil intravenous (IV): May cause fatal respiratory arrest.
  - Halothane, suxamethonium, isoflurane, succinylcholine: can cause malignant hyperthermia and cardiac arrest during anesthesia

SURGERY

- Pacemaker if high-degree AV block present (Becker, Emery-Dreifuss, myotonic dystrophy, occasional limb-girdle dystrophies)
- Low threshold for temporary pacing during surgery due to risk of high grade AV block
- ICDs for patients with malignant arrhythmias

FOLLOW-UP

- Regular follow-up by neurologists
- Regular follow-up by cardiologists (patients need at least regular ECGs and echocardiograms to exclude cardiac involvement)

DISPOSITION

Admission Criteria

- Respiratory complications
- Uncontrolled cardiac failure
- Syncope and sudden cardiac death

Discharge Criteria

Resolution of problems

Issues for Referral

Regular follow-up by cardiologist and cardiac electrophysiologists is advisable for all patients, with regular echocardiograms and ECGs.

PROGNOSIS

- X-linked dystrophinopathies
  - Duchenne
    - Relentless and fatal disease by the second decade
    - Death is due to respiratory and cardiac arrest.
  - Becker
    - Slower progression
    - Cardiac death is more tragic and may happen with mild forms.
    - Adult-onset
    - Isolated right ventricular involvement, and female carriers may be exacerbated during pregnancy.
- Myotonic muscular dystrophy
  - Progression is variable.
  - Sudden cardiac death can happen with minimal disease.

- Emery-Dreifuss and associated disorders
  - Prominent cardiac disease
  - Low threshold for pacing and ICD.
- Limb-girdle muscular dystrophy
  - Slow progression
  - Arrhythmias may require pacing and ICD

COMPLICATIONS
Heart failure, arrhythmias, cardiac arrest, death

PATIENT MONITORING
- Regular monitoring by cardiologists
- Severe heart failure, malignant arrhythmias, and symptomatic conduction disturbances require hospitalization.

REFERENCES
1. Bhakta D, Lowe MR, Groh WJ. Prevalence of structural cardiac abnormalities in patients with myotonic dystrophy type I. *Am Heart J.* 2004;47:224.
2. Duboc D, Meune C, Lerebours G, et al. Effect of perindopril on the onset and progression of left ventricular dysfunction in Duchenne muscular dystrophy. *J Am Coll Cardiol.* 2005;45:855.
3. Emery AE. The muscular dystrophies. *Lancet.* 2002;359:687.
4. Fung KC, Corbett A, Kritharides L. Myocardial tissue velocity reduction is correlated with clinical neurologic severity in myotonic dystrophy. *Am J Cardiol.* 2003;92:177.
5. Hoffman EP, Brown RH Jr, Kunkel LM. Dystrophin: The protein product of the Duchenne muscular dystrophy locus. *Cell.* 1987;51:919.
6. Worton, R. Muscular dystrophies: Diseases of the dystrophin-glycoprotein complex. *Science.* 1995;270:755.

CODES
ICD9-CM
359.1 + 425.8 Cardiomyopathy due to progressive muscular dystrophy

PATIENT TEACHING
Organization:
- Muscular Dystrophy Association USA, National Headquarters, 3300 E. Sunrise Dr., Tucson, AZ 85718; 1-800-572-1717

Activity
As tolerated

Prevention
- Genetic counseling
- Prenatal diagnosis is feasible through amniotic fluid analysis obtained by paracentesis during the second trimester of pregnancy

FAQ
Q: Is muscular dystrophy a single disease?
A: No, the muscular dystrophies are a group of diseases involving the skeletal and cardiac muscles.

Q: Does it occur only in childhood?
A: No, the age of onset can be at any age from 3–35 years.

Q: My child has been recently diagnosed with muscular dystrophy, should I get tested?
A: Yes, you should, as there are some recessive types (milder) that can run in the parents; however, cardiac involvement is more severe.

Q: Can the disease be diagnosed during pregnancy?
A: Yes, it is possible to look for the genetic abnormality in samples obtained from the amniotic fluid.

Q: Does the disease affect only boys?
A: Depending on the type, boys are more commonly and more severely involved in Becker disease; however, females could be involved and become carriers with significant possibility of cardiac involvement.

Q: Is there any relationship between the severity of muscular and cardiac disease?
A: No, cardiac involvement can take place even in so-called "carriers."

Q: What are the manifestations of heart disease in muscular dystrophy?
A: The manifestations include shortness of breath on mild exercise, ankle swelling, palpitations, syncope, and extreme forms of sudden death.

Q: Are there any available treatments for heart disease in muscular dystrophies?
A: Yes, there are treatments for weakness of the heart muscle pump named heart failure; there are also treatments for abnormal heart rhythms in the form pacemakers and ICDs.

M

MYOCARDIAL INFARCTION (DIAGNOSIS AND MANAGEMENT, INCLUDING ALL SUBSET OF ACUTE MI, E.G., STEMI, NON–STEMI)

John A. Riddick
Vineet Kaushik*
Nanette K. Wenger

 BASICS

DESCRIPTION
- Prolonged myocardial ischemia resulting in myocardial injury and necrosis
- Subdivided into ST-segment elevation myocardial infarction (STEMI) and non–ST-segment elevation MI (NSTEMI) that presents with ST-segment depression/nondiagnostic electrocardiogram (ECG)/normal ECG. The distinction is important because the initial therapeutic strategy and clinical course differ.

EPIDEMIOLOGY
- Predominant age: Incidence increases with age.
- Predominant sex: Male > Female

Incidence
Approximately 800,000 people experience acute myocardial infarction (AMI) annually and about 213,000 die.

Pregnancy Considerations
- Rare, estimated incidence 0.01%
- Causes include coronary spasm, dissection, atherosclerosis, thrombosis
- Fibrinolytic therapy relatively contraindicated

RISK FACTORS
Major Risk Factors
- Advancing age
- Sex: Males, postmenopausal females
- Family history of premature coronary atherosclerotic heart disease
- Dyslipidemia: Elevated low-density lipoprotein (LDL) level, low high-density lipoprotein (HDL) level
- Diabetes mellitus
- Smoking
- Hypertension
- Obesity: Particularly central/truncal obesity
- Sedentary lifestyle
- Chronic kidney disease
Other Risk Factors
- Elevated lipoprotein(a)
- Elevated plasma homocysteine
- Hypertriglyceridemia
- Psychosocial factors: Stress, social isolation, depression
- Inflammatory markers: Elevated C-reactive protein
- Prothrombic factors: Elevated fibrinogen

ETIOLOGY
- Coronary atherosclerotic disease (>90%): Acute plaque rupture with thrombus formation
- Coronary vasospasm: Variant/Prinzmetal angina, cocaine
- Coronary emboli: Endocarditis, mural thrombi
- Congenital coronary anomalies
- Thrombotic disease: Hypercoagulable states, sickle cell disease, oral contraceptive use
- Coronary vasculitis: Takayasu, Kawasaki, polyarteritis nodosa, lupus, scleroderma, rheumatoid arthritis, allograft rejection
- Aortic dissection: Proximal type with coronary ostial involvement
- Trauma: Coronary dissection/laceration
- States with oxygen demand exceeding supply: Hypotension, severe left ventricular hypertrophy (LVH), aortic stenosis, anemia, tachycardia

ASSOCIATED CONDITIONS
Peripheral vascular disease, Stroke, Congestive heart failure (CHF)

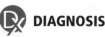 **DIAGNOSIS**

SIGNS AND SYMPTOMS
Signs
- Anxiousness, tachypnea (CHF)
- Diaphoresis, skin pallor, cool, clammy
- Brady-/tachycardia, hypo-/hypertension
- Jugular venous pressure (JVP) elevated with right ventricular (RV) infarction, severe LV failure
- Basilar rales with LV dysfunction
- Soft first heart sound (S1) and second heart sound (S2) with decreased contractility; S3; S4 very common
- Pericardial friction rub
- Systolic murmur at apex; mitral regurgitation from papillary muscle dysfunction/rupture, ventricular septal defect (VSD)
Symptoms
- Chest pain
- Dyspnea
- Pain in abdomen, neck, jaw, arm, back
- Nausea/vomiting
- Diaphoresis

- Palpitations, syncope
- Sudden death
- Cerebrovascular accident (CVA)
- Sudden confusion, weakness
- Severe apprehension

TESTS
Lab
ECG: Less than 10 minutes after arrival; provides the most important initial information to guide management

- Acute ST elevation: ST-segment elevation localizes area of myocardial injury and usually results in Q-wave MI.
  - Exception: posterior: ST depression in leads V_1–V_2, up to V_4; large R wave in V_1
- ST depression/nondiagnostic ECG changes/normal ECG
  - Usually results in non–Q-wave MI (if cardiac biomarkers positive)

Serum Biomarkers

- Creatinine kinase (CK) and MB fraction
  - CK nonspecific; in MM, BB, MB fractions
  - CK-MB sensitive and specific; traditional cardiac enzyme to detect myocardial damage/diagnose MI
  - Elevation onset at 4–6 hours, peak at 14–36 hours (depending on reperfusion therapy), returns to normal at 48–72 hours
- Troponin T and I
  - Elevation onset at 4–6 hours, peak at 24–36 hours (depending on reperfusion therapy), returns to normal in 10–14 days
  - Very sensitive, highly specific
  - Replaced lactate dehydrogenase (LDH) as test of choice to diagnose MI >48 hours from onset
- Myoglobin
  - Elevation onset at 2 hours, returns to normal at 7–12 hours
  - Nonspecific; limited clinical utility lies in early peak

- Complete blood count (CBC) with platelet count early rise in white blood cell (WBC) count in MI, international normalized ratio (INR), partial thromboplastin time (PTT), electrolytes with magnesium, blood urea nitrogen (BUN), creatinine, glucose, lipids, and aPTT

Imaging
Echocardiogram

- Useful to assess wall motion abnormalities; unable to distinguish reliably severe ischemia versus acute infarction versus old infarction
- Information about ejection fraction (EF), mechanical complications

Nuclear Medicine Studies

- Limited use in acute MI, important for postinfarction risk stratification
- Rarely used to diagnose RV infarction or when MI cannot be diagnosed by standard means

CT Scan

- May be helpful as part of "triple rule out": Evaluating for acute coronary syndrome (ACS) pulmonary embolism (PE), or aortic dissection
- Initial studies promising for defining proximal coronary anatomy in NSTEMI; however, radiation, contrast, tachycardia, and arrhythmia issues exist

MRI

- Limited use in acute setting, visualizes proximal coronaries without radiation or contrast concerns but technical issues greater than CT
- Post MI can define wall motion, transmural extent of infarction, presence of LV thrombus, and viability prerevascularization

Cardiac Catheterization
Coronary angiography used in conjunction with primary percutaneous coronary intervention (PCI) ± stenting in acute MI setting

DIFFERENTIAL DIAGNOSIS

- Cardiovascular: Unstable angina, pericarditis, aortic dissection, LVH with repolarization abnormality, early repolarization, Wolfe-Parkinson-White, hypertrophic obstructive cardiomyopathy (HOCM), Brugada syndrome
- Pulmonary: Pulmonary embolus, pleurisy/pneumonia, pneumothorax
- Gastrointestinal: Esophageal disorders (spasm, reflux, rupture), peptic ulcer disease, biliary disease, pancreatitis
- Musculoskeletal: Costochondritis, chest wall pain, cervical disk, or neuropathic pain
- Psychiatric: Somatization or psychogenic pain, panic attack

 TREATMENT

GENERAL MEASURES

- Oxygen: 2 L per minute, reassess if stable >6 hours
- Alleviate pain: Nitrates, morphine
- Alleviate anxiety: Anxiolytics
- Telemetry/cardiac care unit (CCU) monitoring
- Bed rest first 12 hours
- NPO except sips of water until stable
- Stool softener
- Keep plasma K and Mg levels optimal.

M

MEDICATION (DRUGS)

Acute STEMI

Goal: Early reperfusion with fibrinolytic therapy or primary PCI

- Fibrinolytic therapy
  - Indications
    - ST elevation >1 mm in two or more contiguous leads or ST depression >1 mm in true posterior MI
    - New left bundle branch block with history suggesting acute MI
    - Benefit if given <12 hours after symptom onset, greatest benefit < 6 hours
    - Goal: Door-to-needle time <30 minutes
    - Preferred if early presentation (<3 hours) and delay to invasive strategy
  - Contraindications
    - Absolute contraindications: Prior intracranial hemorrhage, known structural cerebral vascular lesion or malignant intracranial neoplasm, ischemic CVA within 3 months (unless <3 hours), suspected aortic dissection, active bleeding or bleeding diathesis (except menses), significant closed-head or facial trauma within 3 months
    - Relative contraindications: History of severe, poorly controlled hypertension or systolic blood pressure >180 mm Hg or diastolic blood pressure >110 mm Hg on arrival, remote cerebrovascular accident or dementia or other intracranial pathology, prolonged CPR (>10 minutes) or major surgery within 3 weeks, recent (2–4 week) history of internal bleeding, noncompressible vascular puncture, prior exposure to streptokinase or anistreplase, pregnancy, PUD, elevated INR
  - Agents available
    - Alteplase, IV bolus 15 mg, infusion 0.75 mg/kg for 30 minutes (max 50 mg), then 0.5 mg/kg not to exceed 35 mg over next 60 minutes to an overall max of 100 mg
    - Reteplase, 10 U IV over 2 minutes; 30 minutes after first dose, give 10 U IV over 2 minutes
    - Streptokinase: 1.5 million U IV over 30–60 minutes
    - Tenecteplase, IV bolus over 10–15 seconds, 30 mg for weight <60 kg; 35 mg for 60–69 kg; 40 mg for 70–79 kg; 45 mg for 80–89 kg; 50 mg for 90 kg or more

- Catheterization/PCI: Alternative to fibrinolytic therapy if performed at experienced center in timely fashion (primary PCI) with goal door-to-balloon <90 minutes, if fibrinolytics contraindicated, with failed fibrinolytics (rescue PCI), cardiogenic shock, or if diagnosis of STEMI uncertain
- Aspirin: Chew 162–325 mg non–enteric-coated then 75–62 mg daily (enteric-coated okay)
- β-Blocker, unless bradycardia or low blood pressure
- Intravenous unfractionated heparin—goal aPTT 1.5 to 2.0 x normal for 48 hours
- Nitrates: Unless suspected RV infarct, low blood pressure or Viagra or Levitra use within past 24 hours (48 hours for Cialis)
- Angiotensin-converting enzyme (ACE) inhibitor: Acutely in <24 hours with anterior MI or CHF with left ventricular ejection fraction (LVEF) <0.40 unless low blood pressure
- Angiotensin receptor blocker (ARB) as above if ACE inhibitor intolerant
- Clopidogrel: If undergoing PCI, loading dose of 300–600 mg followed by 75 mg daily for 1 month minimum if bare metal stent, 3 month for sirolimus drug-eluting stent (DES), and 6 months for paclitaxel DES; continue 12 months after stent in patients not at risk of bleeding
- Hydroxymethylglutaryl coenzyme A (HMG-CoA) reductase inhibitor: Start prior to lipid panel
- Lidocaine: Prophylactic lidocaine not routinely indicated

Acute NSTEMI

- Aspirin
- Intravenous unfractionated heparin or low-molecular-weight heparin (LMWH)
- β-Blocker
- Nitrates
- ACE inhibitor
- Clopidogrel: If early PCI planned some wait for angiography to see if coronary artery bypass grafting (CABG) is required
- Consider IIb/IIIa glycoprotein inhibitor: ST depression, elevated cardiac enzymes, persistent chest pain, hemodynamic instability or early PCI

SURGERY

- PCI: As above
- CABG: In acute setting, reserved for hemodynamic instability or refractory angina not amenable to PCI, or with failed PCI and coronary anatomy amenable to CABG
- IABP: Consider in STEMI with refractory hypotension

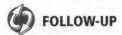 **FOLLOW-UP**

DISPOSITION
Admission Criteria

- CCU monitoring
  - Monitor in CCU 1–3 days depending on course; discharge 4–7 days depending on course (variable clinical practice)
  - Monitor for complications.
- Mechanical/hemodynamic disturbances
  - Heart failure/cardiogenic shock
  - RV infarction
    - Usually in setting of inferior infarction
    - Suspect with hypotension, elevated JVP (Kussmaul sign), clear lungs
    - Maintain RV preload, inotropic support
    - New systolic murmur: Papillary muscle dysfunction, papillary muscle rupture, VSD
    - Cardiac rupture (free wall)
    - Ventricular aneurysm
- Arrhythmias
  - Premature ventricular contractions (PVCs): Usually require no treatment
  - Accelerated idioventricular rhythm occurs with reperfusion, usually requires no treatment
  - Ventricular tachycardia: Lidocaine/direct current (DC) cardioversion
  - Ventricular fibrillation: DC cardioversion
  - Atrioventricular (AV) block: Pacing more often needed with anterior MI than inferior MI
  - Bundle branch blocks
- Recurrent chest pain
  - Recurrent ischemia/infarction
  - Early pericarditis
- LV thrombus with possible embolization
- Dressler syndrome: Late autoimmune pericarditis

PROGNOSIS
- 50% of MI-related deaths within 1 hour of symptom onset, before patient reaches hospital, primarily from ventricular arrhythmias
- Current hospital mortality rate 5–10%
- In-hospital mortality and complication rates higher with STEMI compared with NSTEMI; 2-year mortality rates same in the two groups (up to 30%)
- Main risk factors for serious cardiac events, death: Increased age, EF <40%, recurrent ischemia at rest or with minimal exertion, CHF, VT/VF
- Risk Stratification
  - Estimate EF (echo, multigated acquisition)
  - Stress testing (exercise or pharmacologic with echocardiography, nuclear imaging) versus catheterization prior to discharge (clinical practice varies) to determine need for revascularization
- Electrophysiologic study with VT/VF >48–72 hours into MI for possible ICD
- ICD: EF <0.30 1 month post MI, if EF 0.31–0.40 1 month post MI and nonsustained ventricular tachycardia (NSVT) present consider EP study for possible ICD

REFERENCES
1. Antman EM, Anbe DT, Armstrong PW, et al. ACC/AHA guidelines for the management of patients with ST-elevation myocardial infarction executive summary: A report of the American College of Cardiology/American Heart Association Task Force on Practice Guidelines (Writing Committee to Revise the 1999 Guidelines for the Management of Patients With Acute Myocardial Infarction). *Circulation*. 2004;110:588.

2. Braunwald E, Antman E, Beasley J, et al. ACC/AHA 2002 guideline update for the management of patients with unstable angina and non-ST-segment elevation myocardial infarction-summary article. A report of the American College of Cardiology/American Heart Association Task Force on Practice Guidelines (Committee on the Management of Patients With Unstable Angina). *J Am Coll Cardiol*. 2002;40:1366.

3. Fuster, V et al. ST-segment-elevation: Clinical presentation, diagnostic evaluation, and medical management In: *Hurst's the Heart*, 11th ed. New York: McGraw Hill, 2004;1277–1349.

CODES
ICD9-CM
- 410.9 Acute myocardial infarction, unspecified site
- 410.7 Subendocardial myocardial infarction
- 410.0 Acute myocardial infarction of anterolateral wall

PATIENT TEACHING
Internet Resources
- www.acc.org/clinical/guidelines
- www.americanheart.org
- www.nhlbi.nih.gov

Prevention
Secondary Prevention
- Smoking cessation
- Weight management
- Control blood pressure.
- Control diabetes mellitus.
- Aspirin
- Clopidogrel
- β-Blocker
- HMG-CoA reductase inhibitor: LDL goal <100 mg/dL, <70 mg/dL in high-risk patients
- ACE inhibitor or ARB if ACE-I intolerant
- Consider anticoagulation in selected cases (controversial).
- Aldosterone blockade if already on ACE-I, LVEF <0.40, either DM or CHF present and creatinine <2.5 mg/dL in men or 2.0 in women with K <5.0 mEq/L

Diet
AHA step I diet (<30% total calories from fat with less than one third being saturated fat, low cholesterol)

Activity
Cardiac rehab, exercise prescription

M

MYOCARDITIS

Gary S. Francis
Deepak L. Bhatt
Apur R. Kamdar

 ## BASICS

DESCRIPTION
Myocarditis is an inflammatory condition involving the heart that can be due to a variety of causes, including a direct viral infection.
- There are many kinds of inflammatory myocarditis, including giant cell myocarditis, hypersensitivity myocarditis, viral myocarditis, and eosinophilic myocarditis.
- All are quite unique and have various responses to treatment and natural histories.
- Physicians tend to equate viral myocarditis with myocarditis in general.
- The treatment of viral inflammatory myocarditis is highly variable because of inconsistent responses to immunosuppressive therapy.

EPIDEMIOLOGY
- The epidemiology of viral inflammatory myocarditis is poorly understood.
- It apparently follows cyclical patterns that change over the years.

Incidence
The incidence may vary from decade to decade.

RISK FACTORS
- There are no obvious factors for the development of acute myocarditis.
- It is believed that some patients will develop viral myocarditis following a self-limited viral illness, but the nature of this association is poorly understood.

Pregnancy Considerations
Inflammatory myocarditis can occur during pregnancy, in which case the stress of pregnancy can potentially aggravate the development of heart failure.

ETIOLOGY
- Infectious agents (viruses, bacteria, fungi, parasites, rickettsia, spirochetes)
- Toxins (cocaine)
- Hypersensitivity due to medications (e.g., clozapine)
- Chemotherapy (daunorubicin, doxorubicin)
- Radiation
- Giant cell

ASSOCIATED CONDITIONS
None

DIAGNOSIS

SIGNS AND SYMPTOMS
- Shortness of breath
- Fatigue
- Chest pain
- All of the manifestations of acute and chronic heart failure

TESTS
- Myocardial biopsy of the right ventricle is the most helpful special test.
  - Because of possible sampling error, at least four biopsy samples should be obtained during the procedure.
  - Histopathologic diagnosis of inflammatory myocarditis can be difficult, even by an experienced pathologist.

Lab
There are no specific laboratory procedures, although acute and convalescent titers for viral antibodies may be of some value.

Imaging
Imaging studies such as echocardiography are nonspecific and show either regional or global ventricular dysfunction.

DIFFERENTIAL DIAGNOSIS
- The differential diagnosis of inflammatory myocarditis includes idiopathic dilated cardiomyopathy and acute myocardial infarction.
- The onset of myocarditis can clearly mimic acute myocardial infarction with regional wall motion abnormalities on echocardiography, an increase in serum enzymes, and chest pain.
- Myocarditis can only be diagnosed definitively by tissue analysis.
- When there is suspicion of myocarditis, a myocardial biopsy may be indicated.
- This is somewhat controversial because the treatment of acute inflammatory viral myocarditis is currently poorly defined, and basically consists of treatment for heart failure.
- Nevertheless, some patients will respond to immunosuppressive therapy, including corticosteroids.

TREATMENT

GENERAL MEASURES

Management of inflammatory myocarditis is basically the management of heart failure and therefore includes loop diuretics, angiotensin-converting enzyme inhibitors, β-adrenergic blockers, and in some cases left ventricular assist devices and heart transplantation.

 MEDICATION (DRUGS)

Corticosteroids have been shown to be of no benefit.

SURGERY

Heart transplantation

 FOLLOW-UP

DISPOSITION

Admission Criteria

• Admission and discharge criteria are similar to those for heart failure.

• Patients are usually admitted to the hospital when there is acute severe hemodynamic compromise that requires intravenous diuretics and support with drugs such as nitroprusside and positive inotropic agents.

PROGNOSIS

• Many patients spontaneously improve following the onset of viral inflammatory myocarditis.

• Patients with giant cell myocarditis may have a somewhat worse prognosis than patients with lymphocytic inflammatory myocarditis. Careful follow-up is always indicated.

• Some patients may demonstrate a rapid downhill course and require mechanical support and even heart transplantation.

• Although heart transplantation can be performed in these patients, there can be an exaggerated tendency toward rejection, particularly in the early post-transplantation follow-up phase.

PATIENT MONITORING

As for other etiologies of heart failure

REFERENCES

1. Kilian J, Kerr K, Lawrence C, et al. Myocarditis and cardiomyopathy associated with clozapine. *Lancet.* 1999;354:1841–1845.

2. Rodkey SM, Ratliff NB, Young JB. Cardiomyopathy and myocardial failure. In: Topol EJ, ed. *Comprehensive Cardiovascular Medicine.* Philadelphia: Lippincott Williams & Wilkins, 1998:2593–2594.

3. Wynne J, Braunwald E. The cardiomyopathies and myocarditides. In: Braunwald E, ed. *Heart Disease: A Textbook of Cardiovascular Medicine*, 5th ed. Philadelphia: WB Saunders, 1997:1414–1426.

CODES

ICD9-CM

428.0 Failure, heart, congestive

PATIENT TEACHING

• Patients need to be educated with information about myocarditis, just as they would be for any heart illness culminating in heart failure.

• Patients should be told that there is a higher likelihood of the spontaneous resolution with viral myocarditis compared with other forms of acute heart failure.

• Giant cell myocarditis has a poor prognosis, and affected patients may require transplantation. Granulomas may recur in the transplanted heart but do not appear to lead to severe left ventricular (LV) dysfunction.

• When heart failure is present, patients must be informed about the treatment and expected course of the syndrome.

M

NATRIURETIC PEPTIDES

Rishi R. Vohora
Helge U. Simon*
Gerard P. Aurigemma

 BASICS

DESCRIPTION

A variety of neurohormones, including the group of natriuretic peptides (ANP, BNP), help maintain fluid homeostasis in the healthy individual. These hormones oppose the actions of the renin–angiotensin–aldosterone system in response to short-term perturbations in fluid balance.

Atrial Natriuretic Peptide (ANP)
- 28-amino-acid peptide hormone released from the atria into the circulation
- Main stimulus for release of ANP is atrial stretch

ANP Effects
- Natriuresis is dilation of the afferent glomerular arteriole and constriction of the efferent arteriole, resulting in increased filtration pressure. Sodium reabsorption is inhibited in the collecting duct; both mechanisms cause increased natriuresis.
- Opposes angiotensin effects on aldosterone and renin release, vascular tone, vascular mitogenesis, and renal sodium absorption, further promoting natriuresis; increases vascular permeability
- Antimitotic effect in vitro

- Central nervous system effects: Decreased salt appetite, decreased thirst, decreased corticotropin release
- All of the effects noted previously result in lowered plasma volume and lowered blood pressure.

Brain Natriuretic Peptide (BNP)
- Discovered in brain homogenate
- Secreted in the ventricles, less in the atria
- Similar natriuretic and central effects as those of ANP
- Kidney: Natriuresis nearly as strong as ANP
- Release of BNP is increased in response to high ventricular filling pressures
- BNP circulating concentration is usually less than 20% of ANP, but can exceed levels of ANP in heart failure, making BNP a useful hormone to measure in acute heart failure.

ASSAY
- Initially, immunoradiometric assays were used to measure levels of BNP but were replaced by a "rapid" assay using a fluorescence immunoassay
- Results within 10–15 minutes
- Normal range <100 pg/mL

Marker of Left Ventricular Dysfunction

BNP in Patients with Acute Dyspnea
- In patients presenting to the emergency department, BNP levels >100 pg/mL diagnosed heart failure with a sensitivity of 90% and a specificity of 76%.
- The overall predictive accuracy was 83%, which is as good or superior to a history consistent with heart failure, findings of rales on examination, and cardiomegaly on chest x-ray.
  BNP is also superior to both the Framingham and National Health and Nutrition Examination Survey (NHANES) criteria for heart failure.
- Patients with permanent/paroxysmal atrial fibrillation have significantly higher circulating levels of BNP and therefore a cutoff of at least 200 pg/mL should be used.

BNP as a Prognostic Indicator
- Elevated BNP levels in heart failure are predictors of increased morbidity and mortality. Changes in BNP over time correlate with changes in morbidity and mortality in patients with heart failure.
- BNP may be used as a marker to help gauge efficacy of treatment in heart failure
- Elevated BNP levels in patients presenting with acute coronary syndrome can be used as a predictor for short–term (30 day) and long–term (10 month) morbidity and mortality.

BNP as a Screening Tool for Left Ventricular Dysfunction

- Use of BNP as a biomarker of preclinical ventricular dysfunction is suboptimal as a community-based screening tool.

Potential Sources of Error

- BNP levels increase with age and are increased in females.
- BNP levels are increased in patients with glomerular filtration rate (GFR) <60, regardless of whether they clinically have heart failure. Therefore, monitoring BNP in this subset of patients may not facilitate management of heart failure.
- Young females with stable nonischemic systolic dysfunction (NYHA II–III) can have misleadingly "normal" BNP levels

REFERENCES

1. Anand IS, Fisher LD, Chiang YT, et al. Changes in brain natriuretic peptide and norepinephrine over time and morbidity and mortality in the Valsartan Heart Failure Trial. *Circulation.* 2003;107:1278–1283.
2. Knudsen CW, Omland T, Clopton P, et al. Impact of atrial fibrillation on the diagnostic performance of B-type natriuretic peptide concentration on dyspneic patients. *J Am Coll Cardiol.* 2005;46: 838–844.
3. Levin ER, Gardner DG, Samson WK. Natriuretic peptides. *N Engl J Med.* 1998;339:321–328.
4. Maisel AS, Krishnaswamy P, Nowak RM, et al. Rapid measurement of B-type natriuretic peptide in the emergency diagnosis of heart failure. *N Engl J Med.* 2002;347:161–167.
5. Redfield MM, Rodeheffer RJ, Jacobsen JJ, et al. Plasma brain natriuretic peptide to detect preclinical ventricular systolic or diastolic dysfunction: A community-based study. *Circulation.* 2004;109:3176–3181.
6. Sabatine MS, Morrow DA, de Lemos JA, et al. Multimarker approach to risk stratification in non-ST elevation acute coronary syndromes: Simultaneous assessment of troponin I, C-reactive protein and B-type natriuretic peptide. *Circulation.* 2002;105:1760–1763.
7. Schrier RW, Abraham WT. Hormones and hemodynamics in heart failure. *N Engl J Med.* 1999;341:577–585.
8. Tang WH, Girod JP, Lee MJ, et al. Plasma B-type natriuretic peptide levels in ambulatory patients with established chronic heart failure. *Circulation.* 2003;108:2964–2966.

N

NOONAN'S SYNDROME

Eric D. Fethke
Welton M. Gersony

BASICS

DESCRIPTION
• Noonan syndrome is a Mendelian inherited syndrome characterized by characteristic phenotypic stigmata differentiated from genotype of Turner syndrome (XO).
• System(s) affected: Cardiovascular; Endocrine; Urologic; Otologic; Neurologic; Hematologic
• Synonym(s): Female pseudo-Turner syndrome; Male Turner syndrome; Bonnevie Ullrich syndrome

EPIDEMIOLOGY
• Age at presentation: Fetal to adult; the mean age at diagnosis is approximately 9 years.
• Sex: Male = Female

Prevalence
The overall prevalence is not well established, but is approximately 1/2,000 newborns, with males affected as often as females.

RISK FACTORS
Genetics
• An autosomal-dominant and recessive patterns of inheritance has been established. Many cases may be new stigmata. Normal karyotype.
• Marked genetic heterogeneity
• To date, familial pedigree studies have isolated the locus of Noonan syndrome to several chromosomes, including 12 and 18.
• A large proportion (20–30%) of 1st-generation family members of individuals with Noonan syndrome also are affected with Noonan syndrome.

PATHOPHYSIOLOGY
Depends on associated cardiac defects

ETIOLOGY
Hormonal: Mutations in *PTPN11* resulting in interference with growth hormone and IGF-I signaling in 50% of patients

ASSOCIATED CONDITIONS
• Cardiovascular (50% of cases)
  – Pulmonary valve dysplasia and stenosis is the most common lesion (50–75% of cases)
  – Hypertrophic cardiomyopathy: Typically asymmetric; can be associated with subaortic or subpulmonic stenosis (25–33% of affected individuals)
  – Atrial septal defect (ASD): 27% of cases
  – Tetralogy of Fallot
  – Conduction abnormalities
  – Rarely aortic stenosis and coarctation
• Endocrine/urologic
  – Gonadal dysfunction: Hypofunction of testes in males
  – Cryptorchidism
  – Short stature
  – Renal abnormalities
• Otologic
  – Progressive sensorineural hearing deficits (50% of cases)

• Neuropsychological
  – Mental retardation (25% of cases)
  – Developmental delay
• Hematologic/Oncologic
  – Coagulopathies
  – Chronic myelomonocytic leukemia or "benign" monoclonal gammopathy
  – Malignant schwannoma
• Neurologic
  – Cerebrovascular disease such as moyamoya

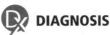

DIAGNOSIS

SIGNS AND SYMPTOMS
• The phenotype varies with the age at presentation
• Fetal
  – Increased nuchal fluid
  – Possible hydrops
  – Pleural effusions
  – Normal karyotype on amniocentesis
  – Brachycephaly or growth retardation
  – Shortened femora
  – Renal abnormalities
• Infant
  – Cardiac abnormalities:
    • Systolic ejection murmur of pulmonary stenosis
    • Ejection click usually not present
    • If left ventricular hypertrophy with outflow obstruction is present, the patient may have typical symptoms of exertional dyspnea, chest pain, palpitations, postural hypotension, or syncope.
  – Edema of hands and feet
  – High arched palate
  – Short or webbed neck
  – Pectus carinatum or excavatum
  – Cubitus valgus
  – Typical facies: Malformed posteriorly rotated ears, antimongoloid palpebral slant, ptosis, broad flat nose
  – Undescended testes with possible hypogonadism
  – Cardiovascular malformations: Predominantly ASD, pulmonary stenosis, and hypertrophic cardiomyopathy may result in symptoms if severe.
• Childhood and adolescence
  – Short stature
  – Developmental delay
  – Characteristic cardiac malformations
  – Sexual maturation delay of approximately 2 years

TESTS
• ECG
  – Isolated pulmonary stenosis or peripheral pulmonary artery stenosis may result in right ventricular hypertrophy.
  – If associated with asymmetric left ventricular hypertrophy, left-axis deviation with left ventricular hypertrophy may be seen.
  – Conduction abnormalities: Typically first-degree atrioventricular block
• Audiometry
  – Sensorineural or conductive hearing losses
• Developmental/psychosocial testing
  – May reveal varying degrees of cognitive, behavioral, and psychosocial deficits

Imaging
• Fetal ultrasonography
  – Subcutaneous edema of nuchal skin folds
  – Generalized fetal edema
  – Renal abnormalities
  – Short femora
  – Cardiac abnormalities
• Transthoracic or fetal echocardiography
  – Pulmonary stenosis, ASD, asymmetric hypertrophic cardiomyopathy, tetralogy of Fallot, rarely aortic stenosis
• Radiographs
  – Chest: Enlarged cardiac silhouette secondary to left or right ventricular hypertrophy
  – Extremity: Bone age studies in association with growth hormone therapy for growth retardation

Diagnostic Procedures/Surgery
• Cardiac catheterization
  – Diagnostic catheterization rarely required
  – Pulmonary stenosis with doming or dysplastic pulmonary valve
  – Hypertrophic cardiomyopathy with possible ventricular outflow tract obstruction

DIFFERENTIAL DIAGNOSIS
• Turner syndrome
• Cardio-facial-cutaneous syndrome
• LEOPARD syndrome
• Costello syndrome
• Neurofibromatosis: In the context of isolated pulmonary stenosis or peripheral artery stenosis, may display right-axis deviation and right ventricular hypertrophy

TREATMENT

GENERAL MEASURES

- Treatment depends on age of diagnosis and presentation to medical attention. All individuals with heart lesions associated with an increased risk for endocarditis should receive appropriate prophylaxis prior to dental or invasive procedures.
- See also: Hypertrophic Cardiomyopathy; Cardiomyopathy, Pediatric
- Prenatal
  - Parental counseling is advised regarding potentially affected systems, especially cardiac and renal. Timing and mode of delivery should be organized through the efforts of a high-risk perinatal team.
- Newborn
  - Patients with fetal hydrops should receive supportive, nutritional, and respiratory care in an experienced center where neonatal, renal, and cardiac care can be provided.
- Infancy and childhood
  - Early recognition of and intervention for cognitive or developmental delays
  - Identification and management of hearing deficits
- Adolescence and adulthood
  - Early evaluation and recognition of growth delay
  - Appropriate referral for management of pubertal delay

 MEDICATION (DRUGS)

First Line

- In symptomatic patients with hypertrophic cardiomyopathy, treatment may include:
  - β-Adrenergic receptor–blocking agents such as propranolol
  - Calcium channel blockers such as verapamil or diltiazem
  - Disopyramide
- Growth hormone therapy beginning as early as 8 years of age for children with growth retardation/short stature

SURGERY

- Cardiac
  - Interventional cardiac catheterization with balloon dilation of pulmonary valvar stenosis or peripheral pulmonary artery stenosis; often poor results for dysplastic pulmonary valve stenosis; surgery usually is required
  - Myotomy or myomectomy for severe left ventricular outflow tract obstruction due to hypertrophic cardiomyopathy
  - Surgical or transcatheter device ASD closure
  - Surgical repair of pulmonary stenosis, tetralogy of Fallot, or other lesions
- Orthopedic
  - Leg-lengthening procedures for short stature
- Otologic
  - Placement of hearing aid devices for sensorineural deficits or myringotomy tubes for conductive hearing loss

 FOLLOW-UP

PROGNOSIS

Overall, the prognosis and outcomes have improved significantly due to early recognition and treatment of associated cardiac malformations and short stature.

Pregnancy Considerations

Pregnancy is possible, but may be of high risk in women with severe manifestations; 50% of offspring of affected mothers or fathers will have Noonan syndrome.

PATIENT MONITORING

- Routine lifelong outpatient visits are recommended, with attention to systems discussed, especially cardiovascular, renal, endocrine, and otologic.
- A well-coordinated multidisciplinary approach is required.

REFERENCES

1. Emmanouilides GC, et al. *Moss and Adams' heart disease in infants, children and adolescents*, 5th ed. Baltimore: Williams & Wilkins, 1995.
2. Ferreira LV, Souza SAL, Arnold IJP, et al. PTPN11 (protein tyrosine phosphatase, nonreceptor type 11) mutations and response to growth hormone therapy in children with Noonan syndrome. *J Clin Endocrinol Metabol*. 2005;90:5156–5160.
3. Grange CS, Heid R, Lucas SB, et al. Anesthesia in a parturient with Noonan syndrome. *Can J Anaesth*. 1998;45:332–336.
4. Harland M, Burch M, McKenna WM, et al. A clinical study of Noonan syndrome. *Arch Dis Child*. 1992;67:178–183.
5. Ishizawa A, Oho S, Dodo H, et al. Cardiovascular abnormalities in Noonan syndrome: The clinical findings and treatments. *Acta Pediatr Jpn*. 1996;38:84–90.
6. Nisbet DL, et al. Prenatal features of Noonan syndrome. Prenatal Diagnosis 1999;19:642–647.
7. Rudolph AM. *Rudolph's pediatrics*, 19th ed. East Norwalk, CT: Appleton & Lange, 1991.

PATIENT TEACHING

Diet

No dietary restrictions

Activity

No restrictions in the absence of cardiac disease

N

OBESITY AND THE HEART

Francisco Lopez-Jimenez
Virend K. Somers

 BASICS

DESCRIPTION

Obesity is defined as excessive body fat. In clinical practice, obesity is defined as a body mass index ≥30.

The most common cause of death in patients with obesity is cardiovascular.

GENERAL PREVENTION

- Obesity is prevented by maintaining a neutral caloric balance.
- Awareness of the total caloric intake and appropriate physical activity can prevent obesity.
- Cardiovascular complications of obesity can be prevented with timely treatment of obesity.

EPIDEMIOLOGY

- Obesity affects men and women of all ages and races.
- Obesity is associated with the development of diabetes mellitus, metabolic syndrome, coronary artery disease, congestive heart failure, diastolic dysfunction, atrial fibrillation, obstructive sleep apnea, systemic and pulmonary hypertension, dyslipidemia, stroke, and sudden death.

Incidence

- The incidence of obesity is rising in both genders and all age groups.
- The increase in the incidence of atrial fibrillation has been partially attributed to the obesity epidemic.

Prevalence

- About two thirds of the U.S. population is either overweight or obese.
- Overweight/obesity is the most prevalent cardiovascular risk factor in patients with myocardial infarction.

RISK FACTORS

- Sedentary lifestyle, low socio-economic status, and family history of obesity
- Patients with morbid obesity or with either the metabolic syndrome or other risk factors are more likely to develop heart disease.

Genetics

- Up to 50% of the variance of weight can be attributed to genetic factors.
- Obesity is considered a polygenic condition with strong environmental interaction.

PATHOPHYSIOLOGY

- The regulation of caloric intake is driven by metabolic signaling and also behavioral factors. Obesity occurs when the "metabolic brain" is overridden by the "cognitive brain."
- Obesity causes insulin resistance, sympathetic nervous system activation, and systemic inflammation; and increases intravascular volume, free fatty acid circulation, renin–angiotensin–aldosterone system activity and leptin levels; and decreases adiponectin levels. All these factors play a role in the development of cardiovascular disease.

ETIOLOGY

- Obesity occurs when caloric intake exceeds caloric expenditure for a long period of time.
- A positive caloric balance of 200 kilocalories a day can result in a 10–15 pound weight gain a year.
- Obesity is believed to cause coronary artery disease through intermediate cardiovascular risk factors such as hypertension, diabetes or hyperlipidemia and also through direct effects of adipocyte-related hormones, increased sympathetic tone, peptides and cytokines.
- Obesity may cause left ventricular dysfunction independently of hypertension and probably due to a direct myopathic effect of fatty tissue.

ASSOCIATED CONDITIONS

Hypertension, diabetes, hyperlipidemia, coronary artery disease, atrial fibrillation, metabolic syndrome, nonalcoholic steatohepatitis, obstructive sleep apnea, pulmonary hypertension, osteoarthritis, depression, gallbladder disease, stroke, sudden death

ALERT

Geriatric Considerations

- Elderly patients may have obesity with normal body mass index because of overall decrease in lean body mass.
- Dietary recommendations for elderly patients must be guided by a dietitian because standard recommendations may lead to malnutrition.
- The safety of weight loss medications in the elderly is not known.

Pediatric Considerations

- The focus of weight management in children should be on increasing physical activity, increasing the intake of vegetables and fruit, and avoiding foods with poor nutritional value.
- Weight loss recommendations for children and adolescents should be implemented with some caution because of the risk for eating disorders, particularly among girls.

Pregnancy Considerations

- Weight loss should not be recommended during pregnancy.
- Weight loss medications or weight loss surgery are contraindicated during pregnancy.

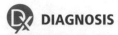 DIAGNOSIS

SIGNS AND SYMPTOMS

- Dyspnea
- Fatigue

History

- Patients usually describe a sedentary lifestyle
- Unrestricted diet
- Family members with obesity

Physical Exam

- Loud P2
- S3 or S4
- Jugular venous distension
- Peripheral edema

TESTS

- Obesity is diagnosed with a weight scale and calculation of body mass index.
- Central obesity is measured with a measuring tape.
- Despite the simplicity, obesity is rarely diagnosed in patients with myocardial infarction.

Lab

- Fasting blood glucose can be elevated, HDL may be low, triglycerides, non-HDL cholesterol, and LDL cholesterol can be elevated.
- ECG may show left ventricular hypertrophy, left atrial dilatation, or poor RR variability. QT may be prolonged.
- Exercise treadmill test may show poor aerobic capacity or signs of myocardial ischemia.

Imaging

- Chest x-ray may show cardiomegaly.
- Transthoracic echocardiography may show left atrial enlargement, left ventricular hypertrophy, diastolic dysfunction, pulmonary hypertension, or right ventricular dysfunction.

DIFFERENTIAL DIAGNOSIS

Conditions associated with volume overload such as congestive heart failure, end-stage renal disease, or liver cirrhosis may be associated with an increased body weight with or without increased body fat.

TREATMENT

GENERAL MEASURES

- Nutritional changes with a 25% decrease in total caloric intake, with emphasis on foods with low caloric density; these are usually vegetables, fruits, soups, and other meals with a low number of calories for each gram of food.
- Attention to portion size
- Increase in nonexercise physical activity such as walking, using stairs, and manual work
- To start a regular exercise program with at least 30 minutes of moderate exercise 5 or more days a week
- Consultation with a registered dietitian can be useful.
- Encouragement to join group-based interventions for weight loss
- Cognitive therapy: Letting patients know their increased risk for cardiovascular complications related to obesity

 MEDICATIONS (DRUGS)

- Orlistat in association with lifestyle changes can induce a weight loss of 3–6 kg in 6 months. Side effects include gastrointestinal symptoms such as diarrhea, flatulence, abdominal discomfort, greasy stools, and deficiency of fat-soluble vitamins.
- Sibutramine, when used in association with lifestyle changes, can induce a weight loss of 4–8 kg for 3–6 months.
- Sibutramine is contraindicated in patients with cardiovascular disease or hypertension.
- Side effects include headache, tachycardia, dry mouth, insomnia, and anxiety.
- Rimonabant (not currently available) induces a loss of 8–12% of body weight, but complete safety profile has not been disclosed.

SURGERY

- Weight reduction (bariatric) surgery should be considered if body mass index $\geq$40, or $\geq$35 if there are comorbidities like diabetes mellitus, hypertension, dyslipidemia, or sleep apnea, all expected to improve with surgery. The roux-en-Y gastric bypass induces an average weight loss of 40–50 kg and is usually maintained in long term.
- Bariatric surgery appears to be relatively safe in patients with coronary artery disease.

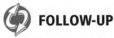 **FOLLOW-UP**

ADMISSION CRITERIA

Patients with obesity who develop cardiovascular complications such as coronary artery disease, congestive heart failure, severe pulmonary hypertension, hypertensive crisis, or atrial fibrillation with rapid ventricular response may require hospital treatment.

Issues for Referral

Referral to a formal weight loss program if general measures have failed.

PROGNOSIS

- Patients who achieve significant weight loss with nonsurgical measures usually regain all weight unless they continue with some maintenance intervention.
- Patients with obesity who do not follow any caloric restriction and do not change lifestyle gain between 2 and 5 kg a year.
- Survival of patients with obesity is reduced.
- Patients with morbid obesity have a life expectancy no better than patients with colon cancer.

COMPLICATIONS

- Coronary artery disease
- Sleep apnea
- Pulmonary hypertension
- Acanthosis nigricans
- Gallbladder disease
- Depression
- Hypertension
- Diabetes
- Hyperlipidemia

PATIENT MONITORING

- Patients with obesity who weigh themselves 3–7 times a week are more likely to succeed at losing weight.
- Food diaries are effective in weight loss programs.

REFERENCES

1. Alpert MA, Terry BE, Mulekar M, et al. Cardiac morphology and left ventricular function in normotensive morbidly obese patients with and without congestive heart failure, and effect of weight loss. *Am J Cardiol*. 1997;80:736–740.
2. James WP, Astrup A, Finer N, et al. Effect of sibutramine on weight maintenance after weight loss: A randomised trial. STORM Study Group: Sibutramine Trial of Obesity Reduction and Maintenance. *Lancet*. 2000;356:2119–2125.
3. Klein S, Burke LE, Bray GA, et al. American Heart Association Council on Nutrition, Physical Activity, and Metabolism. Clinical implications of obesity with specific focus on cardiovascular disease: A statement for professionals from the American Heart Association Council on Nutrition, Physical Activity, and Metabolism: Endorsed by the American College of Cardiology Foundation. *Circulation*. 2004;110:2952–2967.
4. Lopez-Jimenez F, Bhatia S, Collazo-Clavell ML. Safety and efficacy of bariatric surgery in patients with coronary artery disease. *Mayo Clin Proc*. 2005;80:1157–1162.
5. Lopez-Jimenez F, Jacobsen SJ, Reeder GS, et al. Prevalence and secular trends of excess body weight and impact on outcomes after myocardial infarction in the community. *Chest*. 2004;125: 1205–1212.
6. Poirier P, Giles TD, Bray GA, et al. Obesity and cardiovascular disease: Pathophysiology, evaluation, and effect of weight loss: An update of the 1997 American Heart Association Scientific Statement on Obesity and Heart Disease From the Obesity Committee of the Council on Nutrition, Physical Activity, and Metabolism. *Circulation*. 2006;113:898–918.

 MISCELLANEOUS

CODES

ICD9-CM

- 277.7 Metabolic syndrome
- 278.0 Obesity, unspecified
- 278.01 Morbid obesity
- 278.02 Overweight

PATIENT TEACHING

- Recognition of the risks involved with obesity
- Recognition of the amount of excess weight
- Understanding that lifestyle changes are for life

Diet

Caloric restriction

Increase in the Nonprevention

- Recommendations for better nutrition should be extended to the whole family.
- Parents need to understand the consequences of obesity and learn ways to prevent obesity in children.

FAQ

Q: Is BMI accurate for diagnosing obesity?
A: In most cases it is. Elderly patients or patients with chronic conditions may have a decreased muscle mass with a high body fat percent. In those cases, the sensitivity of BMI would be poor to detect obesity.

Q: Is there is a subgroup of patients with obesity at a higher risk for cardiovascular complications?
A: Patients with morbid obesity or with metabolic syndrome are at a much higher risk for cardiovascular complications, as are patients with other associated conditions such as obstructive sleep apnea, hypertension, or dyslipidemia.

Q: From all the common recommendations for lifestyle change, what is the most effective one?
A: Weight loss is hardly achieved unless patients restrict caloric intake. Regular exercise is the best approach to *maintain* a healthy weight but is not effective to achieve significant weight loss.

O

ORTHOSTATIC HYPOTENSION

Husam H. Farah
Rosemary Mehl

 BASICS

DESCRIPTION
Orthostatic hypotension is defined as a decrease in blood pressure of over 20 mm Hg systolic, or 10 mm Hg diastolic, within 3 minutes after standing or during head-up tilt. It is also known as postural hypotension.

EPIDEMIOLOGY
Prevalence
- The prevalence increases with age: 6.6% among individuals 25 to 74 years old, 20% in subjects older than 65 years, 30% among subjects older than 75 years.
- More than 50% of nursing home residents have orthostatic hypotension.

RISK FACTORS
- Age >65
- Systolic hypertension

Genetics
- Most cases are not caused by hereditary illness.
- Heritable causes are rare and include:
  - Autosomal-dominant familial amyloid neuropathy
  - Porphyria
  - Autosomal-recessive familial dysautonomia-Riley-Day syndrome
  - β-Hydroxylase deficiency
  - Aromatic L-amino acid decarboxylase deficiency

PATHOPHYSIOLOGY
- The effect of gravity will shift 400–800 mL of blood from the thoracic to the abdominal cavity upon standing in the normal individual, leading to a decline in the venous return to the heart.
- This leads to a 40% reduction in the stroke volume, which then leads to a fall in the systemic blood pressure.
- This activates the cardiopulmonary, carotid sinus, and aortic arch baroreceptors, leading to sympathetic activation and parasympathetic inactivation. The result is an increase in heart rate (10–15 beats/minute) and peripheral resistance, increasing the diastolic blood pressure by 10 mm Hg with no change in the systolic blood pressure.
- This is followed by neurohormonal changes, with activation of the renin–angiotensin–aldosterone system and vasopressin.
- Normal aging leads to a reduction in the baroreflex sensitivity, resulting in a blunted response to upright posture.
- Normal aging increases the stiffness of the heart, resulting in impaired cardiac relaxation. Any condition that decreases cardiac filling (like reduction of venous return during upright posture) will therefore lead to an exaggerated reduction in the cardiac output.

ETIOLOGY
- Non-neurogenic causes
  - Hypovolemia (blood loss or dehydration)
  - Vasodilation (vigorous exercise or excessive heat)
- Neurogenic causes
  - Drugs
    - Central nervous system–mediated (methyldopa, reserpine, clonidine, barbiturates, amphetamine, anesthetics, minoxidil)
    - Peripheral nervous system–mediated (α-blockers, β-blockers)
    - Combination central and peripheral (tricyclic antidepressants, phenothiazines, levodopa)
    - Autonomic neuropathy (alcohol, vincas)
    - Vascular dilatation (nitrates, hydralazine, angiotensin-converting enzyme inhibitors, angiotensin-II antagonists, potassium channel blockers, calcium antagonists, endothelin antagonists)
  - Metabolic diseases (diabetes mellitus, chronic renal failure, chronic liver disease, vitamin B_{12} deficiency, alcohol-induced, Fabry, Tangiers, porphyria)
  - Inflammatory (Guillain-Barré, transverse myelitis)
  - Infections (syphilis, HIV, Chagas, botulism, tetanus, herpes zoster)
  - Neoplasia (brain tumors, especially third ventricle or posterior fossa, paraneoplastic)
  - Connective tissue disease (rheumatoid arthritis, lupus)
  - Surgery/trauma (sympathectomy, spinal cord transection)
  - Neurally mediated (vasovagal, carotid sinus hypersensitivity, micturition syncope, cough syncope, swallow syncope)
  - Primary chronic autonomic failure syndromes:
    - Multiple system atrophy (MSA)
    - Parkinson disease
    - Multiple cerebral infarcts
  - Secondary neuropathies (congenital growth factor deficiency, familial amyloid neuropathy, Riley-Day syndrome, dopamine β-hydroxylase deficiency, aromatic L-amino acid decarboxylase deficiency)
  - Primary acute and subacute dysautonomias

 DIAGNOSIS

SIGNS AND SYMPTOMS
- May be asymptomatic, especially if longstanding
- Dizziness, visual disturbances, loss of consciousness/syncope, impaired cognition, seizures (cerebral hypoperfusion)
- Classically associated with head-up positional change
- Orthostatic hypotension is more common in the morning, after meals or alcohol.
- A hypotensive response can be delayed: Prolonged standing or a tilt test may be required to elicit signs and symptoms.
- Lower back/buttock pain or suboccipital/paracervical "coathanger" pain (muscle hypoperfusion)
- Angina pectoris
- Oliguria
- Syncope
  - Abrupt drop-attack: no warning symptoms
  - Gradual loss of consciousness: more common
  - Fatigue, lethargy
- Falls (especially in the elderly)
- Blood pressure decreases after 3 minutes in the upright position (usually standing, but may occur with in severely orthostatic individuals)
  - Non-neurogenic causes produce tachycardia and sometimes sweating
  - Neurogenic causes include a decrease in blood pressure without tachycardia

History
A detailed history is very important in making the diagnosis.

Physical Exam
Measurement of blood pressure and heart rate: supine (after resting for 5 minutes), sitting and standing up (after 1 and 3 minutes).

TESTS
May be useful to determine specific suspected cause:
- Magnetic resonance imaging (MRI) (for brain or spinal cord lesions)
- Genetic testing (for familial amyloid neuropathy)
- Sural nerve biopsy for peripheral neuropathy

Lab
Plasma catecholamine measurements in supine and upright positions may help in differentiating certain neurologic conditions.

Diagnostic Procedures/Surgery
- Tilt-table measurement of blood pressure in supine and upright position
- Ambulatory blood pressure monitoring
- Exercise testing or carotid massage may be helpful in determining cause

DIFFERENTIAL DIAGNOSIS
Postural tachycardia syndrome (POTS):
- More common in young patients
- Symptoms occur with tachycardia but without drop in blood pressure.

TREATMENT

GENERAL MEASURES

- Correction of non-neurogenic causes (e.g., hypovolemia) is curative.
- For neurogenic orthostatic hypotension, discontinue medications that may be causative.
- Avoid sudden head-up position changes, prolonged recumbency, straining during micturition/defecation, and vasodilatory stimuli (e.g., alcohol, large meals, overheating, vigorous exercise).
- Head-up tilt (15–30 degrees) at night may increase blood pressure by activation of renin–angiotensin–aldosterone system.
- Ensure adequate fluid and salt intake.
- Identify body positions (leg-crossing, stooping, squatting) that may attenuate hypotension.
- Elastic stockings and abdominal binders may help, but often are not acceptable to patients.
- Water ingestion 30 minutes before getting out of bed and before meals.
- Avoid water ingestion before sleep.
- Frequent small meals (avoid large meals).

SPECIAL THERAPY

Balneotherapy: Alternating exposure of the whole body or extremities to cold and warm water has been proposed. No controlled trials have been performed.

 ## MEDICATION (DRUGS)

- Mineralocorticoids (fludrocortisone) reduce salt loss and expand volume. The dose should be increased slowly. Monitor blood pressure, weight, K, Mg. Avoid in heart failure.
- Sympathomimetics (ephedrine, midodrine) cause vasoconstriction. Use with caution in patients with ischemic heart disease, peripheral vascular disease, or urinary retention.
- Desmopressin reduces nocturnal polyuria.
- Caffeine and octreotide are beneficial in postprandial hypotension.
- Erythropoietin expands red blood cell mass and blood volume in patients with renal failure.
- Prostaglandin synthetase inhibitors (indomethacin), dopamine blockers (metoclopramide), and β-2-blockers prevent vasodilation.
- Dopamine agonists and β-blockers with intrinsic sympathetic activity (pindolol) increase cardiac output.
- DL threo-dihydroxyphenilserine: An amino acid converted to norepinephrine by dopa decarboxylase. Useful in patients with autonomic failure caused by congenital deficiency of dopamine beta hydroxylase.
- Selective serotonin reuptake inhibitors like paroxetine hydrochloride.
- Yohimbine: Acts on presynaptic α_2-adrenoceptors, inhibits norepinephrine reuptake

SURGERY

Cardiac pacemakers are rarely indicated, except in some forms of neurally mediated syncope, such as carotid hypersensitivity.

 ## FOLLOW-UP

PROGNOSIS

- Prognosis is determined by underlying cause rather than the postural hypotension itself.
- In non-neurogenic orthostatic hypotension, treatment of cause and/or reversal of the underlying deficit may be curative.
- Goals of therapy for chronic orthostatic hypotension are to ensure mobility and prevent falls that can cause substantial morbidity and mortality.
- Orthostatic hypotension has been shown to be associated with increased mortality.

PATIENT MONITORING

Ambulatory blood pressure monitoring may be helpful for evaluation of therapeutic measures. At times, however, dissociation between blood pressure and symptoms may occur.

REFERENCES

1. Grubb BP, Kosinski DJ, Kanjwal Y. Orthostatic hypotension: Causes, classification, and treatment. *PACE*. 2003;26:1747–1757.
2. Kaufmann H. Treatment of patients with orthostatic hypotension and syncope. *Clin Neuropharmacol*. 2002;25:133–141.
3. Mathias CJ, Kimber JR. Postural hypotension: Causes, clinical features, investigation, and management. *Annu Rev Med*. 1999;50:317–336.
4. Mukai S, Lipsitz LA. Orthostatic hypotension. *Clin Geriatr Med*. 2002;18:253–268.
5. Oldenburg O, Kribben A, Baumgart D, et al. Treatment of orthostatic hypotension. *Curr Opin Pharmacol*. 2002;2:740–747.
6. Topol E, ed. *Textbook of Cardiovascular Medicine*. Philadelphia: Lippincott Williams & Wilkins, 1998:1807–1831.

CODES

ICD9-CM
458.0 Orthostatic hypotension

PATIENT TEACHING

Education and cooperation are essential for nonpharmacologic preventative measures, as detailed in General Measures.

O

OSTEOGENESIS IMPERFECTA AND THE HEART

Brian C. Jensen
Daniel T. Price

 BASICS

DESCRIPTION

Osteogenesis imperfecta (OI) is a genetic disorder characterized by bones that break easily, often with little or no apparent cause.

- The basic defect is abnormal synthesis of type I collagen molecules.
- Valvular dysfunction and aortic root dilation are associated with this disorder. There are four main types of this disease (Sillence classification):
  - Type I (mild, nondeforming): Mild bone fragility, blue sclera, abnormal dentition (IB), and hearing loss in most; autosomal-dominant inheritance
  - Type II (perinatal lethal): Extreme bone fragility, blue sclera, abnormal dentition; autosomal-recessive inheritance, or sporadic
  - Type III (severely deforming): Severe bone fragility, bluish sclera at birth, abnormal dentition, hearing loss; autosomal-recessive or autosomal-dominant inheritance
  - Type IV (moderately deforming): Variable bone fragility, normal sclera, abnormal dentition (IVB), hearing loss, and autosomal-dominant inheritance

Pregnancy Consideration
Genetic counseling is recommended for prospective parents if one or both are affected by this disorder.

EPIDEMIOLOGY

- There are likely to be between 20,000 and 50,000 cases of OI in the United States.
- Aortic root dilation occurs in 12% of affected individuals.
- Valvular heart disease, predominantly aortic regurgitation, is seen in approximately 2–4% of cases.
- Age
- Several forms of the disease lead to premature death during early childhood.
- Cardiac manifestations noted in patients of all ages.
- Sex
- No apparent gender predominance

Incidence
1/30,000 births

RISK FACTORS
Family history of OI

Genetics
- OI can be inherited in either autosomal dominant or autosomal recessive fashion.
- Sporadic forms also may occur.
- The aortic root dilation appears to segregate in certain families affected by OI.

PATHOPHYSIOLOGY
Most forms of OI are caused by imperfectly formed collagen as a result of a genetic defect in collagen type I.

- Collagen is the major protein of the body's connective tissue.
- In OI, a person has either less collagen or a poorer quality of collagen.
- The dysfunctional collagen results in weakening of the aortic annulus and dilation of the aorta.
- There is no clear association between aortic root dilation and aortic insufficiency.
- The valvular abnormalities appear to be due to a structural defect of the valve tissue rather than a secondary effect from root dilation.
- The degree of aortic root dilation is not related to blood pressure in this population, although hypertension should be treated appropriately in affected individuals.

ASSOCIATED CONDITIONS
Mitral valve prolapse (MVP) has been noted in some surveys of OI, but the inconsistent association with this common disorder may reflect coinheritance of OI and MVP rather than MVP secondary to the collagen defect of OI.

 DIAGNOSIS

SIGNS AND SYMPTOMS
History
- Hearing loss at early age
- History of bone fractures without significant trauma
- Cardiac abnormalities usually are asymptomatic

Physical Exam
- Blue or gray sclera
- Abnormal dentition

TESTS
Skin biopsy is used to determine the amount of collagen present and its structure.

Lab
Genetic testing for *COL1A1* or *COL1A2* 90% sensitive

Imaging
- Echocardiography is used to diagnose valvular abnormalities.
- Aortic root abnormalities also can be detected by computed tomography (CT) scan or magnetic resonance imaging (MRI) of the thorax.

Pathologic Findings
Decreased bone thickness, increased number of bone trabeculae and osteoblasts

DIFFERENTIAL DIAGNOSIS
- The cardiac disorders are generally not the presenting manifestations of OI.
- Dyspnea may be related to mechanical difficulties of respiration (rib fractures, kyphoscoliosis, etc.)
- Frequent bone fractures should trigger consideration of child abuse
- Other connective tissue diseases cause similar cardiac involvement:
  - Marfan disease
  - Cystic medial necrosis
  - Ehlers-Danlos syndrome

TREATMENT

GENERAL MEASURES
- There is no cure for the underlying defect in OI, although gene therapy is under investigation.
- Activity is essential to muscle development, but should be undertaken after consultation with a physician.
- Hypertension should be treated.
- No specific pharmacologic therapy for patients with aortic root dilation without hypertension

 ## MEDICATION (DRUGS)

- β-Blockade has not been advocated to slow progression of aortic root dilation (as is done in Marfan).
- Bisphosphonates may decrease fracture risk.

SURGERY
Surgical therapy for valvular disorders carries higher risk in patients with OI.
- Aortic valve replacement may be undertaken when appropriate if risk is deemed acceptable.
- May be complicated by bleeding problems secondary to platelet dysfunction and capillary fragility
- Poor wound healing of friable tissues due to underlying collagen defect

 ## FOLLOW-UP

DISPOSITION
Admission Criteria
Admission for aortic valve replacement in appropriate individuals is on an elective basis, with discharge based on standard postoperative protocols.

PROGNOSIS
The prognosis for an individual with OI varies greatly depending on the type of OI and severity of defects.
- Type I: Good life expectancy
- Type II: Lethal
- Type III: Decreased life expectancy; few reach adulthood
- Type IV: Good life expectancy

COMPLICATIONS
Possible Complications (Noncardiac)
- Numerous fractures
- Restricted activity
- Short stature
- Brain damage
- The majority of OI patients with cardiac involvement are asymptomatic, and the cardiac conditions rarely are the cause of morbidity and mortality in this disorder.

PATIENT MONITORING
With cardiac valvular involvement, serial echocardiograms and symptoms are followed to determine timing of surgery.

REFERENCES
1. Hortop J, et al. Cardiovascular involvement in osteogenesis imperfecta. *Circulation*. 1986;73:54–61.
2. Rauch F, Glorieux FH. Osteogenesis imperfecta. *Lancet*. 2004;363:1377–1386.
3. Wheeler VR, et al. Cardiovascular pathology in osteogenesis imperfecta type IIA with a review of the literature. *Pediatr Pathol*. 1988;8:55–64.
4. Wong RS, et al. Osteogenesis imperfecta and cardiovascular diseases. *Ann Thorac Surg*. 1995;60:1439–1443.

 ## MISCELLANEOUS

Organization
- Osteogenesis Imperfecta Foundation, 804 W. Diamond Avenue, Suite 210, Gaithersburg, MD 20878; phone (301)947-0083 or (800)981-2663; Fax (301)947-0456; website: http://www.oif.org

CODES
ICD9-CM
765.51 Osteogenesis imperfecta

O

PAGET'S DISEASE AND THE HEART

Gary S. Francis
Deepak L. Bhatt
Apur R. Kamdar

 BASICS

DESCRIPTION

Paget disease is a disorder characterized by excessive resorption of bone and replacement of normal bone marrow with vascular, fibrous connective tissue and coarse, trabecular bone.

- There is increased vascularity of bone and increased blood flow through the cutaneous tissue overlying the involved bone, possibly secondary to local heat production by metabolically hyperactive affected bone.
- For an increased cardiac output to occur in Paget disease, there must be at least a 15% increase in involvement of the skeleton with an increase in alkaline phosphatase.
- The increased cardiac output may precipate heart failure if underlying heart disease is present.
- Augmentation of cardiac output obligated by the increased flow may not be manageable by the diseased heart, leading to heart failure.
- For example, if there is underlying severe aortic stenosis, the added demands placed on the heart by the need for increased flow through new vasculature may lead to clinical deterioration and heart failure.

EPIDEMIOLOGY

- Paget disease is not uncommon, occurring in 3–4% of subjects older than age 40 years.
- White individuals older than age 55 are the group predominantly affected.
- Autosomal-dominant transmission has been described in certain cases.
- Heart failure due to Paget disease is unusual but could easily go unrecognized.

Incidence

There is an increased incidence of Paget disease in first-degree relatives.

RISK FACTORS

There are no known risk factors.

ETIOLOGY

The etiology of Paget disease is unknown.

ASSOCIATED CONDITIONS

- Metastatic calcification
- Headache
- Hearing loss

 DIAGNOSIS

SIGNS AND SYMPTOMS

- Increase in hat size
- Skin warmth (over the skull, tibia)

TESTS

Occasionally bone biopsy is undertaken to exclude other bone disease such as osteomalacia.

Lab

- There is a marked increase in plasma alkaline phosphatase, derived from overactive osteoblasts.
- Urinary hydroxyproline
- Electrocardiogram (ECG) can show atrioventricular (AV) conduction problems or bundle branch block.

Imaging

- The sizes of the affected bones are increased radiographically.
- Echocardiogram may show aortic sclerosis or stenosis, left ventricular dilation, left ventricular hypertrophy (LVH), and mild systolic dysfunction.

DIFFERENTIAL DIAGNOSIS

- There must be a high index of suspicion to diagnose Paget disease.
- Patients may notice that their hat size is increasing.
- The enlarged bones may be painful, deformed, and warm.
- Deafness and nerve compression can occur when it involves the skull.

TREATMENT

GENERAL MEASURES
Treatment for pain may consist of simple analgesics.

MEDICATION (DRUGS)

First Line
- Bisphosphonates may be given to reduce excess bone turnover.
- Calcitonin is also widely used to treat Paget disease.

SURGERY
Fractures of pagetic bone require the usual surgical treatment.

FOLLOW-UP

DISPOSITION
Admission Criteria
As for heart failure of any etiology

PROGNOSIS
As for heart failure of any etiology

PATIENT MONITORING
As for heart failure of any etiology

REFERENCES
1. Heistad DD, Abboud FM, Schnid PG, et al. Regulation of blood flow in Paget's disease of bone. *J Clin Invest*. 1975;55:69.
2. Zipes DP. *Braunwald's Heart Disease: A Textbook of Cardiovascular Medicine*, 7th ed., 2005.

CODES
ICD9-CM
428.0 Failure, heart, congestive

PATIENT TEACHING
As for heart failure of any etiology

P

PARADOXICAL EMBOLISM

Carlos A. Roldan

BASICS

DESCRIPTION

Emboli that originate in the venous system and reach the arterial system via a right-to-left cardiac or extracardiac shunt

- The diagnosis requires four clinical criteria:
  - Venous thrombosis
  - Communication between right and left circulations
  - Right-to-left atrial pressure gradient during the entire or a portion of the cardiac cycle
  - Systemic embolism in the absence of common cardioembolic substrates
- The diagnosis is definite when a thrombus lodged across an intracardiac shunt is shown.
- 50% embolize to lower extremities; 35–40% to brain; and 10–15% to coronary, renal, splenic, retinal, or mesenteric arteries
- ≥2 sites of embolism occur in 25% of patients.
- Pulmonary embolism (PE) is detected in 2/3 of patients and deep venous thrombosis (DVT) in about 40%.
- Patent foramen ovale (PFO) is present in 72% of patients, atrial septal defect (ASD) in 12%, pulmonary arteriovenous fistula in 12%, and ventricular septal defect in 4%.
- Common association of atrial septal aneurysm with PFO

GENERAL PREVENTION
Applicable to prevention of DVT and PE.

EPIDEMIOLOGY
Incidence and Prevalence
- Paradoxical embolism is an uncommon clinical syndrome described in all races, different age groups, and both sexes.
- Its true incidence and prevalence are unknown, but are very low.
- Predominant age: 40 years old
- Predominant sex: Female > Male (2:1)

RISK FACTORS
- High risk: Those with an intra- or extracardiac communication and DVT or PE; association of atrial septal aneurysm with PFO increases risk
- Moderate risk: Those with PFO/ASD and right atrial hypertension due to chronic obstructive pulmonary disease (COPD), right ventricular dysfunction, or atrial fibrillation
- Low risk
  - Those with PFO and normal right atrial pressure who exhibit transient spontaneous or induced (respiration, Valsalva, or coughing) right-to-left atrial pressure gradient
  - Patients with central venous catheters

Genetics
Atrial or ventricular septal defects and other congenital shunts have a genetic etiology.

PATHOPHYSIOLOGY
Migrating venous thrombi through the right heart, which in the presence of an intracardiac shunt and a transient or permanent right to left heart pressure differential migrates into the systemic circulation

ASSOCIATED CONDITIONS
- Intra- or extracardiac communication, DVT, PE, and right atrial hypertension
- In autopsy studies, the prevalence of patent foramen ovale ranges from 22–34%, but most (85%) are 2–5 mm and the minority (15%) are 6–10 mm in diameter (the last more likely to be associated with embolism).
- In patients <55 years of age with systemic embolism, but no cardiac disease, the prevalence of PFO by contrast echocardiography ranges from 25–50%.
- In patients undergoing echocardiography for reasons other than systemic embolism, the prevalence of PFO is 3–15%.
- The prevalence of secundum-type ASD in adults is probably <1%.
- Therefore, paradoxical embolism occurs mostly in association with a PFO.
- Risk factors for DVT and PE include postoperative status, inactivity due to stroke or obesity, myocardial infarction, congestive heart failure (CHF), venous insufficiency, and primary or secondary hypercoagulable states.
- In situ right atrial thrombosis occurs in patients with atrial fibrillation, undergoing right atrial cannulation during cardiopulmonary bypass, or with right atrial catheters.

DIAGNOSIS

SIGNS AND SYMPTOMS
- The signs and symptoms of DVT and PE usually precede those of systemic embolism and are described in other sections of this book.
- Although paradoxical embolism may imply recurrent PE leading to right atrial hypertension, paradoxical embolism also occurs in patients without thromboembolic pulmonary hypertension and rarely in those with normal cardiac pressures.
- The vascular distributions, signs, and symptoms of paradoxical embolism are those of transient ischemic attack, stroke, or peripheral embolism described in the chapter on Arterial Embolism.
- In patients with migraine, especially in those with aura, the prevalence of PFO is twice as common as in those without aura and in healthy controls. If they undergo PFO closure, the migraine headaches improve significantly in frequency, duration, and severity.

History
- Recent bedridden state or long trip
- Conditions associated with pulmonary hypertension (i.e., COPD)
- History of DVT or PE
- History of systemic embolism
- Migraine headaches

Physical Exam
- Can be normal
- Those of pulmonary hypertension/cor pulmonale
  - Jugular venous distension (JVD), prominent *a* and *v* waves
  - Right ventricular heave or lift
  - Accentuated pulmonary closure sound
  - Tricuspid regurgitation

TESTS
Lab
In the absence of traditional risk factors for DVT or PE, congenital or acquired hypercoagulability should be investigated.

Imaging
- Brain CT, MRI/magnetic resonance angiography (MRA), carotid duplex ultrasonography, and angiography
- Transthoracic echocardiography with saline contrast and during Valsalva maneuver or coughing
  - Bubbles seen in the left atrium within the first 3 cardiac cycles suggest a PFO/ASD.
  - Bubbles seen after 3 cardiac cycles suggest a pulmonary arteriovenous communication.
- If systemic embolism has occurred and a PFO or ASD is demonstrated, studies for detection of DVT and PE should be performed.

Pathologic Findings
DVT with or without PE, intracardiac shunt, and evidence of intracardiac thrombi and systemic thromboembolism

DIFFERENTIAL DIAGNOSIS
- Most common causes of cerebral or peripheral thromboembolism are carotid or aortic atherosclerosis, atrial fibrillation, mitral stenosis, prosthetic heart valves, large anterior myocardial infarction, dilated cardiomyopathy, and infective or noninfective endocarditis.
- In patients with systemic embolism and evidence of PFO but no intracardiac thrombi, DVT, or PE, other causes of arterial embolism or thrombosis should be excluded.

TREATMENT

GENERAL MEASURES
- Those related to DVT, PE, and arterial embolism as described elsewhere in this book
- There are no data on primary prevention of paradoxical embolism in patients with known intracardiac shunts, specifically PFO (prevalence of PFO up to 30% of the general population).
- The best treatment for prevention of recurrent paradoxical embolism in patients with PFO or ASD remains undefined. Current alternatives:
  - Anticoagulation
  - Single or dual antiplatelet therapy
  - Percutaneous device closure
  - Surgical closure
- In those without documented DVT, PE, or intracardiac thrombi, antiplatelet and anticoagulant therapy has shown similar benefit.
- To date, there is not a randomized trial comparing medical therapy with percutaneous or surgical closure of defects.

MEDICATION (DRUGS)

First Line
- If DVT or PE is diagnosed, the patient is hemodynamically stable, and risk for cerebral hemorrhagic infarction is low, heparin intravenous (IV) bolus and continuous infusion to a partial thromboplastin time 1.5–2.5 times control is indicated.
- Warfarin is started on days 2–3 and heparin discontinued on day 7–10 or when international normalized ratio (INR) is 2–3.
- If no contraindications, IV thrombolytic therapy should be considered in patients with
  – Recent peripheral thromboembolism
  – Stroke of <3 hours' duration
  – Large pulmonary embolism with hemodynamic compromise or right ventricular dilation or dysfunction without hemodynamic instability
  – Peripheral embolism with jeopardized limb viability
- In patients with suspected paradoxical embolism with PFO with or without associated atrial septal aneurysm and without evidence of DVT or PE, the benefit of antiplatelet or anticoagulant therapy is similar. However, these therapies have not been tested in randomized trials.
- Transcatheter closure of PFO or ASD is an alternative to medical therapy for secondary prevention in patients with paradoxical embolism.
  – Short- and long-term complete closure of the defect is generally >90% (range, 85–96%) and is similar for those with associated atrial septal aneurysm.
  – Periprocedural complications range from 1.5–7.9% and include systemic embolism (1–3%), persistent atrial tachyarrhythmias or sinus node dysfunction (6%), device embolization (<1%), cardiac tamponade (<1%), and thrombus formation on the closure device (<1%).
  – Mortality <1%
  – The recurrence rate of systemic embolism with or without residual shunt ranges from 0–5% over a 12–60 month follow-up.

SURGERY
- In patients with hemodynamically compromising main or proximal pulmonary artery thrombosis who are not candidates for thrombolytic therapy, pulmonary thromboembolectomy, PFO/ASD closure, and inferior vena cava (IVC) interruption via a filter or surgical plication should be considered.
- Recurrent paradoxical embolism despite adequate anticoagulation requires interruption of IVC via filter or surgical plication and closure of the PFO or ASD.
- In patients with peripheral embolism, surgical or percutaneous thromboembolectomy when limb ischemia persists despite anticoagulation.

- In patients with systemic embolism and PFO with or without atrial septal aneurysm and no documented DVT, PE, or intracardiac thrombus, surgical closure of a PFO is an alternative.
  – Complete surgical closure rates are generally >95% (range, 73–100%). Incomplete defect closure is due to incomplete suture of septum primum and secundum or a new iatrogenic defect.
  – Surgical mortality is <1%.
  – Recurrence of systemic embolism occurs in up to 6% of patients.

FOLLOW-UP

Contrast echocardiography to assess for intracardiac shunt after percutaneous or surgical closure

DISPOSITION
Issues for Referral
For secondary prevention, consider referring patient to an experienced center for percutaneous closure of PFO or ASD.

PROGNOSIS
- Limited prospective and longitudinal data
- Patients' clinical course is related to the severity of pulmonary and arterial emboli.
- Stroke in association with recurrent PE portends a poor prognosis.
- Patients with peripheral embolism have better prognosis.
- Most (70%) patients demonstrate full recovery of neurologic or peripheral pulse deficits, whereas 10% have persistent deficits. The remaining 20% die, and PE is the main cause.

COMPLICATIONS
- Limb or organ injury or loss due to embolism
- Persistent shunt and recurrent embolism despite medical therapy or percutaneous or surgical closure of PFO or ASD.

PATIENT MONITORING
Monitoring of warfarin therapy

REFERENCES
1. Chatterjee T, Petzsch M, Ince H, et al. Interventional closure with Amplatzer PFO occluder of patent foramen ovale in patients with paradoxical embolism. *J Interv Cardiol*. 2005;18:173–179.
2. Gasiavelis N, Grinnemo KH, Lindblom D, et al. Surgical closure of patent foramen ovale in patients with suspected paradoxical embolism: Long-term results. *Scand Cardiovasc J*. 2004;38:375–379.
3. Klotz S, Tjan TD, Berendes E, et al. Surgical closure of combined symptomatic patent foramen ovale and atrial septal aneurysm for prevention of recurrent cerebral emboli. *J Card Surg*. 2005;20: 370–374.
4. Kumar S, Khan I, Milton R, et al. Pulmonary and paradoxical embolism in protein C and S deficient patient. *Ann Thorac Surg*. 2005;80: 324–326.
5. Mattle HP, Meier B, Windecker S; PC Trial Group. Practice parameter: Recurrent stroke with patent foramen ovale and atrial septal aneurysm: Report of the Quality Standards Subcommittee of the American Academy of Neurology. *Neurology*. 2004;63:2198–2199.
6. Post MC, Van Deyk K, Werner B. Percutaneous closure of a patent foramen ovale: Single-centre experience using different types of devices and mid-term outcome. *Acta Cardiol*. 2005;60: 515–519.
7. Wahl A, Krumsdorf U, Meier B, et al. Transcatheter treatment of atrial septal aneurysm associated with patent foramen ovale for prevention of recurrent paradoxical embolism in high risk patients. *J Am Coll Cardiol*. 2005;45:377–380.
8. Yasaka M, Otsubo Always, Oe H, et al. Is stroke a paradoxical embolism in patients with patent foramen ovale? *Intern Med*. 2005;44:434–438.
9. Zanchetta M, Rigatelli G, Ho SY. A mystery featuring right-to-left shunting despite normal intracardiac pressure. *Chest*. 2005;128:998–1002.

CODES
ICD9-CM
- 444.9 Paradoxical embolism
- 434.1 Cerebral embolism
- 444.22 Peripheral artery embolism
- 415.1 Pulmonary embolism
- 451.9 Thrombophlebitis

FAQ
- Is the diagnosis of paradoxical embolism or cardioembolism established in a patient with stroke/transient ischemic attack (TIA) and a PFO, but no intracardiac or venous thrombi?
  – No. Other causes of systemic embolism should be investigated.
- Is there indication for primary prevention therapy in patients with PFO?
  – No. No data are available about the value of medical therapy or percutaneous or surgical closure of PFO.
- Is there a superior therapy for secondary prevention in patients with PFO and systemic embolism?
- (i) Antiplatelet versus anticoagulant therapy have revealed similar results; (ii) no randomized and controlled comparison has been made between medical therapy versus percutaneous versus surgical closure of defects.

P

PATENT DUCTUS ARTERIOSUS

Karen Altmann
Welton M. Gersony

 BASICS

DESCRIPTION
Functional closure of the ductus arteriosus usually occurs within the first 24 hours of life. Complete obliteration of the lumen usually is completed in the first weeks of life.

EPIDEMIOLOGY
- In the U.S. as an isolated lesion, a persistent PDA has been estimated to occur in 1/2,000 to 1/5,000 live births and represents 9–12% of all congenital heart lesions.
- Predominant sex: Female > Male

RISK FACTORS
- Prematurity and hypoxemia contribute to persistent patency of the ductus arteriosus.
- Rubella infection early in pregnancy has a high association with persistent patency of the ductus arteriosus.
- Children born at high altitudes have a higher incidence of persistent PDA than do those born at sea level.

Genetics
A genetic factor may be present in some cases. Siblings of patients with a PDA have as high as a 2–4% incidence of having a PDA themselves.

PATHOPHYSIOLOGY
- With persistence of the ductus arteriosus in a neonate, when pulmonary vascular resistance has dropped below the systemic vascular resistance, blood flows from the aorta into the pulmonary artery, resulting in a net left-to-right shunt. This results in an increased volume load on the left atrium and left ventricle. Two major factors control the degree of shunting:
  - Diameter and length of the ductus arteriosus
  - Systemic and pulmonary vascular resistance.
- If the left-to-right shunt is significant, symptoms of pulmonary overcirculation develop.

ASSOCIATED CONDITIONS
PDA can be an isolated lesion or can be associated with virtually all other congenital heart defects.

 DIAGNOSIS

SIGNS AND SYMPTOMS
- Most common signs and symptoms: The clinical findings depend on the magnitude of left-to-right shunt through the PDA and the ability of the heart to manage the extra volume load.
- Premature infants:
  - Diagnosis often made in first week of life, because left-to-right shunt begins early; premature infants usually have low pulmonary vascular resistance from birth.
  - Classical machinery murmur usually is not present.
  - Systolic murmur, which may extend into early diastole, is heard best at the left sternal border in the second and third intercostal spaces.
  - Hyperactive precordium
  - Widened pulse pressure
  - Prominent pulses
  - If a large shunt is present, patients have signs of congestive heart failure (CHF).
- Term infants, older children:
  - Small PDA:
    - Usually not symptomatic
    - Normal first and second heart sounds
    - Murmur usually systolic in infancy and then continuous murmur heard best at second left intercostal space in older child
    - Prominent peripheral pulses
    - Slightly increased arterial pulse pressure
  - Moderate PDA:
    - Patients may have signs of CHF in infancy.
    - Loud continuous murmur with machinery quality at left upper sternal border
    - Increased heart rate
    - Bounding pulses
    - Widened pulse pressure
    - Hyperdynamic precordium
  - Large PDA:
    - Usually have signs of CHF in first few months of life
    - Murmur usually is continuous.
    - Increased heart rate
    - Bounding pulses
    - Widened pulse pressure
    - Hyperdynamic precordium
    - May have mid-diastolic rumble at apex
    - May eventually progress to pulmonary vascular disease and right-to-left shunt if untreated

Physical Exam
The classic finding is the continuous "machinery" murmur at the left upper sternal border (see above).

TESTS
- ECG:
  - Small ductus: ECG is normal.
  - Larger ductus: Increased left ventricular forces, occasionally left atrial enlargement
  - Larger ductus with pulmonary hypertension: Increased biventricular forces

Imaging
- Chest radiograph:
  - The radiographic findings vary in proportion to the degree of left-to-right shunting.
  - With a larger shunt, if cardiomegaly is present, with enlargement of the left ventricle, left atrium, and prominent pulmonary vasculature
- Echocardiography:
  - The ductus is best imaged in a high left parasternal view.
  - Color flow mapping is essential to demonstrate flow through the ductus.
  - Pulsed and continuous wave Doppler are useful for assessing direction of ductal flow and estimating the pulmonary artery pressure.
  - If a significant shunt exists, left atrial and left ventricular dilatation is seen.
  - Echocardiography has a critical role in excluding other significant intracardiac lesions, especially ductal-dependent lesions.

Diagnostic Procedures/Surgery
- Cardiac catheterization
  - Catheterization is rarely needed to make the diagnosis.

Pathologic Findings
The normal ductus arteriosus develops embryologically from the dorsal portion of the left sixth aortic arch. The ductus is a muscular artery with intima, media, and adventitia, but histologically, these layers differ from the adjacent pulmonary trunk and aorta.

DIFFERENTIAL DIAGNOSIS
- The following lesions also cause continuous or to-and-fro murmurs:
  - Venous hum
  - Aortopulmonary window
  - Arteriovenous fistula
  - Ruptured sinus of Valsalva
  - Truncus arteriosus
  - Absent pulmonary valve
  - Ventricular septal defect with aortic insufficiency

TREATMENT

GENERAL MEASURES

- The classic small to large ductus arteriosus should be eliminated, the timing of which is determined by the presence or absence of symptoms.
- The term *silent ductus* refers to echocardiographic findings of a minimal color Doppler shunt diagnostic or is suggestive of a tiny PDA in a patient with no other physical or laboratory evidence of a PDA. In most cases, the echocardiographic study was done for a nonspecific systolic murmur that might well have been classified by a cardiologist as functional without an ultrasonographic study. These patients are often followed without intervention. Although endocarditis with silent ductus specifically is virtually unreported, it may be prudent to nevertheless recommend appropriate antibiotic prophylaxis.

 MEDICATION (DRUGS)

First Line

- Indomethacin has been used successfully to close a PDA in a large proportion of premature infants. It is not effective in term infants.
- Infants with signs of CHF can be managed briefly with anticongestive medications; standard treatment for symptomatic patients is elimination of the ductus arteriosus on an immediate basis.
- A patient with a PDA should receive bacterial endocarditis prophylaxis according to recommended AHA guidelines.

SURGERY

- Using modern surgical techniques, surgical closure has achieved nearly a 100% success rate with almost no mortality risk and low morbidity.
- Neither the size of the patient nor that of the ductus arteriosus is a limiting factor. Although there have been reports of recanalization after ligation alone, and other rare complications (injury to the recurrent laryngeal nerve, injury to the thoracic duct with chylothorax, or accidental ligation of the left pulmonary artery, descending aorta, or carotid artery), surgical ligation or division of the ductus arteriosus has been the standard for more than 60 years.
- More recently, some institutions have begun video-assisted thorascopic ligation of the PDA. This approach may reduce the postoperative convalescence period and may be associated with less chest wall deformity.
  - A potential drawback is greater difficulty controlling intraoperative bleeding. More experience with this procedure will determine the future role it may play in ductal closure.
- Catheter closure:
  - Catheter closure of a PDA was first introduced over 20 years ago and is now accepted as the preferred therapy at most institutions. In patients beyond early infancy, the size of the ductus is not usually a limiting factor for closure. The ductus usually is closed via occluder device or coils.
  - Studies report high success rates with few complications, which include coil embolization, left pulmonary artery stenosis, flow disturbance in the aorta, or hemolysis.

 FOLLOW-UP

PROGNOSIS

- In premature infants, persistent patency of the PDA is common. The great majority will close as the patient matures, but in the context of respiratory distress syndrome, early pharmacologic or surgical intervention often is required.
- Term infants with PDA rarely have spontaneous closure.
- Patients with untreated PDA are at risk for the possible complications listed below.
- The long-term prognosis for children with repaired PDA, and no evidence of vascular disease, is excellent.

COMPLICATIONS

- CHF, usually in young infants with a large ductus arteriosus
- Bacterial endocarditis
- Aneurysm of the ductus arteriosus
- Pulmonary vascular disease

PATIENT MONITORING

The follow-up of patients s/p PDA closure should be tailored to the individual patient, based on symptomatology before repair, evidence of pulmonary vascular disease, and mechanism of PDA closure.

REFERENCES

1. Balzer DT, Spray TL, McMullin D, et al. Endarteritis associated with a clinically silent patent ductus arteriosus. *Am Heart J.* 1993;125:1192.
2. Brook MM, Heymann MA. Patent ductus arteriosus. In: *Moss and Adams' heart disease in infants, children, and adolescents*, 5th ed. Baltimore: Williams & Wilkins, 1995:746.
3. Gersony WM, Peckham GJ, Ellison RC, et al. Effects of indomethacin in premature infants with patent ductus arteriosus: Results of a national collaborative study. *J Pediatr.* 1983;102:895.
4. Kirklin JW, Barratt-Boyles BG. Patent ductus arteriosus. In: *Cardiac surgery*, 2nd ed. New York: Churchill Livingstone, 1993:851
5. Magee AG, Huggon IC, Seed, PT, et al. Transcatheter coil occlusion of the arterial duct: Results of the European Registry. *Eur Heart J.* 2001;22:1817.
6. Moore JW, Levi DS, Moore SD, et al. Interventional treatment of patent ductus arteriosus in 2004. *Catheter Cardiovasc Interv.* 2005;64:91.
7. Pass RH, Hijazi Z, Hsu D, et al. Multicenter USA Amplatzer patent ductus arteriosus occlusion device trial: Initial and one-year results. *J Am Coll Cardiol.* 2004;44:513.
8. Villa E, Eynden FV, Le Bret E, et al. Paediatric video-assisted thorascopic clipping of patent ductus arteriosus: Experience in more than 700 cases. *Eur J Cardiothorac Surg.* 2004;25:387.

P

PECTUS EXCAVATUM, EFFECT ON CARDIAC FUNCTION

Richard Mascolo
Gerard P. Aurigemma

 ## BASICS

DESCRIPTION

- Depression of the sternum, so that the ribs on each side protrude anteriorly beyond the sternum
- This condition is associated with connective tissue disorders such as Marfan's syndrome, Poland syndrome, Pierre Robin syndrome, and scoliosis.
- An increased incidence of mitral valve prolapse, Wolf-Parkinson-White syndrome, and atrial septal defect
- System(s) affected: Musculoskeletal; Cardiovascular; Pulmonary
- Synonym(s): Funnel chest

EPIDEMIOLOGY

Predominant sex: More males affected than females

Incidence

- 0.4–2% of the general population
- Increased incidence in people with a family history

ASSOCIATED CONDITIONS

- Marfan syndrome
- Poland syndrome
- Scoliosis
- Pierre Robin syndrome

 ## DIAGNOSIS

SIGNS AND SYMPTOMS

- Diagnosis by physical examination: Depression of the sternum so that the ribs on each side protrude anteriorly beyond the sternum
- Most patients are asymptomatic. Cardiopulmonary symptoms such as fatigue and decreased exercise tolerance have been reported.
- Heart murmur is evident in 40–50% of cases, most commonly a systolic murmur that mimics pulmonic stenosis. This may be secondary to kinking of the pulmonary artery or changes in the diameter of the right ventricular outflow tract.
- Splitting of the second heart sound is also commonly found.

TESTS

- ECG:
  - Increased left-sided potentials related to leftward displacement of the heart may be seen, as may right ventricular conduction delay.
- Pulmonary function tests:
  - A slightly decreased vital capacity is commonly found, as is an occasional restrictive lung pattern.

Imaging

- Chest radiograph shows the degree of sternal depression.
  - The heart is displaced to the left and rotated.
  - Parasternal soft tissues may be seen as an increased density over the inferomedial portion of the left hemithorax.
  - Occasionally an unusual mediastinal configuration can mimic a mediastinal mass.
- Echocardiogram:
  - Compression of the right atrium or right ventricle may be seen.
  - Morphologic changes in the right ventricle have been reported.
  - These include right ventricle dilatation, rounded apex, sacculations in the free wall, and hypertrophy of the moderator band.

TREATMENT

GENERAL MEASURES
Physicians should be aware of associated conditions and cardiac abnormalities. ECG and echocardiogram should be considered.

SURGERY
- This chest wall deformity can be surgically repaired.
- The majority of people will not have a functional benefit.
- Some case reports suggest symptomatic and hemodynamic improvements.
- Sometimes the defect is repaired for cosmetic reasons.

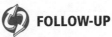 **FOLLOW-UP**

PROGNOSIS
Depends on any other related conditions (e.g., Marfan syndrome)

PATIENT MONITORING
Determined by symptoms and associated conditions

REFERENCES
1. Fraser RG, Pare JA, Pare PD, et al. *Diagnosis of diseases of the chest*. Philadelphia: WB Saunders, 1991.
2. Guller B, Hable K. Cardiac findings in pectus excavatum in children: Review and differential diagnosis. *Chest*. 1974;66:165–171.
3. Mocchegiani R, Bandano L, Lestuzzi C, et al. Relation of right ventricular morphology and function in pectus excavatum to the severity of the chest wall deformity. *Am J Cardiol*. 1995;76: 941–946.
4. Shamberger RC, Welch KJ. Cardiopulmonary function in pectus excavatum. *Surg Gynecol Obstet*. 1988;166:383–391.

PATIENT TEACHING
Diet
No restrictions
Activity
No restrictions

P

PERICARDIAL TAMPONADE

James A. Kong

 BASICS

DESCRIPTION

Pericardial tamponade is defined as fluid accumulation of any nature in the pericardial space resulting in an increase in intrapericardial pressures.

- Tamponade encompasses a spectrum of conditions, from asymptomatic elevation of intrapericardial pressure to hemodynamic compromise with hypotension and electromechanical dissociation (EMD).
- In some instances, tamponade affects only discrete regions of the heart, from loculated effusion or clot.
- The rate of fluid accumulation has important implications for the developing tamponade.
- Acute tamponade develops after rapid accumulation of pericardial fluid. Only 100–200 mL of fluid is required to increase intrapericardial pressures acutely, owing to the limited distensibility of the pericardium.
- Conversely, the more common chronic tamponade develops after gradual accumulation of pericardial fluid. As much as 1–1.5 L of fluid may accumulate in the slowly distending pericardium before tamponade occurs.
- Gradual accumulation allows the pericardium to stretch and compensate for the increasing volume without increasing pressure.
- Physical examination findings may be less reliable in cases of chronic tamponade.
- System(s) affected: Cardiovascular

EPIDEMIOLOGY

Incidence
Unknown

Prevalence
Unknown

RISK FACTORS

Conditions that would predispose to that described previously, including renal failure, a history of chest/mediastinal radiotherapy, and coagulopathy

ETIOLOGY

- When intrapericardial pressure exceeds right ventricular (RV) pressure, RV dysfunction ensues.
- With decreased RV output, left ventricular (LV) output decreases, resulting in systemic hypotension.
- The most common causes of tamponade include trauma, malignancy, uremia, postcardiac surgery, and idiopathic causes.
- Other less common causes include viral syndrome, lupus, rheumatoid arthritis, radiation injury, myocardial infarction, iatrogenic causes (e.g., cardiac catheterization, pacemaker placement), aortic dissection, and infection (e.g., sepsis, tuberculosis, and fungus).
- Rarely, tamponade from pneumopericardium may occur after barotrauma from mechanical ventilation.

 DIAGNOSIS

SIGNS AND SYMPTOMS

- Presentation varies, usually with nonspecific symptoms including dyspnea, fatigue, chest pain, syncope, hypotension, and shock.
- In severe cases, EMD can occur. On physical examination:
  - Tachycardia
  - Tachypnea
  - Clear lungs on auscultation
  - Pulsus paradoxus is a greater than normal decrease in systolic blood pressure with inspiration. It is measured as the difference between the first Korotkoff sound heard intermittently (only at end expiration) and the first Korotkoff sound heard regularly (throughout the respiratory cycle). A difference of >10 mm Hg is abnormal. This finding is nonspecific for tamponade.
  - Beck triad consists of (i) decreased arterial pressure, (ii) increased central venous pressure, and (iii) quiet heart on examination. It is a rare finding, especially in the medical patient with insidious onset of tamponade.
  - Kussmaul sign is the absence of the normally expected decrease, or even a paradoxical increase, in central venous pressure with inspiration.
  - Pericardial friction rub, fever, etc., accompanying the underlying condition leading to tamponade

TESTS

Electrocardiographic findings may include:

- Diffuse low voltage, most helpful when a decrease in voltage is observed on serial tracings
- PR or ST-segment changes consistent with pericarditis
- Nonspecific ST-segment or T-wave changes
- Electrical alternans is periodic variation of the amplitude of the P-QRS complex—rare, but highly specific. Involvement of the QRS complex alone is less specific.

Imaging

- Chest x-ray: A globular heart or rapid changes in the cardiac silhouette on serial radiographs may be seen. However, findings are nonspecific and usually not helpful.
- Transthoracic echocardiography is the most sensitive and specific noninvasive diagnostic test. Characteristic findings by two-dimensional and Doppler studies include:
  - RV collapse in early diastole
  - Right atrial collapse in late diastole
  - Reciprocal respiratory variation in RV and LV diastolic dimension
  - Inferior vena cava plethora with a decrease in the usually observed inspiratory collapse
  - Swinging heart (in the pericardial fluid)
  - Decreased LV filling with inspiration, with increased filling with expiration; reciprocal changes observed for the RV
- Echocardiographic changes may appear before symptoms.
- Transesophageal echocardiography may be helpful in locating loculated effusions or clots that are difficult to visualize by transthoracic examination.

DIAGNOSTIC PROCEDURES/SURGERY

Pulmonary artery catheter monitoring: Equalization of pressures may be observed between the pulmonary arterial diastolic pressure and central venous pressure.

DIFFERENTIAL DIAGNOSIS

- Pericardial tamponade should be considered when hypotension is present and accompanied by the previously noted risk factors.
- Other more common causes of hypotension must be considered, including hypovolemia/hemorrhage, sepsis, tension pneumothorax, massive pulmonary embolus, arrhythmia, myocardial infarction, congestive heart failure or cardiomyopathy, aortic dissection, and constrictive pericarditis.

TREATMENT

GENERAL MEASURES

- Rapid infusion of intravenous fluid may be used for temporary hemodynamic support in preparation for pericardiocentesis.
- Acute tamponade is more likely to respond to intravenous fluid therapy than is chronic tamponade.
- Vasoactive agents are of unproven benefit and should be considered only as a bridge to definitive treatment by drainage.

MEDICATION (DRUGS)

Medical treatment is indicated only for the prevention of recurrent pericardial effusion and may preclude pericardiectomy. Appropriate consultation should be obtained before their use.

First Line
- Intrapericardial steroids: For hemodialysis patients and tamponade due to uremic pericarditis
- Intrapericardial tetracycline or chemotherapeutic agents: for malignant pericardial effusions
- Systemic chemotherapy
  - In small studies and meta-analyses, systemic chemotherapy for prevention of malignant effusions appears superior to pericardiocentesis alone.
  - It does not, however, approach the efficacy of intrapericardial or surgical treatment.
- Precautions
  - Instillation of these agents may cause atrial arrhythmias and ventricular ectopy. Furthermore, tetracycline and chemotherapeutic agents act as sclerosing agents, which may cause pericardial constriction.

SURGERY
- Percutaneous techniques
  - Needle pericardiocentesis
    - Emergent percutaneous drainage of pericardial fluid to relieve intrapericardial pressure
    - Pericardiocentesis should be performed by a skilled and experienced physician.
    - After administration of local anesthesia, a large-bore needle is inserted in the skin via a fifth intercostal or subxiphoid approach and advanced into the pericardial space.
    - Electrocardiographic monitoring and full resuscitative equipment are essential, and single-lead ECG monitoring of the advancing needle may be helpful in avoiding the myocardium.
    - If possible, pericardial fluid may be located echocardiographically prior to needle insertion.
    - Care must be taken not to injure the myocardium or epicardial coronary arteries.
    - Pericardiocentesis may be followed by placement of an indwelling catheter and closed drainage.
    - Continuous drainage is preferred because pericardial effusions may reaccumulate after initial needle drainage.
  - Balloon pericardiotomy
    - A balloon is advanced into the pericardium.
    - Dilation of the balloon creates a potential pathway for drainage of pericardial fluid into the pleural space, without the use of catheter drainage.
    - Complications include pneumothorax and the need for thoracentesis or chest tube.
- Invasive techniques
  - Pericardiotomy (pericardial window)
    - The preferred method of drainage if circumstances allow and wider pericardial excision is not required
    - The pericardium is approached via a xiphisternal or subxiphoid incision. The pericardium is opened and allowed to drain via a small chest tube.
    - This method has the advantage of pericardial biopsy for diagnosis, as well as improved clearance of thicker pericardial fluids (e.g., fibrinous debris or clot).
    - Drainage into the peritoneum is an alternative to tube drainage.
  - Pericardiectomy
    - Indicated when more extensive removal of the pericardium is required
    - Under these circumstances, thoracotomy or median sternotomy approaches are used.

 ## FOLLOW-UP

DISPOSITION
Admission Criteria
- Asymptomatic pericardial effusion requires semiurgent evaluation.
- Hemodynamic instability necessitates immediate treatment by evacuation of the pericardial fluid.

PROGNOSIS
- Variable, depending on the underlying cause and its reversibility
- Development of constrictive pericarditis may lead to impaired cardiac function.

COMPLICATIONS
Inflammation of the pericardium, particularly in infection, may lead to scarring and ultimately pericardial constriction.

PATIENT MONITORING
Follow closely for signs or symptoms of reaccumulation of pericardial fluid.

REFERENCES
1. Ameli S, Shah PK. Cardiac tamponade. Pathophysiology, diagnosis, and management. *Cardiol Clin*. 1991;9:665–674.
2. Cummins RO, ed. *Advanced Cardiac Life Support*. Dallas: American Heart Association, 1997.
3. Moores DWO, Dziuban SW Jr. Pericardial drainage procedures. *Chest Surg Clin North Am*. 1995;5:359–373.
4. Tsang TSM, et al. Diagnosis and management of cardiac tamponade in the era of echocardiography. *Clin Cardiol*. 1999;22:446–452.
5. Vaitkus PT, et al. Treatment of malignant pericardial effusion. *JAMA*. 1994;272:59–64.

 ## MISCELLANEOUS

- See also: Pericarditis, constrictive; Pericardial effusion; Ventricular rupture; Electromechanical dissociation

CODES
ICD9-CM
423.9 Cardiac tamponade

PATIENT TEACHING
Organizations
- American Heart Association National Center, 7272 Greenville Avenue, Dallas, TX 75231;1-800-AHA-USA1; http://www.americanheart.org/
- National Heart Lung and Blood Institute; http://www.nhlbi.nih.gov

Activity
As clinically tolerated

Prevention
Treatment and control of the underlying cause

P

PERICARDITIS, ACUTE

Michael P. Hudson

 BASICS

DESCRIPTION

Acute pericarditis is an inflammation of the pericardium lasting several days to 4–6 weeks. It is characterized by chest pain, pericardial friction rub, serial ECG changes, and pericardial effusion. It is the most common pathologic process involving the pericardium.

EPIDEMIOLOGY

- Predominant age: Occurs at all ages; most frequent in young adults
- Predominant sex: Males > Females
- Coincident chest pain and fever frequently occurring 1–2 weeks after a presumed viral respiratory illness
- Acute pericarditis frequently occurs after injury to the myocardium or pericardium, as seen following cardiac surgery (postpericardiotomy syndrome), trauma, or myocardial infarction (Dressler syndrome).
- Chest pain typically 1–6 weeks following cardiac injury; some episodes may occur months/years later.

Incidence

1/1,000 hospital admissions and 2–5% autopsy series

ETIOLOGY

- Idiopathic
- Viral infection (coxsackie A and B virus, echovirus, adenovirus, mumps, influenza, herpes simplex, HIV)
- Uremia
- Tuberculosis
- Postmyocardial infarction (acute fibrinous pericarditis, Dressler syndrome)
- Postpericardiotomy associated with cardiac surgery
- Neoplasm (carcinoma of lung/breast, lymphoma, melanoma, or acute leukemia)
- Acute bacterial infection (*Streptococcus pneumoniae, Staphylococcus, Neisseria, Legionella, Mycoplasma,* Lyme disease)
- Fungal infection (histoplasmosis, coccidioidomycosis)
- Aortic dissection
- Collagen vascular disease (systemic lupus erythematosus, rheumatoid arthritis, scleroderma, polyarteritis nodosa)
- Drug-induced (procainamide, hydralazine, isoniazid, minoxidil, methylsergide, phenytoin, anthracyclines, beta-lactam antibiotics)
- Radiation
- Hypothyroidism
- Pulmonary embolism
- Trauma

DIAGNOSIS

SIGNS AND SYMPTOMS

- Chest pain/discomfort is typically sharp and localized to the retrosternal or left precordial region with radiation to the back, trapezius ridge, neck, or epigastrium. It is frequently aggravated by inspiration, movement, swallowing, or lying supine, with pain relief or improvement on sitting up or leaning forward. Pain often is absent in slowly developing tuberculous, postirradiation, and neoplastic or uremic pericarditis.
- Fever
- Dyspnea/orthopnea
- Fatigue/weakness
- Near syncope

Physical Exam

- Pericardial friction rub:
  - High-pitched scratching or creaking sound pathognomonic of acute pericarditis
  - Best heard at left sternal border, with patient leaning forward, using stethoscope diaphragm
  - One to three components per cardiac cycle (ventricular systole, atrial systole, early ventricular filling)
  - Frequently missed due to changing location and quality
  - Most often confused with systolic murmurs of mitral or tricuspid regurgitation
  - Correlates poorly with presence and size of pericardial effusion
- Cardiac tamponade:
  - Accompanies 10–15% of patients with acute pericarditis
  - Classic diagnostic quartet is tachycardia, hypotension, jugular vein distension, and pulsus paradoxus.
  - Pulsus paradoxus is augmented decrease (>10–12 mm Hg) in systolic pressure with inspiration.
- ECG features:
  - Abnormal in ≥90% of cases of acute pericarditis
    - Stage 1: Diffuse concave-upward ST-segment elevation involving multiple coronary artery territories with associated PR-segment depression (80%), and absence of pathologic Q-waves or reciprocal ST-segment depression
    - Stage 2: ST-junction returns to baseline accompanied by T-wave flattening
    - Stage 3: Diffuse T-wave inversion observed during recovery period
    - Stage 4: Return of T- waves to normal
  - Other ECG clues of acute pericarditis or large pericardial effusion
    - Low QRS voltage
    - Electrical alternans (<10% acute pericarditis) is regular alteration in the amplitude or configuration of ECG complexes seen with large effusions.
    - Associated atrial arrhythmias or atrial premature beats

TESTS

Lab

- Elevated erythrocyte sedimentation rate (ESR)
- Moderate granulocytosis or lymphocytosis
- Moderate elevations of creatine phosphokinase (CK), creatine phosphokinase MB isoform (CK-MB), or cardiac troponin T or troponin I may occur and reflect accompanying epimyocarditis.
- Other helpful laboratory studies: tuberculin skin test, blood cultures, viral cultures, blood urea nitrogen, creatinine, HIV test, viral cultures, thyroid studies, antinuclear antibody titer, rheumatoid factor, cold agglutinins, and fungal serologies

Imaging

- Little diagnostic value in uncomplicated acute pericarditis
- Enlargement of the cardiac silhouette with occasional "water-bottle" configuration seen with moderate/large effusions
- May demonstrate underlying cause or associated pleural effusion (usually left-sided)
- CT/MRI may confirm pericardial effusion or pericardial thickening and exclude aortic dissection
- Echocardiography:
  - Absence of pericardial fluid does not exclude acute pericarditis.
  - Capable of detecting, localizing, and estimating size of pericardial effusion and guiding pericardiocentesis
  - Pericardial fluid depicted as echo-free space surrounding heart chambers
  - May demonstrate right atrial/right ventricular diastolic collapse or exaggerated inspiratory tricuspid/pulmonic flow with reciprocal mitral flow supporting cardiac tamponade
- Pericardiocentesis and pericardial biopsy:
  - Recommended in cases of cardiac tamponade or to exclude suspected purulent pericarditis

DIFFERENTIAL DIAGNOSIS

- Acute myocardial infarction (MI)
- Myocarditis
- Early repolarization

TREATMENT

GENERAL MEASURES

- Rest, avoidance of vigorous activity, and nonsteroidal anti-inflammatory drugs (NSAIDs) are mainstays.
- Bed rest until chest pain and fever have diminished; frequent observation with vital sign monitoring and repeat echocardiography if a moderate-large effusion is present
- Avoidance of anticoagulation recommended to decrease risk of cardiac tamponade
- If anticoagulation is mandatory (mechanical heart valves), IV heparin preferred over oral anticoagulation
- Hospitalization recommended in following cases:
  - Rule out acute MI
  - Exclude pyogenic process
  - Exclude and observe for cardiac tamponade and hemodynamic compromise
  - Parenteral analgesia for relief of refractory chest pain

 MEDICATION (DRUGS)

- Aspirin (650 mg PO every 4 hours) or indomethacin (25–75 mg PO every 6–8 hours) for analgesia and anti-inflammatory effect
- Morphine or meperidine (PO/IV/IM) may be required for supplemental pain relief.
- Consider oral steroid (prednisone 40–80 mg/day) if chest pain persists beyond 48 hours. Steroid dose may be tapered after 5–7 days and discontinued after 3–6 weeks.
- Chronic/recurrent pericarditis:
  - Reinstitute nonsteroidal anti-inflammatory agents and/or steroids with more gradual tapering over several months.
  - Chronic colchicine (1 mg PO/daily) may improve symptoms and prevent recurrence.
- Etiology-specific therapies:
  - Infectious (streptococcal/staphylococcal): IV β-lactam with or without aminoglycoside or vancomycin; prompt drainage required if signs of tamponade or continued infection
  - Neoplasm: Pericardiocentesis as needed; balloon pericardiostomy, sclerotherapy, or limited subxiphoid surgical window performed for palliation
  - Uremic: Often responds to initiation or intensification of dialysis with surgery reserved for nonresponders or recurrent episodes

SURGERY

- Pericardiocentesis:
  - Increased jugular venous pressure, tachycardia, hypotension, and pulsus paradoxus generally signal cardiac tamponade and need for emergent pericardiocentesis.
  - Intravenous fluids and inotropic drugs may temporarily provide hemodynamic support prior to pericardiocentesis.
- Surgical subxiphoid pericardiotomy (pericardial window) or transthoracic endoscopic pericardiotomy:
  - Limited palliative procedure for patients with poor prognosis
  - Operative mortality = 10%.
  - Procedure of choice for patients with expected long-term survival or loculated pericardial effusions
- Percutaneous balloon pericardiotomy:
  - Palliative option for large pericardial effusions/tamponade
  - Echo- or fluoroscopic-guided insertion of dilating balloon into pericardial sac, creating tear in pericardium

 FOLLOW-UP

PROGNOSIS

- Most episodes are self-limited and resolve within 2–6 weeks.
- Notable complications include recurrent/chronic pericarditis (20%), cardiac tamponade (10–15%), fibrosis or calcification of pericardium (constrictive pericarditis; 5%), effusive-constrictive pericarditis (5%), and arrhythmias, usually supraventricular tachycardias and premature atrial depolarizations.

REFERENCES

1. Chou T. Pericarditis. In: *Electrocardiography in clinical practice*, 3rd ed. Philadelphia: WB Saunders, 1991:219–234.
2. Lorell BH. Pericardial diseases. In: Braunwald E, ed. *Heart disease: A textbook of cardiovascular medicine*, 5th ed. Philadelphia: WB Saunders, 1997:1478–1495.
3. Marriott HJ. Pericardial disease. In: *Bedside cardiac diagnosis*. Philadelphia: JB Lippincott, 1993: 241–246.
4. Permanyer-Miralda G, Sagrista-Sauleda J, Soler-Soler J. Primary acute pericardial disease: A prospective series of 231 consecutive patients. *Am J Cardiol*. 1985;56:623.
5. Spodick DH. The normal and diseased pericardium: Current concepts of pericardial physiology, diagnosis, and treatment. *J Am Coll Cardiol*. 1983;1:240–251.

P

PERICARDITIS, CONSTRICTIVE

Michael P. Hudson

 BASICS

DESCRIPTION

In constrictive pericarditis, a thick, inelastic pericardium encases the heart and restricts diastolic filling, leading to biventricular (right ventricle > left ventricle) diastolic dysfunction, venous engorgement, and diminished cardiac output. Ventricular filling is unimpeded during early diastole but is reduced abruptly by noncompliant pericardium at the end of the first third of diastole. It is typically an indolent, progressive process with symptoms appearing months to years after an acute pericarditis episode or pericardial trauma/surgery.

- Effusive-constrictive pericarditis
  - Accumulation of tense pericardial effusion plus thickened, fibrotic pericardium
  - Hemodynamic features of tamponade before pericardiocentesis, and constriction afterward
  - Diagnosis made by hemodynamic recordings before and after pericardiocentesis with continued elevation of right atrial/central venous pressures after removal of pericardial fluid
  - Definitive treatment is complete pericardiectomy

EPIDEMIOLOGY

- Predominant sex: Male > Female (3:1)
- Predominant age: None; wide age range (8–80 years)

ETIOLOGY

- Idiopathic/unknown (40%)
  - Tuberculosis (10%)
  - Postcardiac surgery (5–10%; incidence after coronary artery bypass grafting 0.3%)
  - Postirradiation (5%)
  - Other postinfectious pericarditis (postviral, bacterial/purulent, fungal/histoplasmosis)
  - Collagen vascular disease [systemic lupus erythematosus, rheumatoid arthritis (RA)]
  - Drug-induced (procainamide, methysergide, hydralazine)
  - Neoplasm
  - Trauma (after pacemaker implantation)
  - Uremic
  - Asbestosis
- Clinical manifestations
  - Dyspnea/orthopnea/cough (78%)
  - Abdominal distention/swelling (68%)
  - Lower extremity edema (54%)
  - Severe weakness and fatigue (25%)
  - Weight loss/anorexia
  - Chest pain (24%)
  - Fever/night sweats

DIAGNOSIS

SIGNS AND SYMPTOMS

- Elevated jugular venous pressure with prominent X and Y venous descents (M- or W-shaped contour)
- Sinus tachycardia with normal or low-normal blood pressure
- Nonpalpable cardiac apical impulse
- Early diastolic pericardial knock with absence of third heart sound (S_3) and regurgitant murmurs
- Kussmaul sign (jugular venous pressure fails to decrease with inspiration)
- Hepatosplenomegaly (>70%)
- Ascites: Often more prominent than lower extremity edema
- Lower extremity edema
- Pulsus paradoxus (uncommon, fewer than one third of cases)
- Peripheral cyanosis
- Muscle wasting/cachexia, particularly of upper extremities

TESTS

- Occult constrictive pericardial disease: Diagnosed when the hemodynamic findings of constriction appear after rapid infusion of 1–2 L saline over 5–10 minutes
- Endomyocardial biopsy: Rarely required; may be needed to exclude infiltrative/restrictive myocardial disease causing restrictive cardiomyopathy
- Electrocardiographic findings
  - Generally nonspecific: Normal electrocardiogram (ECG) rarely observed; low QRS voltage; notched P wave (P mitrale); nondiagnostic ST-T wave abnormalities; atrial fibrillation or flutter
- Catheterization findings
  - Elevation and equalization of pressures: <5 mm Hg difference between mean right atrial pressure, right ventricular diastolic pressure, and pulmonary capillary wedge pressure
  - Prominent X and Y descents on the right atrial and pulmonary artery wedge pressure tracings (M or W configuration)
  - Prominent early left/right ventricular diastolic filling pattern with "dip-and-plateau" waveform ("square-root" sign)
  - Lack of inspiratory decrease in right atrial pressure
  - Modestly elevated right ventricular/pulmonary artery systolic pressure generally <60 mm Hg
  - Right ventricular end-diastolic pressure > 1/3 right ventricular systolic pressure

Lab

Generally nondiagnostic; erythrocyte sedimentation rate may be elevated; hypoalbuminemia and abnormal hepatocellular function tests

Imaging

- Plain-film chest radiography
  - Generally shows normal/small heart size and clear lung fields
  - Calcification of pericardium in 40–50% of cases
  - Best seen on lateral view
  - Calcification predominantly over right atrium/ventricle and in the atrioventricular grooves
  - Prominent right superior mediastinum
  - Left atrial enlargement
- Computed tomography (CT)/Magnetic resonance imaging (MRI)
  - More accurate and useful than echocardiography or chest radiography for detecting thickened pericardium
  - Abnormal pericardial thickness (>3 mm) on thoracic CT or MRI and characteristic hemodynamic changes usually confirm diagnosis.
- Echocardiography
  - Not reliable for detecting a thickened pericardium or excluding diagnosis
  - Small ventricles, dilated atria, and thick pericardium
  - Parallel motion of epicardium and parietal pericardium separated by 1-mm thick echo-free space strongly suggests thickened pericardium (M mode).
  - Numerous suggestive echocardiographic findings may be present: Dilated inferior vena cava/hepatic vein without respiratory variation, abrupt posterior motion of interventricular septum in early diastole (septal bounce), left ventricular (LV) posterior wall flattening, premature opening of pulmonary valve, and marked respiratory variation in diastolic atrioventricular flow velocities (>25% inspiratory decrease in mitral flow velocity).

DIFFERENTIAL DIAGNOSIS

- Every patient with ascites, liver enlargement, and raised jugular venous pressure should be thoroughly investigated for constrictive pericarditis.
- Restrictive cardiomyopathy
- Biventricular congestive heart failure
- Hepatic cirrhosis
- Cor pulmonale
- Tricuspid valve stenosis or regurgitation
- Nephrotic syndrome

TREATMENT

GENERAL MEASURES

Progressive symptoms require confirmatory CT/MRI demonstrating pericardial thickening, right and left cardiac catheterization documenting constrictive physiology, and curative surgical pericardectomy.

 ## MEDICATION (DRUGS)

- Mild symptoms are generally responsive to sodium restriction and diuretic therapy.
- Drugs that slow heart rate may be poorly tolerated.

SURGERY

- Surgical pericardial resection is definitive therapy with 5-year survival of 80%
- Most strongly indicated in NYHA functional class II–III
- Operative mortality is 3–15%
- More extensive calcification, worse functional class (NYHA class IV), LV systolic dysfunction, history of neoplasm, renal insufficiency, and previous pericardial procedure predict poor postoperative survival
- Hemodynamic and symptomatic improvement usually rapid and progressive over several months, with 80–90% survivors achieving NYHA I/II functional class

 ## FOLLOW-UP

PATIENT MONITORING

Progressive disease with minority of patients surviving 5 years without surgical repair

REFERENCES

1. Chou T. Pericarditis. In: *Electrocardiography in Clinical Practice*, 3rd ed. Philadelphia: WB Saunders, 1991:219–234.
2. Lorell BH. Pericardial diseases. In: Braunwald E, ed. *Heart Disease: A Textbook of Cardiovascular Medicine*, 5th ed. Philadelphia: WB Saunders, 1997:1496–1505.
3. Marriott HJ. Pericardial disease. In: *Bedside Cardiac Diagnosis*. Philadelphia: JB Lippincott, 1993:241–246.
4. Mehta A, Mehta M, Jain A. Constrictive pericarditis. *Clin Cardiol*. 1999;22:334–344.
5. Vaitkus PT, Kussmaul WG. Constrictive versus restrictive cardiomyopathy: A reappraisal and update of diagnostic criteria. *Am Heart J*. 1991;122:1431.

CODES

ICD9-CM

- 420.91 Acute idiopathic, pericarditis
- 423.1 Adhesive pericarditis
- 420 Acute pericarditis

P

PERIPHERAL VASCULAR DISEASE

Paul Anaya
Nanette K. Wenger

 BASICS

DESCRIPTION

Peripheral vascular disease is defined as a chronic occlusive arterial disease of the lower extremities. To avoid confusion with disorders of the venous system, the term *peripheral arterial disease* (PAD) is currently the preferred terminology.

EPIDEMIOLOGY

- The prevalence of PAD increases with age, from 3%–6% in persons younger than 60 years of age to >20% in persons older than 70 years of age.
- PAD affects both males and females with a modest male predilection. M:F = 1.4:1. The prevalence among Hispanics and African Americans is higher than among whites, RR = 1.5 and 2.5, respectively.
- PAD coexists with other atherosclerotic diseases, most notably, coronary artery disease (CAD), and is independently associated with an increased risk of all-cause mortality (RR = 3), and mortality from cardiovascular disease (RR = 6.6) [2].
- PAD is considered a CAD risk equivalent.

RISK FACTORS

- Tobacco use
- Diabetes mellitus
- Age
- Hypertension
- Dyslipidemia
- Chronic renal insufficiency

Genetics

Multifactorial

PATHOPHYSIOLOGY

- Most cases of PAD in the United States result from the development of peripheral vascular atherosclerosis.
- Atherosclerosis is a systemic inflammatory disease process affecting all areas of the vasculature. Mechanisms for the development and promotion of atherosclerosis include lipid deposition within the vascular wall, monocyte infiltration and transformation into foam cells, intravascular oxidative stress, vessel wall remodeling, and endothelial dysfunction.
- Plaque rupture leading to platelet activation and acute occlusive thrombosis is an important part of the atherosclerotic process.

ETIOLOGY

- Atherosclerosis
- Inflammatory processes (vasculitis, infection, atherosclerosis)
- Embolism
- *In situ* thrombus formation

ASSOCIATED CONDITIONS

- Coronary artery disease
- Cerebrovascular disease
- Renal insufficiency

 DIAGNOSIS

SIGNS AND SYMPTOMS

- Diminished peripheral pulses
- Cool or mottled extremities
- Nonhealing ulcers (heel, ankle)
- Gangrene
- Intermittent claudication, defined as pain or weakness with walking, which is relieved with rest. The location of the pain/weakness occurs distal to the level of arterial occlusion.
- Lower extremity pain at rest

History

- Up to 40% of persons with PAD have no symptoms. Approximately 10% of patients report symptoms of classic intermittent claudication. The remainder report atypical leg pain symptoms.
- Patients with PAD may not report exertional symptoms because of factors that limit their exercise capacity including older age and comorbid conditions such as pulmonary or cardiac disease or arthritis.

Physical Exam

- Diminished or absent peripheral pulses
- Cool extremities
- Skin discoloration or mottling of the extremities
- Prolonged capillary refill times
- Bruits over large arterial distributions (carotid, abdominal, renal, femoral)
- Abdominal aortic aneurysm

TESTS

Imaging

- Duplex ultrasonography
  - Combines two-dimensional imaging of the vessels with Doppler velocity and flow measurements. Monophasic distal flow is evidence supporting arterial obstruction.
- Conventional lower extremity angiography run-off
- Magnetic resonance imaging (MRI)/magnetic resonance angiography (MRA)
- Computed tomographic angiography

Diagnostic Procedures/Surgery

Ankle brachial Index (ABI): 95% sensitivity, ~100% specific for PAD. Validated against angiography. A normal ABI is 0.9–1.2. An ABI of 0.6–0.9 suggests mild to moderate PAD. An ABI of 0.4–0.6 suggests severe PAD. An ABI of 0.25–0.4 usually correlates with rest pain and/or tissue loss. ABI values greater than 1.2 may indicate vessels that are noncompressible, such as from heavy calcification. This is not uncommon among patients with diabetes or renal disease.

 TREATMENT

GENERAL MEASURES

- Most (60%) of patients with PAD have no progression of symptoms more than 5 years beyond those at initial presentation. The remainder may progress to worsening symptoms or limb loss (<10%). Treatment is dictated more by the fact that PAD is an important marker of coronary heart disease. PAD is associated with a 5-year mortality rate of up to 30%, mostly attributed to coronary heart disease and cerebrovascular disease. Risk of nonfatal myocardial infarction (MI) or stroke is approximately 20% over 5 years. Asymptomatic patients with PAD have the same mortality/morbidity rate as symptomatic patients with PAD. The goals of therapy are (i) secondary prevention of coronary heart disease and cerebrovascular disease, (ii) prevention of limb loss, and (iii) improvement of functional status.
- Considering the important role that tobacco plays in the pathophysiology of peripheral vascular disease, tobacco cessation must be emphasized for both primary and secondary prevention.

MEDICATION (DRUGS)

Antiplatelet therapy: 23% risk reduction in major vascular events in patients with PAD treated with antiplatelet therapy [aspirin (ASA) or extended-release dipyridamole] compared with placebo in the Antithrombotic Trialists' Collaboration. No evidence that combined therapy with ASA and dipyridamole confers additional benefit. Clopidogrel, a thienopyridine derivative, was compared in a prospective, randomized multicenter trial versus ASA in patients with recent stroke, MI, or symptomatic PAD (CAPRI). Results demonstrated a modest but significant reduction in the composite endpoint of MI, cerebrovascular accident (CVA), and vascular death in the group treated with clopidogrel (24% risk reduction versus aspirin). No evidence to support the use of combined therapy of ASA and clopidogrel in patients with PAD in the absence of an acute coronary syndrome. Ticlopidine was superior to placebo with reductions in coronary and stroke events (66% RR reduction) in the Swedish Ticlopidine Multicenter Study. However, serious adverse side effects such as neutropenia and thrombotic thrombocytopenic purpura (TTP) limit its use. All risk reductions (rr) are relative risk reduction unless otherwise specified.

First Line
Oral antiplatelet therapy:
- ASA 160–325 mg daily or clopidogrel 75 mg daily
- Combination of ASA and clopidogrel may be considered with a recurrent vascular event on therapy.

Second Line
- Ticlopidine 250 mg daily
- Lipid lowering: Because PAD is a risk equivalent of coronary heart disease, patients with PAD should be treated similarly to patients with coronary heart disease with aggressive lipid lowering regardless of baseline cholesterol values. Several randomized trials such as the Heart Protection Study and PROVEIT demonstrated significant mortality/morbidity benefit from major adverse cardiovascular events by reducing LDL levels to less than 100 mg/dL. Additional benefit may be derived by lowering low-density lipoprotein (LDL) levels to less than 70 mg/dL. Current recommendations for patients with PAD are to use hydroxymethylglutaryl coenzyme A (HMG-CoA) reductase inhibitors ("statins") as first-line agents for reducing cholesterol to achieve a goal LDL level of less than 70 mg/dL.
- Hypertension control: Optimal control of blood pressure is paramount in the risk-factor modification of a patient with atherosclerotic vascular disease. Angiotensin-converting enzyme (ACE) inhibitors and angiotensin receptor blockers (ARB) may be used as first-line agents because of their association with improved outcomes in both primary and secondary coronary heart disease prevention trials. Diabetics should receive ACE inhibitors or ARB as first-line agents not only for blood pressure control, but for protection against diabetic renal disease. β-Blockers should be used in patients with known coronary heart disease. β-Blockers do not adversely affect walking capacity or exacerbate symptoms of intermittent claudication. Blood pressure goals for patients with PAD should be identical to those for patients with coronary heart disease, that is, <130/<85 mm Hg. Achieving this goal will often require the use of multiple agents, including ACE inhibitors/ARB, β-blockers, diuretics, calcium channel blockers, or hydralazine/nitrates.

- Cilostazol: A phosphodiesterase 3 inhibitor, suppresses platelet aggregation and acts as a direct vasodilator. Several trials have demonstrated improvement in exercise capacity in patients with intermittent claudication. These effects were superior to those seen in patients receiving pentoxifylline or placebo. Use of cilostazol is contraindicated in patients with heart failure.

SURGERY
- Currently no data are available from large prospective randomized, controlled trials comparing the efficacy of revascularization for PAD versus medical therapy. Outcomes following revascularization differ based on the anatomic location of the occlusion in the various segments of the limb arteries). Indications for revascularization include (i) incapacitating symptoms that interfere with work or lifestyle; (ii) limb salvage secondary to limb-threatening ischemia as evidenced by nonhealing ulcers, infection, or rest pain; and (iii) vasculogenic impotence.
- Iliac segment: Percutaneous transluminal angioplasty (PTA) is feasible with localized arterial occlusive disease less than 10 cm in length in the iliac segment. Deployment of intravascular stents improves patency compared with angioplasty alone. Calcified vessels are usually not amenable to PTA, largely due to technical issues leading to an increased risk of vessel rupture or distal embolization. Surgical bypass is recommended for long, irregular iliac artery lesions. Patency rates for PTA range between 60% and 80% at 5 years. Patency rates are better for surgical bypass but at a significantly increased cost. Use of drug-eluting stents in this segment has not been well studied.
- Femoropopliteal segment: Drug-eluting stents (DES) may offer improved patency rates over bare metal stents or PTA alone in the femoropopliteal segment with focal lesions less than 6 cm in length (74% at 2 years). Use of PTA/DES for lesions >6 cm in length in this arterial segment has been associated with lower patency rates. Long-term surgical bypass patency rates are usually better than PTA in this segment.
- Amputation is typically reserved for situations in which tissue loss has progressed beyond limb salvage. It may also be considered if surgical risk outweighs clinical benefit, or when overall life expectancy is very low.

 FOLLOW-UP

For purposes of follow-up, patients may be grouped according to the Fontaine classification scheme:
- I: Mild pain on walking (claudication)
- II: Severe pain on walking relatively shorter distances (intermittent claudication)
- III: Pain while resting
- IV: Loss of sensation to the lower part of the extremity
- V: Tissue loss (gangrene)

DISPOSITION
Issues for Referral
Referral for revascularization: Indications for revascularization include (i) incapacitating symptoms that interfere with work or lifestyle; (ii) limb salvage secondary to limb-threatening ischemia as evidenced by nonhealing ulcers, infection, or rest pain; and (iii) vasculogenic impotence.

REFERENCES
1. Aronow WS. Management of peripheral arterial disease. *Cardiol Rev.* 2005;13:61–68.
2. Bettmann MiA. Atherosclerotic Vascular Disease Conference Writing Group VI: Revascularization. *Circulation.* 2004;109:2643–2650.
3. Faxon DP, et al. Atherosclerotic Vascular Disease Conference Writing Group III: Pathophysiology. *Circulation.* 2004;109:2617–2625.
4. Pasternak RC, et al. Atherosclerotic Vascular Disease Conference Writing Group I: Epidemiology. *Circulation.* 2004;109:2605–2612.
5. Tran H, Anand SS. Oral antiplatelet therapy in cerebrovascular disease, coronary artery disease, and peripheral arterial disease. *JAMA.* 2004;292: 1867–1874.
6. Vita JA. Endothelial function and clinical outcome. *Heart.* 2005;91:1278–1279.
7. Stoyioglou A, Jaff MR. Medical treatment of peripheral arterial disease: A comprehensive review. *J Vasc Intervent Radiol.* 2004;15: 1197–1207.
8. Weitz J, et al. Diagnosis and treatment of chronic arterial insufficiency of the lower extremities: A critical review. *Circulation.* 1996;94: 3026–3049.

CODES
ICD9-CM
443

PATIENT TEACHING
- Smoking cessation
- Exercise rehabilitation: Improves peripheral circulation, walking economy, and overall conditioning
- Foot care: It is important to emphasize properly fitted shoes, daily foot hygiene (washing, emollients to prevent cracks or fissures, nail care), prompt treatment of infections, and use of thick socks and shoe padding to prevent pressure sores.

Activity
Internet resources:
AHA: http://www.americanheart.org
NHLBI: http://www.nhlbi.nih.gov

P

PHEOCHROMOCYTOMA

David Singh
Deborah L. Ekery

 BASICS

DESCRIPTION

Pheochromocytoma is a catecholamine-producing tumor that arises from chromaffin cells of neural crest origin.

- The majority occur in the adrenal glands.
- Approximately 95% arise in the abdomen, 85–90% of which are intraadrenal.
- 10% are extra-adrenal and are sometimes referred to as catecholamine-producing paragangliomas.
- 10% are bilateral.
- 10% are extra-adrenal.
- 10% are malignant.
- 10% are familial.

Pregnancy Considerations

- Maternal and fetal mortality rates are high if maternal pheochromocytoma is not diagnosed antenatally.
- Once diagnosis has been made, the patient should be treated with phenoxybenzamine.
- 1st or 2nd trimester: Tumor should be excised as soon as patient has been adequately pretreated with α-adrenergic blockers.
- 3rd trimester: Patient should be treated with α-blockers until the fetus reaches viability, at which time the baby should be delivered by Cesarean section. The tumor may be removed in the same operation.
- Vaginal delivery is extremely dangerous.
- Magnesium sulfate may be used to control hypertensive emergencies during labor and during resection of the tumor in a pregnant patient.

EPIDEMIOLOGY

Incidence/Prevalence

- Occurs in approximately 0.1–0.6% of patients with hypertension in the United States
- 25% are discovered incidentally by imaging studies for unrelated purposes.
- Predominant age: Sporadic forms are frequently diagnosed in individuals between the ages of 40 and 50; hereditary forms are often diagnosed before the age of 40.
- Predominant sex: Female > Male (slight)
- Predominant race: None

Genetics

5 germline mutations have been linked to familial variants of pheochromocytoma

- *VHL* (associated with von Hippel-Lindau syndrome)
- *RET* (associated with MEN type II)
- *NF1* (associated with Von Reckinghausen disease)
- *SDHB* and *SDHD* (mitochondrial subunit genes coding for succinate dehydrogenase)

ETIOLOGY

- Vast majority occur sporadically.
- Approximately 10% are inherited and are frequently associated with familial syndromes.

ASSOCIATED CONDITIONS

- MEN IIA (Sipple syndrome): Pheochromocytoma, medullary carcinoma of the thyroid, and hyperparathyroidism
- MEN IIB or MEN III syndromes: Pheochromocytoma, medullary carcinoma of the thyroid, mucosal neuromas, ganglioneuromatosis, marfanoid habitus, and other connective tissue disorders
- Neurofibromatosis (von Recklinghausen disease): <5% have pheochromocytomas; central or peripheral neurofibromas and cafu-lait spots are characteristic.
- Cerebelloretinal hemangioblastomatosis (von Hippel–Lindau syndrome): Pheochromocytoma occurs in 10–20%; often bilateral adrenal presentation, and sometimes extra-adrenal; syndrome also associated with retinal angiomas, cerebellar and spinal cord hemangioblastomas, renal cell carcinoma, and pancreatic or renal cysts.
- Paraganglioma syndromes: Associated with germline mutations in succinate dehydrogenase gene
  - Paragangliomas are tumors derived from parasympathetic and sympathetic nervous systems
  - Paragangliomas arising in the head and neck are usually nonfunctioning and are more commonly associated with *SDHD* mutations.
  - The term *catecholamine producing paraganglioma* can be applied to pheochromocytomas of extra-adrenal origin.
  - Paraganglioma syndromes associated with *SDHB* mutations have an increased rate of malignant disease (up to 50%).
- Carney triad (rare): Extra-adrenal pheochromocytoma, gastric leiomyosarcoma, and pulmonary chondroma

℞ DIAGNOSIS

SIGNS AND SYMPTOMS

- Hypertension: The major cardiovascular manifestation of pheochromocytoma
  - Intermittent or sustained; spontaneous or provoked by acute physical stress
  - Classically labile, paroxysmal, and poorly responsive to standard antihypertensive drugs
  - May manifest itself as unusual blood pressure elevations after trauma or surgery
  - Episodes can be precipitated by exercise, palpation of the abdomen, smoking, contrast media, a variety of drugs and hormones, anesthesia, or intraoperative tumor manipulation.
- Tachycardia or reflex bradycardia
- Orthostatic hypotension
- Congestive heart failure: Up to 50% of patients have pathologic evidence of myocarditis or cardiomyopathy, which may be reversed when the tumor is removed.
- Myocardial ischemia/infarction
- Electrocardiographic abnormalities/arrhythmias
- Weight loss
- Pallor
- Hypermetabolism
- Fasting hyperglycemia
- Tremor
- Increased respiratory rate
- Decreased gastrointestinal motility
- Psychosis (rare)
- Flushing (rare)
- Sudden "spells" with headache, palpitations, sweating, nervousness, tremulousness, nausea, and vomiting
- Pain in chest/abdomen
- Weakness/fatigue
- Dizziness
- Heat intolerance
- Paresthesias
- Constipation
- Dyspnea
- Visual disturbances
- Seizures

TESTS

- Clonidine suppression test: Useful for distinguishing excess catecholamine release from pheochromocytoma versus sympathetic activation
  - Failure to suppress norepinephrine or normetanephrine after clonidine administration is highly predictive of pheochromocytoma.
- Vena caval sampling for catecholamines
  - Rarely indicated
  - Occasionally used when tumors cannot be located with other techniques
- Measurement of plasma concentration of neuron-specific enolase: May be useful in differentiating benign from malignant pheochromocytoma
- Electrocardiogram (ECG)
  - Abnormal in up to 75% of patients
  - Abnormalities include T-wave inversion, left ventricular hypertrophy, short P-R interval with narrow QRS complex, supraventricular arrhythmias, and ST-segment elevation or depression
- ECG
  - Left ventricular hypertrophy
  - During a hypertensive crisis, may show systolic anterior motion of anterior mitral valve leaflet, paradoxical septal motion, and proximal excursion of the posterior wall

Lab

- Traditional methods include measurement of plasma and urinary catecholamines, urinary metanephrines, and urinary vanillylmandelic acid (VMA).
- Increasing evidence suggests that measurement of plasma-free metanephrines or urinary fractionated metanephrines (normetanephrine and metanephrine) have the greatest test sensitivity and are adequate for ruling out pheochromocytoma.
  - False positives are frequently associated with the use of drugs known to affect levels of catecholamine and their metabolites (phenoxybenzamine and tricyclic antidepressants most commonly)

Imaging

- Once the diagnosis of pheochromocytoma has been made with biochemical tests, an imaging study should be performed to localize the tumor.
- Computed tomography (CT) scan of the abdomen and pelvis should be performed if tumor location is unknown.
  - Provides precise anatomic information and can detect tumors >0.5 cm in diameter.
  - Theoretical small risk of contrast-induced hypertensive crisis way be prevented by pretreatment with α-blockers.
- Magnetic resonance imaging (MRI) of the adrenals: similar sensitivity to CT
  - Preferred modality for extra-adrenal tumors
  - No α- or β-blockade required
- 123I-metaiodobenzylguanidine (MIBG) scan
  - Uses a radioisotope that localizes to adrenergic tissue
  - Useful in localizing extraadrenal or other difficult-to-find pheochromocytomas
- Arteriography
  - Rarely indicated
  - May precipitate a hypertensive crisis

Diagnostic Procedures/Surgery

Selective adrenal venous sampling: Rarely required and should be reserved for centers with expertise

DIFFERENTIAL DIAGNOSIS

- Hyperadrenergic essential hypertension
- Autonomic dysfunction (postspinal cord injury, Guillain-Barrhypothalamic dysfunction)
- Carcinoid
- Menopausal syndrome
- Panic attacks
- Thyrotoxicosis
- Drugs/medications (e.g., amphetamines, cocaine, monoamine oxidase (MAO) inhibitors, sympathomimetic drugs)
- Alcohol withdrawal
- Migraine or cluster headaches
- Abrupt drug withdrawal (e.g., clonidine or propanolol)
- Hypoglycemia
- Paroxysmal tachycardias
- Acute myocardial infarction or angina pectoris
- Brain tumor or subarachnoid hemorrhage
- Aortic dissection
- Cardiovascular deconditioning
- Menopausal syndrome
- Neuroblastoma in a child
- Diencephalic or temporal lobe seizures
- Toxemia of pregnancy

P

TREATMENT

GENERAL MEASURES

- A team consisting of an internist, anesthesiologist, and surgeon should work together to adequately prepare and follow the patient.
- Because patients can be hypovolemic, sodium intake must be adequate to prevent profound postural hypotension upon initiation of medical therapy and postoperatively; this may require intravenous infusion of saline.
- A β-blocker should not be used prior to adequate α-receptor blockade, because severe hypertension may occur secondary to unopposed α-adrenergic receptor stimulation by circulating catecholamines.

 MEDICATION (DRUGS)

- Phenoxybenzamine
  - A nonspecific α-adrenergic antagonist
  - Should be administered orally beginning at least 7–10 days prior to surgery
  - Initial dose is 10 mg b.i.d. Dosage should be increased to an average of 0.5–1.0 mg/kg daily, administered in two divided doses.
- Prazosin, terazosin, doxazosin
  - Specific α-1-adrenergic antagonists
  - All have the potential to cause severe postural hypotension, so should be given at bedtime

- Labetalol
  - α- and β-antagonist
  - Both oral and intravenous formulations are available.
  - Has higher affinity for β-adrenergic receptors and is therefore less suitable than pure α-blockers
- Metyrosine
  - Competitive inhibitor of tyrosine hydroxylase, the rate-limiting step in catecholamine biosynthesis
  - When used in conjunction with α-antagonists, it may provide more stable blood pressure control.
  - Inhibits catecholamine synthesis in the brain (as well as in the periphery), often causes sedation, and can cause extrapyramidal signs (rare). Central nervous system toxicity may manifest as vivid or frightening dreams and is reversible.
- Calcium channel blockers
- Various chemotherapeutic combinations with or without radiation therapy have been used to treat malignant pheochromocytoma (after aggressive surgical resection).

SURGERY

- Treatment of choice is surgical removal.
- Laparoscopic method preferred for both intra-adrenal and extra-adrenal tumors.
- Medical pretreatment is essential for preventing intraoperative hypertensive complications; drug regimen should be initiated at least 7–10 days prior to surgery (see Medication).
- An intra-arterial line should be placed for continuous blood pressure monitoring.
- Anesthesia should be achieved with halogenated hydrocarbon agents (enflurane or isoflurane), which are unlikely to produce sensitization of the myocardium to catecholamine-induced arrhythmias.
  - Hypertensive emergencies during surgery may be managed with a variety of agents, including phentolamine, sodium nitroprusside, and nicardapine.
- With adequate pretreatment, and an experienced anesthesiologist and surgeon, operative mortality is <1%.

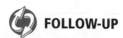
FOLLOW-UP

DISPOSITION
Admission Criteria
Outpatient management except for complications or surgery

PROGNOSIS
- Persistence or recurrence after surgery can occur if the tumor was disrupted or incompletely resected, if a second primary was present and not resected, or if metastatic disease was not appreciated.
- Overall recurrence rate for sporadic pheochromocytoma is estimated at 16%. Patients with familial syndromes or with tumors located in the right adrenal or extra-adrenal sites are more likely to have recurrence
- Long-term survival of patients after the successful removal of a benign pheochromocytoma is essentially the same as for age-matched controls.
- Up to 50% of patients remain hypertensive after successful surgical resection, but are usually easily controlled with medication.

PATIENT MONITORING
- Plasma-free metanephrines should be tested 1–2 weeks postoperatively.
- Patients should be monitored for tumor recurrence for at least 10 years after surgery.

REFERENCES
1. Kaplan NM. Systemic hypertension: Mechanisms and diagnosis. In: Braunwald E, ed. *Heart Disease,* 5th ed. Philadelphia: WB Saunders, 1997:829–830.
2. Keiser HR. Pheochromocytoma and related tumors. In: Degroot LJ, ed. *Endocrinology,* 3rd ed. Philadelphia: WB Saunders, 1995:1853–1877.
3. Lenders JW, Eisenhofer G, Mannelli M, Pacak K. Phaeochromocytoma. *Lancet.* 2005;366:665–675.
4. Radtke WE, Kazmier FJ, Rutherford BD, et al. Cardiovascular complications of pheochromocytoma crisis. *Am J Cardiol.* 1975;35:701–705.
5. Williams GH, Lilly LS, Seely EW. The heart in endocrine and nutritional disorders. In: Braunwald E, ed. *Heart Disease,* 5th ed. Philadelphia: WB Saunders, 1997:1897–1899.

CODES
ICD9-CM
255.6 Pheochromocytoma

PATIENT TEACHING
- Patients should be made aware of symptoms/signs of pheochromocytoma and counseled to notify a physician if these recur after surgical resection.

Organizations
- National Adrenal Diseases Foundation (NADF): 505 Northern Boulevard, Great Neck, NY 11021; (516) 487–4992, www.medhelp.org/nadf/
- American Cancer Society: 1599 Clifton Road NE, Atlanta, GA 30329; (404)320–3333, www.cancer.org
- National Cancer Institute: www.cancer.gov,1-800-4-CANCER
- www.pheochromocytoma.org

P

PICKWICKIAN SYNDROME
Rajesh Dash

BASICS

DESCRIPTION
Pickwickian syndrome (obesity hypoventilation syndrome) is characterized by temporary, recurrent interruptions of respiration during sleep, which results in daytime hypercapnia. The presence of hypercapnea distinguishes it from obesity sleep-apnea hypopnea. Typical features include nocturnal wakefulness, daytime sleepiness, and obesity.
- System(s) affected: Cardiovascular; Pulmonary

EPIDEMIOLOGY
- Predominant age: Middle-aged adults
- Predominant sex: Males > Premenopausal Females, 30:1
  - Approximately 2.5 million people in the United States have sleep apnea.
  - The majority of sleep apnea sufferers are at least 20% over ideal body weight.

RISK FACTORS
- Moderate to severe obesity [body mass index (BMI) >30 kg/m^2]
- Male gender
- Narrowed upper airway/short, thick neck
- Enlarged adenoids or tonsils
- Decreased muscle tone of the soft palate, uvula, and pharynx
- Use of sedative or hypnotic agents
- Alcohol consumption

Pregnancy Considerations
Pregnancy is contraindicated in women with severe pulmonary hypertension.

PATHOPHYSIOLOGY
- Poorly understood interactions between impaired respiratory mechanics, central ventilatory control, and neurohormonal aberrancies
- Postulated role of inadequate leptin levels for given degree of obesity, leading to insufficient ventilatory drive

ETIOLOGY
- Obesity
- Pharyngeal obstruction

ASSOCIATED CONDITIONS
- Coronary artery disease
- Hyperlipidemia
- Diabetes mellitus
- Hypothyroidism
- Obstructive sleep apnea
- Chronic obstructive pulmonary disease
- Degenerative joint disease

DIAGNOSIS

SIGNS AND SYMPTOMS
History
- Daytime sleepiness/somnolence
- Loud nocturnal snoring
- Morning headaches

Physical Exam
- Extreme obesity
- Hypoventilation
- Muscle twitching
- Cyanosis
- Periodic respiration
- In advanced cases: Severe pulmonary hypertension, right ventricular heave, prominent P2 component of the second heart sound, right ventricular failure (elevated jugular venous pressure, hepatomegaly, lower extremity edema)

TESTS
Electrocardiogram (ECG) may reveal right ventricular hypertrophy denoted by tall, peaked P waves in leads II, aVF, V_1 through V_3, clockwise rotation, right axis deviation and R/S ratio in lead V_1 greater than 1, qR pattern in aVr, inverted T waves in leads V_1 through V_4 and the inferior leads.

Lab
- Arterial blood gas: Hypoxia and hypercapnia are common; widened A-a gradient
- Serum bicarbonate: Usually elevated
- Serum phosphorous and creatine phosphokinase (CPK) to rule out other some causes of respiratory muscle weakness
- Complete blood count: Polycythemia common
- Thyroid function testing (hypothyroidism is associated with alveolar hypoventilation)

Imaging
- Chest x-ray: May demonstrate dilation of the main pulmonary artery and its branches, underperfusion of the peripheral pulmonary artery branches, and decreased prominence of the aortic knob due to counterclockwise rotation of the heart on a posteroanterior film; filling of the retrosternal space on a lateral film of the chest
- Echocardiography: Can confirm cor pulmonale and assess pulmonary artery pressures

Diagnostic Procedures/Surgery
- Polysomnography
- Pulmonary function tests to determine if chronic obstructive pulmonary disease (COPD) is contributing to hypoventilation

Pathologic Findings
- Extreme obesity primarily involving the trunk and pharyngeal area
- Small pharyngeal cavity due to redundant palatal tissue, fat deposition in the soft tissues of the pharynx, or superficial fat masses in the neck that compress the pharynx
- Palatal soft tissue edema

DIFFERENTIAL DIAGNOSIS
- Chronic mountain sickness
- Central sleep apnea
- Narcolepsy
- Ondine curse
- Infantile apnea

TREATMENT

GENERAL MEASURES
- Patients with severe hypoxemia, severe hypercapnia, heart failure, syncope, or marked arrhythmias should be hospitalized.
- Weight reduction
- Elevation of the head with pillows or elevation of the head of the bed by 6–8 inches
- Avoid alcohol.
- Avoid sedative and hypnotic agents.
- Continuous positive airway pressure (CPAP), the mainstay of therapy for obesity hypoventilation syndrome and obstructive sleep apnea, promotes eucapnia and reduces daytime drowsiness.
- In patients who do not respond to or tolerate CPAP, trials of bilevel noninvasive positive pressure modalities (NIPPV) should be considered (IPAP, EPAP).

MEDICATION (DRUGS)

- Progesterone: Enhances respiratory drive
- Supplemental oxygen
- Drugs of no proven clinical benefit
  - Theophylline: In low doses and moderate doses causes mild cortical arousal with increased alertness; lowers vascular resistance
  - Protriptyline: Mild alerting and improved attention likely due to enhancement of dopamine-mediated processes
  - Clomipramine: Similar to protriptyline
  - Pemoline: Amphetamine variant that is a central nervous system stimulant; mild alerting, improved attention
  - Nicotine: Mild alerting action with stimulation of the nicotinic receptors in the brain; large concentrations stimulate the respiratory center
- Contraindications
  - Refer to manufacturer's literature.
- Precautions
  - Refer to manufacturer's literature.
- Significant possible interactions
  - Theophylline interacts with a wide variety of medications; refer to manufacturer's literature for specific details.
  - Tricyclic agents, when taken in combination with other antidepressants, can lead to excessive sedation.
    - There are several documented drug interactions with tricyclic agents; refer to manufacturer's literature for further details.
  - Progesterone may increase blood pressure and lower high-density lipoprotein (HDL) in some patients.
- Drugs that may alter laboratory results
  - Diuretics may lead to contraction alkalosis and elevation of bicarbonate levels; excessive intake of antacids may lead to elevated bicarbonate.
- Disorders that may alter laboratory results
  - A diffusion defect, a right-to-left shunt (intracardiac or intrapulmonary), or ventilation-perfusion ratio (V/Q) mismatch can produces a widened A-a gradient.
  - Renal disorders, disorders producing metabolic or respiratory alkalosis, mineralocorticoid excess, and congenital chloridorrhea can lead to elevations in the bicarbonate level.
  - Hemoconcentration, extreme physical exercise, and polycythemia vera lead to an elevated hematocrit.

SURGERY
- Uvulopalatopharyngoplasty
- Tracheotomy

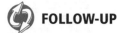 **FOLLOW-UP**

DISPOSITION
Admission Criteria
Intensive care unit (ICU) admission criteria: Worsening hypoxemia, hypercapnia, or respiratory acidosis with pH <7.3, confusion, respiratory muscle failure, intubation, and noninvasive ventilation

Discharge Criteria
- Once patient's acute respiratory and metabolic compromise has resolved, with stable oxygen with or without noninvasive ventilation requirements
- Underlying etiology to obesity-hypoventilation syndrome is being addressed through lifestyle modification, medications, or surgical management.

Issues for Referral
Consider consultation with pulmonary medicine, neurology, physical and rehabilitation medicine, as indicated by patient's clinical status, to help evaluate and manage obesity hypoventilation syndrome.

PROGNOSIS
- Variable, dependent on the degree of obesity, pharyngeal obstruction, pulmonary hypertension, and right ventricular dysfunction
- In cases of overt right ventricular failure with severe pulmonary hypertension, a patient's life expectancy is 6 months to 1 year.

COMPLICATIONS
- Cardiac
  - Systemic hypertension, sinus arrhythmias, extreme bradycardia, sinus arrest, asystole, atrial flutter, atrial fibrillation, ventricular tachycardia, syncope, right ventricular hypertrophy, right heart failure (cor pulmonale), left heart failure
- Respiratory
  - Hypoxemia, hypercarbia, pulmonary hypertension
- Neurologic
  - Morning headaches, excessive daytime sleepiness, slowed mentation, sleepwalking, blackouts, automatic robotlike behavior, bedwetting
- Psychiatric
  - Hallucinations, anxiety, irritability, aggressiveness, jealousy, suspiciousness, irrational behavior, loss of interest in sex
- Hematologic
  - Polycythemia

PATIENT MONITORING
- Depends on the frequency and severity of the patient's complaints
- Hospitalization for oxygen therapy, heart failure management, and arrhythmia management may be necessary in extreme cases.

REFERENCES
1. Berg G, Delaive K, Manfreda J, et al. The use of health-care resources in obesity-hypoventilation syndrome. *Chest*. 2001;120:377–383.
2. Braunwald E. *Heart Disease: A Textbook of Cardiovascular Medicine*, 5th ed. Philadelphia: WB Saunders, 1997.
3. Fauci AS, Braunwald E, Isselbacher KJ, et al. *Harrison's Principles of Internal Medicine*, 14th ed. New York: McGraw-Hill, 1998.
4. Olson AL, Zwillich C. The obesity hypoventilation syndrome. *Am J Med*. 2005;118:948–956.
5. Thoene JG. *Physicians Guide to Rare Diseases*. NJ: Dowden Publishing, 1992.

CODES
ICD9-CM
278.8 Pickwickian syndrome

PATIENT TEACHING
Organizations
- National Organization for Rare Disorders
- American Narcolepsy Association, Inc.
- Narcolepsy and Cataplexy Foundation of America
- Narcolepsy Network
- NIH/National Institute of Neurological Disorders and Stroke

Diet
- Low fat
- Low sodium

Activity
- As tolerated
- Exercise program after physician's approval

Prevention
- Adherence to a low-fat/low-calorie diet
- Regular aerobic/fat-burning exercise
- Tobacco cessation
- Avoid alcohol consumption.
- Avoid sedatives.

FAQ
- The primary treatment for Pickwickian syndrome is weight loss and avoidance of alcohol and sedating agents.
- The gold standard diagnostic test for Pickwickian syndrome is polysomnography.

P

PREGNANCY AND THE HEART

Michael H. Crawford

 BASICS

DESCRIPTION

Maternal blood volume and cardiac output increase up to 50% by 32 weeks of pregnancy and continue at that level until delivery.

- These changes put unique stress on the patient with underlying heart disease and may contribute to the development of certain heart diseases (peripartum cardiomyopathy).
- There are three general patient presentations.
  - Uncorrected congenital heart disease, which can be divided into:
    - Predominant volume loads such as atrial septal defects, patent ductus arteriosus
    - Pressure loads such as pulmonic valve stenosis, coarctation of the aorta, aortic valve disease
    - Complex often cyanotic congenital heart disease such as tetralogy of Fallot
  - Acquired heart disease
    - Most common are rheumatic heart disease, coronary heart disease, and peripartum cardiomyopathy.
  - Corrected congenital or acquired heart disease
    - Common issues here are the patient with a prosthetic valve or partially corrected defects.
- Systems affected: Cardiovascular, Pulmonary

GENERAL PREVENTION

Pregnancy should be avoided with certain heart diseases.

EPIDEMIOLOGY

- Predominant age: Young adults
- Predominant sex: Female
  - Prognosis worsens with heart disease and advancing age of the mother.

Incidence

Maternal heart disease occurs in 1–4% of pregnancies.

RISK FACTORS

Prior pregnancy-associated heart disease increases risk of subsequent pregnancies.

Genetics

Women with congenital heart disease have an increased risk of having children with congenital heart disease.

PATHOPHYSIOLOGY

Increased volume load on the heart

ETIOLOGY

Congenital or acquired

ASSOCIATED CONDITIONS

- Anemia of pregnancy
- Pregnancy-associated hypertension

 DIAGNOSIS

SIGNS AND SYMPTOMS

Clinical presentation of pregnancy complicated by heart disease depends on the underlying disease, its severity, and the stage of pregnancy.

History

- Fatigue and dyspnea, common symptoms of heart disease, are common with normal pregnancies.
- Chest pain from gastroesophageal reflux must be distinguished from angina.
- Palpitations are common during pregnancy (often sinus tachycardia).
- Fever and night sweats are common during normal pregnancy.

Physical Exam

- Alterations in the cardiovascular physical examination due to the normal hemodynamic changes of pregnancy must be distinguished from pathologic changes due to heart disease.
- Normal pregnancy may be associated with:
  - Heart rate in the upper range of normal
  - Systolic blood pressure increases as pregnancy progresses to levels largely determined by the patient's age and parity (increases with both).
  - Higher values for blood pressure are recorded upright or in the left lateral position and the lowest levels in the supine position when the gravid uterus compresses the inferior vena cava and reduces venous return to the heart.
  - An enlarged apical impulse and third heart sound are often present.
  - The first and second heart sounds are often loud and exhibit increased splitting. Fourth heart sounds are rare and suggest the presence of heart disease.
  - Systolic heart murmurs are common in pregnancy and result from the increased stroke volume and hyperkinetic state of pregnancy.
  - A continuous murmur may be heard due to increased blood flow to the breasts (mammary soufflé), and venous hums heard in the aortic area may mimic aortic regurgitation.
  - True diastolic murmurs are rare in pregnancy and suggest heart disease.

TESTS

Confirmation of pregnancy

Lab

- Blood count often shows anemia
- Oxygen saturation reduced in cyanotic congenital heart disease

Imaging

- Use of chest x-rays is of limited value in pregnancy because of the potential hazards of exposing the fetus to radiation.
- Cardiac silhouette is altered by the elevation of the diaphragm, making specific chamber enlargement difficult to diagnose accurately.
- Echocardiography is the diagnostic test of choice.

Diagnostic Procedures/Surgery

- Electrocardiography can be very useful, but a leftward shift in the axis and ST-T wave changes can occur normally in pregnancy.
- Pulmonary artery catheterization can be performed with a flow-directed catheter without the use of fluoroscopy.
- Left heart catheterization can be performed with abdominal shielding and use of a brachial approach to minimize exposure of the fetus to radiation, but should only be performed if the diagnostic information cannot be obtained by other less invasive methods.

Pathologic Findings

Depend on specific heart disease

DIFFERENTIAL DIAGNOSIS

Heart disease versus normal hemodynamic changes of pregnancy

 TREATMENT

GENERAL MEASURES

- Outpatient evaluation and treatment unless the fetus or the mother's life is threatened
- Prompt treatment of infections
- Prevention and treatment of anemia with iron supplements
- Vaginal delivery is generally preferred with pain control to avoid tachycardia and hemodynamic monitoring in selected patients to guide therapy during delivery

MEDICATION (DRUGS)

First Line

- For heart failure
  - Digoxin is safe, but blood levels need to be monitored.
  - Furosemide or other diuretics are safe, but potassium levels need to be monitored.
  - Hydralazine is safe in those patients who do not respond to digoxin and diuretics.

- For arrhythmias
  - Digoxin is useful for controlling the heart rate in supraventricular arrhythmias.
  - β-Blockers can be added if digoxin does not control the heart rate.
  - Verapamil is relatively safe unless heart failure is present.
  - Quinidine is safe in therapeutic doses but can cause abortion at toxic doses.
  - Procainamide is relatively safe.
  - Lidocaine for ventricular tachyarrhythmias is relatively safe.
- For anticoagulation
  - Heparin is preferred because it is not teratogenic, but there is risk of hemorrhage.
- Contraindications
  - Angiotensin-converting enzyme inhibitors increase the incidence of stillbirths and should be avoided. Amiodarone causes fetal hypothyroidism and premature births. Warfarin causes birth defects and fetal death, especially if used in the first trimester.
- Precautions
  - See manufacturer's literature on each product.
- Significant possible interactions
  - Digoxin levels can be increased by concomitant use of calcium channel blockers or quinidine. Many drugs increase warfarin levels.

Second Line
Newer drugs such as angiotensin receptor blockers, type I-C and III antiarrhythmic drugs, and low-molecular-weight heparin have not been used extensively in pregnancy, but may be of use in selected patients.

SURGERY
- When decompensation threatens the mother's life and aggressive pharmacologic therapy is insufficient, surgical correction of any correctable lesions should be considered.
- Risk to the mother is not particularly higher when pregnant, but fetal loss is not uncommon.
- In the case of mitral stenosis, percutaneous balloon valvotomy may be accomplished with less risk to the fetus.
- Cesarean delivery should be reserved for obstetrical reasons because it puts more stress on the heart.

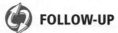 FOLLOW-UP

Depends on the heart condition
- Cardiac physiology does not return completely to normal until lactation has been ceased

DISPOSITION
Admission Criteria
- Heart failure
- Syncope
- Chest pain

Issues for Referral
Patients with suspected heart disease should be referred to a cardiologist.

PROGNOSIS
Maternal mortality rates depend on the underlying cardiac condition.
- Less than 1%
  - Left-to-right shunts at the atrial, ventricular, and ductal levels
  - Pulmonary valve disease
  - Corrected congenital heart disease
  - Bioprosthetic valves
  - Mild to moderate mitral stenosis
- 5–10%
  - Moderate to severe mitral stenosis
  - Mechanical prosthetic valves
  - Aortic stenosis
  - Coarctation of the aorta
  - Uncorrected congenital heart disease
  - Marfan syndrome with normal aorta
- 25–50%
  - Pulmonary hypertension
  - Complicated coarctation of the aorta (aortic stenosis or severe hypertension)
  - Marfan syndrome with dilated aorta

COMPLICATIONS
Fetal abnormalities, fetal death, maternal death, worsening of heart disease (bacterial endocarditis)

PATIENT MONITORING
Pregnant patients with heart disease need frequent visits with the obstetrician and cardiologist, and coordination of delivery plans with an anesthesiologist.

REFERENCES
1. Colman JM, et al. Congenital heart disease in pregnancy. *Cardiol Rev.* 2000;8:166.
2. Elkayam U, et al. Maternal and fetal outcomes of subsequent pregnancies in women with peripartum cardiomyopathy. *N Engl J Med.* 2001;344:1567.

ADDITIONAL READING
Bokhari SW, Reid CL. Heart disease in pregnancy. In: Crawford MH, ed. *Current Diagnosis and Treatment in Cardiology.* New York: McGraw-Hill, 2003.

CODES
ICD9-CM
674.82 Postpartum cardiomyopathy

PATIENT TEACHING
Prenatal care is critical for patients with heart disease.

Diet
Dietary sodium restriction to reduce fluid accumulation; dietary restriction of calories to keep weight gain appropriate

Activity
Restrict activity to decrease the burden on the heart.

Prevention
- Fluid retention, excessive weight gain, and infections should be avoided if possible.
- Antibiotic prophylaxis to prevent bacterial endocarditis is controversial for normal labor and delivery, but should be considered in those at the highest cardiac risk (prosthetic valve, conduits) or with the greatest risk of bacteremia (infected uterus).

FAQ
Q. What is the best drug to treat premature ventricular contractions?
A. There is none. Premature ventricular contractions are common and benign. Reassurance usually suffices.

P

PRIMARY HYPERALDOSTERONISM

Brian C. Jensen
Daniel T. Price

 BASICS

DESCRIPTION
- Increased levels of the hormone aldosterone due to adrenal overproduction
- Hyperaldosteronism is an important, treatable cause of secondary hypertension.

EPIDEMIOLOGY
- Age:
  - Majority of cases occur in middle age (30–50 years).
  - Glucocorticoid-remediable aldosteronism is noted in childhood.
- Sex:
  - Adrenal adenomas are twice as common in women.
  - Idiopathic aldosteronism is more common in men.

Prevalence
- Exact prevalence is unclear, with estimates ranging between 5–13% of hypertensive patients.
  - Higher than previously thought due in part to increased screening.

RISK FACTORS
Genetics
- A genetic form of aldosteronism called *glucocorticoid-remediable aldosteronism* is inherited as an autosomal-dominant trait and is the most common monogenic cause of hypertension.

ETIOLOGY
- Forms of primary aldosteronism:
  - Adrenal adenoma (aldosteronoma), also known as Conn syndrome
  - Idiopathic aldosteronism (bilateral cortical hyperplasia)
  - Unilateral or primary hyperplasia
  - Glucocorticoid-remediable aldosteronism (GRA or familial hyperaldosteronism)
  - Adrenal carcinoma
  - Ectopic aldosterone-producing tumor

 DIAGNOSIS

SIGNS AND SYMPTOMS
- Often asymptomatic
- Hypertension, particularly resistant hypertension
- Headache
- Polyuria, nocturia, and polydipsia
- Muscle cramps
- Serious muscle weakness, paresthesia, tetany, or paralysis resulting from profound hypokalemia can be prominent.
- ECG may show prominent U-waves, cardiac arrhythmias, and premature depolarizations in the setting of hypokalemia.
- Edema usually is absent.

TESTS
Patients with hypertension and hypokalemia, refractory hypertension, or adrenal incidentaloma and hypertension should be screened.

Lab
- Although hypokalemia is the classic finding, patients often are normokalemic.
- Metabolic alkalosis
- Most common screening test: Plasma renin activity (PRA)/Plasma aldosterone concentration (PAC)
  - PAC/PRA >20 ng/dL (or 550 pmol/L) per ng/mL/hr with PAC >15 ng/dL (416 pmol/L) is suggestive of primary aldosteronism.
  - Should be obtained in the morning from seated patient
  - Only spironolactone will confound results.
  - Patients on angiotensin-converting enzyme inhibitor (ACE-I) or angiotensin receptor blocker (ARB) with detectable PRAs are likely have primary aldosteronism.
- If PAC/PRA ratio is suggestive, confirmatory diagnostic testing must be performed.
  - A plasma aldosterone level of <6 ng/dL at the end of 2L saline infusion (infused over 4 hours in the morning) rules out all types of primary aldosteronism.
  - 24-hour urine aldosterone level >14μg (39 nmol) after 3 days of sodium loading (>5,000 mg/day) is diagnostic.
- Percutaneous transfemoral bilateral adrenal vein catheterization and PAC sampling may be used to distinguish unilateral from bilateral process.

Imaging
- All patients diagnosed with primary aldosteronism should undergo imaging to exclude adrenal mass:
  - MRI or CT scan of abdomen is first-line imaging.
    - May miss masses <1cm in diameter
    - "Normal" scan does not exclude bilateral hyperplasia or small mass.
- May also consider scintigraphy with radiolabeled iodocholesterol or 6-β ^{131}iodomethyl-19-norcholesterol after dexamethasone suppression; the uptake of tracer is increased in patients with aldosteronoma and absent in those with idiopathic aldosteronism and usually also in those with adrenal carcinoma. Not widely available or commonly used.

Pathologic Findings
- Aldosteronomas are usually small (<2 cm in diameter), benign, and have a golden yellow color on their cut surfaces.
- Bilateral micronodular or macronodular adrenal hyperplasia is seen in idiopathic aldosteronism.
- Adrenal carcinomas:
  - Larger than the more common, benign aldosteronomas
  - Often produce other adrenal hormones (although they also can secrete only aldosterone)
  - May show evidence of local invasion or distant metastasis

DIFFERENTIAL DIAGNOSIS
- Secondary aldosteronism (high renin)
- Adrenal tumor (multiple corticoid hormone production)
- Bartter syndrome
- Licorice ingestion (due to glycyrrhizinic acid inhibition of 11β-hydroxysteroid dehydrogenase)
- Deoxycorticosterone-producing adenomas
- Defect in cortisol biosynthesis
- Liddle syndrome (autosomal-dominant inherited condition due to defect in β-subunit of sodium channel)

TREATMENT

GENERAL MEASURES

Dietary sodium restriction may be effective in combination with spironolactone or eplerenone.

MEDICATION (DRUGS)

First Line

- Spironolactone or eplerenone. Very important to block the deleterious cardiovascular effects of elevated serum aldosterone levels.
  - Contraindications: Chronic renal failure
  - Precautions: Gastrointestinal symptoms, fatigue, impotence, rash, and gynecomastia (with spironolactone)
  - Interactions: Potential hyperkalemia if used with ACE inhibitor or potassium supplements

Second Line

- Other antihypertensive agents, such as calcium channel blockers or ACE-Is may help with blood pressure control.
- Triamterene and amiloride also are used.
- Glucocorticoid-remediable aldosteronism can be treated with low doses of a glucocorticoid.

SURGERY

- Patients with adrenal adenoma or carcinoma are best treated with removal of the adrenal tumor.
- After surgery, hypertension diminishes markedly or resolves in most of these patients.

FOLLOW-UP

DISPOSITION

Admission Criteria

- Admission with telemetry monitoring may be indicated for severe hypokalemia.
- Admission for diagnostic workup may be appropriate.
- Surgical removal of adrenal tumor requires inpatient hospitalization; laparoscopic removal may shorten hospital stay.

PROGNOSIS

- Surgery is usually curative.
- Medical therapy often is successful, but is limited in men due to side effects of spironolactone (e.g., gynecomastia). Eplerenone, although more expensive, may have a more tolerable side effect profile.
- With idiopathic bilateral hyperplasia, surgery is only indicated if medical therapy is not effective in preventing serious hypokalemia.

COMPLICATIONS

- Elevated circulating aldosterone levels have multiple significant deleterious effects throughout cardiovascular system:
  - Myocardial fibrosis and remodeling due to elevated aldosterone levels
  - Endothelial dysfunction
  - Stroke and cardiac disease secondary to hypertension and vascular disease
  - Metastatic complications in those with carcinoma
  - Side effects of medication in patients not surgically treated

PATIENT MONITORING

- Blood pressure
- CT scans for follow-up of adrenal carcinoma

REFERENCES

1. Ganguly A. Current concepts: Primary aldosteronism. *N Engl J Med*. 1998;339:1828–1834.
2. Stewart PM. Mineralocorticoid hypertension. *Lancet*. 1999;353:1341–1347.
3. Williams GH, Dluhy RG. Diseases of the adrenal cortex. In: Fauci AS, et al. *Harrison's principles of internal medicine*, 14th ed. New York: McGraw-Hill, 1998:2035–2057.
4. Young WF, Kaplan NM, Rose BD. Approach to the patient with hypertension and hypokalemia. UpToDate.
5. Young WF. Primary Aldosteronism: Changing concepts in diagnosis and treatment. *Endocrinology*. 144:2208–2213.

CODES

ICD9-CM

255.1 Primary hyperaldosteronism

PATIENT TEACHING

For patients on medical therapy, instruction regarding dietary sodium intake is important.

P

PROLONGED QT SYNDROME AND PROARRHYTHMIAS

Peter Ott

BASICS

DESCRIPTION

- QT intervals reflect time from onset of cardiac depolarization to completion of repolarization.
- Onset of Q wave (or R wave) to end of T wave on 12-lead electrocardiogram (ECG)
- Do not use U wave unless merged with T wave and/or of high amplitude.
- Corrected for heart rate, many formulas available: Clinically most widely used = Bazett formula: QT (milliseconds) divided by square root of RR (in seconds)
- Prolonged QT interval may cause polymorphic ventricular tachycardia (torsade de pointes). Ventricular tachycardia onset is often preceded by a prolonged RR interval [i.e., post premature ventricular contraction (PVC) pause]

Geriatric Considerations
More susceptible to drug–drug interactions and more prone to electrolyte abnormalities

Pediatric Considerations
In children 1–15 years old, the QT corrected is <0.46.

EPIDEMIOLOGY
Normal QT corrected interval is <0.45 msec in men and <0.47 in women.

RISK FACTORS
- QT interval may be prolonged by electrolyte abnormalities:
  – Hypokalemia
  – Hypomagnesemia
  – Hypocalcemia
- QT interval may be prolonged by various medication groups (see www.qtdrugs.org):
  – Antiarrhythmic drugs
  – Psychotropic drugs
  – Gastrointestinal motility drugs
  – Antibiotic/antifungal drugs
- QT interval may be prolonged in cardiomyopathy

Genetics
- Patients with known long QWT syndrome are at increased risk for prolonged QT interval.
- Patients who develop a long QT interval may be silent carriers of a long QT gene (research ongoing).

PATHOPHYSIOLOGY
- Possible genetic predisposition (genetic mutations in cardiac ion channels)
- Drugs combined with electrolyte shifts
- Drug–drug interaction (inhibition of drug metabolism)
- Bradycardia and female gender

DIAGNOSIS

SIGNS AND SYMPTOMS
- Asymptomatic
- Palpitations
- Syncope
- Sudden death

History
- Careful review of recent drug exposure (prescribed and over the counter drugs)
- Review of family history for syncope or premature sudden death

TESTS
- ECG
- Holter monitor
- Echocardiogram torule out structural heart disease

Lab
- Electrolytes
- Drug level screen if clinically suggested

Imaging
Echocardiogram

Pathologic Findings
Prolonged QTc interval on the 12-lead ECG

DIFFERENTIAL DIAGNOSIS
- QT interval in patients with bundle branch block may be prolonged due to wide QRS complex
- QT interval is difficult to evaluate in patients with a paced QRS complex.

TREATMENT

GENERAL MEASURES
- Discontinue suspected QT-prolonging drug.
- If symptomatic and/or QT interval markedly prolonged, admit for cardiac monitoring.

 MEDICATION (DRUGS)

Replace electrolytes

First Line
Intravenous magnesium suppresses VT

Second Line
Increasing heart rate (by temporary transvenous pacing, or atropine or isoproterenol) shortens QT interval—is indicated in patients with, long QT interval and polymorphic VT, especially if bradycardic.

 FOLLOW-UP

DISPOSITION
Admission Criteria
If symptomatic and/or QT interval markedly prolonged, admit for cardiac monitoring.

Issues for Referral
Cardiac evaluation often needed to rule out congenital long QT syndrome and advise in safety of alternate drug therapy

PROGNOSIS
- Good if QT interval prolongation is diagnosed on time
- Discontinuation/avoidance of responsible medication should resolve QT prolongation.

COMPLICATIONS
Syncope, sudden death

PATIENT MONITORING
Serial ECG and telemetry monitoring until QT interval is normal and precipitating factors (drugs, electrolytes) have resolved

REFERENCES
1. Moss A. Measurement of QT interval and the risk associated with QTc prolongation: A review. *Am J Cardiol*. 1993;72:23B–25B.
2. Tzivoni D, Keren A, Cohen AM, et al. Magnesium therapy for Torsades de Pointes. *Am J Cardiol*. 1984;53:528–530.

PATIENT TEACHING
Avoid QT prolonging drugs (www.qtdrugs.org).

Prevention
- Avoid QT prolonging drugs.
- Serial ECG monitoring

P

PROSTHETIC VALVES

Deryk McDowell
Steven C. Herrmann
Bernard R. Chaitman

BASICS

DESCRIPTION

- 2 classes of heart valves exist: Mechanical prostheses with rigid manufactured occluders, and biologic (tissue) valves with flexible leaflet occluders of animal or human origin.
- Mechanical valves
  - Ball and cage valves
    - Starr-Edwards
  - Tilting disk valve
    - Bjork-Shiley
    - Medtronic Hall
  - Bileaflet
    - St. Jude
    - Duromedics
    - CarboMedics
- Biologic valves
  - Porcine
    - Hancock
    - Carpentier-Edwards
    - Medtronic intact
  - Porcine stentless
    - Toronto stentless
    - Edwards stentless
    - Medtronic Freestyle Valve
  - Pericardial
    - Carpentier-Edwards Bovine
  - Homograft
    - Cadaveric aortic valves
  - Autologous
    - Pulmonary autograft
    - Pericardial autograft
- Complications of prosthetic valves
  - Structural valve deterioration (highest risk with biologic valves)
  - Valve thrombosis and embolism (highest risk with mechanical valves)
  - Nonstructural dysfunction
  - Bleeding events
  - Prosthetic valve endocarditis

Geriatric Considerations

Tissue valves may be the prosthesis of choice in geriatric patients because of the lack of anticoagulation needed.

RISK FACTORS

Risk factors for thromboembolic events in patients with prosthetic valves:

- Mechanical prosthetic valve
- Atrial fibrillation
- Left ventricular (LV) systolic dysfunction
- Previous thromboembolism
- Hypercoagulable states

TREATMENT

GENERAL MEASURES

- In patients with an embolic event in the presence of adequate anticoagulation, antithrombotic therapy should be adjusted as follows:
  - Warfarin, INR 2–3: Warfarin dose should be increased to achieve INR of 2.5–3.5.
  - Warfarin, INR 2.5–3.5: Warfarin dose may need to be increased to achieve INR of 3.5–4.5.
  - Not already on aspirin: Aspirin 80–100 mg/day should be initiated.
  - Warfarin plus aspirin 80–100 mg/day: Aspirin dose may be increased to 325 mg/day if higher dose of warfarin is not achieving the desired clinical results.
  - Aspirin alone: Aspirin dose may need to be increased to 325 mg/day and/or warfarin added to achieve INR of 2.0–3.0.
  - Transesophageal echocardiography should be considered in patients with an embolic event and prosthetic heart valves to evaluate valve function and the possibility of tissue stranding on the prosthesis.
- Antithrombotic therapy in patients requiring noncardiac surgery
  - The risk of increased bleeding during the procedure performed with a patient receiving antithrombotic therapy must be weighed against the risk of thromboembolism caused by stopping antithrombotic therapy.
  - In general, patients on warfarin should stop warfarin 72 hours before the procedure and restart in the afternoon on the day of the procedure or after control of active bleeding.
  - Intravenous heparin or, in some cases, subcutaneous low-molecular weight heparin can be used up to the day of surgery.
  - Patients taking aspirin should stop taking aspirin 1 week before the procedure and restart the day after the procedure or after the control of active bleeding.
  - Therapy should be individualized in unusual circumstances.
- Thrombosis of prosthetic heart valves
  - Patients who have a large clot, those with evidence of valve obstruction, and those in New York Heart Association (NYHA) classes III or IV because of prosthetic thrombosis should undergo early/immediate operation.
  - Thrombolytic therapy for a prosthetic valve obstructed by thrombus is associated with significant risks and is often ineffective; it is reserved for those patients in whom surgical intervention carries high risk and those with contraindications to surgery.
  - Patients with a small clot who are in NYHA functional class I–II and those with left ventricular (LV) systolic dysfunction should have in-hospital, short-term IV heparin therapy. If this is unsuccessful, they may receive a trial of continuous infusion of thrombolytic therapy over several days.

MEDICATION (DRUGS)

- Antibiotic prophylaxis
  - Infective endocarditis: All patients with prosthetic heart valves need appropriate antibiotic prophylaxis against infective endocarditis.
  - Rheumatic carditis: Patients with rheumatic heart disease continue to need antibiotic as prophylaxis against recurrence of rheumatic carditis.
- Antithrombotic therapy
  - All patients with mechanical valves require warfarin therapy.
    - The risk of thromboembolism is 1–2% per year with warfarin therapy and is considerably higher without warfarin therapy.
    - The risk of is greater for valves in the mitral position regardless of whether it is a mechanical or biologic prosthesis.
    - For St. Jude or CarboMedics bileaflet mechanical valves or Medtronic-Hall tilting disk valves in the aortic position, the INR target is 2.5 (range 2.0–3.0).
    - For Starr-Edwards or other disk valves in the aortic position, the INR target is 3.0 (range 2.5–3.5).
    - For patients with any additional risk factors for a thromboembolic event (see above) in combination with an aortic valve prosthesis regardless of type, the INR target is 3.0 (range 2.5–3.5).
    - For any prosthesis in the mitral position, the INR target is 3.0 (range 2.5–3.5).
    - The addition of aspirin (80–100 mg/day) in patients with a mechanical prosthetic valve is a class IIa recommendation.
    - Increasing warfarin to an INR target of 4.0 (range 3.5–4.5) is a class IIa recommendation for high-risk patients who are intolerant of aspirin.
- Bioprosthetic valves
  - The risk of thromboembolism is ~0.7% per year in patients with biologic valves in sinus rhythm.
  - For the first 3 months after implantation, thromboembolic risk is elevated and patients should be treated with warfarin to a target INR of 2.5 (range 2.0–3.0) although some experts suggest aspirin is adequate for bioprosthetic valves in the aortic position.
  - Aortic/mitral valve bioprostheses and no risk factors are treated with aspirin 80–100 mg/day.
  - Aortic/mitral valve bioprostheses and risk factors for thromboembolism are treated with warfarin to target INR of 2.5 (range 2.0–3.0).

SURGERY

- Major criteria for valve selection:
  - The major advantages of a mechanical valve are an extremely low rate of structural deterioration.
  - The disadvantages of mechanical valves are the increased incidence of bleeding due to the need for anticoagulation therapy and the need for meticulous attention to anticoagulation level.
  - The major advantages of a bioprosthesis (whether porcine or pericardial) are a lower bleeding rate and lack of need for anticoagulation therapy.
  - The major disadvantage is the increased rate of structural valve deterioration, especially in young patients and those with end-stage renal disease.
  - In general, mitral valve repair is preferable to mitral valve replacement, provided it is feasible and the appropriate skill and experience are available to perform the procedure successfully.
  - Carefully selected patients with aortic regurgitation (AR) or aortic stenosis (AS) in whom the valve is not calcified are also candidates for valve repair.
  - Pericardial bioprostheses may have a lower rate of structural valve deterioration than porcine bioprostheses in patients ≥65 years of age.
- Recommendations for valve replacement with a mechanical prosthesis:
  - Patients with expected long lifespan (class I)
  - Patients with a mechanical prosthetic valve already in place in a different position than the valve to be replaced (class I)
  - Patients in renal failure, on hemodialysis, or with hypercalcemia (class IIa)
  - Patients requiring warfarin therapy because of risk factors for thromboembolism (class IIa)
  - Patients ≤65 years for AVR and ≤70 years for MVR (class IIa)
  - Valve re-replacement for a thrombosed biologic valve (class IIb)
- Recommendations for valve replacement with a bioprosthesis:
  - Patients who cannot or will not take warfarin therapy (class I)
  - Patients ≥65 years of age needing AVR who do not have risk factors for thromboembolism (class I)
  - Patients considered to have possible compliance problems with warfarin therapy (class IIa)
  - Patients ≥70 years of age needing MVR who do not have risk factors for thromboembolism (class IIa)
  - Valve re-replacement for a thrombosed mechanical valve (class IIb)

- Tricuspid valves
  - The risk of thrombosis is highest in the tricuspid position due to the lower pressure and velocity of blood flow.
  - If tricuspid valve must be replaced, a bioprosthesis is the valve of choice.
    - Fortunately, biologic valves in the tricuspid position exhibit a much slower rate of mechanical deterioration.
- Pregnancy
  - The hypercoagulable state of pregnancy increases the risk of thromboembolism in women who have prosthetic valves.
  - Women with prosthetic heart valves should be counseled against pregnancy. If a woman with a prosthetic valve becomes pregnant, she should be maintained on warfarin to a target INR of 2.5 (range 2.0–3.0). The teratogenic risk to the fetus appears to be less than the risk to the mother if anticoagulation is discontinued.
  - If urgent intervention for a valvular disorder is needed in a pregnant woman, every effort should be made to defer valve replacement until after delivery.
    - Utilization of a pulmonary autograft procedure
    - Balloon valvuloplasty
    - Mitral valve repair
- Reoperation to replace a prosthetic heart valve:
  - Reoperation to replace a prosthetic heart valve is a serious clinical event.
  - It is usually required for moderate to severe prosthetic dysfunction (structural and nonstructural), dehiscence, significant paravalvular regurgitation, and prosthetic valve endocarditis.
  - Reoperation may be indicated for recurrent thromboembolism, severe intravascular hemolysis, severe recurrent bleeding from anticoagulant therapy, thrombosed prosthetic valve, and valve prosthesis–patient mismatch.

 FOLLOW-UP

Patients with prosthetic heart valves should have a transthoracic echocardiogram prior to discharge or at early follow-up from their operation to document the hemodynamics of the valve. This baseline echocardiogram can be used as a reference if changing symptoms might reflect prosthetic valve malfunction.

COMPLICATIONS

- Structural valvular deterioration
- Nonstructural dysfunction
- Valve thrombosis
- Embolism
- Bleeding events
- Prosthetic valvular endocarditis

PATIENT MONITORING

- The first outpatient evaluation after valve surgery usually occurs 3–4 weeks after discharge.
- The workup on this visit should include complete or interval history and physical examination, ECG, chest radiograph, 2-D and Doppler echocardiography, CBC, blood urea nitrogen/creatinine electrolytes, and INR, if indicated.
- Asymptomatic uncomplicated patients thereafter must be followed only at 1-year intervals, at which time a complete history and thorough examination should be performed. ECGs and chest radiograph are not routinely indicated but are valuable in individual patients. The frequency with which 2-D and Doppler echocardiography should be performed in uncomplicated patients is uncertain.
- Once regurgitation is detected, close follow-up with 2-D and Doppler echocardiography every 3–6 months is indicated.
- Any patient with a prosthetic heart valve who does not improve after surgery or who later shows deterioration of functional capacity should undergo appropriate testing, including 2-D and Doppler echocardiography and, if necessary, transesophageal echocardiography and cardiac catheterization with angiography to determine the cause.

REFERENCES

1. Bonow RO, Carabello B, de Leon AC Jr, et al. ACC/AHA 2006 guidelines for the management of patients with valvular heart disease: A report of the American College of Cardiology/American Heart Association Task Force on Practice Guidelines (Writing Committee to Revise the 1998 Guidelines for the Management of Patients with Valvular Heart Disease). American College of Cardiology Web Site. Available at: http://content.onlinejacc.org/cgi/reprint/48/3/e1
2. Fuster V, Alexander RW, O'Rourke RA, eds. *Hurst's The Heart*, 11th ed. New York: McGraw-Hill, 2004.
3. Salem DN, Stein, PD, Al-Ahmed A, et al. Antithrombotic therapy in valvular heart disease—native and prosthetic: The Seventh ACCP Conference on Antithrombotic and Thrombolytic Therapy. *Chest*. 2004;126(3 Suppl): 457S–482S.
4. Zipes D, Libby P, Bonow RO, et al., eds. *Braunwald's Heart Disease: A Textbook of Cardiovascular Medicine*, 7th ed. Philadelphia: Elsevier Saunders, 2005.

P

PULMONARY ATRESIA WITH INTACT SEPTUM

David Brick
Welton M. Gersony

 BASICS

DESCRIPTION
- Atresia of the pulmonary valve with no ventricular septal defect
- The main and branch pulmonary arteries are almost always normal.
  - Forward flow may be present in early fetal life.
  - The ductus arteriosus is usually patent in the neonate for a few days, but when closure occurs, no alternate sources of pulmonary blood flow exist.
  - Pulmonary collateral vessels are not prominent.
- A broad spectrum of coronary artery abnormalities are common, varying from coronary atresia (observed in stillborns) to mild stenoses.
- Myocardial blood flow may depend on right ventricular (RV) sinusoids in some cases.

EPIDEMIOLOGY
- Predominant age: Newborn presentation
- Predominant sex or race: None

Incidence
0.07/1,000 births, 1% of congenital heart disease, 3% of critically ill children

Prevalence
Prevalence decreases due to mortality and is age-dependent.

RISK FACTORS
Genetics
Family history of any congenital heart disease increases probability of pulmonary atresia with intact ventricular septum (PA/IVS). No gene has been specifically identified.

PATHOPHYSIOLOGY
Pulmonary atresia results in no pulmonary blood flow after ductal closure. In untreated patients, severe hypoxia and death result.

ETIOLOGY
Unknown

ASSOCIATED CONDITIONS
Rare

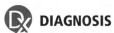 **DIAGNOSIS**

SIGNS AND SYMPTOMS
- Cyanosis
- Tachypnea

History
- Severe cyanosis within 3 days of birth is usual.
- Persistent tachypnea; respiratory distress may develop.
- Murmur may be audible.
- As ductus arteriosus closes, severity of symptoms progresses.
- May have low cardiac output, with myocardial ischemia

Physical Exam
- Severe cyanosis
- Tachypnea
- Normal S1
- Single S2

- May have regurgitant systolic murmur at left lower sternal border due to tricuspid insufficiency

TESTS
ECG:
- Normal sinus rhythm
- Axis 0–120 degrees
- Most often normal axis
- May have right axis if a large RV chamber is present
- Usually decreased RV voltage, V1 and V3R.

Lab
Arterial saturation <70%; less severe hypoxia in patients receiving prostaglandins to keep ductus patent

Imaging
- Chest radiograph
  - Heart size usually is normal, with large right atrium if tricuspid regurgitation is significant. Decreased pulmonary vascular markings are usual, unless ductus is widely patent.
- Echocardiography
  - Documents small to miniscule RV chamber and tricuspid valve and no ventricular septal defect
  - Some cases have large RV chamber.
  - Slightly small to normal pulmonary valve annulus and pulmonary arteries
- Echocardiography (Doppler)
  - Absence of flow across right ventricular outflow tract
  - Assesses severity of tricuspid regurgitation qualitatively and may allow prediction of RV pressure
  - Right-to-left flow across atrial septum
- 3D echocardiography
  - May be benefit in future for defining the potential adequacy of RV chamber
- MRI
  - Gold standard for defining RV volumes in older children. Currently not adequate to determine RV volumes in neonates.
  - Not adequate for replacing cardiac catheterization in defining arterial collaterals and RV sinusoids.

Diagnostic Procedures/Surgery
- Cardiac catheterization
  - Documents atresia of the RV outflow tract
  - Demonstrates size of pulmonary arteries and status of the ductus arteriosus
  - Evaluates for RV-dependent coronary circulation
- RV angiogram can demonstrate filling of coronary arteries retrograde via myocardial sinusoids. Coronary angiogram also is required to observe for stenoses in the coronary circulation.

Pathologic Findings
- Usually slightly small to normal valve annulus with fused leaflets
- Small or miniscule RV chamber with severe myocardial hypertrophy; 20% have large, usually dysfunctional RV; tricuspid valve annulus size correlates with RV size.
- Slightly small but confluent pulmonary arteries; few pulmonary arterial collaterals
- Coronary artery abnormalities are frequent.
- Myocardial function often is abnormal.
- Restrictive atrial communication is rare; foramen ovale is dilated.

- Tricuspid annulus may be large in 5–10% of cases, and tricuspid insufficiency may be present. A few patients with large chambers may have Ebstein deformity.
- Mitral valve abnormalities are rare.

DIFFERENTIAL DIAGNOSIS
The differential diagnosis of a newborn with cardiac cyanosis also includes critical pulmonary stenosis with intact ventricular septum, transposition of the great arteries, total anomalous venous return, tricuspid atresia, Ebstein anomaly, tetralogy of Fallot, and pulmonary atresia with ventricular septal defect (extreme tetralogy variant).

 TREATMENT

GENERAL MEASURES
- Without treatment, prognosis is extremely poor; most neonates die within days.
- Prostaglandin is administered to maintain ductal-dependent pulmonary blood flow. Cardiac catheterization is performed to assess for coronary abnormalities or RV-dependent coronary circulation.

 MEDICATION (DRUGS)

- At birth, virtually all patients require prostaglandin to maintain ductal patency.
- After repair, institute endocarditis prophylaxis.

SURGERY
- The size of the right ventricular chamber and tricuspid valve will determine if a four-chamber repair can be achieved. Several approaches are used to repair, depending on anatomic findings.
- If the tricuspid valve annulus and RV are miniscule, a Blalock-Taussig shunt procedure alone is performed urgently in the neonatal period. These patients will likely undergo multiple operations in childhood, eventually leading to a Fontan type of circulation. (All superior vena cava and inferior vena cava blood flows passively to the lungs, and the left ventricle pumps oxygenated blood to the body.)
- Patients with at least small but not tiny tricuspid valves may undergo surgical valvuloplasty. This is most often performed with an associated Blalock-Taussig shunt for relief of right ventricular outflow tract (RVOT) obstruction. Stenting of the ductus has been used in some patients.
- Some patients may benefit from a transcatheter perforation and valvuloplasty using varying techniques such as laser, radiofrequency, or guidewire perforation, instead of surgical valvuloplasty.
- Patients with RV-dependent coronary circulation eventually may undergo a Fontan procedure that incorporates an RV with systemic pressure into the systemic circulation so that the distal coronary arteries will be perfused. The prognosis often is poor with this type of anatomy.
- For patients with severe coronary artery disease, cardiac transplantation may be the only alternative.
- Late surgery
  - Reopen RVOT later in childhood.
  - Eliminate shunts in patients with good four-chamber anatomy.

– Perform Fontan procedure for patients without functional right ventricle.

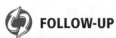 **FOLLOW-UP**

PROGNOSIS

• With no intervention, most patients die in the neonatal period. The remainder die in infancy. Death is due to profound hypoxia and ventricular failure. A few patients with persistent patency of the ductus arteriosus survive into childhood.

• An increased incidence of sudden death occurs among surgically palliated infants, most likely due to left ventricular ischemia or dysfunction and a fatal arrhythmia.

• With intervention, the clinical course depends on the adequacy of the RV. Overall, the 4-year survival rate is 50–90%, depending on complicating factors. Patients with adequate RVs and only one surgical procedure have a better outlook than do patients who have multiple operations and ultimately undergo a Fontan operation. A child with a 2-ventricle repair without coronary disease may have a relatively normal childhood, although exercise tolerance may be decreased.

• As the patient grows, the need for additional surgeries to enlarge the RVOT may be needed. 50% of patients will undergo an additional procedure, but ultimate prognosis may be favorable.

PATIENT MONITORING

• Newborns require close follow-up. All patients require continued monitoring to determine when and if additional surgeries are needed.

• Throughout life, close follow-up is required by a cardiologist well versed in the issues specific to PA/IVS.

• Follow-up should be tailored to the type of repair the patient has undergone.

• Specific issues include:
  – Arterial oxygen saturation and hemoglobin concentration to assess the adequacy of pulmonary blood flow
  – Pulmonary outflow gradients in patients with RVOT repairs
  – Growth of the RV chamber
  – Follow for signs or symptoms of ventricular ischemia

Pregnancy Considerations

• Patients who undergo surgery with 4-chamber anatomy, have normal coronary arteries, and have mild to moderate pulmonary valve stenosis are at low maternal and fetal risk during pregnancy.

• Pregnancy is not recommended for women who have undergone the Fontan procedure, or for those with coronary artery disease or ventricular dysfunction.

REFERENCES

1. Bonow RO, Carabello B, de Leon AC Jr., et al. ACC/AHA guidelines for the management of patients with valvular heart disease: A report of the American College of Cardiology/American Heart Association Task Force on Practice Guidelines (Committee on Management of Patients with Valvular Heart Disease). *J Am Coll Cardiol*. 1998;32:1486–1588.

2. Dyamenahalli U, McCrindle BW, McDonald C, et al. Pulmonary atresia with intact ventricular septum: Management of, and outcomes for, a cohort of 210 consecutive patients. *Cardiol Young*. 2004;14:299–308.

3. Gewillig M, Boshoff DE, Dens J, et al. Stenting the neonatal arterial duct in duct-dependent pulmonary circulation: New techniques, better results. *J Am Coll Cardiol* 2004;43:107–112.

4. Hanley FL, Sade RM, Blackstone EH, et al. Outcomes in neonatal pulmonary atresia with intact ventricular septum. A multi-institutional study. *J Thorac Cardiovasc Surg*. 1993;105:406–427.

5. Humpl T, Söderberg B, McCrindle BW, et al. Percutaneous balloon valvotomy in pulmonary atresia with intact ventricular septum: Impact on patient care. *Circulation*. 2003;108:826–832.

6. Mi YP, Chau AKT, Chiu CSW, et al. Evolution of the management approach for pulmonary atresia with intact ventricular septum. *Heart*. 2005;91:657–663.

ADDITIONAL READING

• Freedom RM. *The natural and modified history of congenital heart disease*. New York: Futura, 2004.

• Gersony W, Rosenbaum M. *Congenital heart disease in adults*. New York: McGraw-Hill, 2002.

CODES

ICD9-CM

746.0 Pulmonary atresia

PATIENT TEACHING

Parents must be informed about the benefits of surgery and possible outcomes with the variations of this lesion.

Activity

Patient's activity should be self-limited, based on cardiac status.

PULMONARY EMBOLISM

Michael H. Crawford

 BASICS

DESCRIPTION
Pulmonary embolism is defined as occlusion of a major pulmonary artery branch by a blood clot originating from the venous system of the body.
- Clinical presentation
  - Acute cor pulmonale: Occlusion of more than two thirds of the pulmonary circulation
  - Pulmonary infarction: Complete occlusion of a distal branch of the pulmonary circulation
  - Unexplained dyspnea: Patients without acute cor pulmonale or pulmonary infarction
- System(s) affected: Pulmonary; Cardiovascular

GENERAL PREVENTION
Avoid prolonged bed rest, inactivity.

EPIDEMIOLOGY
- Predominant age: Increases with advancing age
- Predominant sex: Males affected as often as females

Geriatric Considerations
More common and often fatal.

Pediatric Considerations
Rare

Pregnancy Considerations
Pregnancy increases the risk.

Incidence
250,000 cases/year; 50,000 deaths/year

RISK FACTORS
- Surgery, especially orthopedic, major abdominal, and thoracic
- Immobilization
- Occult cancer (hypercoagulable state)
- Oral contraceptive use
  - Young women on oral contraceptives
- Postpartum
- Obesity
- Advanced age
- Anticardiolipid antibodies (lupus erythematosus)
- Trauma to legs
- Advanced age
- Congestive heart failure

Genetics
Hypercoagulable states (e.g., factor V Leiden deficiency)

PATHOPHYSIOLOGY
Propensity to venous thrombosis and pulmonary embolism increased by venous stasis, altered blood coagulability, and vascular injury (Virchow triad)

ETIOLOGY
See Risk Factors.

ASSOCIATED CONDITIONS
Deep venous thrombosis, Occult cancer, Congestive heart failure, Stroke, Obesity

 DIAGNOSIS

SIGNS AND SYMPTOMS
History
- Acute cor pulmonale
  - Dyspnea
  - Syncope
  - Anxiety
- Pulmonary infarction
  - Pleuritic chest pain
  - Dyspnea
  - Hemoptysis
- Unexplained dyspnea
  - Dyspnea
  - Anxiety

Physical Exam
- Acute cor pulmonale
  - Cyanosis
  - Hypotension
  - Cardiopulmonary arrest
  - Tachypnea
  - Tachycardia
  - Jugular venous distention
  - Third heart sound, right ventricle
  - Right ventricular heave
  - Signs of deep venous thrombosis
- Pulmonary infarction
  - Tachypnea
  - Lungs: Rales, wheezes, or friction rub
  - Signs of deep venous thrombosis
- Unexplained dyspnea
  - Tachycardia
  - Tachypnea
  - Signs of deep venous thrombosis

TESTS
- Acute cor pulmonale
  - Electrocardiogram (ECG); new S1, Q3, T3 pattern, incomplete right bundle branch block or right ventricular ischemia
  - Chest x-ray usually normal
- Pulmonary infarction
  - ECG normal
  - Chest x-ray: Elevated hemidiaphragm, peripheral infiltrate, or small pleural effusion
- Unexplained dyspnea
  - ECG usually normal
  - Chest x-ray normal

Lab
- Acute cor pulmonale
  - Arterial blood gasses: Low po_2, pco_2
- Pulmonary infarction
  - Arterial blood gases; normal or decreased po_2, decreased pco_2, alkalosis
- Unexplained dyspnea
  - Arterial blood gases: Normal or decreased po_2, pco_2
- Plasma D-dimer: High negative predictive value

Imaging
- Computed tomographic scan of pulmonary vasculature and deep veins of legs
- Ventilation-perfusion ratio (V/Q) scan: Most useful if normal or highly suggestive of pulmonary embolism segmental perfusion defects
- Echocardiography: Signs of cor pulmonale
- Ultrasonography of the leg veins to confirm deep venous thromboses

Diagnostic Procedures/Surgery
- Pulmonary angiography: Intraluminal filling defects or arterial cut-offs
- Contrast venography to confirm deep venous thromboses

Pathologic Findings
- Pulmonary infarction
- Pulmonary artery thrombi
- Deep venous thrombosis
- Cor pulmonale

DIFFERENTIAL DIAGNOSIS
- Acute myocardial infarction
- Pneumonia
- Congestive heart failure
- Pericarditis
- Pleurisy
- Anxiety neurosis/panic attacks

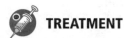 **TREATMENT**

GENERAL MEASURES
- Hospitalization, in the intensive care unit if unstable
- Oxygen as necessary
- Ventilatory assistance if needed
- Graduated leg compression stockings for deep venous thrombosis
- Emotional support (unexpected acute illness)

Diet
Nothing special

Activity
Bed rest with leg movement exercises; ambulation as soon as possible

MEDICATION (DRUGS)

First Line
- Intravenous heparin 5,000–10,000 units, followed by a continuous infusion to keep the partial thromboplastin time 1.5–2.5 times normal for at least 5 days
- Warfarin PO beginning 12–24 hours after heparin for at least 6 weeks
- Warfarin dose adjusted to increase the international normalized ratio (INR) to 2.0–3.0 times normal (1.0)
- Thrombolytic therapy is indicated for patients with hemodynamic instability, right heart failure, massive pulmonary embolism, or extensive deep venous thrombosis: Streptokinase 250,000 U over 30 minutes followed by 100,000 U per hour for 24 hours or recombinant tissue plasminogen activator (rt-PA) 100 mg over 2 hours.

Contraindications
- The major contraindication to anticoagulation or thrombolytic therapy is active bleeding.
- Recent hemorrhagic stroke, intracranial disease or head trauma, a high risk of bleeding (recent surgery), and significant thrombocytopenia are contraindications to thrombolytic therapy.

Precautions
- If the partial thromboplastin time and INR are adjusted appropriately, the risk of major hemorrhage can be minimized.

Significant Possible Interactions
- Many drugs alter the metabolism of warfarin, making management by a specialized clinic desirable.

Second Line
Low-molecular-weight heparin given subcutaneously every 12 hours is an alternative to intravenous heparin and warfarin.

SURGERY
- Pulmonary thrombectomy by catheter or surgery for rare patient unresponsive to medical therapy or with chronic pulmonary hypertension from prior pulmonary embolism
- Inferior vena cava filter to prevent further thromboemboli in patients unresponsive to, refractory to, or contraindicated for medical therapy

 ## FOLLOW-UP

Calf-deep venous thrombosis (DVT) can be treated with anticoagulants for 6 weeks; more central veins for 3 months. However, patients with ongoing risk of DVT probably should be treated indefinitely.

DISPOSITION
Admission Criteria
All with suspected pulmonary embolism

Discharge Criteria
- Resolution of symptoms
- Achieve adequate anticoagulation

Issues for Referral
Need for thrombolysis or invasive procedure

PROGNOSIS
- With appropriate therapy, hospital mortality rate is less than 10%.
- Long-term prognosis is determined by coexisting disease, residual pulmonary function, and level of pulmonary pressures.

COMPLICATIONS
- Pulmonary infarction
- Chronic pulmonary hypertension
- Right heart failure

PATIENT MONITORING
The INR must be followed carefully in a patient on chronic warfarin.

REFERENCES
1. Aklog L, et al. Acute pulmonary embolectomy: A contemporary approach. *Circulation*. 2002;105:1416.
2. Sukhija R, et al. Electrocardiographic abnormalities in patients with right ventricular dilation due to acute pulmonary embolism. *Cardiology*. 2006;105:57–60.

ADDITIONAL READING
Goldhaber SZ. Pulmonary embolic disease. In: Crawford MH, ed. *Current Diagnosis and Treatment in Cardiology*, 2nd ed. New York: McGraw-Hill, 2003.

 ## MISCELLANEOUS

See also: Thrombosis, deep vein

CODES
ICD9-CM
415.1 Pulmonary embolism and infarction

PATIENT TEACHING
- Avoidance of prolonged immobilization
- Weight loss

Prevention
- Graduated compression stockings in susceptible patients (surgical patients)
- Periodic ambulation during long airplane or car trips
- Chronic warfarin or low-molecular-weight heparin therapy for high-risk patients
- Inferior vena cava interruption for high-risk patients

FAQ
- Does normal arterial blood gases rule out pulmonary embolism? No, arterial blood gases and the alveolar arterial oxygen gradient are not useful for excluding the diagnosis of pulmonary embolism.
- Does postmenopausal hormone replacement therapy (HRT) increase the risk of venous thromboembolism? Yes, three large studies have now shown that HRT can increase the risk 2–4 times.

P

PULMONARY HYPERTENSION, PRIMARY AND SECONDARY

B. Robinson Williams III
Pradyumna E. Tummala*
Nanette K. Wenger

 BASICS

DESCRIPTION
Pulmonary hypertension is defined as elevation of pulmonary arterial pressures to a mean of 25 mm Hg at rest or 30 mm Hg during exercise due to intrinsic abnormalities of pulmonary vasculature [primary pulmonary hypertension (PPH)] or secondary causes including lung disease, chronic elevations of pulmonary venous pressures as a result of left heart disease (secondary pulmonary hypertension, SPH), and rare syndromes such as veno-occlusive disease and pulmonary capillary hemangiomatosis.

EPIDEMIOLOGY
PPH
• Female predominance (2.5:1); mean age 35 years

Prevalence
2 per million for PPH

RISK FACTORS
Female sex

Pregnancy Considerations
High risk to mother and fetus due to associated hemodynamic stresses, particularly in immediate postpartum period; oral contraceptives not recommended because they may exacerbate pulmonary hypertension

Genetics
Autosomal-dominant transmission in 6% of PPH, with one chromosomal locus mapped to 2q31–q32

ETIOLOGY
(Revised World Health Organization Classification of Pulmonary Hypertension, 2004)
Group I. Pulmonary arterial hypertension
• Idiopathic (primary)
• Familial
• Associated with significant venous or capillary involvement
  – Pulmonary veno-occlusive disease
  – Pulmonary-capillary hemangiomatosis
• Persistent pulmonary hypertension of the newborn
• Also see section entitled Associated Conditions
Group II. Pulmonary venous hypertension
• Left-sided atrial or ventricular heart disease
• Left-sided valvular heart disease
Group III. Pulmonary hypertension associated with hypoxemia
• Chronic obstructive pulmonary disease
• Interstitial lung disease
• Sleep-disordered breathing
• Alveolar hypoventilation disorders
• Chronic exposure to high altitudes
• Developmental abnormalities

Group IV. Pulmonary hypertension due to chronic thrombotic disease, embolic disease, or both
• Thromboembolic obstruction of proximal pulmonary arteries
• Thromboembolic obstruction of distal pulmonary arteries
• Pulmonary embolism (tumor, parasites, foreign material)
Group V. Miscellaneous
• Sarcoidosis, pulmonary Langerhans cell histiocytosis, lymphangiomatosis, compression of pulmonary vessels (adenopathy, tumor, fibrosing mediastinitis)

ASSOCIATED CONDITIONS
• Collagen vascular disease (e.g., CREST syndrome), Congenital systemic-to-pulmonary shunts, Portal hypertension, HIV infection, Drugs and toxins (e.g., anorexigens, rapeseed oil, L-tryptophan, methamphetamine, cocaine)
• Other conditions: Thyroid disorders, Glycogen storage disorders, Gaucher disease, Hereditary hemorrhagic telangiectasia, Hemoglobinopathies, Myeloproliferative disorders, Splenectomy

 DIAGNOSIS

SIGNS AND SYMPTOMS
• Symptoms: Dyspnea, fatigue, dizziness, chest pain, cough, hoarseness, hemoptysis, orthopnea, effort syncope, edema, increased abdominal girth, palpitations
• Signs/physical examination findings: Tachypnea, tachycardia, elevated jugular venous pressure with large A wave and large V wave if significant tricuspid regurgitation present, prominent right ventricular impulse, right ventricular third heart sound (S_3) or fourth heart sound (S_4) that increase with inspiration, loud pulmonic component (P2) of S_2 or single S_2, murmur of tricuspid regurgitation or pulmonic insufficiency, hepatomegaly, ascites, peripheral edema
• Findings or signs associated with underlying pulmonary disease (wheezes, rales, decreased excursion and air movement), and left heart disease, including those of mitral or aortic valve disease and dilated cardiomyopathy/left ventricular failure (murmur, S_3)

TESTS
• Special tests to consider to rule out secondary causes of pulmonary hypertension, depending on the history and physical examination findings, include the following with Doppler study:
• Echocardiography to rule out left heart disease
• Ventilation-perfusion (V/Q) scan to rule out chronic pulmonary embolism
• Spiral computed tomographic scan to confirm pulmonary emboli and assess pulmonary parenchyma
• Pulmonary function tests to rule out severe obstructive or restrictive patterns
• Sleep study to rule out sleep apnea
• Screen for collagen vascular diseases (scleroderma, systemic lupus erythematosus, polyarteritis nodosa)
• Screen for infectious etiologies: HIV, schistosomiasis, filariasis (highly recommended in excluding causes of SPH)

Diagnostic Procedures/Surgery
Investigations to confirm pulmonary hypertension and identify the causes include the following:
• Electrocardiogram (ECG): Right axis deviation, right atrial abnormality, right ventricular hypertrophy
• Chest x-ray: Enlarged central pulmonary arteries, enlarged right atrium/ventricle, possible "pruning" of pulmonary vasculature, findings of left heart disease, including left atrial or ventricular enlargement
• Echocardiography with Doppler: Right atrial/ventricular enlargement, right ventricular hypertrophy/dysfunction, elevated posteroanterior (PA) pressures, tricuspid/pulmonic insufficiency; may diagnose dilated cardiomyopathy, aortic and mitral valve disease, intracardiac shunts
• Right heart catheterization to assess right ventricular and pulmonary arterial pressures and pulmonary capillary wedge pressure (should be <15 mm Hg in PPH), to rule out intracardiac shunts, and to assess for response to pharmacologic challenge
• Consider CT or V/Q scan if history and screening suggest thromboembolic disease.

Pathologic Findings
Histologic findings common to all forms of PPH include intimal fibrosis, increased medial thickness, pulmonary arteriolar occlusion, and plexiform lesions.

TREATMENT

GENERAL MEASURES

SPH

Three mechanisms contribute to development and worsening of SPH: (i) transmittance of high pulmonary venous pressures from left heart disease; (ii) pulmonary endothelial dysfunction from elevated pressures, hypoxemia, and acidosis; and (iii) remodeling/hypertrophy of pulmonary arterial vasculature over time due to elevated pressures and hypoxemia. Whereas the latter is irreversible, the first two have some reversibility. Treatment should aim to alter these factors:

- Treatment of left heart failure with diuretics, angiotensin-converting enzyme inhibitors, β-blockers, aldosterone antagonists, digoxin, inotropes, and valve repair or replacement
- Treatment of hypoxemia and acidosis in hypoventilation syndromes with oxygen, continuous positive airway pressure, and mechanical ventilation
- Treatment of lung disease with bronchodilators, antibiotics, steroids, and smoking cessation
- Prevention of recurrent venous thromboembolic events with anticoagulants and/or vena caval filter
- Pulmonary thromboendarterectomy for chronic pulmonary emboli and proximal pulmonary arterial occlusion

PPH

Treatment includes:

- Supplemental oxygen to treat hypoxemia and vasoconstriction
- Vasodilator therapy if patient demonstrates a significant hemodynamic response (20% decrease in pulmonary artery pressure or pulmonary vascular resistance)
  - Calcium channel blockers (nifedipine 30–240 mg PO daily or diltaizem 120–900 mg mg PO daily)
  - Intravenous prostacyclin (epoprostenol), given as a continuous intravenous infusion (2–20 ng/kg/minute)
  - Treprostinil, a prostacyclin analog, administered by continuous subcutaneous infusion
  - Iliprost, an inhaled prostacyclin analog (2.5 or 5.0 μg 6–9 times daily)
  - Bosentan, an oral endothelin-receptor antagonist (62.5–250 mg b.i.d.)
  - Sildenafil, an oral phosphodiesterase inhibitor (20–80 mg t.i.d.)
- Diuretics to treat right heart failure
  - Furosemide (40–500 mg/day) and spironolactone (25–100 mg/day) for ascites, edema, dyspnea
  - Closely monitor to avoid hypotension from overdiuresis (even in presence of edema, jugular venous distension) due to need for higher filling pressures with severe right ventricular failure.

- Inotropes such as dobutamine (2.5–7.5 mcg/kg/min) or milrinone (0.35–0.75 μg/kg/minute), either as temporary measure to improve right ventricular performance or chronically for patients with severe right ventricular failure refractory to above therapy
- Chronic anticoagulation with warfarin [target international normalized ratio (INR) 2.0–3.0] to prevent pulmonary emboli in presence of severe right heart failure appears to improve survival.
- Consider percutaneous atrial septostomy in normoxemic patients to improve left ventricular filling and cardiac output (at the expense of slightly worsening oxygenation from right-to-left shunt).
- Consider lung transplantation or heart–lung transplantation (with coexistent left-sided heart disease).

Diet
Sodium, fluid restrictions to control heart failure

Activity
- As tolerated without symptoms
- Optimize exercise tolerance in a cardiac rehabilitation program.
- Avoid high levels of activity (e.g., competitive sports).

 MEDICATION (DRUGS)

See SPH and PPH sections in General Measures.

SURGERY
Consider percutaneous atrial septostomy, lung transplantation, heart–lung transplantation, inferior vena caval filter placement, and pulmonary thromboendarterectomy (see section on General Measures).

FOLLOW-UP

DISPOSITION
Admission Criteria
Admission for patients with NYHA class IV symptoms or class II/III symptoms who require major dose adjustments of vasodilators, diuretics, inotropes under hemodynamic monitoring; discharge when stable on same medical, dietary, activity regimen as at home

PROGNOSIS
- PPH
  - Survival depends on clinical presentation; median survival is 2.5 years.
  - Prognosis markedly improved if the patient responds to vasodilator therapy (up to 95% survival at 5 years)
  - Most deaths due to heart failure, sudden death (arrhythmia, pulmonary emboli), pneumonia, and other common causes of death
- SPH: Depends on nature/reversibility of left heart disease

PATIENT MONITORING
- Close frequent follow-up due to increased mortality rate
- Pneumococcal, influenza vaccines
- Monitor INR (2.0–3.0) on warfarin therapy

REFERENCES
1. Farber HW, Loscalzo J. Pulmonary arterial hypertension. *N Engl J Med*. 2004;351:1655–1665.
2. Galie N, et. al. Sildenafil citrate therapy for pulmonary arterial hypertension. *N Engl J Med*. 2005;353:2148–2157.
3. Higenbottam T, Stenmark K, Simonneau G. Treatments for severe pulmonary hypertension. *Lancet*. 1999;353:338–340.
4. Humbert M, Sitbon O, Simonneau G. Treatment of pulmonary arterial hypertension. *N Engl J Med*. 2004;351:1425–1436.
5. Lawrence EC, Brigham KL. Chronic cor pulmonale. In: Fuster V, Alexander RW, O'Rourke RA eds. *Hurst's the Heart,* 11th ed. New York: McGraw-Hill, 2004.
6. Rubin LJ: Primary pulmonary hypertension. *N Engl J Med*.1997;336:111–117.
7. Rubin, LJ. Pulmonary hypertension. In: Fuster V, Alexander RW, O'Rourke RA eds. *Hurst's the Heart,* 11th ed. New York: McGraw-Hill, 2004.

CODES
ICD9-CM
- 416.0 Primary pulmonary hypertension
- 416.8 Other chronic pulmonary heart diseases: Pulmonary hypertension, secondary

PATIENT TEACHING
Internet Resources:
- Pulmonary Hypertension Association website: volunteer support organization and source of information for patients with primary and secondary pulmonary hypertension. http://www.phassociation.org

P

PULMONARY REGURGITATION

Joseph Pollizi
Steven C. Herrmann
Bernard R. Chaitman

 BASICS

DESCRIPTION
Pulmonic regurgitation (PR) is incompetence of the pulmonary valve resulting in retrograde flow from the pulmonary artery to the right ventricle during diastole.

Pregnancy Considerations
Well tolerated in the absence of pulmonary hypertension (PH)

EPIDEMIOLOGY
- Trivial and mild cases of PR are common findings in both adolescents and adults.
- Childhood cases of significant PR usually are associated with other congenital heart defects; isolated cases of severe PR are rare.
- Most cases of significant PR diagnosed in adulthood are due to pulmonary causes.

Prevalence
Uncommon

PATHOPHYSIOLOGY
Isolated PR causes right ventricular overload and is well tolerated for many years, unless it is associated with, or complicated by, PH and subsequent right ventricular failure.

ETIOLOGY
- The most common causes are related to either dilation of the pulmonary valve ring or the pulmonary artery itself.
  - Dilation of the pulmonary valve ring: Secondary to PH of any cause
  - Dilation of pulmonary artery: May be idiopathic or due to connective tissue disorders such as Marfan's syndrome
- The second most common cause is infective endocarditis.
- Pulmonic valve lesions: Congenital malformation alone, such as malformed or absent leaflets, or more commonly associated with other congenital anomalies, particularly tetralogy of Fallot, ventricular septal defect, and pulmonary valve stenosis
- Less common causes include trauma, iatrogenic causes (induced during surgical treatment of tetralogy of Fallot, congenital pulmonary, stenosis repair, or pulmonary catheter placement), carcinoid syndrome, rheumatic involvement, and syphilis.

 DIAGNOSIS

SIGNS AND SYMPTOMS
- Patients usually present with signs and symptoms of right heart failure that include swelling of feet, shortness of breath without much orthopnea, leg edema, ascites, hepatomegaly, venous distention (increased jugular venous pressure) and, in longstanding cases, splenomegaly.
- PR caused by endocarditis may have septic emboli.

Physical Exam
- Physical examination may reveal palpable systolic pulsations in the left parasternal area due to hyperdynamic right ventricular function and a palpable PA due to dilation in the second left intercostal space (ICS).
- A pulmonic tap due to pulmonary valve closure is usually easily heard at the second left ICS in patients with severe PH and PR.
- On auscultation, wide splitting of S2 may occur, due to a prolonged right ventricular ejection period, and P2 may be loud in the presence of PH.
- The diastolic murmur of PR is low-pitched and heard at the left third and fourth parasternal border.
- A nonvalvular systolic ejection click and mid-systolic ejection murmur, most prominent in the second left ICS, also may be appreciated in severe PR due to enhanced right ventricular output.
- In the presence of right ventricular failure, a right-sided S3 or S4 often is heard in the 4th ICS at the left parasternal area, which augments with inspiration.
- Graham Steell murmur is the diastolic murmur of PR usually heard in the presence of severe PH, with systolic pulmonary artery pressures exceeding 55 mm Hg. It is a high-pitched, diastolic, blowing decrescendo murmur that starts immediately after P2 and is most prominent at the left parasternal area in the second to fourth ICS. The Graham Steell murmur is augmented by inspiration and reduced by Valsalva maneuver.

TESTS

Imaging
- Radiologic/angiographic
  - Chest radiograph: Both the pulmonary artery and right ventricle are usually enlarged, but these signs are not specific.
  - Right heart catheterization may show elevated right ventricular end-diastolic pressure with or without PH.
  - PR may be visualized by opacification of the right ventricle following injection of the pulmonary artery with contrast agent.
  - Contrast CT and cardiac MRI can show dilation of the right ventricle and pulmonary artery.
  - Fluoroscopy can demonstrate an enlarged, pulsatile pulmonary artery.
  - Injection of contrast into the pulmonary artery results in opacification of the RV through the incompetent pulmonic valve.
- Echocardiography
  - In patients without pulmonary hypertension, the ECG usually shows a rsR configuration in the right precordial leads, suggesting right ventricular diastolic overload pattern.
  - In patients with PI and pulmonary hypertension, the ECG usually shows evidence of right ventricular hypertrophy.
  - Right ventricular dilation and right ventricular hypertrophy noted, if PH is present.
  - Diastolic flattening of the septum characteristic of volume overload may be evident.
  - Pulsed-width Doppler of the pulmonic valve inflow is often elevated in the presence of severe PR and has a shorter acceleration time in the presence of PH.
  - Doppler of the PR jet can estimate both mean pulmonic pressure and PA diastolic pressure.
  - Color Doppler is accurate in detecting and assessing the severity of PR.
  - Notching of the posterior leaflet of the pulmonic valve by M-mode and absence of the A-component of the pulmonic valve is noted in patients with PI and pulmonary hypertension.
- MRI
  - Cardiac MRI may aid in determining the degree of pulmonary artery dilation, evaluation of right ventricular function, and assessment of the regurgitant jet.

Lab
Nonspecific

DIFFERENTIAL DIAGNOSIS
Aortic regurgitation

TREATMENT

GENERAL MEASURES
- Isolated PR is seldom severe enough to require specific treatment.
- Treatment of the primary condition responsible for PR usually ameliorates PR.

 ## MEDICATION (DRUGS)

- Cardiac glycosides in the presence of right ventricular dilatation and failure
- Diuretics in the presence of volume overload
- Precautions: Hypokalemia induced by loop diuretics may potentiate digoxin toxicity and arrhythmias.

SURGERY
PI is rarely severe enough to require therapy and often improves after management of the causes of pulmonary hypertension (mitral valve surgery) or treatment of endocarditis. Patients with tetralogy of Fallot and severe PI may require surgical intervention with prosthetic valve replacement in the presence of right-sided heart failure.

PROGNOSIS
Usually well tolerated over a long course; also depends on treatment of the primary problem

PATIENT MONITORING
No recommendation for follow-up for isolated PR

REFERENCES
1. Bonow RO, Carabello B, de Leon AC Jr, et al. ACC/AHA 2006 guidelines for the management of patients with valvular heart disease: A report of the American College of Cardiology/American Heart Association Task Force on Practice Guidelines (Writing Commitee to Revise the 1998 Guidelines for the Management of Patients With Valvular Heart Disease). American College of Cadiology Web Site. Available at: http://content.onlinejacc.org/cgi/reprint/48/3/e1
2. Bouzas B, Chang AC, Gatzoulis MA. Pulmonary insufficiency: Preparing the patient with ventricular dysfunction for surgery. *Cardiol Young.* 2005;15: 51–57.
3. Braunwald E, ed. *Heart disease: A textbook of cardiovascular medicine,* 7th ed. Philadelphia: DP Zipes, 2005.
4. Feigenbaum H, ed. *Echocardiography,* 6th edition. Baltimore: Williams & Wilkins, 2005.

 ## MISCELLANEOUS

CODES
ICD9-CM
424.3

PATIENT TEACHING
Diet
Low-sodium diet in the presence of right heart failure and fluid overload

Activity
No limitation until severe PH or reduced cardiac output due to right heart failure

Prevention
Routine use of antibiotics is not recommended in the absence of complex valvular lesions.

P

PULMONARY STENOSIS, ADULT

Joseph Polizzi
Steven C. Herrmann
Bernard R. Chaitman

 BASICS

DESCRIPTION
Pulmonic valve stenosis (PS) is an obstruction to right ventricular outflow at the level of the pulmonary valve secondary to abnormal valve morphology. The lesion may range from isolated valvular stenosis to severe atresia of the pulmonary outflow tract.

Pregnancy Considerations
Isolated mild or moderate pulmonary stenosis is rarely a significant impediment to successful pregnancy.

EPIDEMIOLOGY
Usually seen in children with associated congenital heart disease, including abnormalities of the right ventricle, tricuspid valve, and coronary arteries; however, it also may present as an isolated finding. The diagnosis of PS also may be made in adults by auscultation of a systolic murmur, fatigue, lightheadedness, dyspnea, or right-sided heart failure.

Prevalence
The congenital form is the most common form, but overall it is an uncommon finding.

PATHOPHYSIOLOGY
The high resistance of the valve leads to an increased pressure gradient between the right ventricle and pulmonary circulation, and can result in right-sided heart failure.

ETIOLOGY
- Peripheral pulmonary artery stenosis: Localized or diffuse; commonly associated with supravalvular aortic stenosis, infantile hypercalcemia, and rubella syndrome (in association with patent ductus arteriosus).
- Pulmonary valve stenosis: Commonly isolated lesion (7% of all congenital heart lesions); also occurs as part of Noonan's syndrome, tetralogy of Fallot, and rubella syndrome, and rarely acquired as part of carcinoid syndrome or rheumatic inflammation.
- Pulmonary infundibular stenosis: Rare as isolated lesion and usually associated with a ventricular septal defect (VSD) or tetralogy of Fallot, or in association with pulmonary valve stenosis.
- Pulmonary subinfundibular stenosis: Rarest form described and usually occurs as part of right-sided obstructive cardiomyopathy.
- Compression from outside: Cardiac tumors and aneurysm of sinus of Valsalva

 DIAGNOSIS

SIGNS AND SYMPTOMS
- The effect of pulmonary stenosis depends on severity of obstruction, the presence of associated right ventricular function, and the presence or absence of other associated lesions.
- Common symptoms are dyspnea, fatigue (low cardiac output), and lightheadedness. Severe pulmonic stenosis may lead to chest discomfort from right ventricular angina due to hypertrophy. Orthopnea and paroxysmal nocturnal dyspnea are not reported.
- The symptoms of right ventricle failure (leg edema, ascites, jaundice, etc.), cyanosis in patients with right-to-left shunt (associated ASD or patent foramen ovale), and retarded growth in children also may be present.
- Rarely will pulmonic stenosis present with the signs and symptoms of endocarditis.

Physical Exam
- Physical signs may include rounded plump face with isolated pulmonary stenosis, characteristic facies of Noonan's and William's syndrome, prominent A-waves in the venous pulse, and a left parasternal heave, suggestive of right ventricular hypertrophy.
- Auscultation reveals pulmonary ejection click in patients with valvular pulmonary stenosis and ejection systolic crescendo–decrescendo murmur, usually best heard at the left second to fourth intercostal space (ICS).
- With mild stenosis A2 and P2 are well heard and widely split, but as stenosis becomes severe, P2 is delayed and softer and may be inaudible.
- In patients with a pliable pulmonic valve, an ejection click may be heard, which softens with inspiration. The duration between tricuspid valve closure and the ejection click shortens with increasing severity of the pulmonic valve.
- With peripheral pulmonary artery stenosis, P2 may be very loud.

TESTS
Imaging
- Radiographic/angiographic
  - Chest radiograph may show a normal cardiac silhouette and normal lung fields if the stenosis is mild to moderate. In severe disease, post-stenotic dilation of the pulmonary artery may be seen, with oligemic lung fields, right ventricular hypertrophy, and right atrial enlargement.
  - Cardiac catheterization confirms pressure gradient across stenotic pulmonary valve, and digital subtraction or selective pulmonary angiography defines exact location, extent, and distribution of lesions in patients with peripheral pulmonary artery stenosis.
- Echocardiography
  - Congenital pulmonary stenosis usually is characterized by fusion of valve cusps and an incompletely formed raphe, resulting in a domelike structure with a narrowed orifice.
  - 2-D echo in adults shows thickened pulmonic valve leaflets with decreased excursion, with bowing or doming in systole. Right ventricular hypertrophy may be seen.
  - Poststenotic pulmonary dilatation is frequently evident, but its presence does not correlate with severity.
  - Typically, the valve annulus is normal in size.
  - Pulse Doppler can be useful in defining the exact location of the stenosis.
  - The severity of the stenosis is best defined by Doppler assessment of the pulmonic valve velocities.
  - If serial stenotic lesions are present, Doppler only provides an estimate of the most severe stenosis.
- ECG
  - In mild pulmonic stenosis, ECG may be normal.
  - In moderate to severe stenosis, ECG may show right atrial abnormality, P-pulmonale, incomplete or complete right bundle branch block, right axis deviation, and right ventricular hypertrophy.

Pathologic Findings
Most patients with stenosis have a conical or dome-shaped pulmonary valve formed by fusion of valve leaflets.

DIFFERENTIAL DIAGNOSIS
- Aortic valve or subaortic stenosis
- VSD
- Ebstein anomaly
- Atrial septal defect (ASD)

TREATMENT

GENERAL MEASURES
- Mild pulmonary stenosis is a benign disease and usually does not require any treatment or intervention.
- Symptomatic patients with pulmonary stenosis and asymptomatic patients with moderate to severe stenosis (peak-to-peak gradient of >50 mm Hg) may be treated with balloon valvuloplasty, which is the procedure of choice for a typically domed, thickened valve with fused commissures.
- Patients with dysplastic pulmonary stenosis tend to have less favorable results with balloon valvuloplasty. It may be attempted prior to surgery, with varying success. It may reduce the gradient and delay the need for surgery.

SURGERY
Surgery's is required for a dysplastic valve, as seen in Noonan syndrome, or in patients with subinfundibular or peripheral pulmonary artery stenosis.

 ## FOLLOW-UP

PROGNOSIS
- Very good for patients with mild pulmonary stenosis
- Long-term data not available on balloon valvuloplasty but mid-term data (10 years) suggest results similar to surgical valvuloplasty, with little or no recurrence over a 22- to 30-year period.

PATIENT MONITORING
- ECG and echocardiography in patients with mild pulmonary stenosis (gradient <29 mm Hg) at interval of every 5 to 10 years
- ECG and echocardiography in patients with moderate to severe pulmonary stenosis (gradient >30 mm Hg) at interval of every 3 years

REFERENCES
1. Almeda FQ, Kavinsky CJ, Pophal SG, et al. Pulmonic valvular stenosis in adults: Diagnosis and treatment. *Catheter Cardiovasc Interven.* 2003;60:546–557.
2. Bonow RO, Carabello B, de Leon AC Jr, et al. ACC/AHA 2006 guidelines for the management of patients with valvular heart disease: A report of the American College of Cardiology/American Heart Association Task Force on Practice Guidelines (Writing Commitee to Revise the 1998 Guidelines for the Management of Patients With Valvular Heart Disease). American College of Cadiology Web Site. Available at: http://content.onlinejacc.org/cgi/reprint/48/3/e1
3. Braunwald E, ed. *Heart disease: A textbook of cardiovascular medicine*, 7th ed. Philadelphia: DP Zipes, 2005.
4. Elkayam U, Bitar F. Valvular heart disease and pregnancy part I: Native valves. *J Am Coll Cardiol.* 2005;46:223–230.
5. Feigenbaum H, ed. *Echocardiography*, 6th ed. Baltimore: Lippincott Williams & Wilkins, 2005.
6. Graham TP, Driscoll DJ, Gersony WM, et al. Task Force 2: Congenital heart disease. *J Am Coll Cardiol.* 2005;45:1326–1333.
7. Vricella LA, Kanani M, Cook AC, et al. Problems with the right ventricular outflow tract: A review of morphologic features and current therapeutic options. *Cardiol Young.* 2004;14:533–549.

 ## MISCELLANEOUS

CODES
ICD9-CM
424.3

PATIENT TEACHING
Very low risk for infective endocarditis, except probably patients with severe pulmonary stenosis

Diet
Low-sodium diet in patients with fluid overload

Activity
Applicable on patients with right ventricle failure

P

PULMONARY STENOSIS, PEDIATRIC

Constance J. Hayes
Welton M. Gersony

 BASICS

DESCRIPTION
Pulmonary stenosis (PS) is defined as obstruction to outflow from the right ventricle due to obstruction at the level of the pulmonary valve, the right ventricular (RV) outflow tract, or the branch pulmonary arteries.

EPIDEMIOLOGY
- Predominant age: Congenital; murmur is heard shortly after birth
- Predominant sex: Male = Female

Incidence
- Valvar PS occurs in 8–12% of patients with congenital heart disease.
- Infundibular stenosis with an intact ventricular septum is rarely seen and accounts for only 5% of all cases of RV outflow tract obstruction.
- Peripheral pulmonary artery stenosis (PPS) occurs in several forms, from a single obstructive lesion in the branch pulmonary arteries, to multiple lesions along the right and left pulmonary arteries, to branch pulmonary artery hypoplasia. It is rarely an isolated lesion.
  - Neonatal PPS is often noted but is almost always transient.

Prevalence
Second most common congenital heart lesion

RISK FACTORS
None

Genetics
- Noonan syndrome
  - 50% of patients have heart disease.
  - 75% have valvar PS with thickened dysplastic pulmonary valve leaflets.
- Williams syndrome
  - 50% of the patients have cardiac defects; PPS is reported.
- Rubella syndrome
  - 50–80% have heart disease, with PPS and patent ductus arteriosus being the most common lesions.

PATHOPHYSIOLOGY
- RV pressure is elevated secondary to obstruction to RV cardiac output.
- RV hypertrophy is proportional to degree of obstruction.
- In PPS there is flow acceleration at the acute angle of the bifurcation of the pulmonary artery into right and left branches or along the peripheral pulmonary arteries.

ETIOLOGY
Congenital

 DIAGNOSIS

SIGNS AND SYMPTOMS
- Valvar PS, mild
  - Systolic murmur is heard soon after birth.
  - The patient is asymptomatic.
- Valvar PS, moderate
  - Asymptomatic
- Valvar PS, severe
  - Mild cyanosis may be present.
- Critical valvar PS
  - Presents in the neonatal period
  - The infant is cyanotic, and may be in distress.
- PPS in the neonate
  - Asymptomatic

History
Congenital

Physical Exam
- Valvar PS, mild
  - Quiet precordium, normal second heart sound
  - Grade 2/6 short ejection systolic murmur at upper left sternal border
  - Variable systolic ejection click heard at left mid sternal border.
- Valvar PS, moderate
  - Grade 3/6 longer ejection systolic murmur extends to second heart sound at upper left sternal border
  - Ejection click is often heard
- Valvar PS, severe
  - Systolic thrill may be palpated at the upper left sternal border
  - Long ejection systolic murmur obscures the second heart sound.
  - Mild cyanosis may be present.
- Critical valver PS
  - Neonatal presentation
  - Long systolic ejection murmur
  - Cyanosis results from right-to-left shunting across the foramen ovale.
  - RV pressure is systemic or greater.
  - If cardiac output is compromised (in the most severe cases), murmur may be diminished.
- PPS in the neonate
  - Short grade 2/6 mid-systolic murmur at cardiac base
  - Murmur radiates to axillae and back.

TESTS
- Electrocardiogram (ECG) and chest x-ray (CXR)
- Valvar PS, mild
  - ECG is normal.
  - CXR reveals normal heart size and pulmonary vascular markings.
- Valvar PS, moderate
  - ECG reveals right-axis deviation with right ventricular hypertrophy proportional to the amount of obstruction.
  - CXR reveals prominent main pulmonary artery segment secondary to poststenotic dilation of the pulmonary artery. Heart size is normal.

- Valvar PS, severe
  - ECG shows severe RV hypertrophy with strain pattern.
  - CXR reveals mild cardiomegaly and may show diminished pulmonary vascular markings.
- Critical valvar PS
  - ECG reveals marked right-axis deviation and right ventricular hypertrophy with strain.
  - CXR reveals cardiomegaly with diminished pulmonary vascular markings.
  - PPS
  - ECG findings vary with degree of RV hypertrophy; usually normal in neonate.
  - CXR is normal.

Imaging
- Echocardiography reveals abnormal, thickened pulmonary valve leaflets that dome in systole.
- Gradient is estimated by Doppler:

Severity	RV-PA gradient
Mild	<40 mm
Moderate	41 to 59 mm
Severe	>60 mm

Diagnostic Procedures/Surgery
- Valvar PS, mild
  - No further procedures indicated.
  - Lesion does not progress.
- Valvar PS, moderate
  - Cardiac catheterization with balloon valvuloplasty if RV hypertrophy is present
- Valvar PS, severe
  - Balloon valvuloplasty; if unsuccessful in neonate with critical PS or with dysplastic valve, cardiac surgery necessary to open valve

Pathologic Findings
- Valve may be domed, bicuspid, or tricuspid.
- The orifice size varies from a pinhole to several millimeters in diameter, depending on the amount of obstruction.

DIFFERENTIAL DIAGNOSIS
- Valvar PS in the asymptomatic child must be differentiated from an atrial septal defect (ASD).
  - The murmur is similar, but with an ASD there is a right ventricular impulse, a wide and fixed split second heart sound, and a mid-diastolic flow murmur over the tricuspid valve.
  - There is mild cardiomegaly and the pulmonary vascular markings are increased on chest x-ray; the echocardiogram demonstrates the defect in the atrial septum.
- In the cyanotic infant with critical PS, tetralogy of Fallot reveals a similar picture.
- The echocardiogram demonstrates the large ventricular septal defect that is part of tetralogy of Fallot.

TREATMENT

GENERAL MEASURES
- Valvar PS, mild
  - No intervention required. There is no need for cardiac catheterization.
  - The lesion does not tend to progress.
- Valvar PS, moderate
  - Elective cardiac catheterization with anticipated balloon valvuloplasty
- Valvar PS, severe
  - Cardiac catheterization with interventional balloon valvuloplasty is recommended on an urgent basis.
- Critical valvar PS
  - Urgent balloon valvuloplasty is recommended. Prior to the procedure, the infant should be stabilized with a prostaglandin infusion, and any acidosis should be corrected.

First Line
- Bacterial endocarditis prophylaxis
- Prophylaxis is recommended by the AHA for all patients with PS. The incidence of bacterial endocarditis (BE) is negligible (5.6/10,000 patient-years).

SURGERY
- If valvuloplasty fails, emergent surgery to open the valve is necessary.
- PPS may or may not be amenable to surgery or catheter intervention.
  - Neonate—PPS is self limiting.

PROGNOSIS
- Valvar PS, mild
  - Prognosis is excellent and normal lifespan is anticipated.
- Valvar PS, moderate
  - Mild restriction of physical activity; can participate in low-intensity competitive sports; following relief of the stenosis, unrestricted activity may be pursued 2–4 weeks after successful valvuloplasty.
  - If surgery is used, unrestricted activity may be pursued 3 months later, the prognosis is excellent.
- Valvar PS, severe
  - Moderate restriction of physical activity; following relief of the obstruction, unrestricted activity is permitted 6 months later; prognosis is very good.
- PPS: Variable, depending on severity
  - Neonatal: Excellent; murmur disappears, examination is normal

PATIENT MONITORING
- Valvar PS, mild
  - Follow as outpatients every 1–2 years with clinical examination, ECG, and periodic echocardiograms; there is no need for restriction in physical activity.
- Valvar PS, moderate
  - Follow as outpatients once or twice a year to assess progression of the stenosis.
- Valvar PS, severe
  - Moderate restriction prior to valvuloplasty/surgery; 6 months later, with evidence of relief of the obstruction, unrestricted activity is permitted.
  - Although rarely a significant finding, patients with severe pulmonary regurgitation and significant RV enlargement following intervention can participate in low-intensity competitive sports.

REFERENCES
1. Fyler DC, ed. *Nadas' pediatric cardiology.* Philadelphia: Hanley & Belfus, 1992:459–470.
2. Garson A Jr, Bricker JT, McNamara DG. *Science and Practice of Pediatric Cardiology.* Vol. 2. Philadelphia: Lea & Fibiger, 1990:1382–1420.
3. Gersony WM, Hayes CJ, et al. Bacterial endocarditis in patients with aortic stenosis, pulmonary stenosis, or ventricular septal defect. In the report of the Second Natural History Study of Congenital Heart Defects (NHS-2). *Circulation.* 1993;(87 Suppl):121–126.
4. Graham, TP, Driscoll, DJ, et al. Task Force 2: Congenital heart disease. *JACC.* Vol 45, No. 8, 2005;45:1326-1333.
5. Hayes CJ, Gersony WM, et al. Results of treatment of patients with pulmonary stenosis. In the report of the Second Natural History Study of Congenital Heart Defects (NHS-2). *Circulation.* 1993;(87 Suppl):28–37.

CODES
ICD9-CM
746.02

P

RADIATION HEART DISEASE

Cheryl Russo

 BASICS

DESCRIPTION

- Radiation-induced heart disease may involve:
  - Pericardium: Effusion, scarring, constriction or tamponade; pericarditis is the most common cardiac manifestation of radiation injury.
  - Myocardium: Myocardial infarction (MI) and left ventricular failure
  - Coronary arteries: Plaque formation, thrombosis, acute MI, and vessel rupture
  - Conduction system: Arrhythmias and conduction disorders
  - Heart valves: Mitral regurgitation (MR)
- Damage may present acutely or as long as 20 years after radiation exposure. It may be difficult to differentiate from clinical presentation of malignancy.

EPIDEMIOLOGY

- 10% of all patients requiring drainage of pericardial effusions have radiation-induced heart disease. Most are commonly associated with:
  - Hodgkin lymphoma: Mantle field therapy associated with 5–20% incidence of pericarditis
  - Non-Hodgkin lymphoma
  - Breast carcinoma: <5% incidence of pericarditis
  - Other thoracic tumors, including thymoma and tumors of the lung and esophagus (15% incidence of pericarditis)

RISK FACTORS

- Radiation dose, volume of heart in radiation field, radiation fractionation, treatment duration, radiation source, anterior weighting of radiation
- Mediastinal radiation for Hodgkin disease exposes a larger proportion of the heart than treatment of breast carcinoma. Consequently, fewer cardiac complications occur in treatment of the latter, which can tolerate higher doses and longer duration of radiation.

ETIOLOGY

- Pericardial disease:
  - Direct damage (fibrosis of the parietal pericardium), hypersensitivity, vasculitis (fibrinous exudate results from damaged vessels)
- Myocardial disease:
  - Acute changes include inflammation and endothelial damage.
  - Delayed changes include patches of fibrosis and scarring leading to interstitial myocardial fibrosis, usually of the anterior left ventricular and right ventricular walls.
- Coronary artery disease (CAD):
  - Endothelial damage
- Conduction system:
  - Secondary to ischemic fibrosis
- Heart valves:
  - Distortion secondary to fibrosis near valve rings

ASSOCIATED CONDITIONS

- Pericardial disease:
  - Pericardial effusions, chronic constrictive pericarditis (effusion organizes and adheres)
- Myocardial disease:
  - Restrictive cardiomyopathy
- CAD:
  - Premature atherosclerosis

 DIAGNOSIS

SIGNS AND SYMPTOMS

- Pericardial disease:
  - Acute pericarditis/effusion: Usually not clinically evident. Symptoms include pain and malaise. Signs include fever, friction rub, and ECG abnormalities.
  - Delayed pericarditis: May present as asymptomatic pericardial effusion with pleural effusions on chest radiograph; 50% of patients have dyspnea, jugular venous distension, and pulsus paradoxus.
- Myocardial disease:
  - Results from constriction and severe heart failure
  - May not be evident until after failed pericardiectomy
- CAD:
  - Angina, acute MI

TESTS

- Pericardiocentesis: Effusion may be serous, serosanguineous, or hemorrhagic, with a high protein and lymphocyte content.
- Right heart catheterization

Lab

Pericardial fluid: Routine infectious disease studies, and cytology to rule out malignant cells

Imaging
- Pericarditis/pericardial effusions:
  - ECG: ST-segment elevation throughout the precordium
  - Chest radiograph: Pleural effusions with delayed pericarditis
  - Echocardiography: Pericardial fluid accumulation

DIFFERENTIAL DIAGNOSIS
- Pericardial disease:
  - Effusion must be differentiated from that of malignancy. Effusions are usually larger, with tamponade more likely in malignant accumulations.
  - Viral pericarditis
  - Effusion secondary to radiation-induced hypothyroidism
- Myocardial disease:
  - Viral cardiomyopathy, drug-induced cardiomyopathy
- CAD:
  - Ischemic heart disease

TREATMENT

GENERAL MEASURES
According to presentation

MEDICATION (DRUGS)

- Nonsteroidal anti-inflammatory drugs (NSAIDs) to control pain associated with early inflammation or effusion
- Corticosteroids reserved for use in severe pain

SURGERY
- Pericardial effusions with hemodynamic compromise may require pericardial decompression/window, or pericardectomy for constrictive pericarditis.
- Operative mortality 21% versus 8% in idiopathic disease.
- Bypass surgery may be complicated by internal mammary artery damage or mediastinal fibrosis.

FOLLOW-UP

PROGNOSIS
- Acute pericarditis usually terminates abruptly, is not treatment-limiting, and does not predict chronic changes.
- Pleural effusion treated surgically with a window has a late constriction rate near 75%.
- After pericardectomy, the 5-year survival rate is 51% (versus 83% in nonradiation patients).
- Restrictive cardiomyopathy carries a poor prognosis.

PATIENT MONITORING
Asymptomatic pericardial effusions may be followed by physical examination and serial echo.

REFERENCES
1. Lorell BH. Pericardial diseases in heart disease. In: Braunwald E, ed. *A textbook of cardiovascular medicine*, 5th ed. Philadelphia: WB Saunders, 1997:1484–1534.
2. Selwyn AP. The cardiovascular system and radiation. *Lancet*. 1983;2:152–154.
3. Stewart JR, Fajardo LF, Gillette SM, et al. Radiation injury to the heart. *Int J Radiat Oncol Biol Phys*. 1995;31:1205–1211.

PATIENT TEACHING
Organization: American Heart Association National Center, 7272 Greenville Avenue, Dallas TX 75231; 1-800-AHA-USA1; www.americanheart.org

R

REMODELING

Gerard P. Aurigemma

 BASICS

DESCRIPTION

- The term *remodeling* is most commonly used in connection with a progressive change in shape of the left ventricle (LV) in response to alterations in load or ischemic damage. More recently, surgical procedures have been undertaken to favorably affect remodeling in patients with dilated cardiomyopathy.
- The LV has the remarkable ability to remodel in order to compensate for alterations in load. The physiologic principle underlying such remodeling is known as the law of Laplace, which dictates that the force borne per unit myocardium, or LV afterload (wall stress, sG), is directly proportional to pressure, directly proportional to ventricular size, and inversely proportional to wall thickness. Thus:
  $$\sigma = P\, r/th$$
  where σ is afterload (wall stress), P is systolic pressure, r is LV cavity radius, and th is wall thickness. Moreover, end-systolic stress is the force that limits systolic ejection. Accordingly, high wall stress will be associated with reduced systolic ejection performance, even in instances where the intrinsic contractile function of the LV is normal.

PATHOPHYSIOLOGY

Cardiac remodeling is an expected finding in chronic valvular heart disease.

- Aortic regurgitation: Ventricular volume is increased as a result of aortic valve incompetence; systolic pressure is increased due to increased forward stroke volume in the face of normal or diminished peripheral vascular resistance. Chronic severe aortic regurgitation is often associated with eccentric hypertrophy.
- Mitral regurgitation: Ventricular volume is increased as a result of chronic mitral valve incompetence, thus contributing, by the Laplace relationship, to increased afterload. By contrast, in acute severe mitral regurgitation, afterload is reduced. Systolic pressure is usually normal. This valvular lesion is generally associated with eccentric hypertrophy, with a lower relative wall thickness (RWT) than seen in chronic aortic regurgitation.
- Aortic stenosis: The important hemodynamic impairment is severe pressure overload, occasioned by the marked increase in intracavitary systolic pressure. In the fully adapted LV, increased wall thickness permits normalization of afterload; LV cavity size is normal to slightly diminished. Severe aortic stenosis would be expected to be associated with concentric hypertrophy.

- Without compensatory ventricular remodeling, afterload "excess" in these three settings would be associated with a diminution in systolic function. However, in chronic valvular regurgitation, the ventricle remodels by series replication of sarcomeres to better bear the increased force associated with a larger circumference. These changes permit ejection of larger volumes of blood and maintenance of normal ejection fraction despite increased heart size and systolic pressure. These same principles of cardiac remodeling also apply to patients with longstanding hypertension, although ventricular systolic pressures are not expected to be as high as those encountered in severe valvular aortic stenosis. Increases in wall thickness, which often accompany hypertension, normalize wall stress and can keep ejection fraction in the normal range. Ganau and co-workers analyzed a group of untreated middle-aged hypertensive patients and characterized these individuals into 1 of 4 categories:
  - Normal (roughly 52% of the population)
  - Eccentric hypertrophy (28%)
  - Concentric hypertrophy (8%)
  - Concentric remodeling (12%)
- A review of other studies in the literature suggests that the proportion of hypertensive patients with hypertrophy is roughly 20%, although the prevalence varies considerably depending on race, age, and the prevalence of obesity. Patients with concentric hypertrophy appear to have a worse prognosis than those with eccentric hypertrophy; those with concentric remodeling, in one study, fared less well than patients with normal mass index and geometry.
- Remodeling in ischemic heart disease
- In many, if not the majority, of patients dying of acute myocardial infarction, pathologic evidence of infarct expansion is found. Following the initial infarction, remodeling of LV may be observed. The process comprises myocyte necrosis and subsequent elongation of the infarct zone (infarct expansion). In time, due to altered load on the noninfarcted LV, dilation and dysfunction may ensue. Factors that predispose to infarct expansion and subsequent remodeling include size of the infarction, Q-wave infarction, anterior/apical location, and persistent infarct-related artery occlusion. The pioneering series of studies by Pfeffer and Pfeffer, culminating in the Survival and Ventricular Enlargement (SAVE) study, demonstrated that remodeling could be attenuated by use of angiotensin-converting enzyme inhibitors.

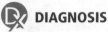 **DIAGNOSIS**

IMAGING

- Echocardiography provides a noninvasive method to assess cardiac remodeling in all forms of heart disease. Hearts can be characterized by whether hypertrophy is present and by the geometry or shape of the LV. Simple M-mode echocardiographic measurements of LV size and wall thickness in diastole are used to estimate the mass (weight) and to characterize LV shape.
- LV mass is estimated by an anatomically validated formula:
  $$\text{LV mass} = 0.8\, \{1.04\,[(STd + LVIDd + PWTd)]^3 - LVIDd^3]\} + 0.6g$$
  LV mass, computed from this formula, should be indexed to some measure of body size, either height or body surface area. Hypertrophy is defined as an LV mass index exceeding the value represented by the mean plus two standard deviations of a normal population. Indexation to height will characterize some obese subjects as having hypertrophy, and some clinicians therefore prefer this method of indexation. It has been repeatedly demonstrated that left ventricular hypertrophy carries an ominous prognosis, even when controlling for age and cardiac risk factors.
- The LV can also be characterized by its ratio of wall thickness to cavity size; this measure, the RWT provides an estimate of LV shape. When the RWT exceeds 0.45 (the value that represents mean plus two standard deviations of a normal population), concentric geometry is said to be present.
  $$RWT = 2 \times PWTd/LVIDd$$

Thus any population can be subcategorized as to whether hypertrophy is present and whether the geometry is concentric or eccentric (high LV mass index, normal RWT). The term *concentric remodeling* has been used to describe the subpopulation of individuals with normal LV mass index but concentric geometry. Some literature suggests that hypertensives with concentric remodeling have a worse prognosis than those with normal mass and geometry; other work suggests that these individuals have mild impairment of systolic function.

TREATMENT

SURGERY

The rationale underlying LV volume reduction surgery is the aforementioned Laplace relationship, which predicts a decrease in end-systolic stress (and an increase in systolic function) with reduction in cardiac size. Batista has reported favorable impact of such surgery (partial left ventriculectomy) on symptom status in patients with class IV patients with low ejection fractions (<20%). It stands to reason that mitral valve repair in patients with severe mitral regurgitation, to the extent that heart size is reduced by removal of the regurgitant leak, might achieve some of the same benefits.

REFERENCES

1. Aurigemma GP, Gaasch WH, Villegas B, et al. Noninvasive evaluation of left ventricular volume, mass, and systolic function. *Curr Probl Cardiol.* 1995;20:6:361–440.

2. Bach DS, Bolling SF. Improvement following correction of secondary mitral regurgitation in end stage cardiomyopathy with mitral annuloplasty. *Am J Cardiol.* 1996;78:966–971.

3. Batista RJ, Santos JL, Takeshita N, et al. Partial left ventriculectomy on left ventricular function in end stage heart disease. *J Cardiol Surg.* 1996;11:96–102.

4. Casale PN, Devereux RB, Milner M, et al. Valve of echocardiographic measurement of LV mass in predicting cardiovascular morbid events in hypertensive men. *Ann Intern Med.* 1986;105:173–178.

5. Devereux R, Reichek N. Echocardiographic determination of left ventricular mass in man. Anatomic validation of the method. *Circulation.* 1977;55:613–618.

6. Ganau A, Devereux R, Roman M, et al. Patterns of LV hypertrophy and geometric remodeling in essential hypertension. *J Am Coll Cardiol.* 1992;19:1550–1560.

7. Goldfine H, Aurigemma GP, Zile MR, et al. Left ventricular length-force-shortening relations before and after surgical correction of chronic mitral regurgitation. *J Am Coll Cardiol.* 1998;31:180–185.

8. Hutchins GM, Bulkley BH. Infarct expansion versus extension: Two different complications of acute myocardial infarction. *Am J Cardiol.* 1978;41:1127–1133.

9. Levy D, Garrison RJ, Savage D, et al. Prognostic implications of echocardiographically determined left ventricular mass in the Framingham heart study. *N Engl J Med.* 1990;322:1561–1666.

10. McKay RG, Pfeffer MA, Pasternak RC, et al. Left ventricular remodeling after myocardial infarction: A corollary to infarct expansion. *Circulation.* 1986;74:693–696.

11. Pfeffer JM, Pfeffer MA, Fletcher PJ, et al. Progressive ventricular remodeling in rat with myocardial infarction. *Am J Physiol.* 1991;260:H1406.

12. Pfeffer MA, Braunwald E. Ventricular remodeling after myocardial infarction: Experimental observations and clinical implications. *Circulation.* 1990;81:1161–1170.

13. Pfeffer MA, Braunwald E, Moye LA, et al. Effect of captopril on mortality and morbidity in patients with left ventricular dysfunction after myocardial infarction: Results of the survival and ventricular enlargement trial. *N Engl J Med.* 1992;27:669–677.

14. Ross J Jr. Afterload mismatch in aortic and mitral valve disease. *J Am Coll Cardiol.* 1985;5:811–826.

15. Sadler D, Aurigemma GP, Williams DW, et al. Systolic function in hypertensive men with concentric remodeling. *Hypertension.* 1997;30:777–781.

R

RENAL ARTERY STENOSIS
Jason S. Reingold
David S. Bader

 BASICS

DESCRIPTION
Renal artery stenosis (RAS) is a narrowing of the main renal artery and/or its major branches. This results in two major clinical syndromes, ischemic nephropathy and hypertension, and also increased the patient's cardiovascular (CV) mortality risk.

EPIDEMIOLOGY
- Age <20: Fibromuscular dysplasia (FMD; female predominance)
- Age >45: Atherosclerosis (male predominance)

Prevalence
- 5% of the general population (estimation is difficult due to lack of reliable screening tests)
- Up to 10–45% in patients with acute, severe, or refractory hypertension

RISK FACTORS
- Extremes of age (<20 and >55)
- White race compared to African Americans
- Coexisting atheromatous disease [coronary artery disease (CAD), peripheral vascular disease (PVD), cerebrovascular accident (CVA)]
- Tobacco use
- Diabetes mellitus

PATHOPHYSIOLOGY
Decrease in renal perfusion activates the renin–angiotensin system, thereby leading to hypertension.

ETIOLOGY
- Atherosclerosis: 90% of cases, usually involves the proximal 1/3 of the renal artery; progressive
- FMD: <10% of cases, most involve the media of distal renal artery

ASSOCIATED CONDITIONS
- Atherosclerosis
- Diabetes mellitus
- Malignant hypertension with flash pulmonary edema
- Ischemic nephropathy

 DIAGNOSIS

HISTORY
- Hypertension in persons <20 or >50 years of age
- Atherosclerotic disease elsewhere
- Hypertension: Acute onset or resistant to drug therapy
- Azotemia following initiation of therapy with angiotensin-converting enzyme (ACE) inhibitors
- Recurrent episodes of acute pulmonary edema or unexplained heart failure

Physical Exam
- Abdominal bruit (40%);
- Hemorrhagic (grade III or IV) retinopathy

TESTS
Lab
- Azotemia (with bilateral kidney involvement or following ACE-I initiation)
- Hypokalemia
- Proteinuria
- Elevated plasma renin activity: Sensitivity 50–80%, improved to 75–100% with administration of Captopril

Imaging
Noninvasive testing: generally less sensitive with more false negative studies, especially for the detection of FMD and bilateral stenosis
- Nonstimulated renal ultrasound: Identifies "salvageable" kidneys, up to 25% false-negative rate
- Captopril-stimulated renal ultrasound: Sensitivity 92%, specificity 93%, assesses hemodynamic significance of stenosis; limited utility in bilateral stenosis and severe renal impairment
- Duplex ultrasonography: Provides both anatomic and functional assessment, high positive and negative predictive values in a high-risk population (97%); time consuming and highly operator dependent; resistive index adds prognostic data for clinical response
- Magnetic resonance angiography with gadolinium: Sensitivity of 97% and specificity of 93% for stenoses >50%; better for atherosclerosis than FMD; no functional or clinical response data
- Spiral computed tomography (CT) with contrast injection: Sensitivity 98%, specificity 94%; undesirable for patients with renal insufficiency, does not provide functional or clinical response data

Diagnostic Procedures/Surgery
Renal angiography with digital subtraction: The gold standard with sensitivity 88%, specificity 90%; test is invasive and requires a high contrast load; best for FMD

DIFFERENTIAL DIAGNOSIS
Intrinsic arterial stenosis
- Renal artery infarction
- Embolus—cholesterol or atherosclerosis
- Vasculitis: Takayasu arteritis or polyarteritis nodosa
- Radiation-induced fibrosis
- Extrinsic arterial stenosis
- Tumor (e.g., pheochromocytoma)
- Cysts
- Neurofibromatosis

 TREATMENT

GENERAL MEASURES
Screening is based on pretest probability and only recommended if there is a plan to intervene
- Low suspicion for RAS: No further evaluation, even with noninvasive imaging due to low positive predictive value
- Moderate suspicion for RAS: Noninvasive testing with high sensitivity depending on local experience
- High suspicion for RAS: Renal arteriogram or renal vein renin

 MEDICATION (DRUGS)

- Many patients with this diagnosis can be treated successfully with medications alone.

First Line
- ACE inhibitors (with unilateral stenosis)
- Thiazide diuretics (in combination with other agents or for bilateral stenosis)
- Statins for atherosclerosis

Second Line
Calcium channel blockers (theoretical maintenance of glomerular filtration rate (GFR) due to afferent arteriole dilation)

SURGERY
Extremely limited randomized clinical trial data in regards to patient selection and outcomes
- Surgery: Aortorenal bypass rarely done except for individuals <60 with clearly progressive end organ disease
- Percutaneous angioplasty with stenting: Evolving as new standard of care with better patency and restenosis rates
  - DRASTIC (2000): No significant difference between balloon angioplasty and medical therapy alone in terms of blood pressure, daily drug doses, or renal function
  - Future trials: STAR, ASTRAL, CORAL to better study cardiac and renal outcomes

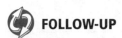 **FOLLOW-UP**

PROGNOSIS

Without intervention: 4-year survival is 21% lower compared to patients without renal artery stenosis. With angioplasty intervention:

- FMD: 58–80% have normalization of diastolic blood pressure (DBP) without meds, 35–75% are improved (15% decrease in DBP but still requiring medications); 7–10% fail (<15% decrease in DBP).
- Atherosclerosis: 15–22% have normalization of DBP without meds, 57–75% are improved, and 10–21% fail; restenosis rate in atheromatous disease is 19–25%, and 35% if the lesion is ostial

COMPLICATIONS

Procedural: Distal embolization, contrast nephropathy

PATIENT MONITORING

All patients should be followed closely for worsening hypertension, medication side effects, progressive atrophy of the kidney distal to the stenosis, and development of or worsening azotemia.

REFERENCES

1. Leier CV. Renal disorders and heart disease. In: Braunwald E, ed. *Heart Disease: A Textbook of Cardiovascular Medicine*, 5th ed. Philadelphia: WB Saunders, 1997:1914–1938.
2. Pohl MA. Renal artery stenosis, renal vascular hypertension, and ischemic nephropathy. In: Schrier RW, Gottschalk CW, eds. *Diseases of the Kidney*, 6th ed. Boston: Little, Brown, 1997:1367–1423.
3. Safian RD, Textor SC. Renal artery stenosis. *N Engl J Med*. 2001;344:431.
4. Van Jarrsveld BC, et al. The effect of balloon angioplasty on hypertension in atherosclerotic renal artery stenosis: DRASTIC. *N Engl J Med*. 2000; 342:1007.
5. Vasbinder GV, Nelemans PJ, Kessles AG. Diagnostic tests for renal artery stenosis: A meta-anaylsis. *Ann Intern Med*. 2001;135:401.
6. Zalunardo N, Tuttle KR. Atherosclerotic renal artery stenosis. *Curr Opin Nephrol Hypertens*. 2004;13:613.
7. Zoccali C, Mallamaci F, Finocchiaro P. Atherosclerotic renal artery stenosis: Epidemiology, outcomes, and clinical prediction rules. *J Am Soc Nephrol*. 2002;13:S179.

ADDITIONAL READING

- Bax L, et al. The benefit of stent placement and blood pressure and lipid lowering for the prevention of progression of renal dysfunction: STAR-study. *J Nephrol*. 2003:16:807.
- Slovut D, Olin JW. Fibromuscular dysplasia. *N Engl J Med*. 2004;350:1862.
- Textor SC. Pitfalls in imaging for renal artery stenosis. *Ann Intern Med*. 2004;141:730.

CODES
ICD9-CM
- 440.1 Renal artery stenosis
- 401.9 Hypertension
- 402.01 Malignant hypertension

R

RENAL FAILURE AND THE CARDIOVASCULAR SYSTEM

Ian S. Harris
David S. Bader

 BASICS

DESCRIPTION
- Renal failure is a syndrome characterized by a reduction in the glomerular filtration rate (GFR), regardless of cause, retention of nitrogenous waste products and alteration of extracellular fluid, electrolyte, and acid–base homeostasis. It may be subdivided into acute renal failure (ARF), which typically occurs over a period of hours to days, and chronic renal failure, or chronic kidney disease (CKD), which is characterized by a progressive decline in GFR over a period of at least 3 months. End-stage renal disease (ESRD) is said to be present when irreversible loss of renal function occurs, such that renal replacement therapy (RRT) is necessary.
- Cardiac disease is the major cause (>40%) of mortality and a major cause of morbidity in patients with ESRD. Cardiac arrest due to ventricular arrhythmias and acute myocardial infarction (MI) due to accelerated atherosclerosis, and congestive heart failure (CHF) with volume overload are the most common major cardiovascular events.
- Pericarditis and valvular disease also are prevalent.
- The coexistence of CKD and chronic heart failure has been termed the *cardiorenal syndrome* and represents an increasingly important and prevalent entity and therapeutic challenge.

EPIDEMIOLOGY
- The predominant age group is ≥65 years old.
- Males > Female
- Blacks > Whites > Asians

Incidence
- Acute renal failure occurs in 2–5% of hospitalized patients.
- Acute renal failure occurs in 4–15% of patients after cardiopulmonary bypass.
- Approximately 20,000 patients develop ESRD in the U.S. each year.

Prevalence
- In the U.S., approximately 11 million patients have CKD, and approximately 270,000 patients are currently undergoing dialysis; an additional 100,000 patients are living with a functional renal transplant.
- By 2010, the number of patients undergoing RRT is estimated to reach 600,000.

RISK FACTORS
Among patients with renal failure, a greater prevalence exists of the conventional cardiac risk factors:
- Diabetes
- Hypertension
- Tobacco
- Hyperlipidemia
- Male gender
- Family history of coronary artery disease (CAD)
- Obesity
- Metabolic abnormalities

PATHOPHYSIOLOGY
Causes of acute renal failure may be classified as prerenal, intrinsic renal, or postrenal.
- Prerenal ARF is caused by a reduction in effective renal blood flow. In patients with cardiac disease, this may be a consequence of the disease process or of treatment.
  - Overdiuresis
  - Low-output state/cardiogenic shock
- Intrinsic ARF results from injury to the glomeruli, renal blood vessels, tubules, or interstitium.
  - Acute tubular necrosis can occur from prolonged hypotension, as in cardiac arrest, or as a consequence of exposure to radiocontrast agents.
  - Acute glomerulonephritis with rapidly progressive renal failure may complicate infective endocarditis.
  - Renal embolism/atheroembolism may complicate cardiac catheterization.
- Ureteral or bladder outlet obstruction may result in postrenal ARF.

ETIOLOGY
- Diabetes
- Hypertension
- Renovascular disease
- Glomerulonephritis
- Polycystic kidney disease
- Other urologic causes

ASSOCIATED CONDITIONS
- Anemia: Diminished myocardial oxygen supply; increased cardiac workload
- CHF
  - Approximately 35% of ESRD patients
  - Both systolic and diastolic LV dysfunction
  - Probability of developing pulmonary edema requiring hospitalization after the initiation of dialysis is 10% per year.
- Left ventricular hypertrophy (LVH): Closely linked with hypertension, anemia, and pulmonary edema
- Dyslipidemia: Elevated triglycerides and lipoprotein (a); lowered high-density lipoprotein (HDL) cholesterol
- Hypertension: Either as a cause of renal failure or secondary to ESRD
- Pericarditis: Approximately 10% of hemodialysis patients
- Valvular heart disease:
  - Aortic calcification 30–55%
  - Hemodynamically significant aortic stenosis 10%
  - Mitral calcification 25–50%
  - Calcific mitral stenosis: Rare
  - Mitral regurgitation: Common

 DIAGNOSIS

SIGNS AND SYMPTOMS
- The diagnosis of an acute coronary syndrome may be difficult in patients with renal failure.
- Classical angina pectoris may not be present, as in the case of diabetic nephropathy.
- Silent ischemia may be present (15–35%).
- Many patients have nonatherosclerotic ischemic heart disease with typical symptoms of angina pectoris, but with patent coronary arteries.
- Baseline ECG abnormalities secondary to LVH or electrolyte abnormalities are prevalent, limiting accurate assessment of myocardial ischemia.

TESTS
Lab
- Cardiac troponin T and creatinine kinase (CK) and MB fraction are often elevated in patients with renal failure, without evidence of myocardial ischemia/injury (false positive).
- Cardiac troponin I is a sensitive marker of myocardial ischemia/injury in renal failure. However, the kinetics of its elimination are altered, resulting in a more prolonged elevation of serum concentration.
- Cardiac catheterization is the gold standard for defining coronary vasculature. This may lead to contrast-induced nephropathy (CIN), defined as an increase in creatinine of ≥1.0 mg/dL.
  - Incidence ~10%
  - Begins within 24–48 hours
  - Peaks in 3–5 days
  - Return to baseline creatinine in 7–10 days
  - Need for temporary dialysis is uncommon.
  - Potential risks for developing CIN:
    - Pre-existing renal insufficiency
    - Diabetes
    - Volume depletion
    - Age
    - CHF/volume overload
    - Hypertension
    - Dose of contrast (>50 cc)
    - High osmolarity contrast agent (controversial)
- Exercise ECG test: Limited role due to high prevalence of abnormal baseline ECGs
- Exercise and dipyridamole nuclear imaging tests:
  - High incidence of abnormal resting nuclear images in patients with ESRD
  - False-positive results with diffuse myocardial hypertrophy (may mimic a lateral wall MI)
  - Overall specificity 70–75%, sensitivity 80–88%, positive predictive value 70–75%
  - Exercise or dobutamine echocardiography: Limited data available; promising for the evaluation of CAD in renal failure

TREATMENT

GENERAL MEASURES

- Medical management of patients with renal failure and CAD follows the same general guidelines that have been established for patients with normal renal function.
- Specific attention is focused on the dosing of medications and careful monitoring of renal function.
- Dialysis
  - Advantages
    - Normalizes intravascular volume
    - Controls blood pressure
    - Corrects metabolic abnormalities
    - May improve LV systolic function
  - Disadvantages
    - Arteriovenous fistula increases cardiac output and may lead to high-output failure.
    - Higher risk of infective endocarditis
    - Dialysis-related hypotension
  - ECG abnormalities and dysrhythmias during dialysis
    - Decreased T-wave amplitude
    - Increased QRS amplitude
    - Prolonged or shortened QTc interval
    - Ischemic-like ST-segment and T-wave abnormalities
    - Atrial fibrillation/flutter (28%)
    - Ventricular ectopy (27%)
    - Nonsustained ventricular tachycardia (20%)
  - Peritoneal dialysis in CAD has the theoretic advantage of avoiding extremes in intravascular volume and electrolyte shifts, improved blood pressure control, avoidance of high-output states, and providing more constant acid–base equilibrium.
- Special therapy
  - Strategies for reducing the risk of radiocontrast-induced nephropathy:
    - Acetylcysteine
    - Hydration using an isotonic bicarbonate-containing solution (150 mEq/L $NaHCO_3$, 3 cc/kg/hr x 1 hr before contrast administration, followed by 1 cc/kg/hr x 6h after contrast administration).

MEDICATION (DRUGS)

Many cardiac medications are renally excreted. See standard references for a listing of renally excreted medications.

SURGERY

- Coronary artery bypass
  - Perioperative mortality rate of up to 10% in patients on dialysis
  - Dialysis can be performed on the day prior to surgery and immediately postoperatively or intraoperatively. Both approaches are safe and effective.
  - Risks for increased mortality and morbidity in patients with renal failure:
    - Creatinine >2 mg/dL
    - Elevated blood urea nitrogen (linear relationship)
    - Acidosis
    - Electrolyte abnormalities
    - Fluid retention
  - Relative immunocompromise leading to infection
  - Bleeding secondary dysfunctional platelets
- Percutaneous transluminal coronary angioplasty and coronary stenting:
  - Similar approach to the nonuremic patient
  - Initial technical results are as good, but restenosis rates may be higher.

FOLLOW-UP

PROGNOSIS

- Patients with ischemic heart disease (IHD) and ESRD have up to 50% greater mortality than patients with ESRD alone.
- LVH, LV dilatation, and systolic dysfunction confer greater mortality independent of age, sex, diabetes, and IHD.
- Patients with CHF at baseline or at initiation of therapy for ESRD have a reported median survival of 36 months, versus 62 months in those without CHF.
- Patients with recurrent CHF have a median survival of 29 months, versus 45 months in those without recurrent CHF.

PATIENT MONITORING

Standard guidelines for patients with established CAD are followed. Serum creatinine should be checked 2–4 days after initiating or altering potentially nephrotoxic medications (e.g., angiotensin-converting enzyme inhibitors [ACE-Is]).

REFERENCES
1. Boerrigter G, Burnett JC Jr. Cardiorenal syndrome in decompensated heart failure: Prognostic and therapeutic implications. *Curr Heart Fail Rep.* 2004;1:113–120.
2. Boudoulas H, Leier CV. Renal disorders and cardiovascular disease. In: Braunwald E, ed. *Heart disease: A textbook of cardiovascular medicine*, 6th ed. Philadelphia: WB Saunders, 2001: 2280–2297.
3. Foley RN, Harnett JD, Parfrey PS. Cardiovascular complications of end-stage renal disease. In: Schrier RW, Gottschalk CW, eds. *Diseases of the kidney*, 6th ed. Boston: Little, Brown, 1997: 2647–2660.
4. Hochrein J. The heart and the renal system. In: Topol EJ, ed. *Comprehensive cardiovascular medicine*. Philadelphia: Lippincott-Raven, 1998: 987–1000.
5. Kotlyar E, Keogh AM, Thavapalachandran S, et al. Prehydration alone is sufficient to prevent contrast-induced nephropathy after day-only angiography procedures: A randomised controlled trial. *Heart Lung Circ.* 2005;14:245–251.
6. Zagler A, Azadpour M, Mercado C, et al. N-acetylcysteine and contrast-induced nephropathy: A meta-analysis of 13 randomized trials. *Am Heart J.* 2006;151:140–145.

CODES

ICD9-CM

- 586 Renal failure
- 593.9 Renal insufficiency
- 414.01 Coronary artery disease

PATIENT TEACHING

Instructions regarding dietary regimen to optimize fluid and electrolyte status, particularly in those with CHF

R

REYNAUD'S SYNDROME

Shannon M. Dunlay

 BASICS

DESCRIPTION
- Primary Raynaud
- Secondary Raynaud is associated with another condition (rheumatologic, infection, drug, endocrine)
- Raynaud syndrome was originally described as cold-induced digital vasospasm.
  - Has been implicated in systemic vasospasm
  - Can produce vasospasm in heart, lung, kidney
- Associated with myocardial infarction (MI) in normal coronaries
- Implicated in cold-induced coronary vasospasm or "coronary Raynaud syndrome"
- Possible association with Prinzmetal angina

EPIDEMIOLOGY
- Raynaud phenomenon occurs in 3–5% of the population.
- MI with normal coronaries occurs in 2–12% of cases.
- Vasospastic angina is implicated in 10% of MI in Asian population, other populations less prevalent.
- Inducible ischemia is present on cold-stress myocardial scintigraphy in 57% patients with primary Raynaud syndrome.

RISK FACTORS
- Associated connective tissue disease [scleroderma, systemic lupus erythematosus (SLE), polymyositis]
- Genetic link between Raynaud migraine and coronary artery disease found in epidemiologic studies

PATHOPHYSIOLOGY
- Not fully elucidated
- Primary Raynaud syndrome associated with abnormal α-adrenergic response
- May involve cycle of repeated vasospasm with reperfusion endothelial injury resulting in chronic ischemia and vascular fibrosis

ETIOLOGY
- Raynaud syndrome is an exaggerated response to cold or stress.
- Possible immunologic, inflammatory, neurologic components to response

ASSOCIATED CONDITIONS
- Migraine headache
- Connective tissue diseases:
  - Systemic scleroderma
  - SLE
  - Polymyositis/dermatomyositis
  - Rheumatoid arthritis

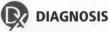 **DIAGNOSIS**

SIGNS AND SYMPTOMS
- Ischemic chest pain symptoms in response to cold in patient with history of Raynaud syndrome or connective tissue disease:
  - Substernal chest pressure
  - Other symptoms: Radiation to arms/neck, associated dyspnea, diaphoresis, nausea

History
- Past history of connective tissue disease
- Prior cold, painful, white fingers in response to cold (digital Raynaud syndrome)
- Prior history of angina/coronary artery disease (CAD)

Physical Exam
- Cardiac exam
- Digital exam: Digital pitting scars, ulcers, nailfold capillary microscopy

TESTS
- EKG: Examine for changes consistent with coronary ischemia:
  - ST elevation or depression
  - T-wave inversions
  - Q-waves indicative of prior MI
- Cold-induced transient MI has been demonstrated with dipyridamole testing.

DIFFERENTIAL DIAGNOSIS
- CAD-associated angina
- Other variant angina (Prinzmetal, cocaine-induced spasm)
- Nonischemic chest pain (pericarditis, musculoskeletal, pulmonary)

TREATMENT

- Initial stabilization:
  - Remove from cold.
  - Treat chest pain according to ischemic chest pain protocol.
  - If known variant angina/Raynaud syndrome, consider use of calcium channel blocker or vasodilator such as nitroglycerin.

 FOLLOW-UP

Appropriate cardiology and rheumatology follow-up should be established.

REFERENCES

1. Ammann P, Marschall S, Kraus M, et al. Characteristics and prognosis of myocardial infarction in patients with normal coronary arteries. *Chest*. 117:333–338.
2. Braunwald E, ed. *Heart disease: A textbook of cardiovascular medicine*, 5th ed. Philadelphia, PA: WB Saunders; 1996.
3. Candell-Riera J, Armadans-Gil L, Simeon CP, et al. Comprehensive noninvasive assessment of cardiac involvement in limited systemic sclerosis. *Arthritis Rheumatism*. 39:1138–1145.
4. Gordon MM, Madhol R. Fatal myocardial necrosis. *Ann Rheumat Dis*. 58:198–199.
5. Ho M, Belch J. Raynaud's phenomenon: State of the art 1998. *Scand J Rheumatol*. 27:319–322.
6. Lekakis J, Mavrikakis M, Emmanuel M. Cold-induced coronary Raynaud's phenomenon in patients with systemic sclerosis. *Clin Exper Rheumatol*. 16:135–140.
7. Riemakasten G, Opitz C, Audring H. Beware of the heart: The multiple picture of cardiac involvement in myositis. *Rheumatology*. 1999;38(11):1153–1157.
8. Williams FM, Cherkas LF, Spector TD, et al. A common genetic factor underlies hypertension and other cardiovascular disorders. *BMC Cardiovasc Dis*. 2004;4(1):20.

CODES
ICD9-CM
- 443.0 Raynaud syndrome
- 413.1 Prinzmetal angina/variant angina

NURSING CONSIDERATIONS
Nursing Diagnosis
- Chest pain
- Raynaud phenomenon

Key Outcomes
MI

Nursing Interventions
Ensure that patient is chest pain–free; provider should be notified if patient has recurrent chest pain.

Monitoring
Appropriate monitoring via telemetry and for recurrent chest pain should be performed on all patients presenting with chest pain thought to be due to myocardial ischemia.

PATIENT TEACHING
Prevention and avoidance of triggers is key for patients with Raynaud syndrome.

Prevention
- Avoid exposure to cold.
- Stress reduction
- Avoid sympathomimetic drugs and caffeine.

R

RHEUMATIC FEVER

Deryk McDowell
Steven C. Herrmann
Bernard R. Chaitman

BASICS

DESCRIPTION
- Rheumatic fever (RF) is a systemic disease with multiorgan involvement. None of its manifestations, except for carditis, leads to permanent damage. In 1944, the Jones criteria were introduced to guide the diagnosis of acute rheumatic fever (ARF). Those criteria were modified in 1956, revised in 1965 and 1984, and then updated in 1992. They are divided into major and minor criteria.
- Major criteria
  - Carditis
    - A pancarditis that involves the endocardium, myocardium, and/or pericardium
    - Carditis occurs in 40–50% of the initial attacks of RF. It is the most specific finding of acute RF.
    - Valvulitis is the most characteristic component of rheumatic carditis, and the mitral valve is almost always affected. Myocarditis and pericarditis in the absence of valvulitis is not likely due to RF.
    - Severity is variable and can result in death from cardiac failure; however, predominant effect is subsequent scarring of the heart valves.
    - Carditis is more apt to recur if RF occurs in patients who have had carditis in the initial attack, thus increasing the risk of severe residual heart disease.
  - Arthritis
    - Mainly affects large joints and is typically asymmetrical and migratory.
    - Occurs in about 75% of patients during the acute stage of the disease; most common manifestation of acute RF but the least specific.
    - Joints are left without sequelae.
  - Chorea (Sydenham chorea or St. Vitus dance)
    - Characterized clinically by purposeless movements, motor weakness, and emotional instability.
    - Occurs in approximately 20% of patients with acute RF.
    - The latent period between streptococcal infection and chorea is 1–6 months. As a result, by the time the chorea is manifest, antibodies and acute phase reactants are normal.
    - Symptoms typically persist for up to 2 weeks then resolve spontaneously.
  - Subcutaneous nodules
    - Seen rarely in acute RF (<3% of cases)
    - Range in diameter from 0.5–2 cm; occur on the extensor surface of bony prominences
    - Occur with severe carditis
  - Erythema marginatum
    - Occurs in about 5% of patients with acute RF
    - An area of erythema with an advancing edge and clearing center
    - Transient and found mainly over the trunk and inner aspects of the thighs and arms
    - Nonpruritic and blanches on pressure
- Minor criteria
  - Fever
  - Arthralgia
  - Elevated acute phase reactants (ESR, CRP)
  - Prolonged PR interval

- Laboratory evidence indicating acute infection
  - Erythrocyte sedimentation rate (ESR) is almost always elevated (>60 mm/h). Congestive heart failure lowers ESR, but not to normal levels.
  - C-reactive protein
  - CBC usually demonstrates a moderate anemia. Leukocyte count is increased to moderate degree.

Pregnancy Considerations
ARF tends to recur during pregnancy.

EPIDEMIOLOGY
- Due to a causal relationship, the epidemiology of RF is identical to that of group A streptococcal pharyngitis.
- Predominant age: School-age group has the highest attack rate.

Incidence
- Incidence of RF in the U.S. is estimated at <2 cases per 100,000 population.
- In developing countries, the risk of acute RF is >100 cases per 100,000 population.

Prevalence
- RF is still the predominant cause of heart disease in children.
- In the U.S., RF maintains its position as the leading cause of postnatally acquired heart disease in children.

RISK FACTORS
- Lower standards of living, especially overcrowding
- Lower socioeconomic status
- Lack of access to adequate health care

Genetics
- The incidence of RF after streptococcal pharyngitis in patients who have suffered previous episodes of RF is approximately 50%. When this is compared with the 3% occurrence rate in virgin hosts, it suggests some host factors that increase susceptibility to the disease.
- Some epidemiologic studies indicate a familial predisposition to the disease.
  - A specific B-cell alloantigen has been described in almost all patients with RF (99%) compared with only 14% in control subjects.
  - Susceptibility also has been linked to HLA DR-1, -2, -3, and -4 haplotypes in various ethnic groups.

PATHOPHYSIOLOGY
- Despite extensive study, the exact pathogenesis of acute RF remains ill-defined.
- It is most likely caused by an autoimmune reaction induced by similarity of certain streptococcal antigens to various human tissues.
  - Epitopes are shared between cardiac myosin and streptococcal M proteins.
  - Structural similarities also exist between streptococcal M proteins and heart valves, sarcolemmal membrane proteins, synovium, and articular cartilage.

ETIOLOGY
The evidence that group A streptococcus is the agent causing RF is indirect but strong.
- Immunologic evidence: Initial as well as recurrent attacks of RF do not occur without a streptococcal antibody response.

- Clinical evidence: Septic sore throat preceding ARF and its recurrences has been recognized clinically for over 100 years.
- Prophylactic evidence: Convincing evidence is provided by the prevention of RF by penicillin therapy.

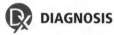 DIAGNOSIS

SIGNS AND SYMPTOMS
- Signs and symptoms of congestive heart failure (CHF) in cases of carditis
- The unequivocal signs of carditis in a patient with RF are:
  - An organic heart murmur that was not previously present
  - Pericardial friction rub or effusion
  - Cardiac enlargement with or without heart failure
- Arthralgia and arthritis
- Chorea
  - Involuntary, uncoordinated, purposeless movements.
  - The tongue is affected, with an inability to keep it protruded.
  - The handgrip often is unsustained (milkmaid hands).
  - Flexion of the wrist together with dorsiflexion of the interphalangeal joints gives "silver fork" deformity.
- Skin manifestations: Subcutaneous nodules and erythema marginatum
- Fever

Physical Exam
See Valvular heart disease.

TESTS
- No specific clinical, laboratory, or radiological test can by itself confirm the diagnosis of acute RF. The diagnosis of acute RF is made on clinical grounds based on presence of evidence of a previous group A streptococcal infection and the Jones criteria.
- Evidence of an antecedent group A streptococcal infection is required to entertain the diagnosis of acute RF.
- In the presence of evidence suggesting a prior group A streptococcal infection, then the following are suggestive of a high likelihood of acute RF:
  - The presence of 2 major criteria
  - The presence of 1 major and 2 minor criteria

Lab
- Elevated acute phase reactants are nonspecific.
- ESR is useful for monitoring the course of disease, because it typically returns to normal as rheumatic activity ebbs.
- Evidence should exist of a prior group A streptococcal infection to confirm the diagnosis of RF. This can come in the form of:
  - Recovery of the organism on culture
  - Elevated or rising antistreptococcal antibody titers, such as antistreptolysin O and antideoxyribonuclease B. These titers may remain elevated for weeks or months.

Imaging
Echocardiography might allow earlier diagnosis.

Pathologic Findings

2 main lesions characterize RF.

- Exudative-degenerative lesion
  - Consists of edema of the ground substance and fragmentation of collagen fibers as well as cellular infiltrate
  - Persists for 2–3 weeks and responds to anti-inflammatory agents
- Proliferative lesion (Aschoff nodule)
  - The myocardial nodule is usually oval in shape.
  - A paravascular aggregation of large multinucleated cells is present, with basophilic cytoplasm.
  - Many of them have a characteristic owl-eye nucleus.
  - The origin of those nodules is controversial.

DIFFERENTIAL DIAGNOSIS

- Fever and arthritis
  - Juvenile rheumatoid arthritis
  - Infective endocarditis
  - Sickle cell anemia
  - Polyarthritis
  - Immune complex disease
- Carditis
  - Functional murmurs
  - Myocarditis
  - Pericarditis
  - Mitral valve prolapse

TREATMENT

GENERAL MEASURES

Bed rest is recommended because it tends to lessen joint pain.

MEDICATION (DRUGS)

First Line

Therapy for acute RF is targeted toward eradicating the presence of group A streptococci from the host and relieving symptoms of inflammation and carditis.

- Antistreptococcal antibiotic therapy
- Penicillin G Benzathine: 600,000 units for patients weighing <60 pounds (IM once)
  - Penicillin G: 1,200,000 units for patients weighing >60 pounds
  - Penicillin V 500mg BID orally for 10 days
  - Erythromycin, clarithromycin, or azithromycin are used for penicillin-allergic patients.
- Aspirin or salicylates
  - Indicated in patients with arthritis; usually results in rapid resolution of symptoms and signs
  - Usual dosage is 90–120 mg/kg/day divided, given at 4-hour intervals.
  - If joint pain persists for 24 hours after initiation of salicylate therapy, diagnosis of RF should be questioned.
  - Patients without carditis are treated for 1 month or until clinical or laboratory evidence of resolution.
  - Dose should be tapered to prevent a rebound of inflammatory manifestations

- Corticosteroids
  - Prednisone 1–2mg/kg/day is the usual dose.
  - Reserved for patients with severe carditis accompanied by CHF
  - No evidence that it terminates the disease or prevents residual heart damage
- Diuretics, digoxin, and afterload reduction are indicated for CHF due to acute RF. Digoxin should be used cautiously, because toxicity may occur with conventional dosing in the presence of myocarditis.

Second Line

- Sulfadiazine
  - 0.5 g once daily for patients weighing <60 pounds
  - 1 g once daily for patients weighing >60 pounds
- Erythromycin: 250 mg PO b.i.d.
- For individuals allergic to penicillin:
  - Erythromycin: 20–49 mg/kg/day (PO for 10 days)
  - Azithromycin (PO for 5 days)
    - 500 mg on 1st day
    - 250 mg/day for the next 4 days

FOLLOW-UP

- Penicillin G Benzathine: 1,200,000 units every 4 weeks for patients weighing >60 pounds IM every 4 weeks
- Penicillin V 250 mg b.i.d. PO
- Duration of treatment depends on severity of disease.
  - RF with carditis or residual cardiac lesion: ≥10 years since the last episode at least until the age of 40 years
  - RF with carditis but no residual cardiac lesion: 10 years or until adulthood, whichever is longer
  - RF without carditis: 5 years or until the age of 21 years, whichever is longer
- Endocarditis prophylaxis: Patients with a history of rheumatic valvular heart disease require lifelong short-term antibiotic prophylaxis to prevent infective endocarditis prior to surgical or dental procedures.
  - In general, antibiotic regimens used for secondary prevention of RF are inadequate for the prevention of endocarditis.
  - Current guidelines recommend clindamycin, azithromycin, or clarithromycin for endocarditis prophylaxis in patients who are taking penicillin for secondary prevention of RF.

PROGNOSIS

The presence or absence of carditis is an important determinant of the course and prognosis of ARF.

COMPLICATIONS

- Rheumatic valvular heart disease
- CHF
- Recurrent ARF

PATIENT MONITORING

- Patients should be monitored closely for evidence of heart failure.
- The sedimentation rate as well as C-reactive protein can be followed as a marker of activity.

REFERENCES

1. Bonow RO, Carabello B, de Leon AC Jr, et al. ACC/AHA 2006 guidelines for the management of patients with valvular heart disease: A report of the American College of Cardiology/American Heart Association Task Force on Practice Guidelines (Writing Commitee to Revise the 1998 Guidelines for the Management of Patients With Valvular Heart Disease). American College of Cadiology Web Site. Available at: http://content.onlinejacc.org/cgi/reprint/48/3/e1
2. Carapetis JR, McDonald M, Wilson NJ. Acute rheumatic fever. *Lancet.* 2005;366:155–168.
3. Dajani AS, Taubert KA, Wilson W, et al. Prevention of bacterial endocarditis: Recommendations by the American Heart Association. *JAMA.* 1997;277: 1794.
4. Zipes D, Libby P, Bonow RO, et al., eds. *Braunwald's heart disease: A textbook of cardiovascular medicine*, 7th ed. Philadelphia: Elsevier Saunders, 2005.

MISCELLANEOUS

See also: Individual valvular heart diseases

CODES

ICD9-CM

391.0

PATIENT TEACHING

Diet

Low-sodium diet if heart failure is evident

Activity

- Patients must remain in bed during the acute febrile episode.
- Light activity can be allowed once the acute febrile episode is over.
- Patients with carditis should have rest until the signs of cardiac inflammation subside.

Prevention

- Primary prevention: Prompt recognition and treatment represent primary RF prevention.
- Secondary prevention: For patients who have had a previous episode of RF, continuous antistreptococcal prophylaxis results in secondary prevention.

R

RHEUMATOID ARTHRITIS AND THE HEART

Cheryl Russo

 BASICS

DESCRIPTION

Cardiac manifestations include the following:
- Pericarditis: A spectrum from asymptomatic disease to cardiac compression
- Valvular disease, usually regurgitation; in order of decreasing prevalence, mitral, aortic, tricuspid, and pulmonary
- Coronary arteritis (rarely causes significant dysfunction)
- Myocarditis
- Conduction pathway disease (most commonly first-degree heart block)
- Aortic arch disease
- Pulmonary hypertension

EPIDEMIOLOGY
- Pericarditis
  - Most common cardiac lesion in rheumatoid arthritis (RA) patients
  - 11–50% of patients have pericarditis.
  - <1% develop cardiac compression
- Valvular
  - At autopsy, rheumatoid granulomata involve valves in 3–5% of patients.
  - Echocardiography reveals 13% with mitral valve abnormalities.
- Coronary arteritis
  - At autopsy, up to 20% of RA patients have coronary arteritis.
- Myocarditis
  - Up to 20% of patients have nonspecific, focal myocarditis.
- Conduction disease
  - Up to 10% of patients have various degrees of heart block.
- Aortic arch disease
  - At autopsy, up to 5% of patients have involvement.
  - Complicated by aneurysm formation

RISK FACTORS
Pericarditis is associated with acute disease with other extra-articular involvement, usually in seropositive patients.

ETIOLOGY
- In general, disease is fibrinous, granulomatous, and complement mediated.
- Pericarditis
  - Fibrinous pericarditis
  - Fibrinous adhesions
  - Rheumatoid granuloma/nodular type changes
- Valvular disease
  - Nonspecific valvulitis with diffuse thickening and fibrosis
  - Spares peripheral portions of the valve
  - May be identical to rheumatoid nodule versus nongranulomatous valve inflammation
- Vascular disease
  - Involvement usually limited to smaller intramyocardial arteries
  - Pulmonary vasculitis
- Cardiomyopathy
  - Drug-induced
  - Myocarditis

ASSOCIATED CONDITIONS
- Pleural effusion (found in half of patients with pericarditis and cardiac compression)
- Pericardial effusion
- Bacterial endocarditis (rarely, in association with valvular disease)

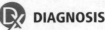 **DIAGNOSIS**

SIGNS AND SYMPTOMS
- Cardiac disease is often clinically inconspicuous and rarely life threatening.
- Often "silent heart disease" with 3 alterations typical of RA patients in absence of symptoms: Posterior pericardial effusion, aortic root alterations, valvular thickening
- Pericarditis: Chest pain, peripheral edema, orthopnea, friction rub, pericardial effusion (edema, dyspnea, tamponade, pulsus paradoxus)

TESTS
Pericardiocentesis: Pericardial fluid reveals low glucose, low complement, variable white blood cell stain, culture, and sensitivities (acid-fast bacillus, fungal)

Lab
Tests for rheumatoid arthritis
- Rheumatoid factor, inflammatory indices (erythrocyte sedimentation rate, C-reactive protein)

Imaging
- ECG: 1st-degree atrioventricular block, precordial ST segment elevation with pericarditis
- Echocardiography: Pericardial effusion, valvular disease, cardiomyopathy

DIFFERENTIAL DIAGNOSIS
- Pericardial disease
  - Pericarditis (infectious, idiopathic)
  - Pericardial effusion (infectious, inflammatory, idiopathic, neoplastic, radiation-induced)
- Valvular disease
  - Endocarditis
  - Liebman-Sachs
  - Mitral valve prolapse
  - Acute valvular incompetence
- Myocardial disease
  - Ischemic
  - Drug-induced
  - Alcohol-related
  - Infiltrative disorders

TREATMENT

GENERAL MEASURES
- Pericarditis: Usually resolves with aggressive medical therapy for RA [steroids, nonsteroidal anti-inflammatory drugs (NSAIDs), disease-modifying agents]
- Cardiomyopathy: Appropriate heart failure medicines

 MEDICATION (DRUGS)

- NSAIDs
- Corticosteroids
- Disease-modifying agents
- Immunosuppressives

SURGERY
- Pericardial effusion with compression: Pericardiocentesis, surgical decompression/window
- Constrictive pericarditis: Pericardiectomy
- Valvular: Rarely, involvement produces hemodynamic valve incompetence requiring valve replacement.

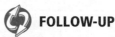 FOLLOW-UP

DISPOSITION
Admission Criteria
Follows clinical presentation

PROGNOSIS
Pericarditis: Favorable, although marker for decreased survival

PATIENT MONITORING
Pericarditis: Watch for recurrence (15%) or pericardial effusion.

REFERENCES
1. Coblyn JS, Weinblatt ME. Rheumatic diseases and the heart. In: Braunwald E, ed. *A textbook of cardiovascular medicine*, 5th ed. Philadelphia: WB Saunders, 1997:1776–1778.
2. Corrao S, Salli L, et al. Cardiac involvement in rheumatoid arthritis: Evidence of silent heart disease. *Eur Heart J*. 1995;16:253–256.
3. Mione S, Valentini G, Giunta A, et al. Cardiac involvement in RA: An echocardiographic study. *Cardiology*. 1993;83:234–239.

PATIENT TEACHING
Organization: Arthritis Foundation, 1330 West Peachtree Street, Atlanta, GA 30309; www.arthritis.org

R

SARCOIDOSIS AND THE HEART

Cheryl Russo

 BASICS

DESCRIPTION

Cardiac involvement occurs in 25% of patients with systemic sarcoidosis and includes the following:

- Congestive heart failure (CHF): Right-sided secondary to pulmonary disease; left-sided includes systolic and diastolic disease; global versus segmental abnormalities
- Chest pain: Associated with abnormal functional study and normal angiogram
- Pericardial disease: Rare, yet may be complicated by constriction or tamponade
- Valvular disease: Secondary to papillary muscle involvement
- Conduction abnormality: Complete heart block is the most common clinical manifestation of cardiac involvement; right and left bundle branch block also may be seen.
- Ventricular arrhythmias: Ventricular tachycardia is the second most common presentation.
- Ventricular aneurysms: More common on the left than the right
- Coronary artery damage involving the intramural arteries

EPIDEMIOLOGY

Incidence

- CHF: 30–40%
- Valvular involvement: <3%
- Complete heart block: 25%
- Ventricular tachycardia: 20% (11–50%)
- Ventricular aneurysm: 8–10%

RISK FACTORS

Chronic steroid use may increase the rate of ventricular aneurysm. Ventricular aneurysms increase the risk of ventricular tachycardia.

ETIOLOGY

- No HLA type association
- Japanese disease with clinical variations: Higher incidence of sudden death and more infiltrative disease with associated high amount of replacement fibrosis
- Noncaseating granulomas involve the left ventricular free wall most often, followed by the ventricular septum, right ventricle, papillary muscle, right atrium, and left atrium.
- Surrounding involvement compresses/narrows the lumen of intramural arteries, producing chest pain. It serves as a focus for abnormal automaticity in ventricular arrhythmias. Replacement fibrosis narrows ventricular walls, increasing risk of aneurysm.

ASSOCIATED CONDITIONS

- Hypercalcemia: Secondary to sarcoidosis
- Hypokalemia: Secondary to steroids

 DIAGNOSIS

SIGNS AND SYMPTOMS

- Must have high clinical suspicion.
- Only 50% of patients with cardiac involvement of sarcoidosis are identified premortem.
- Physical examination for multiorgan involvement: Skin involvement (lupus pernio [rash on nose, cheek, hands], erythema nodosum), hepatomegaly, lymphadenopathy, pulmonary involvement (dyspnea)
- Presentation ranges: Asymptomatic with abnormal chest radiograph, fever, weight loss
- Cardiac presentations include complete heart block (syncope), ventricular tachycardia, heart failure, sudden death, and chest pain.

TESTS

- Kveim-Siltzbach test, pulmonary function test, ophthalmologic examination to determine extent of sarcoid involvement
- Exercise stress test, Holter monitor for patients with cardiac involvement
- Endomyocardial biopsy: 20–30% yield secondary to patchy disease or lower right ventricle involvement

Lab
- Serum calcium
- Angiotensin-converting enzyme (ACE) level: Elevated in 80% patients with sarcoidosis

Imaging
- ECG: Arrhythmia, conduction abnormalities
- Chest radiograph: Right heart enlargement, pulmonary infiltrate, hilar adenopathy, pericardial effusion
- Echocardiography: Septal thickening, pericardial effusion, ventricular dysfunction, valve regurgitation, ventricular aneurysm
- Gallium scan: Active disease in lung and extrathoracic locations

DIFFERENTIAL DIAGNOSIS
- Heart failure: Ischemic heart disease; other infiltrative disease (amyloid)
- Chest pain: Acute myocardial infarction (MI); pericarditis
- Conduction abnormalities: Ischemic heart disease; medication-induced block

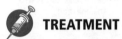
TREATMENT

GENERAL MEASURES
- Correlate with presentation.
- Pacemaker, defibrillator, heart failure medications, antiarrhythmic medications (caution with calcium and potassium abnormalities)

MEDICATION (DRUGS)

Steroids are associated with aneurysm formation, yet are known to change the course of the disease when started early.

SURGERY
- Cardiac transplantation
- Valvular repair

FOLLOW-UP

DISPOSITION
Admission Criteria
- Determined by clinical presentation
- Heart failure, arrhythmia, conduction abnormalities

PROGNOSIS
- In general, the mortality rate of sarcoidosis alone is low, but very high with cardiac involvement.
- Average survival with clinically significant disease is 1–2 years.
- Major causes of death are as follows:
  - Sudden death (approaches 65% with significant disease)
  - Heart failure
    - Pulmonary fibrosis
    - Pulmonary hemorrhage secondary to aspergilloma

PATIENT MONITORING
- Physical examination
- ECG
- Holter monitor
- Echocardiography

REFERENCES
1. Shammas RL, Movahed A. Sarcoidosis of the heart. *Clin Cardiol*. 1993;16:462–472.
2. Sharma OP, Maheshwari A, Thaker K. Myocardial sarcoidosis. *Chest*. 1993;103:253–258.

PATIENT TEACHING
Organization: American Lung Association, 1740 Broadway, New York, NY 10019-4374; (212)315–8700, www.lungusa.org

SCLERODERMA AND THE HEART

Christopher K. Dyke

 BASICS

DESCRIPTION

Scleroderma is a multisystem disorder of unknown etiology characterized by cutaneous and visceral tissue fibrosis. There are two subsets:

- Diffuse or progressive systemic sclerosis (SSc) includes early and serious visceral involvement.
- Limited sclerosis (CREST; calcinosis, Raynaud phenomenon, esophageal dysmotility, sclerodactyly, and telangiectasia) is associated with a long delay in visceral involvement. Survival is closely linked to the visceral involvement of the disease.
- Conduction System Disease
  - Common and often represents first manifestation of cardiac disease; may precede cutaneous lesions
  - Electrocardiographic abnormalities reported in up to 50% in some series (nonspecific ST-T wave, low voltage, right and left ventricular hypertrophy)
  - Pseudoinfarction patterns have been observed on electrocardiogram (ECG) in the posteroapical and anteroseptal regions
  - Various degrees of heart block as well as rhythm disturbances (supraventricular tachycardia, ventricular tachycardia, bradyarrhythmias) are common.
  - Fibrosis of sinoatrial node (most common), atrioventricular atrioventricular (AV) node, or His-Purkinje system seen at autopsy
  - Pericardium
  - Pericarditis is common in systemic sclerosis (up to 70% of autopsy series)
  - Effusion has been demonstrated on echocardiography in up to 40% of patients, whereas only one third are symptomatic; reports of pericardial tamponade have been infrequent
  - No evidence of immune complexes or complement activation in pericardial fluid has been found.
  - Found in limited scleroderma and mixed connective tissue disease, but not as frequent as diffuse SSc
  - Constrictive pericarditis reported as a single case
  - Pericardial disease does not appear to affect overall mortality in SSc

- Myocardium
  - Symptoms of myocardial involvement are usually those of CHF, although clinically evident myocardial disease is not common.
  - Cardiomyopathy attributable to myocardial fibrosis is found in less than 10% of the diffuse variant.
  - Myocarditis has been described but is considered rare.
  - Postmortem lesions are seen in up to 80% and affect all chambers of the heart without coronary artery involvement.
- Valvular Heart Disease
  - Rarely produces lesions that affect only valvular tissue (other etiology should be sought if valvular disease present)
- Coronary Artery Disease
  - Involvement appears limited to the microvasculature due to changes in small arteries and arterioles leading to "intramyocardial Raynaud phenomenon" as supported by catheterization studies demonstrating normal arteries with reduced perfusion and delayed runoff.
  - Myocardial perfusion defects are common in diffuse scleroderma.
  - Echocardiographic and reversible perfusion abnormalities have been demonstrated in up to 70% of patients when exposed to a cold stimulus, but the clinical significance remains unclear.
  - Angina, myocardial infarction, and sudden death have been described.
- Pulmonary Hypertension
  - More common with limited disease variant
  - In one report, 67% of patients with SSc who underwent cardiac catheterization had evidence of at least mild pulmonary hypertension.

EPIDEMIOLOGY

- Women are affected 3 times as often as men.
- SSc is more frequent and severe in young black women.
- Rarity of disease and lack of a specific diagnostic test may contribute to an underestimation of incidence and prevalence.

Incidence

The incidence of scleroderma increases with age and peaks in the 3rd to 5th decades of life.

Prevalence

- 13.4 to 75 per 100,000 persons
- The highest reported prevalence per ethnic group is found among the Choctaw Native Americans.

RISK FACTORS

Some studies have shown an association with HLA-DR1, -DR2, -DR3, and -DR5. Environmental factors associated with SSc and sclerodermalike illnesses include coal and gold mining (silica dust), polyvinyl chloride, benzine, toluene, and rapeseed oil.

ETIOLOGY

Unknown

ASSOCIATED CONDITIONS

CREST, myopathy, symmetric polyarthritis, renal failure, sicca syndrome, hypothyroidism, trigeminal neuralgia, and impotence

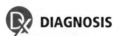 **DIAGNOSIS**

SIGNS AND SYMPTOMS

Dyspnea, orthopnea, paroxysmal nocturnal dyspnea, palpitations, angina pectoris, distant heart sounds, elevated jugular venous pressure, pulsus paradoxus, precordial murmur, friction rub, pulmonary rales

TESTS

- Primary evaluation of the cardiac status should be a 12-lead ECG and 24-hour ECG monitoring, followed by a thallium scan if indicated.
- Holter monitoring increases diagnostic yield of ECG abnormalities and is more sensitive compared with exercise or resting 12-lead ECG.

Lab
- Antinuclear antibody is found in up to 95% of patients.
- Erythrocyte sedimentation rate may be elevated.
- Hypergammaglobulinemia [immunoglobulin (IgG)] is found in approximately 50% of patients.
- Rheumatoid factor in low titer is present in 25% of patients.

Imaging
- Echocardiography is best for suspicion of pericarditis and pericardial effusion.
- Nuclear perfusion studies often demonstrate myocardial perfusion deficits of unknown clinical significance.

Pathologic Findings
- Range from focal myocardial involvement with contraction band necrosis to diffuse fibrotic replacement of both ventricles. These lesions occur in the absence of intraluminal coronary artery disease. An abnormal immune response has been indicated.
- It is suggested that contraction band necrosis in the myocardium is secondary to vascular spasm of the coronary arteries, which is similar to Raynaud phenomenon occurring in the distal extremities.

DIFFERENTIAL DIAGNOSIS
- In early disease, SSc may initially be confused with other connective tissue diseases such as rheumatoid arthritis, systemic lupus erythematosus, polymyositis, or MCTD.
- Because SSc has numerous cardiac manifestations, the differential diagnosis includes the potential etiologies for each respective manifestation.

 TREATMENT

GENERAL MEASURES
SSc cannot be cured, but treatment of involved organ system can relieve symptoms and improve function.

 MEDICATION (DRUGS)

- In uncontrolled studies, D-penicillamine reduced skin thickening and prevented the development of significant organ involvement.
- Glucocorticoids are indicated in those patients with inflammatory myositis or pericarditis, but high doses of steroids may play a role in precipitating renal crisis.
- Antiplatelet therapy may play a role in the treatment of SSc, but despite the therapeutic rationale, low doses of aspirin or dipyridamole did not show any benefit in a 2-year double-blind study.
- If a Raynaud-like phenomenon occurs in the heart, vasodilator or sympatholytic agents may play a role. Angiotensin-converting enzyme inhibitors are attractive not only as vasodilators, but may block angiotensin-induced myocardial fibrosis that has been shown in rabbits. These agents have experimental support demonstrating a decrease in perfusion abnormalities in patients with SSc.

SURGERY
Heart–lung or single-lung transplantation may be a therapeutic option in those patients with severe symptomatic pulmonary hypertension without other significant systemic involvement.

 FOLLOW-UP

PROGNOSIS
The course of SSc is variable. Patients with limited scleroderma have a good prognosis. Prognosis is generally worse in patients with diffuse SSc, particularly when the onset occurs at an older age. In addition, males have a worse prognosis. Death occurs most often from cardiac, renal, or pulmonary involvement. The 10-year mortality rate has been estimated at 55% in patients with diffuse disease and 75% in those with limited disease. ECG evidence of heart involvement has been found to be associated with higher mortality.

PATIENT MONITORING
Routine history and physical examination will direct further diagnostic testing. Routine ECG may detect early cardiac involvement because conduction abnormalities often represent the first manifestation of SSc in the heart.

REFERENCES
1. Anvari A, Graninger W, Schneider B, et al. Cardiac involvement in systemic sclerosis. *Arthritis Rheum.* 1992;35:1356–1361.
2. Botstein GR, LeRoy EC. Primary heart disease in systemic sclerosis (scleroderma): Advances in clinical and pathologic features, pathogenesis, and new therapeutic approaches. *Am Heart J.* 1981;102:913–919.
3. Oram S, Stokes W. The heart in scleroderma. *Br J Med.* 1961;23:243–259.
4. Sackner MA, Heinz ER, Steinberg AJ. The heart in scleroderma. *Am J Cardiol.* 1966;17:542–559.
5. Topol EJ. *Cardiovascular Medicine*. Philadelphia: Lippincott Williams & Wilkins, 1998:912–915.

CODES
ICD9-CM
Underlying Disease
- 710.1 Systemic sclerosis (includes CREST, progressive systemic sclerosis, and scleroderma)

Specific Manifestations
- 416.8 Pulmonary hypertension (secondary), unspecified
- 422.90 Acute myocarditis, unspecified
- 423.9 Pericardial disease, unspecified

PATIENT TEACHING
Organizations
- Scleroderma Foundation: www.scleroderma.org
- Clinical Trials Listing Service: www.centerwatch.com

SEPSIS AND THE HEART

Vasanth Vedantham
Jarvis W. Lambert

 BASICS

DESCRIPTION

- Sepsis is a systemic inflammatory response, typically to infection, characterized by hypotension and multiorgan failure due to the release of inflammatory mediators.
- Sepsis syndromes are classified according to the severity of hemodynamic and metabolic abnormalities (definitions below).
- Systemic inflammatory response syndrome (SIRS)
  - Temp $>38°C$ or $<26°C$
  - HR >90 bpm
  - RR >20 breaths/min or $P_aCO_2 <32$ mm Hg
  - WBC $>12,000$ /mm^3, WBC $<4,000$ /mm^3, or $>10\%$ band forms
- Sepsis: SIRS plus evidence of infection
- Severe sepsis: Sepsis plus organ dysfunction, evidence of tissue hypoperfusion, or hypotension
- Septic shock: Severe sepsis plus hypotension and hypoperfusion despite adequate volume resuscitation
- Myocardial depression most often accompanies severe sepsis and septic shock, but can be seen in any of the sepsis syndromes. Typical cardiac abnormalities identified in septic patients are as follows:
  - Cardiac index is elevated, and often an early period of hyperdynamic function occurs.
  - Subsequently, LV end-diastolic dimension increases, ejection fraction decreases, but cardiac index remains high.
  - Myocardial dysfunction usually peaks within a few days of onset and resolves within 7–10 days in survivors.
  - To some degree, these changes may be protective and adaptive, because patients who do not exhibit left ventricular dilatation have, on average, a worse prognosis than patients who do.

EPIDEMIOLOGY

- Septic shock is the most common cause of death in intensive care units in the U.S.
- 750,000 cases of sepsis occur per year, with 200,000 deaths per year in the U.S.
- Many of these patients develop cardiac dysfunction (at least 25%).

Incidence

- Sepsis: 240.4/100,000
  - Mortality rate: 18%

RISK FACTORS

- Increased risk with increasing age
- Sex: Male > Female
- Nonwhite race
- Immunosuppression (bone marrow suppression, splenectomy, etc.)

PATHOPHYSIOLOGY

- Sepsis
  - In adults with systemic infections, products and toxins of micro-organisms activate host immune cells.
  - Host immune cells synthesize pro-inflammatory mediators [cytokines, such as tumor necrosis factor (TNF) and interleukin-6 (IL-6)].
  - Inflammatory cascade and counter-regulatory cascade cause systemic physiologic abnormalities, such as:
    - Activation of coagulation cascade
    - Systemic vasodilation
    - Increased vascular permeability
- Myocardial dysfunction in sepsis:
  - A circulating factor or factors, myocardial depressing substances (MDSs), leads to myocardial dysfunction in sepsis.
  - MDSs trigger changes in cellular metabolism that lead to decreased contractility by decreasing intracellular calcium.
  - MDSs trigger increases in intracellular nitric oxide (NO), which promotes myocardial relaxation.
  - These changes generally reverse within 7–10 days in patients who survive.

ETIOLOGY

- The etiology of myocardial depression in sepsis is incompletely understood and is the subject of intense, ongoing investigation, largely in animal models. As stated in Pathophysiology, MDSs lead to cellular changes. Well-studied mechanisms have included:
  - Likely causes
    - Endotoxin: Not the direct cause of myocardial depression, but it may contribute indirectly by inducing MDS.
    - Inflammatory mediators: TNF-α and IL-1b can produce myocardial depression *in vivo* and in culture.
    - Arachidonic acid metabolites: May play roles as secondary mediators downstream of cytokines
    - Catecholaminergic signaling and NO are cellular mediators of decreased contractility and increased relaxation.
  - Unlikely causes
    - Myocardial ischemia is not believed to be involved in the myocardial dysfunction of sepsis.
      - Myocardial blood flow is increased in septic humans.
      - In animals, no reduction occurs in available high-energy phosphates in sepsis.

ASSOCIATED CONDITIONS

Other causes of a systemic inflammatory response syndrome are:

- Trauma
- Pancreatitis
- Burns

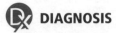 **DIAGNOSIS**

SIGNS AND SYMPTOMS

Sepsis is a heterogeneous disease with varied clinical presentations and complex, fluctuating hemodynamics. Classic features of the initial presentation include:

- Fever or hypothermia
- Respiratory distress
- Tachycardia
- Hypotension with warm extremities (early) or cool, mottled extremities (late)
- Altered mental status
- Oliguria
- Focal signs and symptoms of infection

History

- Hypotension
- Warm or cool periphery depending on hemodynamic state

TESTS

Assessment of myocardial function in patients with sepsis is accomplished with a combination of laboratory, electrocardiographic, and imaging modalities, each of which can add useful information to help guide therapy.

Lab

- In sepsis, widespread metabolic abnormalities may be present [electrolytes, creatinine, blood urea nitrogen (BUN), lactate, etc.].
- BNP may be elevated in patients with myocardial depression.
- Troponin-I often is elevated and indicates some degree of myocardial injury.
- Electrocardiogram often exhibits nonspecific ST-segment and T-wave changes.

Imaging

Echocardiography

- May initially reveal hyperdynamic function
- Subsequently reveals increase in LV diastolic dimension and decrease in ejection fraction
- Usually the pattern of myocardial systolic dysfunction is global.
- Right ventricular dysfunction often occurs as well.
- Diastolic function in septic patients is the subject of ongoing investigation, but given increase in LV distensibility, it is likely that diastolic dysfunction actually improves in septic patients.

Diagnostic Procedures/Surgery

Occasionally, pulmonary artery catheterization is helpful, although several randomized trials have not shown overall benefit to its routine use. The hemodynamics in septic patients can vary greatly, but the features of classic distributive shock are:

- Elevated cardiac index (often despite myocardial dysfunction) assuming adequate volume resuscitation
- Low systemic vascular resistance
- Pulmonary capillary wedge pressure normal to slightly elevated if adequate volume resuscitation

DIFFERENTIAL DIAGNOSIS

Other causes of myocardial depression due to coexisting cardiac disease always must be considered.

TREATMENT

GENERAL MEASURES

Early goal-directed therapy has emerged as a paradigm for the treatment of septic shock, and can be applied when sepsis is complicated by myocardial depression. In general, myocardial contractility should be a target of therapy only when cardiac output is insufficient to meet total body demand despite adequate volume resuscitation, oxygen-carrying capacity, oxygenation, and mean arterial pressure. The stepped approach to therapy is as follows:

- Establish control over airway, ventilation, and oxygenation.
- Establish central venous access and continuous measurement of central venous pressure (CVP).
- Aggressive fluid resuscitation's goal is CVP 8–12 mm Hg to optimize filling pressures.
- Institute broad-spectrum antibiotics and begin search for cause of sepsis (without delaying subsequent steps).
- Transfuse blood products to maintain hematocrit >30%.
- Use peripheral vasoconstrictors (norepinephrine, phenylephrine) to achieve mean arterial pressure >65 mm Hg.
- Follow central venous oxygen saturation (CVO_2) as a surrogate for total body oxygen supply/demand mismatch.
- If CVO_2 <70% despite HCT >30%, MAP >65 mm Hg, and CVP 8–12 mm Hg, add inotropic agents (dobutamine).
- Perform cosyntropin challenge and add corticosteroids if appropriate.
- Determine whether therapy with recombinant human activated protein-C is appropriate, and institute if it is.
- If CVP and CVO_2 data do not suffice to guide therapy because LV filling pressures and cardiac output are in doubt:
  - Consider pulmonary artery catheter insertion (controversial; several randomized trials have shown no improvement in outcome, although patient selection remains a concern in these studies).
  - Consider echocardiography (clinical utility has not been established in trials, but widely used as an adjunctive test to estimate LV function, cardiac output, and filling pressures).
  - The early institution of nutritional support (enteral preferred to parenteral when possible) leads to improved outcomes.

 MEDICATION (DRUGS)

- Directed at sepsis and septic shock in general:
  - Broad-spectrum antibiotics
  - Vasoconstrictors
  - Corticosteroids when endogenous stress response inadequate
  - Recombinant human activated protein-C in selected patients (controversial)
- Directed specifically at myocardial depression in septic shock:
  - Inotropic agents when cardiac output insufficient to meet total body oxygen demand
- Drugs that have been proven ineffective in randomized trials:
  - Ibuprofen
  - N-Acetylcysteine
  - Nitric oxide synthase inhibitors (N-mono-methyl-L-arginine) increase mortality in sepsis.
  - TNF-α inhibitors (can improve LV function but has no effect on mortality)

 FOLLOW-UP

PROGNOSIS

Cardiac factors associated with a worse prognosis in septic patients include:

- Lack of LV end-diastolic dilatation
- Persistent hyperdynamic profile
- Increased heart rate

PATIENT MONITORING

Sepsis, especially when complicated by myocardial dysfunction, requires monitoring in an intensive care unit.

REFERENCES

1. Court O, Kumar A, Parrillo JE, et al. Clinical review: Myocardial depression in sepsis and septic shock. *Crit Care*. 2002;6:500.
2. Krishnagopalan S, Kumar A, Parillo JE, et al. Myocardial dysfunction in the patient with sepsis. *Curr Opin Crit Care*. 2002;8:376.
3. Kumar A, Haery C, Parrillo JE. Myocardial dysfunction in septic shock. I: Clinical manifestation of cardiovascular dysfunction. *J Cardiothor Vasc Anesth*. 2001;15:364.
4. Kumar A, Krieger A, Symeoneides S, et al. Myocardial dysfunction in septic shock. II: Role of cytokines and nitric oxide. *J Cardiothor Vasc Anesth*. 2001;15:485.

ADDITIONAL READING

- Martin G, Mannino DM, Eaton S, et al. The epidemiology of sepsis in the United States from 1979 through 2000. *N Engl J Med*. 2003;348:1546.
- Rivers E, Nguyen B, Havstad S, et al. Early goal-directed therapy in the treatment of severe sepsis and septic shock. *N Engl J Med*. 2001;345:1368.

CODES
ICD9-CM
785.59 Sepsis

PATIENT TEACHING
Diet
Early institution of nutritional support (enteral preferred to parenteral when possible) leads to improved outcomes.

SEXUAL DYSFUNCTION AND THE HEART

Timothy James (T. J.) Paterick
Timothy Paterick

 BASICS

DESCRIPTION
Erectile dysfunction (ED) is defined as the inability of the male to achieve or maintain an erection sufficient for sexual intercourse.

GENERAL PREVENTION
- Ideal body weight
- Regular aerobic exercise
- Prevention of endothelial dysfunction through risk factor modification

EPIDEMIOLOGY
- Massachusetts Male Aging Study (MMAS) revealed that 52% of 1,290 men aged 40 to 70 had some degree of dysfunction and 10% had total absence of erectile function.
- MMAS revealed a deleterious epidemiologic link between coronary artery disease, diabetes, and erectile dysfunction.

Incidence
The overall incidence rate is estimated at 26 cases per 10,000 man-years; the rate increases with age and the presence of such factors as lower level of education, diabetes, heart disease, and hypertension. New cases of specific disease (ED) per population at risk expressed as percentage.

Prevalence
ED affects as many as 30 million men in the United States.

Geriatric Considerations
- The prevalence and incidence is higher in the elderly.
- Higher incidence of predisposing risk factors for ED in the elderly
- Higher sensitivity to the medications that cause ED in the elderly

Risk Factors
- Age: Men >40 years.
- Hypertension with or without treatment (>140/40)
- Diabetes mellitus (fasting blood glucose <125 mg 70%)
- Family history of heart disease in primary relative: Male <55 years
- Elevated low-density lipoprotein (LDL) cholesterol/triglycerides (>100 mg/dl)
- Low high-density lipoprotein (HDL) cholesterol (<40 mg/dl)
- Cigarette smoking/passive smoking
- Central obesity associated with the metabolic syndrome
- Physical inactivity
- Elevated homocysteine, lipoprotein (a), C-reactive protein, fibrinogen, factor VIII, factor VII

Genetics
Close link between ED and vascular disease; therefore, polygenic inheritance with clustering of the risk factors in families

PATHOPHYSIOLOGY
With sexual stimulation nitric oxide (NO) is released into the corpora cavernosa from nonadrenergic–noncholinergic autonomic nerves and the vascular endothelium. NO stimulates the enzyme guanylate cyclase to produce cyclic guanosine monophosphate (cGMP), which ultimately causes relaxation in the vascular smooth muscle of the arteries, arterioles and sinusoids of the corpora cavernosa, which then fills with blood like a sponge fills with water. The blood is trapped in the penis (tumescence). A frequent underlying cause of ED is lack of cGMP.

ETIOLOGY
- Unknown; associated with the risks contributing to atherosclerosis
- Causes include alcohol, anticholinergics, antidepressants, antihypertensives (thiazide diuretics, reserpine, β-blockers, methyldopa, hydralazine), cancer chemotherapeutics, clofibrate, gemfibrozil, digoxin, statins, H2 receptor antagonists, and tranquilizers. Other causes include:
  - Hypogonadism, hypothyroidism, hyperthyroidism, pituitary tumor, hyperprolactinemia
  - Cerebrovascular accidents, multiple sclerosis, nerve damage postprostate surgery, neuropathies, spinal cord injuries
  - Peyronie disease, priapism, trauma
  - Atherosclerosis and associated risk factors, vascular surgery, venous leaks
  - Psychogenic

ASSOCIATED CONDITIONS
- Vascular disease (coronary, cerebral and peripheral)
- Diabetes mellitus
- Elevated lipids (total cholesterol >240, HD >60 was protective)
- Smoking
- Hypertension
- Obesity
- Sedentary lifestyle

 DIAGNOSIS

SIGNS AND SYMPTOMS
- ED is common and increases with age
- Cigarette smoking, diabetes, hypertension, hyperlipidemia, cerebral, coronary and peripheral vascular disease, obesity, and sedentary lifestyle are all associated with ED.
- Side effect of various drugs
- Depression, anxiety, and marital discord

History and Physical Exam
- Directing questions regarding vascular disease, smoking, diabetes, hypertension, dyslipidemia, neuropathy, hypertensive medications, and sexual function
- Examination with an eye toward vascular disease and hypertension, manifestations of diabetes (end-organ damage: retinopathy, neuropathy and nephropathy)

TESTS
- Blood pressure measurement
- Electrocardiogram (ECG) and stress testing to identify coronary and peripheral ischemia
- Carotid ultrasound
- Ophthalmologic examination

Lab
Fasting lipid profile with serum homocysteine, lipoprotein (a), C-reactive protein, glycosilated Hg, and urinary protein analysis

Imaging
- Noninvasive
  - Chest x-ray: Calcification of coronary arteries and aorta
  - Ultrasound to evaluate carotid arteries, peripheral vessels, and abdominal aorta for plaque and aneurysm
  - Electron beam CT: Quantify coronary artery calcification to identify plaque burden and location.
- Invasive
  - Angiography
  - Intravascular ultrasound to evaluate lesion characteristics
  - Transesophageal echocardiography to evaluate proximal coronary artery plaque burden and atheromatous disease of the aorta

Therapeutic Procedures
- Angioplasty of carotid/coronary/peripheral systems or surgery
- High-risk group for ED.
- Careful questioning regarding sexual function in this subset of patients to establish diagnosis of ED and risk factor reduction as well as treatment options

TREATMENT

GENERAL MEASURES

- Stress reduction, tobacco cessation, dietary changes, lifestyle changes to increase exercise and maintain ideal body weight, treatment of hypertension, lipid analysis and treatment (LDL <100)
- Diet should be low saturated fat, low cholesterol, low sodium; recommend American Heart Association step 1 and step 2 diets
- Weight reduction/physical activity: Aerobic activity for 30 minutes at a minimum of 3 times per week

SPECIFIC MEASURES

- The management of sexual dysfunction in patients with cardiovascular disease is based in part upon estimated risk for adverse cardiovascular events.
- In 2005, the Second Princeton Consensus Panel on sexual activity and cardiac risk published recommendations for the initiation or resumption of sexual activity in patients with cardiovascular disease.
- Low risk: No symptoms and less than 3 cardiovascular risk factors; a sedentary lifestyle is considered a risk factor, coronary revascularization without evidence of exercise-induced ischemia, mild valvular disease
- Low-risk patients can be safely encouraged to initiate or resume sexual activity or to receive treatment for sexual dysfunction.
- Intermediate risk: No symptoms and 3 or more risk factors (excluding gender), moderate stable angina, a recent myocardial infarction (>2 weeks and <6 weeks) in patients who have not undergone revascularization, asymptomatic left ventricular (LV) dysfunction with ejection fraction <40% or NYHA class 2 heart failure, peripheral vascular disease or recent stroke or transient ischemic attack (TIA).
- Intermediate-risk patients should receive further evaluation in order to stratify into a low- or high-risk category. This is best achieved with stress testing and consultation with cardiologist.
- High risk: Unstable angina, uncontrolled hypertension, class 3 or 4 NYHA heart failure, myocardial infarction within 2 weeks, complex arrhythmias, hypertrophic cardiomyopathy (HCM), moderate to severe valvular disease (particularly aortic stenosis).
- High-risk patients should be stabilized by appropriate medical and surgical therapy and further risk stratified before resuming sexual activity or being treated for sexual dysfunction.
- An important component of the treatment of sexual dysfunction in all patients is correction of reversible causes and to risk stratify to achieve a low-risk status so sexual activity can be resumed or available treatment options pursued.

MEDICATION (DRUGS)

- PDE-5 inhibitors: The phosphodiesterase-5 inhibitors (sildenafil, vardenafil, and tadalafil) are widely used in the treatment of ED in men and can have important effects in men with cardiovascular disease. Most of the published data is related to sildenafil (Viagra).

- Sildenafil
  - Improves ED in patients with stable ischemic heart disease (this was illustrated in a report with 357 men with stable chronic disease; sildenafil improved erection in 70% as compared to 20% with placebo)
  - Effective in men with high blood pressure, diabetes, and psychogenic causes of ED.
  - Decreases blood pressure, and it can interact with nitrates.
  - PDE-5 inhibitors (sildenafil, vardenafil, and tadalafil) should not be used with nitrates in any form.
  - Dilates epicardial coronary arteries and in patients with coronary artery disease improved endothelial dysfunction and inhibits platelet activation
  - Among patients with exercise-induced ischemia, sildenafil has an intermediate effect between nitrates and placebo.
- Vardenafil and tadalafil (Levitra and Cialis)
  - More potent and selective PDE-5 inhibitors than sildenafil
  - As effective as sildenafil in the treatment of ED
  - Tadalafil has a longer duration of action; thereby allowing greater spontaneity in sexual activity.

OTHER THERAPIES

There are no specific cardiovascular effects of androgen replacement therapy, penile prosthesis, or vacuum-assisted erection devices.

FOLLOW-UP

- After risk stratification to a low-risk status and initiation of drug therapy or other therapies, the follow up is yearly with the primary care physician assuming no side-effects.
- Routine follow-up should include reinforcement of exercise and prevention of endothelial dysfunction through risk-factor modification.
- Symptoms of heart disease should prompt cardiology consultation, and recurrence of ED should prompt urology consultation.

REFERENCES

1. Cheitlin MD, et al. ACC/AHA expert consensus document. Use of sildenafil (Viagra) in patients with cardiovascular disease. American College of Cardiology American Heart Association. *J Am Coll Cardiol*. 1999;34:1850.
2. DeBusk R, et al. Management of sexual dysfunction in patients with cardiovascular disease: Recommendations of the Princeton Consensus Panel. *Am J Cardiol*. 2000;86:175.
3. Derby CA, et al. Modifiable risk factors and erectile dysfunction: Can lifestyle changes modify risk? *Urology*. 2000;56:302.
4. Feldman HA, et al. Erectile dysfunction and coronary risk factors: Prospective results from the Massachusetts Male Aging Study. *Prev Med*. 2000;30:328.
5. Feldman HA, et al. Impotence and its medical and psychosocial correlates: Results of the Massachusetts Male Aging Study. *J Urol*. 1994;151:54.
6. Kloner, RA. Cardiovascular effects of the 3 phosphodiesterase-5 inhibitors approved for the treatment of erectile dysfunction. *Circulation*. 2004;110:3149.
7. Kloner RA, Hutter AM, Emmick JT, et al. Time course of the interaction between tadalafil and nitrates. *J Am Coll Cardiol*. 2003;42:1855.
8. Kostis JB, Jackson G, Rosen R, et al. Sexual dysfunction and cardiac risk (the Second Princeton Consensus Conference.) *Am J Cardiol*. 2005;96:313.
9. Mittleman MA, Maclure M, Glasser DB. Evaluation of acute risk for myocardial infarction in men treated with sildenafil citrate. *Am J Cardiol*. 2005;96:443.
10. Pickering TG, Shepard AM, Puddy I, et al. Sildenafil citrate for erectile dysfunction taking antihypertensive therapy. Sildenafil Study Group. *Am J Hypertens*. 2004;14:70.

CODE

ICD9-CM

607.84 Erectile dysfunction

PATIENT TEACHING

- Encourage exercise, ideal body weight, and risk factor modification of endothelial dysfunction.
- Discuss side effects of prescribed medication and indications for follow-up. Stress the importance of immediate follow-up if cardiovascular symptoms occur.
- Review the interaction between PDE-5 inhibitors and nitrates; also discuss the effect of PDE-5 inhibitors and blood pressure.
- Encourage yearly follow-up for comprehensive medical evaluation, review of risk factors, and discussion of potential side effects.

FAQ

Q: What associated conditions increase the likelihood of ED?
A: (i) vascular disease, (ii) diabetes, (iii) smoking, (iv) obesity, (v) sedentary lifestyle, (vi) abnormal lipid profile
Q: What medication is absolutely contraindicated for simultaneous use with the PDE-5 inhibitors?
A: Nitrates in any form
Q: What is the most essential component to establish the diagnosis of ED in the primary care setting?
A: Careful questioning regarding sexual function in patient with a high burden of risk factors for endothelial dysfunction

SICKLE CELL DISEASES AND THE HEART

Brian C. Jensen

 BASICS

DESCRIPTION

- Sickle cell diseases are characterized by the presence of sickle- or crescent-shaped erythrocytes in the peripheral blood. Abnormally shaped red blood cells become rigid and lodge in capillaries, preventing the flow of oxygen to tissues and organs.
- Sickle cell diseases include sickle cell anemia, sickle cell-hemoglobin C disease, and sickle cell-thalassemia disease.
- The majority of the 50,000 persons in the U.S. with sickle cell disease are African Americans, although aboriginal South Asians, Italians, Greeks, and other persons of Mediterranean ancestry are also afflicted.
- System(s) affected: Cardiovascular; Respiratory; Skeletal; Hematologic; Skin; Immunologic; Renal; Gastrointestinal; Genitourinary; Nervous

Geriatric Considerations
Unusual in light of the high early mortality

Pediatric Considerations
Common

EPIDEMIOLOGY
- Predominant age: Children and young adults
- Predominant sex: Male = Female

Pregnancy Considerations
- A relatively high rate of preterm birth, small-for-gestational-age infants, and fetal loss occurs during pregnancy.
- Increases the risk of a sickle crisis
- May aggravate a patient's anemia
- Increased risk of gestational hypertension
- On average, the maternal mortality rate is 1.6%.

Prevalence
- Homozygotes (approximately 0.6% of blacks in the U.S.) have sickle cell anemia.
- Heterozygotes (8–13% of blacks) carry the sickle cell trait and generally are not anemic; however, sickling has been demonstrated *in vitro*.
- 40% of the population in some areas of Africa carries the sickle cell trait. The trait appears to confer protection against malaria.

RISK FACTORS
Genetics
Sickle cell disease is inherited in an autosomal recessive fashion. Hemoglobin-β subunit position 6 has valine substituted for glutamic acid.

PATHOPHYSIOLOGY
Cardinal features are hemolytic anemia and vaso-occlusion.
- Polymerization of sickle hemoglobin leads to reduced deformability of RBCs.
- Abnormalities in coagulation, WBCs, and vascular endothelium also contribute.
- These factors result in vasculopathy and vascular occlusion with resultant organ damage.
- Average half-life of sickle RBCs is 4 days.

ETIOLOGY
- In the deoxygenated state, hemoglobin polymerizes abnormally, deforming RBC membrane.
- Iron in free heme promotes formation of reactive oxygen species, which further damage RBC membranes.
- Reduced nitric oxide bioavailability leads to endothelial dysfunction.
  - L-Arginine (NO substrate) deficiency
  - Increased plasma arginase levels
  - Increased NO consumption by free plasma hemoglobin and reactive oxygen species
  - Impaired release of RBC nitric oxide

ASSOCIATED CONDITIONS
- Sickle cell–thalassemia
- Hemoglobin SC disease
- Hemoglobin C disease

 DIAGNOSIS

SIGNS AND SYMPTOMS
- Infants/toddlers/children
  - Onset of symptoms typically occurs in the first 3 years after birth
    - Hemolytic anemia
    - Acute attacks of pain in the chest, abdomen, limbs, and joints
    - Pallor of the tongue and lips
    - Dactylitis, "hand-foot" syndrome
    - Irritability
    - Crying
    - Poor eating habits
    - Splenomegaly
    - Hepatomegaly
    - Jaundice
    - Scleral icterus
    - Cardiac murmurs
    - Cognitive impairment and premature stroke
    - Abnormal bone development
- Adolescents/young adults
  - Severe pain
  - Delayed puberty
  - Progressive anemia
  - Leg ulcers
  - Nosebleeds
  - Dental disease
  - Renal disease
  - Aseptic necrosis of the femoral head
  - Retinal lesions
  - Splenic infarct and autosplenectomy (predisposes to infection)
  - Priapism
- Individuals 20 years old and older
  - Chronic pain syndromes
  - Leg ulcers
  - Retinitis
  - Gallbladder disease
  - Iron overload from multiple transfusions
  - Cardiac manifestations

- Cardiomegaly is common.
  - Striking left atrial and biventricular enlargement and interventricular septal hypertrophy often develop.
    - Right ventricular hypertrophy with eventual right heart failure, especially in the setting of pulmonary hypertension
    - Left ventricular enlargement secondary to chronic anemia and vascular occlusions
    - Normal to increased cardiac contractility
    - Reduced maximum cardiac output at maximum exercise
    - Decreased peripheral vascular resistance secondary to peripheral vasodilatation, microvascular arteriovenous shunts, and decreased blood viscosity
    - Increased resting cardiac output with a hemoglobin level below 7 g/dL of blood
  - Myocardial infarction (MI) is relatively uncommon (although it may occur in the absence of atherosclerosis due to vasculopathy and vascular occlusion).
  - Late manifestations could be associated with iron overload from chronic transfusion
- Pulmonary manifestations
  - Pulmonary vascular congestion/pulmonary edema secondary to cardiac failure
  - Pulmonary hypertension is common and is secondary to pulmonary infarction (from focal pulmonary sickling or thromboembolism) and veno-occlusive disease.
  - Cor pulmonale
  - Dyspnea
  - Reduced vital capacity
- Neurologic complications
  - Stroke and cognitive impairment

History
- Dyspnea on exertion and decreased exercise capacity are common.
- Although chest pain is common and MI is uncommon, ECG always should be obtained.

Physical Exam
Abnormalities result from cardiac structural changes, pulmonary hypertension, and high flow state.
- Hyperdynamic precordium
- Normal to mildly increased heart rate; tachycardia should raise suspicion of myocardial dysfunction or an acute decrease in hemoglobin
- Paradoxical splitting of the second heart sound
- Prominent third heart sound
- Ejection click due to pulmonary artery dilatation
- Systolic flow murmurs associated with anemia
- Patients with severe anemia and resultant high flow may develop diastolic cardiac murmurs and dilatation of the aortic ring.

TESTS
- The diagnosis of sickle cell anemia is made by serum electrophoresis:
  - The homozygous state is denoted by the presence of only hemoglobin S with variable amounts of hemoglobin F.
  - The heterozygous state is denoted by the presence of both hemoglobin A and S (with more A than S present).
- Prenatal screening for at-risk parents

Lab
- Normocytic anemia
- Wide RDW
- Reticulocytosis of 10–40%
- Baseline leukocytosis makes WBC count less reliable index of infection.
- Thrombocytosis usually is present.
- Bone marrow is hyperplastic, with a predominance of normoblasts. The bone marrow may become aplastic during "sickle crisis" or severe infection.
- Serum bilirubin usually is elevated.
- Fecal and urinary urobilinogen levels also are elevated.
- The erythrocyte sedimentation rate is generally low.

Imaging
- ECG may show right or left ventricular hypertrophy.
- Chest radiography may reveal cardiomegaly and enlarged pulmonary arteries. Infiltrates are present in acute chest syndrome.
- Echocardiography may confirm cor pulmonale, MI, pulmonary hypertension, left ventricular hypertrophy, and valvular abnormalities.

Pathologic Findings
Arterial occlusions and infracted tissue

DIFFERENTIAL DIAGNOSIS
- Hemoglobin SC disease
- Hemoglobin SB thalassemia
- Hemolytic uremic syndrome

TREATMENT

GENERAL MEASURES
- Ideally, infants will be screened and identified at birth.
- Counseling, comprehensive care, and psychosocial support
- Pain control
- Annual transcranial Doppler to screen for cerebrovascular accident (CVA) in children
- Blood transfusions should be administered only when clearly indicated:
  - Straight transfusions if Hgb <9, exchange transfusions if Hgb >11
  - Accepted indications for blood transfusion include:
    - Cardiopulmonary symptoms, particularly when the hemoglobin level is <5 g/dL.
    - High-output failure
    - Hypoxemia with PO_2 <65 mm Hg
    - Severe infection
    - Sepsis

- Cerebral vascular accident
- Organ failure
- Prior to general anesthesia
- Prior to surgery
- Recalcitrant leg ulcers
- Pregnancy
- Priapism
- Crises should be managed with aggressive IV fluid hydration, analgesics, and supplemental oxygen.

MEDICATION (DRUGS)

- Pneumococcal vaccine and prophylactic penicillin for infants
- Hydroxyurea decreases pain crises, acute chest presentations, and increases mortality.
- Folic acid 1 mg/day
- Erythropoietin may enhance erythropoiesis.
- Inhaled nitric oxide has vasodilatory and antisickling properties and may be clinically useful.
- Danazol may enable sickle cell erythrocytes to flow through very small capillaries.
- Angiotensin-converting enzyme inhibitors (ACE-Is) may help slow progression of renal disease.
- Sildenafil may be effective in treating pulmonary hypertension.
- Analgesia

SURGERY
- Allogeneic bone marrow transplantation is the only currently available treatment that can cure sickle cell disease.
- Gene transfer therapy has the potential to provide marked improvement in or cure of patients with sickle cell disease.

FOLLOW-UP

ADMISSION CRITERIA
- Pulmonary embolus
- Sickle crisis
- Heart failure

Discharge Criteria
Resolution of problem

Issues for Referral
Transfusion should be undertaken with the assistance of a trained hematologist.

PROGNOSIS
- The lifespan of patients with homozygous hemoglobin S (sickle cell disease) has increased to >50 years.
- Causes of death include infections, multiple pulmonary emboli and pulmonary hypertension, thrombosis of a vital vascular bed, and renal failure.

COMPLICATIONS
- Organ failure
- Congestive heart failure
- Severe pulmonary hypertension
- Cardiac arrest
- Stroke
- Limb ischemia

PATIENT MONITORING
- Depends on the frequency and severity of the patient's symptoms
- Children should be screened regularly for organ damage.

REFERENCES
1. Bonds, DR. Three decades of innovation in the management of sickle cell disease: The road to understanding the sickle cell disease phenotype. *Blood Rev.* 2005;19:99–110.
2. Claster S, Vichinsky EP. Managing sickle cell disease. *Br Med J.* 2003;327:1151–1155.

CODES
ICD9-CM
282.60

PATIENT TEACHING
Organizations
- National Organization for Rare Disorders (NORD)
- National Association for Sickle Cell Disease, Inc.
- NIH/National Heart, Lung and Blood Institute (NHLBI)
- Cooley's Anemia Foundation, Inc.
- The Canadian Sickle Cell Society
- March of Dimes Birth Defects Foundation
- National Center for Education in Maternal and Child Health (NCEMCH)

Diet
Ensure adequate nutrition and hydration.

Activity
As tolerated

Prevention
- Antibiotics (prophylactic penicillin until the age of 6 years)
- Pneumococcal vaccine
- Haemophilus influenzae type b vaccine
- Regular check-ups
- Avoid becoming chilled.
- Dress warmly.
- Eat balanced meals.
- Ensure ample sleep.
- Practice deep breathing 5 minutes before going to sleep.

FAQ
Q: What is acute chest syndrome (ACS)?
A: The diagnosis of ACS requires the identification of a new infiltrate on chest radiograph associated with one or more new symptoms: Fever, cough, dyspnea, or hypoxia. In older patients with sickle cell, this diagnosis must not be confused with acute coronary syndrome (ACS).
Q: Is there any cure for sickle cell disease?
A: Bone marrow transplantation has been used rarely to cure sickle cell disease in humans. Gene therapy has been successfully applied in mice.

SILENT MYOCARDIAL ISCHEMIA

Joshua M. Larned
Gerard P. Aurigemma*
Nanette K. Wenger

 BASICS

DESCRIPTION

- Silent ischemia is defined as objectively documented myocardial ischemia, occurring without associated angina or an anginal equivalent. One of the first studies to establish the importance of silent myocardial ischemia was the Framingham Heart Study, which demonstrated that 1/3 of patients with a new myocardial infarction (MI) during routine ECG had no antecedent symptoms. The incidence of myocardial silent ischemia not associated with MI is likely to be much less. A precise incidence of silent ischemia in asymptomatic patients is not known. Some smaller studies permit an estimate of the incidence of silent ischemia. Such studies suggest that 25–45% of patients with documented myocardial ischemia have evidence of myocardial ischemia during daily activities; most of these episodes are asymptomatic. Most episodes of silent ischemia occur with minimal or no physical exertion.
- Possible mechanisms for silent ischemia include:
  - Defective angina warning system
  - Presence of a higher pain threshold
  - Shorter duration of ischemic episodes
- It is difficult to ascertain the mechanism of silent ischemia in an individual patient. Most have underlying atherosclerotic coronary artery disease (CAD) but coronary artery vasospasm appears to play a part. Whether decreases in coronary supply versus increases in coronary flow demand are the primary inciting stimulus for silent ischemia has not been established; it is likely that this varies from patient to patient. This is supported by the fact that both β-adrenergic blockers (which primarily act by lowering heart rate and blood pressure but do not improve myocardial perfusion) and nonrate-lowering calcium channel blockers (which likely act primarily to improve myocardial perfusion) both reduce the number of silent ischemia episodes.

GENERAL PREVENTION

- No defined role for screening exists beyond established methods of coronary heart disease (CHD) risk-assessment and prevention.
- Smoking cessation
- Diet
- Exercise
- Stress reduction

EPIDEMIOLOGY

- Asymptomatic patients unknown. Prevalence increases with major CHD risk factors.
- Symptomatic patients:
  - Post-MI 15–30%
  - Unstable angina 30–40%
  - Stable angina 25–50%

RISK FACTORS

- Traditional CHD risk factors
- CHD and CHD-equivalent disease
- Mental stress

PATHOPHYSIOLOGY

- Reduced coronary blood flow
- Increased myocardial oxygen demand
- Endothelial dysfunction
- Elevated catecholamine levels
- Defective pain response to ischemia
- Circadian variability

ETIOLOGY

- Coronary atherosclerotic heart disease
- Coronary artery vasospasm

ASSOCIATED CONDITIONS

End-stage renal disease on hemodialysis

 DIAGNOSIS

SIGNS AND SYMPTOMS

History

- Symptoms may be absent or nonspecific.
- Angina (stable or unstable)
- History of MI
- Symptoms of congestive heart failure (CHF) may be present.

Physical Exam

- Vital signs may be normal or reveal hypertension, tachycardia.
- Findings may be associated with typical findings for CHD or CHF.
- Findings may be associated with CHD-equivalent disease (diabetes, stroke, peripheral vascular disease).

TESTS

- Exercise testing
  - Ischemic ST-segment changes during submaximal or maximal stress is diagnostic.
  - Exercise treadmill testing (ETT) has low specificity in:
    - Asymptomatic patients
    - Women
    - Patients with abnormal resting ECGs
    - Patients on medicines that alter repolarization (e.g., digitalis)
- Ambulatory ECG monitoring
  - Diagnostic if flat or downsloping ST-depression 1 mm or greater with gradual onset and offset for 1 minute
- Nuclear imaging with pharmacologic/nonpharmacologic stress
  - Adjuvant test of choice in asymptomatic patients with a positive ETT
- Exercise echocardiography
- Dobutamine stress echocardiography
- Electron beam computed tomography
  - Coronary calcium scores predict asymptomatic individuals at risk for CHD but have not been definitively shown to independently predict silent ischemia.

 TREATMENT

GENERAL MEASURES

No ideal therapy exists. Present treatment is directed toward underlying pathophysiology.

 MEDICATION (DRUGS)

- β-Blockers
- Calcium channel blockers
- Nitrates
- HMG-CoA reductase inhibitors
- Combination therapy

First Line

β-Blockers:

- Atenolol Silent Ischemia Trial (ASIST)
  - 306 patients with mild or no angina randomized to Atenolol 100 mg vs. placebo
  - Statistically significant reduction in number and duration of ischemic episodes on 48-hour ambulatory ECG monitoring
  - Greater event-free survival
  - Increased time to first event

Second Line

Calcium channel blockers:

- Amlodipine, long-acting nifedipine, and long-acting diltiazem have been shown to reduce silent ischemic episodes up to 68%.

SURGERY

- Coronary revascularization
  - Asymptomatic Cardiac Ischemia Pilot (ACIP)
    - 558 patients randomized to angina-guided medical therapy, ischemia-guided medical therapy, or revascularization using coronary artery bypass graft (CABG) or percutaneous transluminal coronary angioplasty (PTCA)
    - CABG superior to PTCA in reducing silent ischemia seen on Holter monitoring at 12 weeks
    - Revascularization superior to medical therapy in reducing total mortality at 2 years
- Revascularization should be considered in the context of coronary anatomy, left ventricular function, diabetes, and individual considerations.

FOLLOW-UP

DISPOSITION
- Post-MI
  - DANAMI- Trial
    - 1,000 patients treated with thrombolytics for acute MI developed spontaneous angina or inducible ischemia on predischarge exercise testing. 56% demonstrated silent ischemia.
    - Revascularization at 2–10 weeks post-MI reduced recurrent MI, unstable angina, mortality
- Coronary arteriography should be considered in patients with silent ischemia post-MI, although optimal management has yet to be determined.

PROGNOSIS
- Asymptomatic patients
  - Multiple Risk Factor Intervention Trial
    - 12,866 men with two or more risk factors had increased risk for cardiac-related death if silent ischemia evoked by ETT.
- Stable angina
  - 107 patients with chronic stable angina prospectively followed with ambulatory ECG during a 2-year period:
    - Increased overall mortality if silent ischemia documented
- Post-MI
  - Silent ischemia post-MI associated with a higher frequency of adverse cardiac events.

REFERENCES
1. Bourassa M, Pepine C, Forman S, et al. Asymptomatic cardiac ischemia (ACIP) study: Effects of coronary angioplasty and coronary artery bypass surgery on recurrent angina and ischemia. *J Am Coll Cardiol*. 1995;26:606–614.
2. Crawford MH, Bernstein SJ, Deedwania PC, et al. ACC/AHA guidelines for ambulatory electrocardiography: Executive summary and recommendations. *Circulation*. 1999;100:886–893.
3. Davies RF, Goldberg D, Forman S, et al. Asymptomatic cardiac ischemia (ACIP) study two-year follow-up. Outcomes of patients randomized to initial strategies of medical therapy versus revascularization. *Circulation*. 1997;95:2037–2043.
4. Davies RF, Habibi H, Klinke WP, et al. Effect of amlodipine, atenolol, and their combination on myocardial ischemia during treadmill exercise and ambulatory monitoring. *J Am Coll Cardiol*. 1995;25:619–625.
5. Deedwania PC, Carbajal EV. Silent ischemia during daily life is an independent predictor of mortality in stable angina. *Circulation*. 1990;81:748–756.
6. Deedwania PC, Carbajal EV. Silent myocardial ischemia—a clinical perspective. *Arch Int Med*. 1991;151:2373–2382.
7. Deedwania PC, Carbajal, EV, Nelson JR, et al. Anti-ischemic effects of atenolol versus nifedipine in patients with coronary artery disease and ambulatory silent ischemia. *J Am Coll Cardiol*. 1991;17:963–969.
8. Deedwania PC. Should asymptomatic subjects with silent ischemia undergo further evaluation and follow-up? *Int J Cardiol*. 1994;44:101–103.
9. Gottlieb SO, Gottlieb SH, Achuff, et al. Silent ischemia on Holter monitoring predicts mortality in high-risk postinfarction patients. *JAMA*. 1988;259:1030–1035.
10. Gottlieb SO, Wesifelt ML, Ouyant P, et al. Silent myocardial ischemia as a marker for early unfavorable outcomes in patients with unstable angina. *N Engl J Med*. 1986;314:1214–1219.
11. Madsen JK, Grande P, Saunamaki K, et al. Danish multicenter randomized study of invasive versus conservative treatment in patients with inducible ischemia after thrombolysis in acute myocardial infarction (DANAMI). *Circulation*. 1997;96:748–755.
12. Multiple Risk Factor Trial Intervention Research Group. Exercise electrocardiogram and coronary heart disease mortality in the Multiple Risk Factor Intervention Trial. *Am J Cardiol*. 1985;55:16–24.
13. Narula AS, Jha V, Bali HK, et al. Cardiac arrhythmias and silent myocardial ischemia during hemodialysis. *Ren Fail*. 2000;22:355–368.
14. Pepine CJ, Cohn PF, Deedwania PC, et al. Effects of treatment on outcome in mildly symptomatic patients with ischemia during daily life. The Atenolol Silent Ischemia Study. *Circulation*. 1994;90:762–768.
15. Stone PH, Krantz DS, McMahon RP, et al. Relationship among mental stress-induced ischemia and ischemia during daily life and during exercise: The Psychologic Investigators of Myocardial Ischemia (PIMI) study. *J Am Coll Cardiol*. 1999;33:1476–1484.
16. Theroux P, Baird M, Juneau M, et al. Effect of diltiazem on symptomatic and asymptomatic episodes of ST segment depression occurring during daily life and during exercise. *Circulation*. 1991;84:15–22.
17. Tzivoni D, Gavish A, Zin D, et al. Prognostic significance of ischemic episodes in patients with previous myocardial infarction. *Am J Cardiol*. 1988;62:661–664.

CODES
ICD9-CM
- 414.0 Coronary atherosclerosis
- 414.9 Ischemic heart disease NOS

Snomed
- 233823002 silent myocardial ischemia (disorder)

PATIENT TEACHING
Internet resources:
- National Heart, Lung, and Blood Institute; http://www.nhlbi.nih.gov
- American Heart Association; http://www.americanheart.org
- Centers for Disease Control; http://www.cdc.gov/cvh

SINGLE VENTRICLE AND TRICUSPID ATRESIA

Allan J. Hordof
Welton M. Gersony

 BASICS

DESCRIPTION

This condition is characterized by a univentricular atrioventricular (AV) connection resulting in a single functioning ventricular chamber. Tricuspid atresia is a form of single ventricle, but is often classified as a separate congenital heart defect.

- The AV connections include a single-inlet ventricle associated with atresia of one of the AV valves (tricuspid atresia, mitral atresia), a double-inlet ventricle, and a common-inlet ventricle with an unbalanced AV connection. The latter is associated with AV septal defects (AV canal).
- The ventricular morphology is subdivided into dominant left ventricle, dominant right ventricle, and indeterminate ventricular morphology.
- The great-vessel position may be normal, levo-transposed, dextro-transposed, or doublet-outlet malposed.
- Pulmonary outflow obstruction common.
- Coarctation of the aorta also may occur in some forms of single ventricle.
- System affected: Cardiovascular

EPIDEMIOLOGY

- Predominant age: Most patients present in early life in the neonatal or early infancy period. They present with cyanosis due to inadequate pulmonary blood flow (the majority) or congestive heart failure due to unobstructed pulmonary blood flow.
- Predominant sex: Male predominance in tricuspid atresia with transposition of the great vessels

Incidence

- It has been reported that single-ventricle variants make up 1.1% of patients with congenital heart disease.
- Dominant left ventricular morphology makes up the majority, accounting for 74–84%.
- A subset includes patients with asplenia and polysplenia associated with dextrocardia, abdominal heterotaxy, and a complex constellation of associated congenital heart lesions.

Prevalence

- Tricuspid atresia is the third most common form of cyanotic congenital heart disease, with prevalence in clinical series of 0.3–3.7%.
- The prevalence rate in autopsy series is 2.9%. Tricuspid atresia occurs in 1/15,000 live births.

RISK FACTORS

Genetics

- Most often multifactorial
- Some lesions associated with 22q deletions or other chromosomal syndromes

PATHOPHYSIOLOGY

- All forms of single ventricle are associated with mixing of systemic and pulmonary venous return.
- Degree of arterial desaturation depends on pulmonary blood flow limitation by pulmonary outflow obstruction or pulmonary vascular disease and/or the presence or absence of elevated pulmonary venous pressures.

ETIOLOGY

Congenital

ASSOCIATED CONDITIONS

- Pulmonary outflow obstruction common
- Coarctation of the aorta also may occur in some forms of single ventricle.
- Anomalous pulmonary venous connections
- Subaortic obstruction

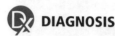 **DIAGNOSIS**

SIGNS AND SYMPTOMS

- The majority of patients with obstruction to pulmonary blood flow secondary to pulmonary atresia or other forms of severe pulmonary outflow obstruction present in the newborn period or early infancy with severe cyanosis and hypoxemia secondary to restrictive pulmonary blood flow.
- Patients with unobstructed pulmonary blood flow and/or significant AV valve insufficiency present in early infancy with signs and symptoms of congestive heart failure:
  – Tachypnea
  – Tachycardia
  – Hepatomegaly
    • Poor feeding
    • Failure to thrive
    • Mild cyanosis

History

See Signs and Symptoms.

Physical Exam

- Systolic ejection murmur of pulmonary stenosis; or rarely, continuous murmur of ductus arteriosus or collateral blood flow
- Nonspecific systolic murmur and/or systolic murmur of AV valve insufficiency at the lower left sternal border and /or apex; diastolic flow murmur at the apex
  - Tachycardia
  - Gallop rhythm
  - Tachypnea
  - Hepatomegaly
  - Patients with associated coarctation of the aorta have diminished or absent pulses in the lower extremities and may present with low cardiac output syndrome and cardiogenic shock.

TESTS

- Oximetry: Dependent on pulmonary blood flow; usually varies from 60% to 90%
- ECG
  - Tricuspid atresia with normal great arteries: Short PR interval, left superior axis, and absent right ventricular forces
  - AV discordance with l-transposition of the great arteries: AV conduction abnormalities, including complete AV block
  - Asplenia and polysplenia syndromes with abnormal situs; abnormal P-wave morphology
  - Other single ventricles: Abnormal R-wave progression in precordial leads, although findings variable and nonspecific

Lab

Howell-Jolly bodies in asplenia syndrome and chromosome abnormalities in some patients (e.g., Downs syndrome)

Imaging

- Chest x-ray
  - Findings are dependent on pulmonary blood flow:
    - Pulmonary atresia or moderate to severe pulmonary stenosis: Heart size normal with normal to decreased pulmonary vascular markings
    - Unobstructed pulmonary blood flow, moderate to severe cardiomegaly with increased pulmonary vascular markings
  - Additional abnormalities
    - Situs inversus or heterotaxy, dextrocardia or mesocardia, pulmonary venous obstruction; lungs have ground glass appearance with linear reticular pattern
- Echocardiography and magnetic resonance imaging (MRI)
  - Echocardiography and/or MRI may diagnose and elucidate characteristics of the most complex single-ventricle variant. The segmental approach demonstrates:
    - Abdominal and atrial situs
    - Type and mode of AV connections
    - Morphology and function of the main ventricular chamber
    - Ventriculoarterial connections and relationships
    - Systemic and pulmonary venous connections
    - Status of the atrial septum
    - Status of pulmonary valve and arteries
    - Status of aortic arch, AV valves and bulboventricular septum
    - Fetal echocardiography identifies a significant number of these complex defects.

- Cardiac catheterization
  - Hemodynamic parameters
    - Systemic arterial saturation
    - Degree of intracardiac shunts
    - Pulmonary arterial pressure and resistance
    - Gradients between the main ventricle and pulmonary artery and ascending aorta
    - Gradient between ascending and descending aorta
    - Intra-atrial gradients
    - Gradient between pulmonary capillary wedge pressure and ventricular end-diastolic pressure
    - Gradients between main and branch pulmonary arteries
  - Angiography parameters
    - Pulmonary arterial architecture
    - Systemic and pulmonary venous return
    - Presence of aorticopulmonary collaterals
    - AV valve function
    - Ventricular function
    - Status of the bulboventricular foramen and aortic arch

Pathologic Findings

- Ventricular morphology
  - Single left ventricle
  - Single right ventricle
  - Undifferentiated ventricle
- AV valves
  - Double-inlet ventricle
  - Single-inlet ventricle with either tricuspid or mitral atresia or severe hypoplasia
  - Common AV valve with AV septal defect

- Pulmonary outflow tract: Atretic or severely stenotic, unobstructed
- Aortic Arch Normal Coarctation of Aorta
  - Interrupted aortic arch
  - Anomalous pulmonary venous connection
  - Subaortic obstruction

DIFFERENTIAL DIAGNOSIS
The differential diagnosis is dependent on the associated anatomic lesions.
- Patients with obstruction to pulmonary blood flow
  - Tetralogy of Fallot
  - Pulmonary atresia with ventricular septal defect (VSD)
  - Transposition of the great arteries with VSD and pulmonary stenosis
  - Double-outlet right ventricle with VSD and pulmonary stenosis
- Patients with unobstructed pulmonary blood flow
  - Complete AV septal defect (AV canal)
  - Truncus arteriosus
  - Transposition of great arteries with large VSD
  - VSD with coarctation of the aorta
  - Total anomalous pulmonary venous return
  - Double-outlet right ventricle with VSD
  - Hypoplastic left heart syndrome
  - Interrupted aortic arch with large VSD

TREATMENT

GENERAL MEASURES
Treatment depends on associated cardiac defects and age of presentation.
- Severe pulmonary stenosis or pulmonary atresia: Emergent establishment of an aorticopulmonary connection via pharmacologic (prostaglandin E1) and subsequent surgical shunt
- Unobstructed pulmonary blood flow: Medical treatment for congestive heart failure and subsequent surgical treatment to control pulmonary blood flow

MEDICATION (DRUGS)

- Treatment of heart failure with digitalis, diuretics, and afterload reducing agents.
- Treatment of arrhythmias with antiarrhythmic agents, pacemakers, or implantable cardioverter–defibrillator (ICD).
- Treatment with anticoagulants as required by anatomic and physiologic status.

First Line
- Severe pulmonary stenosis or pulmonary atresia in the neonatal period treated with intravenous prostaglandin E1 to establish patency of the ductus arteriosus
- Unobstructed pulmonary blood flow and congestive heart failure treated with digitalis and diuretics; may have associated coarctation of aorta requiring prostaglandin E1 and pressors to maintain cardiac output

SURGERY
- Palliative surgery
  - Neonatal and early infancy
    - Systemic to pulmonary artery shunts (primarily modified Blalock-Taussig procedure) or central shunt for patients with inadequate pulmonary blood flow

- Atrial septectomy in patients with a restrictive atrial septal defect and stenosis or atresia of the left AV valve
- Repair of coarctation of the aorta
- Pulmonary artery banding for patients with unobstructed pulmonary blood flow and pulmonary artery hypertension to control pulmonary blood flow and pulmonary artery resistance
- Repair of total anomalous pulmonary venous connection
  - Late infancy and early childhood
    - Bidirectional Glenn or HemiFontan (superior vena cava to pulmonary artery anastomosis) increases effective pulmonary blood flow without increased volume load on ventricle.
    - Repair of branch pulmonary artery stenosis
    - Relief of subaortic stenosis
- Later surgery
  - The Fontan procedure with passive filling of the pulmonary arteries from the systemic venous system is the definitive surgical option, which may be fenestrated or nonfenestrated. The procedure has undergone modifications to either a lateral tunnel or external conduit Fontan.
  - Interventional catheterization
    - Balloon or stent atrial septostomy
    - Coil embolization of aorticopulmonary collaterals or venous collaterals
    - Balloon dilation and stenting of stenotic pulmonary arteries
    - Balloon dilation and stenting of coarctation of the aorta
    - Device closure of fenestration

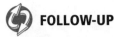 **FOLLOW-UP**

PROGNOSIS

Physiology of the Fontan procedure predisposes patients to long-term complications:

- Progressive exercise intolerance
- Progressive ventricular dysfunction
- Chronic recurrent pleural effusions
- Chronic atrial arrhythmias, especially atrial flutter and intra-atrial re-entrant tachycardia
- Ventricular arrhythmias
- Sinus and AV node dysfunction
- Thromboembolic events
- Protein-losing enteropathy
- Although the operative mortality rate is in the 5–10% range and postoperative survival for 20 years is not uncommon, many of the survivors require chronic therapy for long-term complications, including anticongestive therapy, antiarrhythmic therapy, pacemakers, ICD, and anticoagulation.
- Chronic intractable arrhythmias require ablation, pacemakers, ICD, or surgery.
- Late failure of the Fontan circulation has resulted in the need for revision of the Fontan with arrhythmia surgery or cardiac transplantation.

COMPLICATIONS

See Prognosis.

PATIENT MONITORING

- Patients who have had a completed Fontan procedure must be considered as chronic cardiac patients for life.
- These patients require monitoring for heart failure, arrhythmias, thromboembolic events, protein losing enteropathy (PLE), and failure of the Fontan circulation.

Pregnancy Considerations

Pregnancy can cause marked deterioration in the status of a Fontan patient.

REFERENCES

1. Airan B, Sharma R, Choudhary SK, et al. Univentricular repair: Is routine fenestration justified? *Ann Thorac Surg.* 2000;69:1900–1906.
2. Anderson RH, Becker AE. Historical review. In: Anderson RH, Crupi G, Parenzan L, eds. *Double Inlet Ventricle*. Tunbridge Wells, UK: Castle House, 1987.
3. Béeri E, Maier SE, Landzberg MJ, et al. In vivo evaluation of Fontan pathway flow dynamics by multidimensional phase-velocity magnetic resonance imaging. *Circulation.* 1999;98:2873–2882.
4. Bridges ND. Early and medium-term outcomes after the fenestrated Fontan operation. *Adv Cardiac Surg.* 1999;11:221–231.
5. Cecchin F, Johnsrude CL, Perry JC, et al. Effect of age and surgical technique on symptomatic arrhythmias after the Fontan procedure. *Am J Cardiol.* 1995;76:386–391.
6. Choussat A, et al. Selection criteria for Fontan procedure. In: Anderson RH, Shinebourne EA, eds. *Pediatric Cardiology*, 1977. Edinburgh, UK: Churchill Livingstone, 1978.
7. de Leval MR, Kilner P, Gewilling M, et al. Total cavopulmonary connection: A logical alternative to atriopulmonary connection for complex Fontan operations. Experimental studies and early clinical experience. *J Thorac Cardiovasc Surg.* 1988;96:682–695.
8. Gentles TL, Mayer JE Jr, Gauvreau K, et al. Fontan operations in five hundred consecutive patients: Factors influencing early and late outcome. *J Thorac Cardiovasc Surg.* 1997;114:376–391.
9. Jayakumar KA, Addonizio LJ, Kichuk-Chrisant MR, et al. Cardiac transplantation after the Fontan or Glenn Procedure. *J Am Coll Cardiol.* 2004;44:2065–2072.
10. Mahle WT, Wernovsky G, Bridges ND, et al. Impact of early ventricular unloading on exercise performance in preadolescents with single ventricle Fontan physiology. *J Am Coll Cardiol.* 1999;34:1637–1643.
11. Mavroudis C, Backer CL, Deal BJ, et al. Total cavopulmonary conversion and maze procedure for patients with failure of the Fontan operation. *J Thorac Cardiovasc Surg.* 2001;122:863–871.
12. Mertens L, Hagler DJ, Sauer U, et al. Protein losing enteropathy after the Fontan operation: An international multicenter study. PLE study group. *J Thorac Cardiovasc Surg.* 1988;115:1063–1073.
13. Petrossian E, Reddy VM, McElhinney DB, et al. Early results of the extracardiac conduit Fontan operation. *J Thorac Cardiovasc Surg.* 1999;117:688–696.
14. Rychik J, Spray TL. Strategies to treat protein-losing enteropathy. *Semin Thorac CV Surg.* 2002;5:3–11.
15. Shekerdemian LS, Bush A, Shore DF, et al. Cardiopulmonary interactions after Fontan operations: Augmentation of cardiac output using negative pressure ventilation. *Circulation.* 1997;96:3934–3942.
16. Van Praagh R, Plett JA, Van Praagh S. Single ventricle: Pathology, embroyology, terminology, and classification. *Hertz.* 1979;4:113–150.

CODES
ICD9-CM

- 745.3 Single Ventricle
- 746.1 Tricuspid Atresia

SINUS OF VALSALVA ANEURYSM

Chris Vaccari
Craig M. Brodsky
Nanette K. Wenger

 BASICS

DESCRIPTION
A sinus of Valsalva aneurysm is a congenital or acquired diverticulum of the coronary sinus that, when ruptured, creates a fistula between the aorta and a cardiac chamber, typically the right ventricle.
- Right coronary sinus most commonly affected (65–85%); noncoronary sinus affected in 20–30% of cases
- Left coronary sinus rarely affected, <5% of cases

EPIDEMIOLOGY
- 3.5% of patients with congenital heart disease that require surgery
- Age 20–40 years (presentation in childhood rare)
- Males > Females (3:1)
- Increased incidence in Asian populations

RISK FACTORS
- Congenital heart disease
- Male gender

ETIOLOGY
- Lack of continuity between aortic media and annulus fibrosis of the aortic valve
- Causes
  - Congenital: Lack of fusion of media of aorta with annulus fibrosis of aortic valve
    - May be associated with connective tissue diseases (e.g., Marfan syndrome and Ehlers-Danlos syndrome) or other congenital heart diseases (e.g., common supracristal ventricular septal defect with right sinus aneurysm, atrial septal defect, and aortic coarctation)
  - Acquired: Syphilis, rheumatoid heart disease, atherosclerosis, trauma, endocarditis

ASSOCIATED CONDITIONS
Associated conditions present in 50–70% of cases
- Congenital heart disease
  - Ventricular septal defect
  - Atrial septal defect
  - Coarctation of aorta
  - Aortic stenosis
  - Tetralogy of Fallot
- Connective tissue disease
  - Marfan syndrome
  - Ehlers-Danlos syndrome
- Acquired diseases
  - Aortic valve regurgitation
  - Endocarditis
  - Rheumatoid heart disease
  - Syphilitic aortitis

 DIAGNOSIS

SIGNS AND SYMPTOMS
- Asymptomatic prior to rupture, but rarely causes compression of coronary arteries with anginal symptoms
- With rupture, abrupt onset of chest pain
Congestive heart failure symptoms secondary to acute volume overload (e.g., dyspnea, orthopnea, edema, weakness, and fatigue)
- Fistula signs (e.g., bounding pulses; increased pulse pressure; loud continuous murmur, accentuated in diastole, heard best along lower left sternal border; parasternal thrill, hyperdynamic apex)

TESTS
Electrocardiogram (ECG)
- Normal (approximately 20%)
- Sinus tachycardia with rupture
- Conduction disturbances (including bundle branch blocks)
- Ventricular hypertrophy (left and/or right)

Lab
Blood cultures if endocarditis is suspected

Imaging
- Chest x-ray
  - Cardiomegaly
  - Pulmonary edema with acute rupture
- Ultrafast computed tomography (CT) scan
  - Visualizes the aneurysm
- Transthoracic echocardiography
  - 2-D echocardiography demonstrates aneurysm in multiple views.
  - Doppler studies demonstrate flow between the aortic sinus and the chamber into which fistula empties. In the majority of cases, fistula is located between the right coronary cusp and right ventricle. It may also be located between the noncoronary cusp and the right atrium.
  - Contrast echocardiography may demonstrate fistula.
- Transesophageal echocardiography
  - Enhances visualization of fistula
  - Aids in planning surgical approach, management
  - Magnetic resonance imaging (MRI) may demonstrate aneurysm
- Cardiac catheterization
  - Aortography may demonstrate aneurysm or fistula.
  - Sampling of oxygen saturations reveals step up at level of communication.

Classification
- Type A (ruptured)
- Type B-I (unruptured and asymptomatic)
- Type B-II (unruptured and symptomatic)
- Type C (extracardiac)

DIFFERENTIAL DIAGNOSIS
Rupture can present as abrupt onset of dyspnea, chest pain, weakness, and fatigue. Other cardiovascular disorders can present similarly.
- Congestive heart failure
- Aortic regurgitation
- Aortic dissection

 TREATMENT

GENERAL MEASURES
Acute rupture is an emergency requiring admission to the intensive care unit. Diagnostic procedures are indicated to define the exact location of the aneurysm, as well as associated conditions. Immediate surgical consultation is indicated because most ruptured sinus of Valsalva aneurysms require surgical intervention.
- Adequate oxygenation
- Afterload reduction with medical therapies listed in subsequent text
- Diuresis if pulmonary congestion present
- Antibiotics for endocarditis if present

MEDICATION (DRUGS)

First Line
- Angiotensin-converting enzyme (ACE) inhibitors are the standard of care for congestive heart failure that may result from a ruptured sinus of Valsalva aneurysm. Angiotensin receptor blockers (ARBs) with ACE intolerance (cough).
- Contraindications
  - ACE inhibitors: Known allergy, progressive renal failure, renal artery stenosis, hypotension
  - Diuretics: Hypotension
- Precautions
  - ACE inhibitors: May cause cough, cause or aggravate renal failure with renal artery stenosis, increase serum potassium levels
  - Diuretics: Loop diuretics may cause nephrotoxicity, ototoxicity; may deplete potassium, magnesium levels, predisposing to arrhythmias

Second Line
- Nitrates plus hydralazine
- Sodium nitroprusside
- Anticoagulation for asymptomatic aneurysms
- Treatment of coexistent arrhythmias

SURGERY
- Cardiac surgery treatment of choice for ruptured aneurysm
- Operative techniques include simple plication, patch repair, aortic root replacement and aortic valve replacement, and reimplantation of coronary arteries
- Rarely, percutaneous closure devices have been successful if surgery is not an option.

 FOLLOW-UP

For unruptured aneurysm without symptoms, clinical follow-up every 6 months with repeated imaging
- No guidelines on size of asymptomatic aneurysm that warrants surgical intervention

Admission Criteria
- Chronic sinus of Valsalva aneurysm does not require hospital admission.
- Acute rupture of sinus of Valsalva aneurysm requires admission to an intensive care unit.

PROGNOSIS
- Ruptured sinus of Valsalva aneurysm carries a grave prognosis unless surgically repaired.
- Repaired aneurysms carry an 85% ± 7.4% long-term survival rate.

COMPLICATIONS
- Acute rupture
- Pulmonary edema with respiratory failure
- Circulatory collapse with shock
- Endocarditis
- Aortic valve regurgitation

REFERENCES
1. Botefeu J-M, Moret PR, Hahn C, et al. Aneurysms of the sinus of Valsalva: Report of seven cases and review of the literature. *Am J Med.* 1978;65:18–24.
2. Cheitlin MD, Alpert JS, Armstrong WF, et al. ACC/AHA guidelines for the clinical application of echocardiography. *Circulation.* 1997;95:1686–1744.
3. Chiang CW, Lin FC, Fang B-R, et al. Doppler and two-dimensional echocardiographic features of sinus of Valsalva aneurysm. *Am Heart J.* 1988;116:1283–1288.
4. Feigenbaum H. Diseases of the aorta. In: Feigenbaum H, ed. *Echocardiography,* 5th ed. Baltimore: Williams & Wilkins, 1994:646–647.
5. Lewis BS, Agathangelou NE. Echocardiographic diagnosis of unruptured sinus of Valsalva aneurysm. *Am Heart J.* 1984;107:1025–1027.
6. McKenny PA, Shemin RJ, Wiegers SE. Role of transesophageal echocardiography in sinus of Valsalva aneurysm. *Am Heart J.* 1992;123:228–229.
7. Nakamura K, Suzuki S, Satomi G. Detection of ruptured aneurysm of sinus of Valsalva by contrast two dimensional echocardiography. *Br Heart J.* 1981;45:219–221.
8. Takach TJ, Reul GJ, Duncan JM, et al. Sinus of Valsalva aneurysm or fistula: Management and outcome. *Ann Thorac Surg.* 1999;68:1573–1577.
9. Vural KM, Sener E, Tasdemir O, et al. Approach to sinus of Valsalva aneurysms: A review of 53 cases. *Eur J Cardiothorac Surg.* 2001;20:71–76.
10. Webb GD, Smallhorn JF, Therrien J, et al. Congenital heart disease. In: Braunwald E, ed. *Heart disease: A Textbook of Cardiovascular Medicine,* 7th ed. Philadelphia: Elsevier Saunders, 2005:1535–1536.

CODES
ICD9-CM
441.9 Aortic aneurysms

Diet
Diet may be regular unless on a special diet or NPO for another disorder. Sodium restriction with congestive heart failure (CHF).

Activity
- Activity should be limited to bed rest for ruptured aneurysm.
- Activity as tolerated for nonruptured or repaired aneurysm

SITUS INVERSUS

Kimara L. Targoff
Welton M. Gersony

 BASICS

DESCRIPTION

- Situs inversus is a mirror-image inversion of the atrial or visceral right/left position.
- Situs solitus is determined by thoracoabdominal asymmetry with left-sided structures, including the cardiac apex, a bilobed lung, the stomach, and the spleen, and right-sided structures including the vena cava, a trilobed lung, and the larger liver lobe. In the context of situs solitus, patients can have:
  - Dextrocardia (heart in the right hemithorax) = isolated dextrocardia
  - Levocardia (heart in the left hemithorax) = normal anatomy
- Situs inversus refers to a total mirror-image reversal of this asymmetry. In the context of situs inversus, patients can have:
  - Dextrocardia (heart in the right hemithorax) = situs inversus totalis
  - Levocardia (heart in the left hemithorax) = isolated levocardia
- Situs ambiguous (abdominal heterotaxy) is a combination of situs solitus and situs inversus that usually occurs with major anomalies of the heart and great vessels, biliary tract and liver, and with malrotation of the bowel. Patients with situs ambiguous generally have asplenia (right atrial isomerism) or polysplenia (left atrial isomerism).

EPIDEMIOLOGY
Incidence
- The incidence of situs inversus with dextrocardia is 1/7,000 to 1/8,000.
- The incidence of situs solitus with dextrocardia is less common and ranges from 1/2,500 to 1/29,000.
- Patients with dextrocardia and situs inversus totalis most often do not have congenital heart disease (CHD).
- >90% of patients with dextrocardia and situs solitus have CHD.
- Close to 100% of patients with isolated levocardia have CHD.
- 20–25% of patients with situs inversus totalis have Kartagener syndrome or primary ciliary dyskinesia (PCD). This syndrome includes ciliary dyskinesia leading to bronchiectasis, sinusitis, and infertility.

RISK FACTORS
Genetics
Increasing evidence emerges of familial cases that are governed by both autosomal and X-linked genes with dominant and recessive expression patterns such as CRYPTIC, LEFTYA, and ZIC3.

PATHOPHYSIOLOGY
Varies with associated CHD.

ETIOLOGY
- Teratogens associated with situs inversus in the fetus include maternal diabetes and retinoic acid.
- However, situs inversus usually occurs sporadically.

Pregnancy Considerations
- Males with Kartagener syndrome are infertile secondary to the dysfunctional dynein in the microtubules of the cilia and spermatozoa.
- Although females with Kartagener syndrome are able to conceive, they have impaired fertility resulting from dyskinesia of the fallopian tubes.

ASSOCIATED CONDITIONS
- Dextrocardia and situs inversus (situs inversus totalis)
  - Atrioventricular discordance
  - Ventricular septal defect
  - Corrected transposition of the great arteries (TGA)
  - Complete TGA
  - Double outlet right ventricle
  - Pulmonary stenosis or atresia
  - Right aortic arch
- Levocardia and situs inversus (isolated levocardia)
  - Atrioventricular canal
  - Total anomalous pulmonary venous connection
  - Pulmonary stenosis or atresia
  - Asplenia or polysplenia occurs in approximately 80% of these patients
- Situs ambiguous (abdominal heterotaxy)
  - Asplenia (right atrial isomerism):
    - Malrotation of the bowel
    - Midline liver
    - Right-sided stomach
    - Bronchopulmonary malformations
    - Conotruncal defects
    - Atrioventricular canal
    - Univentricular atrioventricular connection
    - Anomalous pulmonary venous connection
    - Cardiac malformations are generally more severe than in polysplenia
  - Polysplenia (left atrial isomerism)
    - Malrotation of the bowel
    - Inverted liver with larger lobe on the left side
    - 2 or more spleens along greater curvature of the stomach
    - Extrahepatic biliary atresia
    - Bronchopulmonary malformations
    - Atrial septal defects
    - Ventricular septal defects
    - Bilateral superior vena cava
    - Partial anomalous pulmonary venous connection
    - Intrahepatic interruption of the inferior vena cava with azygous or hemiazygous continuation

 DIAGNOSIS

SIGNS AND SYMPTOMS
- Asymptomatic patients may be diagnosed through incidental findings at the time of a chest roentgenogram.
- Depending on severity of an associated CHD, the patient may present with:
  - Cyanosis
    - Complete TGA
    - Pulmonary atresia
    - Total anomalous pulmonary venous return
  - Respiratory distress
    - Ventricular septal defect
    - Double outlet right ventricle
    - Atrioventricular canal
  - Murmur
    - Pulmonary stenosis
    - Corrected TGA with tricuspid valve regurgitation

Physical Exam
- Cardiac impulse and heart sounds are found on the right side of the chest in the setting of dextrocardia.
- Palpation of the abdomen may reveal a left-sided liver edge and a right-sided spleen tip or, with situs ambiguous, a midline liver.
- Additional physical examination findings depend on the particular associated cardiac lesion.

TESTS

Lab
- In the patient with situs inversus, laboratory tests should be unremarkable unless abnormalities are found related to specific forms of CHD.
- ECG
  - Situs inversus with dextrocardia demonstrates inversion of normal atrial and ventricular forces.
  - The P-wave axis is shifted rightward and inferiorly secondary to atrial inversion.
  - Nonsinus atrial rhythm is common.

Imaging
- Chest roentgenogram can reveal the location of the liver and the stomach. In addition, the situs of the lungs can often be visualized.
- Echocardiography is essential to determine abdominal situs, systemic venous connections to the heart, atrioventricular (AV) and ventriculoatriol (VA) connections. In addition, the associated lesions of septal defects, valvar abnormalities, and abnormal pulmonary venous connections should be clarified.
- Ultrasound, MRI, or CT can be used to further delineate the visceral anatomy and rule out the possibility of abdominal situs ambiguous.

Diagnostic Procedures/Surgery
Cardiac catheterization and angiography are usually unnecessary for diagnosis and management of patients with situs inversus. However, these invasive procedures may be helpful to determine additional hemodynamic and anatomic data in complicated cases.

DIFFERENTIAL DIAGNOSIS
The differential diagnosis of situs inversus depends on the nature of the particular associated lesions. A broad spectrum of clinical presentations exists, ranging from the asymptomatic patient to the cyanotic newborn with pulmonary atresia or total anomalous pulmonary venous connection.

 TREATMENT

GENERAL MEASURES
- No treatment is required for the patient with asymptomatic situs inversus without heart disease or Kartagener syndrome.
- For patients with significant heart disease, such as total anomalous pulmonary venous connection or transposition of the great arteries, stabilization at the time of birth may require mechanical ventilation, inotropic support, and diuresis.

 MEDICATION (DRUGS)

- Medical therapy is not indicated in the asymptomatic patient with situs inversus. However, for patients who are symptomatic from associated CHDs, various medical regimens are recommended:
  - Prostaglandin E_1 to maintain patency of the ductus arteriosus
  - Diuretics and inotropes in the context of pulmonary overcirculation

SURGERY
- Surgical repair must needs to be tailored to the particular type of cardiac lesion (i.e., arterial switch for TGA).
- Patients with Kartagener syndrome who develop severe respiratory insufficiency may require bilateral lung transplant.

 FOLLOW-UP

PROGNOSIS
- Patients with situs inversus without significant cardiac defects have a normal life expectancy.
- Following cardiac surgical repair, routine monitoring should include evaluation of cardiac function, exercise tolerance, and rhythm disturbances.
- Specific prognosis depends on the severity of the cardiac defect(s).

REFERENCES
1. Aylsworth AS. Clinical aspects of defects in the determination of laterality. *Am J Med Gen.* 2001;101: 345–355.
2. Garson A, Jr., Bricker JT, Fisher DJ, et al. *The science and practice of pediatric cardiology,* 2nd ed. Baltimore: Lippincott Williams & Wilkins, 1998.
3. Kathiriya RS, Srivastava D. Left-right asymmetry and cardiac looping: Implications for cardiac development and congenital heart disease. *Am J Med Gen (Semin Med Genet).* 2000;97:271–279.
4. Moss AJ, Adams FH, Emmanouilides GC, eds. *Heart disease in infants, children, and adolescents,* 6th ed. Baltimore: Lippincott Williams & Wilkins, 2000.
5. Tonkin ILD. The definition of cardiac malpositions with echocardiography and computed tomography. In: Friedman WF, Higgins CB, ed. *Pediatric cardiac imaging.* Philadelphia: WB Saunders, 1984;157–187.

CODES
ICD9-CM
759.3 Situs inversus

PATIENT TEACHING
- Patients should be aware of the diagnosis of situs inversus to reduce the risk of missing a location-specific symptom, such as for appendicitis.
- If a family history of situs abnormalities is possible, patients should be referred to a geneticist for further evaluation and counseling.

SLE AND THE HEART

Christopher K. Dyke

 BASICS

DESCRIPTION

Systemic lupus erythematosus (SLE) is an autoimmune disease with a wide array of cardiac manifestations, including pericarditis, myocarditis, valvular heart disease, coronary artery disease (CAD), conduction system disease, antiphospholipid antibody syndrome, and hypertension.

- Pericardium
  - Pericarditis most common cardiovascular manifestation of SLE
  - Pericarditis may occur at any time during active disease, and may be persistent or recurrent.
  - Tamponade is a rare complication but may be the presenting feature.
  - Constrictive pericarditis noted but unusual
- Myocardium
  - The existence of lupus-related cardiomyopathy remains controversial.
  - Clinically evident heart failure is infrequent.
- Valvular heart disease
  - Libman-Sacks lesion: A small verrucous vegetation adherent to the endocardium
- Coronary artery disease
  - Atherosclerotic, thrombotic, embolic or inflammatory (arteritis)
  - Typically, medium-sized arteries are affected.
  - Accelerated atherosclerosis on corticosteroid therapy
  - Severe coronary disease is often associated with pericardial and valvular disease.
- Conduction system disease
  - Small vessel vasculitis may injure nodal or other conducting tissue.
  - Infiltration of sinus or atrioventricular nodes by fibrous or granulation tissue
  - Degrees of heart block and bundle branch block have been described, but complete heart block is rare.
  - Atrial fibrillation and flutter may be associated with pericarditis.
- Antiphospholipid antibody syndrome
  - Valvular disease most common manifestation
  - Valvular involvement may correlate with anticardiolipin levels and SLE duration.
  - Anticardiolipin antibody levels associated with myocardial infarction and graft occlusion
  - Intra-atrial and ventricular thrombi are rare manifestations.
- Hypertension
  - Associated with renal disease and corticosteroid therapy

EPIDEMIOLOGY

- Predominant sex: Females > Males (5:1)
- Predominant age: 15–40 years
- Predominant race: African Americans and Hispanics affected more often than whites
- Pericardium
  - Clinically apparent in 20–30% of larger series, and up to 39% of echocardiographic studies
  - Pericardial effusions occur in up to 42% by echocardiography.
- Myocardium
  - Most clinical studies suggest about 8% affected.
- Valvular heart disease
  - Valvular thickening most common abnormality [50% on transesophageal echocardiography (TEE)], with equal frequency on mitral and aortic valves
  - Vegetations in 43% and located on the basal, middle, or tip of leaflets, and predominantly on the atrial side of the mitral valve or on the vessel side of the aortic valve
  - Libman-Sacks lesions in 60% prior to use of steroids, 35% at autopsy once steroid use common
  - Importantly, valvular lesions have been reported to resolve, change, or develop new abnormalities.
- Coronary artery disease
  - The frequency of clinically recognizable CAD is reported to be between 6.1% and 8.9% in adults.
  - Thallium scans in asymptomatic individuals with SLE have reported perfusion defects in up to 39%.
  - The frequency of coronary atherosclerosis in autopsy series is as high as 45%.
- Antiphospholipid antibody syndrome
  - Incidence of antiphospholipid antibodies is up to 50%.

Prevalence

- The prevalence of SLE is 1/2,000 individuals.
- Autopsy series report a prevalence of cardiovascular involvement that averages nearly 70%.
- Estimates of clinically apparent disease range from 23–60% with an average of 29%.
- The prevalence of cardiac disease diagnosed by echocardiography is reported to be as high as that in autopsy series.

RISK FACTORS

SLE is a disease of unknown etiology in which tissues are damaged by pathogenic autoantibodies and immune complexes. These abnormal immune responses probably depend on interactions between susceptibility genes and environment.

Pregnancy Considerations

- Antiphospholipid antibody syndrome is characterized by recurrent pregnancy loss.
- Association between maternal lupus and congenital heart block in offspring regardless of maternal disease activity

ASSOCIATED CONDITIONS

- Pleuritis has been noted to accompany pericarditis.
- In a single report, association between lupus myocarditis and peripheral myositis
- Cardiomyopathy and pulmonary hypertension associated with antiphospholipid antibody syndrome

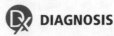 **DIAGNOSIS**

SIGNS AND SYMPTOMS

Almost any symptom or sign that could be attributed to cardiac disease may occur in a patient with SLE, including the following:

- Inspiratory chest pain, recumbent chest pain relieved by sitting, dyspnea, orthopnea, paroxysmal nocturnal dyspnea, palpitations, angina pectoris, nausea/emesis, diaphoresis, fever, distant heart sounds, elevated jugular venous pressure, pulsus paradoxus, precordial murmur, friction rub, pulmonary rales

TESTS

Lab

- Positive antinuclear antibody (ANA) test is not specific for SLE.
- Antibodies to double-stranded DNA (dsDNA) and to Smith are relatively specific for SLE.
- Determining the complete autoantibody profile of each patient helps predict clinical subsets.
- High levels of ANA and anti-dsDNA and low levels of complement usually reflect disease activity.
- CH_{50} levels are the most sensitive measure of complement activation.

Imaging

Echocardiography

- Particularly helpful in diagnosing cardiac manifestations of SLE.
- TEE is more sensitive for detecting valvular verrucae.

Pathologic Findings

- Valvular heart disease
  - Small verrucous vegetation that is adherent to the endocardium
  - Ventricular surface of the mitral valve is most commonly affected, but the verrucae can be located on both surfaces of the leaflets of all four valves.
  - Rarely, lesions may become large, approaching 10 mm.
  - Microscopic: Proliferating endothelial cells and myocytes with chronic inflammatory cells
  - Granulomatous formation, fibrosis, necrosis, and hematoxylin bodies also present
  - Immunoglobulins and complement found on the endoluminal surface of vessels from verrucae
  - Pericardium
  - No pathologic hallmarks of lupus pericarditis
  - Histologic: Fibrinous exudate, fibrinoid necrosis, and hematoxylin bodies
  - Chronic: Obliteration of pericardial space with fibrous adhesions
  - Pericardial fluid: Antinuclear antibodies, lupus erythematosus (LE) cells, immune complexes, and a reduced complement level
- Myocardium
  - No gross lesions
  - Role of endomyocardial biopsy unclear but helpful if alternative diagnosis identified
  - Histologic: Perivascular and interstitial mononuclear cell infiltration, focal fibrinoid necrosis, and infrequent hematoxylin bodies
- Coronary artery disease
  - Arteritis lesions display polymorphonuclear cells in all vascular layers, leading to edema, narrowing, and occasionally to obstruction.
  - Autopsy findings reveal focal or diffuse obstruction of smaller intramural coronary arteries by hyaline deposits and intimal proliferation.

DIFFERENTIAL DIAGNOSIS

Because SLE has numerous cardiac manifestations, the differential diagnosis includes the potential etiologies for each respective manifestation.

TREATMENT

GENERAL MEASURES

The treatment of lupus is generally initiated or modified according to its clinical features.

- Valvular heart disease
  - Antibiotic prophylaxis not evidence-based but should be considered
  - Infective endocarditis should be ruled out in febrile patients.
  - Antiplatelet therapy not evidence-based but suggested to reduce potential cardioembolic complications
  - Anticoagulant therapy suggested following hemispheric cerebrovascular accident after vasculitis ruled out
  - No consensus on the use of steroids to treat verrucous endocarditis
  - Valve replacement has been performed in the mitral and aortic positions but with a high mortality rate (25%).
- Pericardial disease
  - Asymptomatic, hemodynamically insignificant effusions are not treated.
  - Symptomatic, uncomplicated pericarditis generally responds to nonsteroidal antiinflammatory drugs.
  - More severe cases may be treated with corticosteroids.
  - Hemodynamically significant effusions treated with percutaneous drainage or pericardial window
- Myocardial disease
  - A prolonged 3- to 6-month course of steroid therapy or other immunosuppressants used for myocarditis
- Coronary artery disease
  - Steroid therapy reported to reverse coronary arteritis, but steroids should be tapered after stabilization

FOLLOW-UP

PROGNOSIS

- The treatment of SLE and its complications has improved dramatically over the last 30 years.
- However, the morbidity and mortality associated with the cardiovascular complications of SLE are increasing and are reported to be the third most common cause of death in SLE patients.
- Mortality is correlated with serologic activity.

PATIENT MONITORING

- Serologic tests for disease activity
- Echocardiogram when clinically indicated

REFERENCES

1. Doherty NE, Siegel RJ. Cardiovascular manifestations of systemic lupus erythematosus. *Am Heart J.* 1985;110:1257–1265.
2. Ginzler EM. Clinical manifestations of disease activity, its measurement, and associated morbidity in systemic lupus erythematosus. *Curr Opin Rheumatol.* 1991;3:780–788.
3. Mandell BF. Cardiovascular involvement in systemic lupus erythematosus. *Semin Arthritis Rheum.* 1987;17:126–141.
4. Roldan CA, Shively BK, Crawford MH. An echo-cardiographic study of valvular heart disease associated with systemic lupus erythematosis. *N Engl J Med.* 1997;335:1424–1430.
5. Topol EJ. *Cardiovascular Medicine.* Philadelphia: Lippincott Williams & Wilkins, 1998:912–915.

CODES
ICD9-CM
Underlying disease
- 710.0 Systemic lupus erythematosus
- 795.79 Antiphospholipid antibody syndrome

Specific manifestations
- 424.91 Endocarditis
- 422.90 Acute myocarditis, unspecified
- 423.9 Pericardial disease, unspecified
- 404.90 Hypertension, cardiorenal disease, unspecified

PATIENT TEACHING
Organizations
- Lupus Foundation of America (LFA): www.lupus.org
- National Library of Medicine: http://www.nlm.nih.gov/medlineplus/lupus.html
- Lupus Canada: www.lupuscanada.org
- Clinical Trials Listing Service: www.centerwatch.com

SLEEP DISTURBANCE AND THE HEART

Quynh A. Truong

 BASICS

DESCRIPTION
Sleep-disordered breathing (SDB) can be classified as:
- Obstructive sleep apnea (OSA)
  - Characterized by repetitive upper airway obstruction associated with apnea or hypopnea during sleep, leading to oxygen desaturations resulting from anatomic obstruction of the upper airway and periodic apneic episodes
- Central sleep apnea (CSA) or sleep hypoventilation syndrome
  - Defined by cyclical Cheyne-Stokes respiration, linked with anomalies of central control
- "Mixed apneas"
  - Combination of OSA and CSA
  - Usually begins as central and then becomes obstructive as respiratory effort is restored
- Systems affected: Cardiovascular, Pulmonary, Neurologic

GENERAL PREVENTION
Weight loss

EPIDEMIOLOGY
- Predominant age: Middle age; peak incidence in middle age
- Predominant sex: Male

Incidence
Occurs in 5–15% of population

Geriatric Considerations
- Incidence increases with weight increase
- Incidence increase with age due to changes in oropharyngeal collapsibility

Pediatric Considerations
Rare

Prevalence
- Almost 15 million Americans
- Up to 1/3 of older men
- High prevalence in congestive heart failure (CHF) population
  - Up to 2/3 of clinically stable outpatients with CHF have sleep-disordered breathing.
  - 11–40% have CSA
  - 30–58% have OSA
- Remains commonly underdiagnosed

RISK FACTORS
- Male sex
- Advanced age
- Obesity

PATHOPHYSIOLOGY
- Nocturnal sympathetic activation and increase in left ventricular post-charge leading to hypertension and cardiac dysfunction
- Autonomic abnormalities with interaction of chemoreceptor and baroreceptor reflexes by hypoxia and hypercapnia leading to increased basal heart rate, R-R interval variability, and increase blood pressure variability
- Proinflammatory and prothrombotic factors leading to coronary artery disease, pulmonary arterial hypertension, and strokes

ETIOLOGY
- OSA (two components):
  - Obstruction results from prolapse of the soft palate or tongue base during inspiration.
  - Apnea results from medullary hyporeactivity to hypercapnia and hypoxia.
- CSA
  - Due to loss of ventilatory motor output

ASSOCIATED CONDITIONS
- Obesity
- Systemic hypertension
- Pulmonary hypertension
- Congestive heart failure
- Cardiac arrhythmias
- Stroke
- Coronary artery disease
- Myocardial infarction

 DIAGNOSIS

SIGNS AND SYMPTOMS
- Heavy snoring with periodic cessation of breathing
- Frequent awakenings
- Cheynes-Stokes respiration
- Excessive daytime sleepiness (daytime hypersomnolence)
- Morning headache
- Insomnia
- Fatigue
- Nocturnal angina
- Paroxysmal nocturnal dyspnea
- Obesity
- Nocturnal desaturation
- Cognitive deficits
- Systemic hypertension
- Pulmonary hypertension and right heart failure
- Cardiac arrhythmias, including:
  - Sinus bradycardia
  - Sinus arrest
  - Asystolic episodes
  - Premature atrial or ventricular contractions
  - Atrial fibrillation
  - Ventricular tachycardia
- Congestive heart failure
- Ischemic stroke or transient ischemic attacks
- Myocardial ischemia or infarction

History
Progressive decline in exercise tolerance, worsening heart failure symptoms, which are refractory to conventional pharmacologic therapies for CHF

Physical Exam
- Obesity
- If right heart failure has developed:
  - Right heart enlargement
  - Increased pulmonic second sound
  - Increased jugular venous distention
  - Tricuspid regurgitation heard at left sternal border
  - Peripheral edema

TESTS
- ECG may show:
  - Right ventricular hypertrophy with right axis deviation
  - Right atrial enlargement (P waves >2.5 mV in lead II)

Lab
Suggestive but not diagnostic:
- Arterial blood gas may show high pco_2 and low po_2.
- High serum bicarbonate
- High hemoglobin and hematocrit
- Elevated BNP (brain natriuretic peptide)

Imaging
Echocardiography may show:
- Elevated pulmonary artery systolic pressure, tricuspid regurgitation, and right atrial enlargement
- Severe pulmonary hypertension may show right ventricular enlargement with reduced right ventricular (RV) systolic function, and pulmonicregurgitation.

Diagnostic Procedures/Surgery
- Small ambulatory oximeters
- Formal polysomnogram (PSG) sleep study is the gold standard.
- Right heart catheterization may show elevated pulmonary artery pressure if pulmonary hypertension is present.

DIFFERENTIAL DIAGNOSIS
- Obesity–hypoventilation syndrome (Pickwickian syndrome)
- Tracheal stenosis
- Neuromuscular disorders
- Parenchymal lung disorders

 TREATMENT

GENERAL MEASURES
- Continuous positive airway pressure (CPAP) improves symptoms of CSA and attenuates obstructive component of OSA. Requires formal fitting of the nasal CPAP mask by respiratory therapist.
  - Use nightly to be effective.
  - Improves nocturnal oxygenation
  - Decreases pulmonary artery pressure and improves ejection fraction
  - Lowers norepinephrine levels
  - Increases 6-minute walk distance
  - Improves quality of life, although no mortality benefit
- Nasal bilevel positive airway pressure (BiPAP) also effective for CSA
- Nocturnal oxygen therapy may improve saturation in CSA but not effective for OSA
- Tongue restraining device (special dental guards), if tongue is main source of obstruction
- Atrial overdrive pacing (remains controversial)
- Weight loss

MEDICATION (DRUGS)

- No pharmacologic therapies are available for treatment of sleep apnea.
- Modafinil (Provigil) can be used as adjuvant therapy to improve wakefulness and decrease excessive sleepiness (not to substitute conventional nasal CPAP treatment).
- Avoid sedatives, tranquilizers, "sleeping pills," and alcohol, since these may interfere with breathing.
- Tailor pharmacologic therapy to treat hypertension, heart failure, and pulmonary hypertension.

SURGERY

- In OSA patients who fail (or are noncompliant with) CPAP therapy, surgical measures may be considered.
- Tracheostomy is the most effective surgical procedure but remains a radical and unfavorable option for many patients.
- Other surgical options for OSA:
  - Uvulopalatopharyngoplasty (UPPP) surgery has ~50% success rate.
  - Geniohyoid (jaw) advancement is limited to few specialized surgical centers).
  - Laser palatoplasty is approved for snoring only (lacking data as treatment of SDB).

 ## FOLLOW-UP

DISPOSITION
Set up for home CPAP at bedtime.

Admission Criteria
- Right heart failure due to pulmonary hypertension
- Congestive heart failure requiring intravenous (IV) diuretics
- Cardiac arrhythmias

Discharge Criteria
Improvement or resolution of admission criteria

Issues for Referral
- Sleep specialist for formal sleep study and management of CPAP
- Cardiologist for congestive heart failure workup and management
- Pulmonary hypertension specialist if pulmonary artery pressures are elevated

PROGNOSIS
- Successful treatment of OSA may improve the symptoms of right heart failure and pulmonary hypertension, but will not reverse the disease process.
- Early recognition and treatment are critical to prevent development of the irreversible sequelae of OSA.

COMPLICATIONS
Congestive heart failure, pulmonary hypertension and right heart failure, myocardial infarction, stroke, arrhythmias, and even sudden death.

PATIENT MONITORING

- Recognition and correction of the side effects associated with CPAP use improves compliance with therapy. Some common problems related to the use of CPAP include the following:
  - Claustrophobia
  - Intolerance to pressure
  - Discomfort from improper fit of CPAP mask
- Weight loss may improve symptoms of OSA in obese patients.

REFERENCES

1. Badr MS. Central sleep apnea. *Prim Care*. 2005;32:361–374.
2. Ballard RD. Sleep and medical disorders. *Prim Care*. 2005;32:511–533.
3. Bradley T, et al. Continuous positive airway pressure for central sleep apnea and heart failure. *N Engl J Med*. 2005;353:2025–2033.
4. Coleman J. Complications of snoring, upper airway resistance syndrome, and obstructive sleep apnea syndrome in adults. *Otolaryngol Clin North Am*. 1999;32:223–234.
5. Cooper VL, et al. Interaction of chemoreceptor and baroreceptor reflexes by hypoxia and hypercapnia—a mechanism for promoting hypertension in obstructive sleep apnoea. *J Physiol*. 2005;568:677–687.
6. Cormican LJ, et al. Sleep disordered breathing and its treatment in congestive heart failure. *Heart*. 2005;91:1265–1270.
7. Davidson TM, et al. The sse of ENT-prescribed home sleep studies for patients with suspected obstructive sleep apnea. *Ear Nose Throat J*. 1999;78:754–766.
8. Elwood P, et al. Sleep disturbance, stroke, and heart disease events: Evidence from the Caerphilly cohort. *J Epidemiol Community Health*. 2006;60:69–73.
9. Ferrier K, et al. Sleep-disordered breathing occurs frequently in stable outpatients with congestive heart failure. *Chest*. 2005;128:2116–2122.
10. Parish JM, et al. Obstructive sleep apnea and cardiovascular disease. *Mayo Clin Proc*. 2004;79:1036–1046.
11. Phillips B. Sleep-disordered breathing and cardiovascular disease. *Sleep Med Rev*. 2005;9:131–140.
12. Piper AJ, Stewart DA. An overview of nasal CPAP therapy in the management of obstructive sleep apnea. *Ear Nose Throat J*. 1999;78:776–790.
13. Sakakibara M, et al. Effectiveness of short-term treatment with nocturnal oxygen therapy for central sleep apnea in patients with congestive heart failure. *J Cardiol*. 2005;46:53–61.
14. Simantirakis EN, et al. Atrial overdrive pacing for the obstructive sleep apnea-hypopnea syndrome. *N Engl J Med*. 2005;353:2568–2577.
15. Yaggi HK, et al. Obstructive sleep apnea as a risk factor for stroke and death. *N Engl J Med*. 2005;353:2034–2041.

 ## MISCELLANEOUS

See also: Pulmonary hypertension; Congestive heart failure

CODES
ICD9-CM
- 780.53 Hypersomnia with sleep apnea NOS
- 780.57 Sleep apnea NOS
- 327.20 Organic sleep apnea, unspecified
- 327.26 Sleep related hypoventilation/hypoxemia in conditions classifiable elsewhere
- 786.04 Cheyne-Stokes breathing

PATIENT TEACHING
- Educate the patient about the symptoms of OSA.
- Encourage patients to comply with CPAP.

Diet
- Calorie restriction
- Low salt (if heart failure present)

Activity
Exercise should be encouraged to aid weight loss.

Prevention
Obesity, especially in males, should be avoided.

FAQ
Q: When and how should sleep apnea be treated?
A: Significant episodes are >10 seconds in duration. Usually five or more of such episodes per hour require treatment. Formal PSG sleep study is the definitive test for diagnosis. Weight loss and breathing-assisted devices (CPAP or BiPAP) are first line in therapy.
Q: Are there medications to take as an alternative to CPAP?
A: No pharmacologic therapy is currently available for treatment of sleep apnea.
Q: What if the nasal CPAP mask is uncomfortable?
A: A respiratory therapist should fit the nasal mask formally. Nasal pillows (or "Adam circuit") are a smaller alternative to the mask.
Q: Will I need CPAP for the rest of my life?
A: There is currently no device-free "cure" for SDB. Surgical options have limitations (see previous text).

STEAL SYNDROME

Julie J. Ramos
Andrew B. Chung*
Nanette K. Wenger

 ## BASICS

DESCRIPTION
- Steal syndrome is vascular insufficiency secondary to dysfunction of arterial blood flow autoregulation rather than solely due to static flow-limiting occlusions.
- System(s) affected: Cardiovascular; Cerebrovascular; Musculoskeletal; Gastrointestinal

GENERAL PREVENTION
- Smoking cessation
- Hypertension management
- Glycemic control
- Lipid management

EPIDEMIOLOGY
- Predominant age: Increasing incidence after age 35
- Predominant sex: Male > Female
- Age-related factors:
  - Pediatric: More associated with congenital vascular anomalies
  - Adult: More associated with atherosclerotic vascular disease

Incidence
- Common
- Vascular diseases of medium-sized branching arteries
  - Atherosclerosis
  - Endothelial dysfunction
- Coronary artery steal
- Vertebral artery steal
- Subclavian artery steal

RISK FACTORS
- Cigarette smoking
- Hypertension
- Diabetes
- Dyslipidemia
- Male sex
- Family history
- Advanced age

PATHOPHYSIOLOGY
- Stimulus: Increased metabolism
- Response: Arteries dilate to meet higher metabolic demands.
- Normal: Minimal pressure decreases at distal branch points where organs and muscle groups compete for blood flow.
- Abnormal: Inability to vasodilate fully with increased demand
  - Low "vascular reserve"
- Anatomic stenosis: Physical stricture with normal vessel wall, atherosclerosis
- Endothelial dysfunction
- Steal syndrome prerequisites:
  - Abnormal supplying artery
  - Abnormal branch defaulting to at least 1 relatively normal arterial branch

ASSOCIATED CONDITIONS
Atherosclerotic vascular disease

 ## DIAGNOSIS

SIGNS AND SYMPTOMS
- Myocardium: Angina pectoris
- Vertebral arteries: Transient neurologic deficits
- Skeletal muscle: Claudication
- Intestinal segments
  - Postprandial abdominal pain
  - Bowel obstruction

Physical Exam
- Palpation for unequal pulses
- Measurement of unequal blood pressures
- Bruits on auscultation

TESTS
Simultaneous pressure tracings via intra-arterial catheters

Imaging
- Occlusive plethysmography
- Vascular ultrasonography with Doppler
- Magnetic resonance angiography
- Radiographic contrast angiography
- Radionuclide perfusion imaging

DIFFERENTIAL DIAGNOSIS
- Fixed obstructive lesions
  - Normal arterial wall architecture
  - Atherosclerosis
  - Kink or bend
- Steal syndrome: Unbalanced competition for limited vascular reserve

 ## TREATMENT

GENERAL MEASURES
- Oxygen
- Reduce metabolic demands.
- For angina pectoris:
  - β-Adrenergic blockade
  - Nitroglycerin to decrease preload
- For transient cerebrovascular ischemia:
  - Bed rest
  - Lower head of bed.
- For claudication:
  - Physical exertion should be discontinued.
- For gastrointestinal symptoms:
  - Nasogastric suctioning
  - NPO status for bowel rest
  - Nitroglycerin may overcome endothelial dysfunction.
  - Correct anemia if significant.

 ## MEDICATION (DRUGS)

- Antiplatelet agents, such as aspirin, clopidogrel
- Lipid-lowering medications, such as HMG-CoA reductase inhibitors
- β-Adrenergic blockers, such as metoprolol
- Nitroglycerin to ameliorate spasm caused by endothelial dysfunction
- Calcium channel blockers to prevent subsequent episodes
- Others: Aggressive medical treatment of other underlying atherogenic conditions, such as hypertension and diabetes
- Contraindications: Pre-existing allergy or intolerance
- Precautions: Refer to manufacturer's profile for each drug.
- Significant possible interactions:
  - β-Adrenergic blockers combined with nondihydropyridine calcium channel blockers can result in bradyarrhythmias.
  - Nitroglycerin should not be administered within 24 hours of sildenafil or vardenafil or 48 hours of tadalafil use.

SURGERY
- Vascular bypass surgery
- Percutaneous angioplasty ± stenting

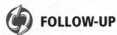

FOLLOW-UP

PROGNOSIS
- Progression to fixed occlusive vascular disease with:
  - Tissue infarction
  - Intractable symptoms
- Medical therapy can potentially slow/halt progression.

COMPLICATIONS
Acute thrombotic occlusion leading to tissue infarction

PATIENT MONITORING
Close regular visits to assess gradually progressive symptoms that may indicate failure of medical therapy or endovascular intervention

REFERENCES
1. Cai H. NAD(P)H oxidase–dependent self-propagation of hydrogen peroxide and vascular disease. *Circulation Res*. 2005;96:818–822.
2. Casserly IP, Sachar R, Yadav JS, eds. *Manual of peripheral vascular intervention*. Philadelphia: Lippincott Williams & Wilkins, 2005.
3. Davignon J, Ganz P. Atherosclerosis: Evolving vascular biology and clinical implications role of endothelial dysfunction in atherosclerosis. *Circulation*. 2004;109:III-27–III-32.
4. Fuster V, Alexander RW, O'Rourke RA, et al., eds. *Hurst's the heart*, 11th ed. New York: McGraw-Hill, 2004.
5. Harrison DG, Cai H. Endothelial control of vasomotion and nitric oxide production. *Cardiol Clin*. 2003;21(3):289–302.
6. Ishikawa M, Stokes KY, Zhang JH, et al. Cerebral microvascular responses to hypercholesterolemia: Roles of NADPH oxidase and P-selectin. *Circulation Res*. 2004;94:239.
7. Kloner RA. Cardiovascular effects of the 3 phosphodiesterase-5 inhibitors approved for the treatment of erectile dysfunction. *Circulation*. 2004;110:3149–3155.
8. Rossum AC, Steel SR, Hartshorne MF. Evaluation of coronary subclavian steal syndrome using sestamibi imaging and duplex scanning with observed vertebral subclavian steal. *Clin Cardiol*. 2000;23(3):226–229.
9. Weber C. Platelets and chemokines in atherosclerosis: Partners in crime. *Circulation Res*. 2005;96:612–616.
10. Werner GS, Figulla HR. Direct assessment of coronary steal and associated changes of collateral hemodynamics in chronic total coronary occlusions. *Circulation*. 2002;106:435–440.

MISCELLANEOUS

CODES
ICD9-CM
- 413 Angina pectoris
- 413.9 Angina, unspecified
- 435.1 Vertebral artery steal
- 435.2 Subclavian steal
- 557.9 Bowel ischemia (transient)
- See also: Stable Angina Pectoris; Claudication; Transient Cerebrovascular Ischemia; Ischemic Bowel

PATIENT TEACHING
- Risk factors for endothelial dysfunction:
  - Cigarette smoking
  - Dyslipidemia
- Risk factors for progression of atherosclerotic disease:
  - Internet resource: http://www.theheart.org

Diet
Low-fat/low-cholesterol diet

Activity
Rest as needed.

Prevention
- Smoking cessation
- Regular exercise
- Maintain ideal body weight.
- Low-fat and low-cholesterol diet
- Surveillance for hypertension, diabetes, and dyslipidemia

STEM CELLS AND THE HEART

Benjamin Prentiss
Gerard Aurigemma

BASICS

DESCRIPTION

- Stem cells are pluripotent cells from which all cells within an organism are derived.
- Embryonic stem cells have long been known to have the capacity to differentiate into cells of other organs and even other germ layers. Populations of stem cells have been identified in adult organisms, and these cells also carry this high degree of plasticity.
- Adult stem cells have been found in numerous adult human tissues, including organs that were once believed to be postmitotic, like the brain and heart. Through signaling methods not yet completely understood, these stem cells can be activated to differentiate into the tissues in which they reside, or even migrate throughout the body and differentiate into other tissues.
- Cytokines such as stem cell factor and granulocyte colony stimulating factor are known to markedly increase the number of circulating heart stem cells.

The Heart's Response to Physiologic and Pathologic Stress

- The ability of the heart to adapt to disease processes by myocyte regeneration is a controversial topic. This concept applies to a wide spectrum of diseases of the heart, including hypertension, atherosclerosis, and heart failure.
- There has been a longstanding paradigm that the heart has a limited ability to sustain and adapt to diseases that affect the cardiac myocytes. This belief is founded on the premise that postnatal maturation only allows for hypertrophy of existing myocytes as an adaptive response to disease. When the mechanism of hypertrophy is exhausted, progressive organ failure ensues.
- Evidence refuting the dogma of the heart as a terminally differentiated organ exists, however, and is gaining acceptance. Numerous findings indicate that the heart responds to many physiologic and pathologic conditions by forming new myocytes.

- Studies have demonstrated that new myocytes are formed continuously to replace aging, apoptotic myocytes, as is seen in many self-renewing organs. These processes are increased in pathologic states, and an imbalance between cell growth and death is likely a factor in determining the onset of organ dysfunction and failure.
- Undifferentiated cells expressing surface antigens similar to those found in hematopoietic stem cells have been identified in the human heart. These cells have been signaled to differentiate to multiple cell lines *in vitro*. Whether a resident population, present since birth, or as a blood-borne population, infiltrating the heart because of molecular signaling, these primitive stem cells are present at levels suggestive of a mechanism of continuous renewal of cardiac myocytes.
- Self-renewing organs have their stem cells clustered in specific areas called *niches*. Cardiac stem cells have been found in niches located primarily in areas of lower mechanical stress, including the atria and apex.

Myocardial Repair by Primitive Bone Marrow Cells

• Generation of *de novo* myocardium and vascular structures has been demonstrated in experimental *in vivo* models using bone marrow cells implanted next to infarcted myocardium. Within 9 days of implantation, the primitive bone marrow cells formed numerous small cardiac myocytes and functional vasculature that extended into the zone of infarction, improving the cardiac performance.

• Systemic infusion of stem cell factor and granulocyte colony stimulating factor (a protocol for reconstituting hematopoietic system of irradiated mice) was shown to also cause reconstitution of infarcted myocardium. This method also produced an improvement in cardiac structure and function.

Myocardial Repair by Cardiac Stem Cells

It has been demonstrated in animal models that, when provided with the proper cytokine stimulation (insulin-like growth factor-1, and hepatocyte growth factor), resident cardiac stem cells have reconstituted infarcted ventricular tissue.

Chimerism of Transplanted Hearts

When male patients have been transplanted with female donor hearts, cells containing a Y chromosome have been identified in the myocardium, arterioles, and capillaries of the donor heart, indicating migration from the recipients' body. When transplanted hearts were compared to control hearts, markedly increased numbers of primitive stem cells were identified in the transplanted organs, indicating active processes of regeneration.

Hyperplasia as Well as Hypertrophy

Studies of human hearts with aortic stenosis, in which there is a markedly increased work load placed on the myocardium, have demonstrated intense new formation of myocyte cells from stemlike cells found in the myocardium. These results suggest that cardiac myocyte hyperplasia plays a significant role in the development of hypertrophy.

REFERENCES

1. Lanza R, et al. *The Handbook of Stem Cells*. Burlington, MA.: Elsevier Academic Press, 2004.
2. Mattson MP, Van Zant G. *Stem Cells: A Cellular Fountain of Youth*. Elsevier Science B.V., 2002.
3. Quaini F, Urbanek K, Beltrami AP, et al. Chimerism of the transplanted heart. *N Engl J Med*. 2002;346:5–15.
4. Turkson K, ed. *Adult Stem Cells*. Totowa, NJ. Humana Press, 2004.

SUDDEN DEATH

Peter Ott
Andrew E. Epstein

 ## BASICS

DESCRIPTION

Sudden death is defined as the natural, sudden, unexpected loss of consciousness and death of a person in previously stable condition, with or without known heart disease. It is usually assumed to be a consequence of a ventricular arrhythmia, but bradycardia and noncardiac causes such as pulmonary embolism may be the etiology.

- Synonyms
  - The following have been used interchangeably but are not synonymous:
    - Cardiac arrest (refers to collapse due to ventricular tachycardia or fibrillation)
    - Ventricular tachycardia followed by ventricular fibrillation is the usual cause of sudden death.

Pregnancy Considerations

Pregnancy may precipitate ventricular arrhythmias in long QT syndrome.

EPIDEMIOLOGY

There are 350,000 sudden, unexpected deaths each year in the United States. Persons of any age may be affected.

RISK FACTORS

- Same as in coronary artery disease (cigarette use, hyperlipidemia, and hypertension)
- Electrocardiographic abnormalities, often determined by ambulatory monitoring, including premature ventricular contractions and nonsustained ventricular tachycardia, left ventricular hypertrophy, nonspecific ST-T wave changes, intraventricular conduction delays, increased QT dispersion, T-wave alternans, and decreased heart rate variability
- Decreased functional capacity
- Increased age
- Higher heart rate
- Obesity
- Low left ventricular ejection fraction
- Low vital capacity
- Inducible ventricular tachycardia in high-risk patient (after myocardial infarction, low left ventricular ejection fraction)

ETIOLOGY

- Coronary artery disease is the most common cause, and is not specifically a genetic disease, although there are genetic components.
- There are some clearly inherited disorders of rhythm and conduction such as the long QT syndrome, Brugada syndrome, congenital complete heart block, myotonic dystrophy, Kearn-Sayre syndrome, and, rarely, arrhythmogenic right ventricular dysplasia.
- Cardiomyopathies, both hypertrophic and dilated, are associated with an incidence of sudden, arrhythmic death.

ASSOCIATED CONDITIONS

See Risk Factors.

 ## DIAGNOSIS

SIGNS AND SYMPTOMS

By definition, the unexpectedness makes prodromal symptoms not a necessary component of the syndrome.

- New or worsening chest discomfort, dyspnea, palpitations, or fatigue over weeks or months may be present.
- 40–50% of all persons who die suddenly have seen a physician in the preceding month because of symptoms not necessarily recognized as being related to the heart.

TESTS

- Electrocardiogram (ECG) (in the setting of myocardial infarction)
- Cardiac enzymes [creatine kinase (CK), CK with MB fraction, troponin]
- Echocardiogram
- Coronary and left ventricular angiography
- Cardiac magnetic resonance imaging (MRI) (useful in diagnosing arrhythmogenic right ventricular dysplasia)
- Exercise test with perfusion imaging (to assess ischemia)
- Electrophysiologic study
- Many other tests may be appropriate depending on the clinical circumstances. For example, if pulmonary embolus is suspected, ventilation-perfusion imaging, spiral computed tomographic (CT) scanning, or pulmonary angiography can be considered. If intracranial hemorrhage is suspected, cerebral MRI or CT scanning would be indicated.

Lab

- Cardiac enzymes may identify myocardial infarction.
- If infarction has occurred, the chance for recurrence is low.
- Myocardial infarction as a cause of cardiac arrest would prompt evaluation of coronary anatomy.

Pathologic Findings

- Coronary artery disease usual substrate
- Cardiomyopathy, either hypertrophic or dilated
- Anomalous coronary artery
- Pulmonary embolus
- Cerebral hemorrhage

DIFFERENTIAL DIAGNOSIS

- The cause of sudden, unexpected collapse and death within 1 hour of symptom onset is often elusive.
- Although such events are usually presumed to be cardiac in origin, many other catastrophic events can present with a similar time course, such as pulmonary embolism, aortic rupture, and intracerebral hemorrhage.
- Sometimes postmortem examination can define the cause of sudden death, but even then, the cause cannot always be determined.

 ## TREATMENT

GENERAL MEASURES

- Prompt resuscitation
- Management of airway, circulation, and brain

 ## MEDICATION (DRUGS)

- Avoid drugs that cause QT prolongation in patients with a history of torsade de pointes ventricular tachycardia, and long QT syndrome.
- Amiodarone is indicated if drug treatment strategy is chosen. For cardiac arrest not due to a reversible cause, implantable defibrillators provide a greater chance for long-term survival than does drug therapy.
- β-Blockers decrease risk of sudden death in patients recovering from myocardial infarction.
- β-Blockers, angiotensin-converting enzyme (ACE) inhibitors, and aldactone reduce total mortality in patients with heart failure.
- Class IC drugs are contraindicated when coronary artery disease is present. Class IA drugs are also known to cause proarrhythmia.

SURGERY

Surgical interventions are dictated by the cause of the cardiac arrest.

- If there is severe coronary artery disease, coronary revascularization is indicated.
- If profound bradycardia is documented, a pacemaker should be implanted.
- If ventricular fibrillation or tachycardia is documented, implantation of an implantable defibrillator should be considered.

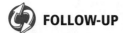 **FOLLOW-UP**

DISPOSITION
Admission Criteria
- The resuscitation rate in the field is usually <10%.
- If a survivor makes it to the hospital, admission is obviously the only option.
- Even survivors to admission have a high in-hospital mortality rate and often disability if they are discharged alive.

PROGNOSIS
- Outcome depends on the underlying substrate. In the absence of acute myocardial infarction, the chance for recurrent cardiac arrest if sudden death was due to ventricular fibrillation or tachycardia is about 30% at 1 year.
- In the AVID trial, 1,013 patients with sudden death or hemodynamically unstable VT were randomized to either implantable cardioverter–defibrillator (ICD) or amiodarone therapy. The ICD group had a 30% relative risk reduction in total mortality.

PATIENT MONITORING
- Assess changes in functional capacity and cardiac symptoms that may be warning of changing ischemic substrate.
- If drug therapy is chosen, assess compliance, drug levels, effect on ECG, and changes in myocardial substrate.
- Device follow-up if implantable defibrillator chosen
- Control of coronary risk factors and prevention of acquired heart disease
- Correct ischemia (surgical or percutaneous revascularization, β-blockade).
- Improve left ventricular function (ACE inhibitors in coronary artery disease).
- If amiodarone is used, follow chest x-ray, thyroid and liver function, and ECG.
- Avoid proarrhythmic drugs.
- Identification of high-risk groups by noninvasive (ECG, signal averaged ECG, heart rate variability, baroreflex depression) and invasive (electrophysiologic study) assessment

REFERENCES
1. Akhtar M, Myerburg RJ, Ruskin JN, eds. *Sudden Cardiac Death: Prevalence, Mechanisms, and Approaches to Diagnosis and Management*. Philadelphia: Williams & Wilkins, 1994.
2. Dunbar SB, Ellenbogen K, Epstein AE, eds. *Sudden Cardiac Death: Past, Present and Future*. Armonk, NY: Futura, 1997.
3. Goldschlager N, Epstein AE, Naccarelli G, et al. Practical guidelines for clinicians who treat patients with amiodarone. *Arch Intern Med*. 2000;160:1741–1748.
4. Poole JE, Bardy GH. Sudden cardiac death. In: Zipes DP, Jalife J, eds. *Cardiac Electrophysiology: From Cell to Bedside*. Philadelphia: WB Saunders, 1995:812–832.
5. AVID trial. *N Engl J Med* 1997;337:1576–1583.

 MISCELLANEOUS

See also: Defibrillators, implantable; Premature ventricular contractions; Torsade de pointes Ventricular tachycardia; Ventricular fibrillation; Ventricular tachycardia; Brugada syndrome; Long QT syndrome

CODES
ICD9-CM
- 427.41 Ventricular fibrillation
- 427.5 Cardiac arrest

PATIENT TEACHING
- Genetic testing and counseling, if indicated (e.g., for patients with long QT syndrome or Brugada syndrome)
- Avoidance of drugs that may be proarrhythmic, such as QT-prolonging drugs in patients with long QT syndrome
- Recommendations for diet and activity are specific for the individual patient affected.

SYNCOPE, ADULT

Marcus Williams
Jonathan Langberg
Samer Garas
Nanette K. Wenger

 BASICS

DESCRIPTION
- Transient loss of consciousness usually accompanied by loss of postural tone
- Precipitated by variety of disorders ranging from benign to fatal

EPIDEMIOLOGY
- 5–20% of adults experience a syncopal episode by age 75.
- 6% of emergency room visits, 3% of hospital admissions
- Evaluation, treatment for syncope in 1 million people annually
- Incidence increases with age.
- Prognosis worsens with increasing age.
- Most common causes
  - Neurally mediated (including vasovagal)
  - Orthostatic
  - Arrhythmia-related
  - Seizure

Pregnancy Considerations
- Relatively common, evaluate carefully
- Due to aortocaval compression by enlarged uterus decreasing venous return

RISK FACTORS
- Increasing age
- Cardiac disease
- History of neurologic disease
- Peripheral neuropathy

ETIOLOGY
- Any condition leading to decreased cerebral blood flow
- No etiologic diagnosis established in 30–50% of patients

ASSOCIATED CONDITIONS
- Cardiac disorders, including arrhythmias
- Neurologic disorders
- Chronic illness

DIAGNOSIS

SIGNS AND SYMPTOMS
History and physical examination identify up to 50% of probable causes.

History
Careful interview of patient, witnesses, medical personnel should be undertaken regarding:
- Situation (description of setting, events leading to episode)
- Prodrome (palpitations, dizziness)
- Period of unconsciousness (time-course, behavior)
- Residual symptoms (postevent sensations)
- Past medical history
- Medications
- Family history: Sudden death, syncope
- Drugs, alcohol

Physical Exam
- Check orthostatic blood pressure: Approximately 8% occurrence
- Check blood pressure in each arm.
- Cardiac examination, including bedside maneuvers (e.g., Valsalva, carotid sinus massage), murmur of aortic stenosis, HC

TESTS
- Electrocardiogram (ECG): Recommended for all patients with syncope
- Finger stick glucose: Rule out hypoglycemia
- Echocardiography: Useful for suspected organic heart disease such as aortic stenosis, HC
- Exercise testing: Consider with exertional syncope, signs of ischemia
- Electroencephalography: Performed with history suggesting seizure disorder
- Ambulatory ECG monitoring: History suggesting arrhythmia versus loop event monitoring for recurrent syncope
- Tilt table: If neurocardiogenic syncope suspected
- Electrophysiology: After consultation with cardiology, suspected ventricular arrhythmia

Lab
- Routine laboratory testing not recommended
- Only as specifically suggested by history, physical examination

Imaging
- No routine imaging studies unless suggested by history, physical examination
- Brain imaging [usually with computed tomography (CT) scan] if focal neurologic signs noted
- Carotid or transcranial Doppler indicated if bruits present or history suggests vertebrobasilar insufficiency. Carotid disease generally does not cause syncope.

DIFFERENTIAL DIAGNOSIS
- Neurocardiogenic: Vasovagal, situational: Cough, micturition, defecation, swallowing
- Orthostatic
- Cardiac
  - Arrhythmic: Bradyarrhythmia [sinus node disease, atrioventricular (AV) block, pacemaker malfunction, drug induced], tachyarrhythmia (ventricular, supraventricular), carotid sinus hypersensitivity
  - Obstructive: Aortic stenosis, hypertrophic cardiomyopathy
- Neurologic: Seizures
- Vascular: Subclavian steal
- Psychiatric: Conversion disorder, hyperventilation
- Metabolic: Hypoglycemia
- Medications: Antidepressants, antihypertensives, analgesics
- Unknown

TREATMENT

GENERAL MEASURES
- Vary, based on etiology of syncope
- Acutely, recumbent position, head down
- Avoid dehydration.
- Volume expansion: Increase salt and water intake.
- Avoid precipitating factors and drugs.
- Recognize prodrome.
- Learn adaptive maneuvers.
- Cardiology consultation if further workup indicated; cardiac catheterization, electrophysiology study
- Consider neurology consultation if significant neurologic disease is documented.

 MEDICATION (DRUGS)

- Vary with diagnosis
- Empiric drug therapy may increase recurrence.
- For vasovagal syncope
  - Fludrocortisone
  - β-Blockers
  - α-Agonists: midodrine
  - Anticholinergic agents
  - Serotonin reuptake inhibitors
  - Methylxanthines
  - Magnesium
  - Clonidine

SURGERY
The following surgical measures may be considered after electrophysiology consultation and testing:
- Pacemaker
- Implantable cardioverter–defibrillator (ICD)
- Catheter ablation

 FOLLOW-UP

DISPOSITION
Admission Criteria
- Most patients do not benefit from hospitalization.
- Consider hospitalization for elderly patients, suspected arrhythmia.
- Consider admission
  - Severe orthostatic hypotension
  - Unexplained syncope with injury
  - New neurologic findings
  - Concomitant conditions requiring therapy
  - Structural heart disease
  - Frequent syncope

PROGNOSIS
- Negative evaluation usually denotes favorable long-term prognosis.
- 45–50% do not experience recurrence.
- No recurrence over several years associated with good prognosis
- Prognosis worsens with increasing age.
- Mortality risk based on etiology; highest mortality with associated structural heart disease

PATIENT MONITORING
Follow-up depends on therapy chosen (e.g., pacemakers, ICDs need regular follow-up with measurement of function and battery life).

REFERENCES
1. Boudoulas H, Nelson SD, Schaal FS, et al. Diagnosis and management of syncope. In: Alexander RW, et al., eds. *Hurst's the Heart,* 11th ed. New York: McGraw-Hill, 2004.
2. Linzer M, Yang E, Estes M, et al. Diagnosing syncope part I. *Ann Intern Med.* 1997;126: 989–996.
3. Linzer M, Yang E, Estes M, et al. Diagnosing syncope part II. *Ann Intern Med.* 1997;127:76–86.
4. Olahansky B. Evaluating syncope: How to do it efficiently and safely. *J Crit Illness.* 1999;14: 423–430.

CODES
ICD9-CM
780.2

PATIENT TEACHING
- Lifestyle changes to prevent recurrence
- High-salt diet in certain situations: Orthostatic, neuropathy
- Restrict driving until cause of syncope is identified and treated.
- Other restrictions based on frequency, etiology (e.g., job restrictions)

SYNCOPE, PEDIATRIC

Robert H. Pass
Welton M. Gersony

 BASICS

DESCRIPTION
Syncope is defined as a sudden transient loss of consciousness and postural tone with recovery of sensory perception shortly thereafter (<1 minute).
- Associated physical trauma to the affected patient as a result of the episode is common.
- Consciousness usually returns with assumption of the supine position.
- Episode reflects a transient decrease in cerebral perfusion pressure.
- Rarely life-threatening in children and adolescents
- System(s) affected: Cardiovascular, Neurologic, Musculoskeletal
- Synonym(s): For neurocardiogenic syncope, vasovagal, common faint, neurally mediated, and benign syncope

GENERAL PREVENTION
For patients with neurocardiogenic syncope, recognition of signs and symptoms preceding a syncopal episode will often allow prevention of such episodes.

EPIDEMIOLOGY
- Represents 3% of emergency room visits and 6% of hospitalizations for adults in the United States
- Far less frequent in childhood
- Predominant age: Uncommon in children; increasing frequency through adolescence
- Predominant sex: Males = females

Incidence
Roughly 20% of children will have a syncopal episode by age 15.
- Larger percentage will have presyncopal sensations.

Prevalence
Not well described in children

RISK FACTORS
- For neurocardiogenic syncope: Prolonged recumbency, physical exhaustion, and pregnancy
- Breath-holding spells in infancy are usually neurocardiogenic in nature.
- For other forms of syncope: Presence of Wolff-Parkinson-White (WPW) syndrome on resting electrocardiogram (ECG), arrhythmogenic right ventricular dysplasia (ARVD), prolongation of the QT interval on ECG or family history of such, presence of massive ventricular hypertrophy or family history of sudden death in hypertrophic cardiomyopathy, or serious electrolyte abnormalities

Pregnancy Considerations
Represents a risk factor for neurocardiogenic syncope in adults

Genetics
Variable depending on etiology

PATHOPHYSIOLOGY
Common pathway for all forms of neurocardiogenic syncope is stimulation of the medullary vasodepressor region via the Bezold-Jarisch reflex.

ETIOLOGY
- Most common etiology is neurocardiogenic (23–93% of all childhood syncope)
- Major forms of neurocardiogenic form include vasodepressor, cardioinhibitory, and mixed response.
- Other potential etiologies include bradycardias (sinus bradycardia or atrioventricular block), serious ventricular arrhythmias (e.g., long QT syndrome), supraventricular arrhythmias, or congenital lesions associated with reduced antegrade flow such as aortic stenosis, cardiomyopathy, coronary arterial anomalies, severe pulmonary stenosis, and cardiac tumors.

 DIAGNOSIS

SIGNS AND SYMPTOMS
Most common signs and symptoms:
- Light-headedness or visual changes are often noted prior to loss of consciousness (neurocardiogenic).
- When neurocardiogenic in etiology, consciousness returns rapidly with assumption of supine position.
- When syncope is due to arrhythmogenic mechanism (e.g., Long QT Syndrome (LQTS), supraventricular tachycardia, and ventricular arrhythmias), often preceded by palpitations or rapid or irregular heart beat; length of syncopal period may be longer than neurocardiogenic
- For patients with syncope due to arrhythmia, ECG/Holter monitoring may offer clues to etiology such as presence of WPW, ventricular or atrial ectopy, or prolongation of the QT interval.

History
- Neurocardiogenic (vasovagal, neurally mediated, common faint)
- Commonly seen on hot/humid day, on rapidly arising from supine or seated position, in setting of poor nutrition or hydration
- Standing upright for long periods with venous pooling in lower extremities
- History of light-headedness with arising from supine position
- Positive family history of neurocardiogenic syncope often present.

Physical Exam
- For patients with neurocardiogenic syncope, presence of orthostatic changes should be assessed, with this exception: Physical examination is often not useful in diagnosis.
- Patients with congenital heart defects can have multiple findings on auscultation (see chapters on specific heart defects).

TESTS
- ECG
  - Atrial and ventricular ectopy may be noted.
  - Presence of ventricular pre-excitation (e.g., WPW) should be assessed.
  - Atrioventricular conduction should be reviewed (PR interval).

- Assessment of precordial voltages and ST-T wave changes in assessing for hypertrophic cardiomyopathy should be made (may be more sensitive than even echocardiography for this diagnosis).
  - QTc interval should be measured in all cases.
  - 24-hour ambulatory Holter should be screened for ectopy.
  - Home event recording can be useful to detect infrequent arrhythmic events.
- Head-up tilt-table test
  - Rarely performed in cases where history and etiology are not clear. Test can be repeated with isoprenaline infusion, although specificity decreases with this addition.
- Electrophysiologic study
  - Performed in patients with syncope and WPW; otherwise, performed when the etiology is unclear and arrhythmia is suspected either by history or common association (e.g., tetralogy of Fallot)
- Exercise stress study
  - Should be performed in all patients with exercise-induced syncope as well as patients with activity-related arrhythmias; often used to assess ventricular ectopy response to high-catechol state in patients with ventricular arrhythmias

Lab
- Complete blood count and electrolytes (including magnesium, calcium, and glucose); blood and urine for toxicology in cases of potential ingestion or illicit drug use
- Genetic testing is successful in identifying ~65% of patients with LQTS; all genetic mutations have not, however, been identified thus far.

Imaging
Echocardiography
- Used primarily to rule out congenital heart disease and cardiomyopathies; also useful to assess ventricular function

Diagnostic Procedures/Surgery
- Cardiac catheterization
  - May be necessary to diagnose congenital heart disease
  - Right ventricular (RV) angiography may help in diagnosis of arrhythmogenic right ventricular dysplasia (although not very sensitive)
- Cardiac magnetic resonance imaging (MRI)
  - Demonstrated relatively sensitive for diagnosis of ARVD

Pathologic Findings
For various congenital heart lesions, refer to specific AHA Consult Book chapters. Thinned out, fat-infiltrated RV outflow tract is noted in arrhythmogenic RV dysplasia.

DIFFERENTIAL DIAGNOSIS
Neurologic disorders (e.g., seizure disorder, neuropathies, brain arteriovenous malformations), metabolic disorders (e.g., diabetic ketoacidosis), anemia or ingestions/illicit drug usage

TREATMENT

GENERAL MEASURES

- For neurocardiogenic syncope, care is most often outpatient. For most other forms, hospitalization for evaluation/observation or intervention may be necessary.
- Self-awareness of symptoms prior to fainting is important to prevention of neurocardiogenic episodes.
  - When symptoms are felt, patients should either sit or assume a supine position.
  - Adequate hydration is the cornerstone of prevention of episodes.
- Rule of thumb is that patients are adequately drinking when the urine is entirely clear (and not concentrated).
- When the previously noted measures are carefully followed, they are 95% effective in prevention of further neurocardiogenic syncopal episodes.

MEDICATION (DRUGS)

First Line

Drug therapy is not usually required for neurocardiogenic syncope. For those cases in which it is required, the following are occasionally prescribed:

- Mineralocorticoid steroid therapy (e.g., fludrocortisone) has been demonstrated useful in certain patients to increase intravascular volume and reduce episodes.
- β-Blockade had proven efficacious in some patients with this disorder.
- Methylxanthines have been advocated as treatment for patients with more cardioinhibitory symptomatology.
- Disopyramide has anticholinergic and negative inotropic effects that have been demonstrated efficacious in certain tilt-table studies.
- For patients with arrhythmic etiologies, antiarrhythmic therapy (tailored to the individual arrhythmic substrate) is indicated.
- β-Blockers; LQTS patient should all be treated with β-blockers as this has been definitively demonstrated to reduce syncope and death via arrhythmia in all series in children and adults.
- Contraindications
  - For patients with WPW, use of digoxin and verapamil is limited in patients younger than 1 year of age and absolutely contraindicated in patients older than 1 year of age.
- Precautions
  - Refer to manufacturer's profile of each drug.

SURGERY

- Pacemaker implantation is indicated in cases of bradycardia and may be indicated in rare cases of neurocardiogenic syncope with a predominant cardioinhibitory component.
- Also demonstrated effective in prevention of ventricular arrhythmias in certain forms of LQTS
- Automatic internal cardioverter–defibrillator (AICD) implantation is indicated in patients with documented ventricular arrhythmias unresponsive to or unprotected by medication.
- The role of ICD implantation in children with high risk diseases such as hypertrophic cardiomyopathy or LQTS is still controversial and not fully yet elucidated, but their use in this population is growing with improved ease of implantation.
- Stellate gangliectomy has been demonstrated efficacious in certain forms of LQTS in some series.
- Surgery for treatment of associated congenital lesions may be indicated.

FOLLOW-UP

- Close regular visits for assessment of symptoms and change in such with therapy is indicated.
- Follow-up for various other conditions causing syncope other than neurocardiogenic are reviewed in individual chapters on separate conditions.

PROGNOSIS

- For patients with neurocardiogenic syncope, symptoms usually improve as patients age, with fewer episodes in late adolescence and early adulthood. This may represent self-education at avoidance of activities that induce episodes or recognition of preceding symptoms with subsequent appropriate preventive measures.
- Arrhythmia course is highly variable and is largely related to efficacy of drug or other (e.g., radiofrequency catheter ablation, AICD) therapy.
- Incidence of atrial arrhythmias following Fontan or Mustard/Senning palliation for congenital heart disease increases with time from operation. Episodes or recognition of preceding symptom complexes with subsequent appropriate preventive measures.

COMPLICATIONS

- Bodily musculoskeletal injury due to falls is common.
- Brain injury due to hypoperfusion of the brain in the setting of prolonged, severe arrhythmias can occur.

PATIENT MONITORING

Close regular visits for assessment of symptoms and change in such with therapy is indicated.

REFERENCES

1. Fogoros RN, ed. *The Evaluation of Syncope in Electrophysiologic Testing*, 2nd ed. Cambridge, MA: Blackwell, 1995.
2. Kanter RJ. In: Gillette, Garson, eds. *Syncope in Clinical Pediatric Arrhythmias*. Philadelphia: WB Saunders, 1999.
3. Maron BJ. Ten common questions about hypertrophic cardiomyopathy and misconceptions. *Cardiol Rev.* 2005;13:59–60.
4. Priori SG, Schwartz PJ, Napolitano C, et al. Risk stratification in the long-QT syndrome. *N Engl J Med.* 2003;348:1866–1874.
5. Rickers C, Wilke NM, Jerosch-Herold M, et al. Utility of cardiac magnetic resonance imaging in the diagnosis of hypertrophic cardiomyopathy. *Circulation.* 2005;112:855–861.
6. Wiley TM, O'Donoghue S, Platia EV. Neurocardiogenic syncope: Evaluation and management. *Cardiovascular Review and Reports.* 1993;14:15–25.
7. Wolff GS, Young ML, Tamer DF. In: Deal, Wolff, Gelband, eds. *Syncope: Diagnosis and Management in Current Concepts in Diagnosis and Management of Arrhythmias in Infants and Children.* New York: Futura, 1998.

PATIENT TEACHING

- Educate patients with neurocardiogenic syncope to appreciate and note the anticipatory feelings of light-headedness that precede syncopal episodes in order to take appropriate actions (supine position, head between knees, etc.) to avoid syncope.
- For other conditions, understanding the importance of compliance with medical regimen is critical.

Diet

For patients with neurocardiogenic syncope, high-salt diets with adequate hydration are indicated.

Activity

- For patients with aortic outflow obstruction, decreased isometric exercise is indicated.
- Certain LQTS patients may have episodes of torsade de pointes triggered by high catecholamine level activities, and in these patients activity that is associated with high catecholamine levels should be curtailed.

Prevention

For patients with neurocardiogenic syncope, recognition of signs and symptoms preceding a syncopal episode will often allow prevention of such episodes.

FAQ

Q: What is the natural history of neurocardiogenic syncope in childhood?
A: Most children will ultimately "outgrow" this condition; although symptoms may persist, most recognize, over time, the signs and symptoms and avoid activities that enhance the chance of recurrence.

SYPHILITIC HEART DISEASE

Jesse P. Jorgensen
Mark Steiner*
Nanette K. Wenger

 BASICS

DESCRIPTION
Syphilitic heart disease results from involvement of the cardiovascular system by the spirochete *Treponema pallidum* subspecies *pallidum*. Manifestations include aortitis, coronary ostial stenosis, aortic aneurysm, and aortic regurgitation.

GENERAL PREVENTION
- Primary prevention: Safe sex practices, single-dose intramuscular (IM) penicillin or oral azithromycin during incubation stage
- Secondary prevention: Early diagnosis, treatment, and notification of sexual contacts

EPIDEMIOLOGY
- Transmission occurs via sexual contact (most common), placental (congenital syphilis), close contact with an active lesion, accidental direct inoculation (e.g., needlestick), and blood transfusion.
- Most infections occur in the 15–30 age group.
- Greatest disease burden in developing countries and Eastern Europe

Incidence
- Worldwide, 12.2 million new cases per year
- In the United States, fewer than four cases per 100,000 people per year
- Increased incidence in the 1970s and 1980s associated with unprotected homosexual sex
- Most recent peak in 1990 in African American heterosexual men and women, associated with exchange of sex for crack cocaine in urban areas

Prevalence
- 31,575 total cases in United States in 2000, down from 575,593 in 1943
- Prevalence much higher in African Americans
- Cardiovascular syphilis now rare in developed countries as a result of effective antibiotic therapy

RISK FACTORS
- Unprotected sexual activity
- Immunocompromised host

PATHOPHYSIOLOGY
- The spirochete penetrates mucocutaneous tissues, enters lymphatics and/or the bloodstream, and becomes widely disseminated within days.
- Syphilis is a chronic, systemic illness classified by progressive stages:
  - Incubation: Asymptomatic, with replication of spirochetes and subclinical immune response, lasts 3 weeks
  - Primary: Appearance of chancre, then disappears in 4–6 weeks

- Secondary: Spirochetes widely disseminated, high bacterial load, affects skin and multiple organ systems, develops 6–8 weeks after chancre heals and lasts 2–6 weeks
- Latent: Clinically silent period after secondary stage, detectable only by serologic testing
- Tertiary/Late: Slowly progressive inflammatory disease affecting 1/3 of untreated patients
  - Symptoms appear 3–10 years to decades following infection
  - Neurologic and cardiovascular disease
  - Granuloma-like lesions called *gummas* in skin, liver, bones, and spleen
- Spirochete invasion of the vasa vasorum causes endarteritis obliterans and results in ischemic injury of the aortic media.
  - Medial necrosis and elastic tissue destruction lead to aortitis and aneurysm formation.
  - Since density of vasa vasorum is greatest in the ascending aorta and arch, these areas are most commonly affected.
  - Other large arteries, such as temporal artery, may also be involved.
  - Symptomatic cardiovascular involvement develops in 10% of untreated patients with latent syphilis, 10–40 years after infection.
  - Anatomic evidence of aortitis is found at autopsy in up to 50% of untreated patients.

ASSOCIATED CONDITIONS
- Coinfection with HIV is common, due to common mode of acquisition and enhanced transmission of each condition on the other
- Course of syphilis is accelerated and more malignant
- Accounts for most cases of tertiary syphilis in developed countries
- Serologic tests altered, either as failure to develop in response to infection or remaining falsely elevated following adequate therapy

ALERT
Pregnancy Considerations
Congenital syphilis results from vertical transmission *in utero*
- Risk highest during early stages, but may occur in women with cardiovascular syphilis
- Cardiovascular syphilis as a late complication of congenital syphilis is rare.
- Mainstay of prevention is early maternal treatment, minimizing risk of fetal transmission.
  - Penicillin appropriate for stage as recommended for nonpregnant patients
- Infant treated with parenteral penicillin, regardless of maternal treatment status

 DIAGNOSIS

SIGNS AND SYMPTOMS
Primary
- Chancre: Red, painless dermal papule that develops at the site of inoculation and ulcerates
- Inguinal lymphadenopathy: Painless, rubbery, nonsuppurative; develops soon after chancre

Secondary
The signs and symptoms of secondary syphilis are notoriously protean and highly variable, may affect any organ systems.
- Constitutional: Fever, headache, arthralgias, malaise, weight loss
- Skin: Macular rash developing into papular over months, involving trunk, palms, soles, and flexor surfaces of extremities
- Condyloma latum
- Generalized lymphadenopathy
- Gastrointestinal: Hepatitis and gastritis
- Neurologic: Headache, aseptic meningitis, nerve disorders, cerebrovascular accident
- Musculoskeletal: Periostitis, arthritis
- Ocular: Uveitis, iritis
- Renal: Glomerulonephritis, nephritic syndrome
- Cardiac: Myocarditis

Tertiary
- Gummatous disease: Skin nodules, portal hypertension, painless testicular swelling
  - Gumma may involve the myocardium; involvement at the base of the interventricular septum may result in damage to the conduction system and atrioventricular block.
- Neurosyphilis: Tabes dorsalis, paresis, psychosis, dementia, cerebrovascular accident, meningitis, spinal cord disease
- Aortitis often occurs in association with neurosyphilis, may be asymptomatic
- Aortic aneurysm: Pain from erosion of ribs or vertebral bodies, hoarseness, cough, dysphagia, pulsation in sternoclavicular joint
  - Develops in 5–10% of patients with aortitis
  - May be asymptomatic with incidentally discovered dilated, calcified aorta on chest x-ray
  - Usually saccular, occasionally fusiform
  - 10% of syphilitic aneurysms involve the abdominal aorta, infrarenal involvement rare
  - Dissection is rare, owing to transverse scarring of the aortic media
- Aortic regurgitation: Diastolic murmur, peripheral "water-hammer" pulses, bisferiens pulse, left ventricular hypertrophy and enlargement, congestive heart failure
  - Develops in 20–30% of patients with aortitis from extension to the sinuses of Valsalva, resulting in dilation of the aortic root and valve ring
  - Aortitis does not involve the valve cusps or subvalvular structures

- Coronary ostial stenosis: Angina pectoris or, rarely, myocardial infarction
  - Develops in 25–30% of patients with aortitis, which predisposes to development of atherosclerosis in the aortic root
  - Atheromatous disease in the aortic root may envelop and obstruct the coronary ostia
  - Most patients have associated aortic regurgitation
  - At the start of the 20th century, exceeded coronary atherosclerotic disease as a cause of angina pectoris

TESTS
Cardiac catheterization/angiography: Coronary ostial stenosis
Lab
- Nontreponemal (reaginic tests)
  - Venereal Disease Research Laboratory (VDRL) test
  - Rapid plasma reagin (RPR) test
  - Automated reagin test (ART)
- Specific treponemal tests
  - Fluorescent antibody absorption (FTA-ABS) test
  - *T. pallidum* hemagglutination (TPHA and MHA-TP) assay
  - Treponemal immobilization (TPI) test
- Dark-field microscopic examination of fluid from chancre
- All patients with cardiovascular syphilis should have serologic cerebrospinal fluid (CSF) examination.
- Laboratory Problems
  - VDRL and RPR tests should gradually become nonreactive following successful therapy, but may remain positive in some patients, especially those with HIV.
  - RPR/VDRL test may be nonreactive during latent and tertiary phase.
  - Antibody test results always positive; negative results exclude late syphilis.
  - Causes of false-positive tests: Other infectious diseases (tuberculosis, subacute bacterial endocarditis, leprosy, etc.), early HIV, hepatitis, systemic lupus erythematosus, pregnancy, and others

Imaging
- Electrocardiogram (ECG): Left ventricular hypertrophy, occasional atrioventricular (AV) or conduction disease
- Chest x-ray: Cardiac enlargement, linear calcification and dilation of the ascending aorta
  - Linear calcification is rarely seen with atherosclerotic disease of the aorta.
- Echocardiogram: Aortic regurgitation, aortic dilation with aortic root enlargement, aortic aneurysm, left ventricular hypertrophy, left ventricular enlargement
- Computed tomography (CT) or magnetic resonance angiography (MRA): Aortic aneurysm

Pathologic Findings
- Obliterative endarteritis of the vaso vasorum
- Staining with direct immunofluorescent antibody, immunoperoxidase antibody, or silver stain

DIFFERENTIAL DIAGNOSIS
- Collagen vascular diseases
- Aortitis, AR from other causes

TREATMENT

GENERAL MEASURES
- Prevention with safe sexual practices
- Patient education
- Early treatment of primary syphilis

MEDICATION (DRUGS)

- Parenteral penicillin is the preferred therapy for all stages, including cardiovascular syphilis.
- Azithromycin, doxycycline, or tetracycline for penicillin-allergic patients
- Whereas early syphilis and neurosyphilis respond dramatically to antibiotics, the impact of antibiotic therapy on progression of disease after aortitis has developed is not clear.
- Precautions
  - Jarisch-Herxheimer reaction: Systemic reaction occurring 1–2 hours after initial treatment with effective antibiotics
    - Abrupt onset of fever, chills, myalgias, headache, flushing, tachycardia, and mild hypotension
    - Usually self-limited, lasts 12–24 hours
    - May be treated or prevented with anti-inflammatory agents (e.g., aspirin or steroids); prophylaxis prior to antibiotic therapy should be considered in patients with cardiovascular syphilis to prevent acute decompensation

SURGERY
- Consideration for surgical repair of syphilitic aneurysms and aortic regurgitation is same as for patients without syphilis
- Rare surgical resection of large gumma

FOLLOW-UP

PROGNOSIS
- High likelihood of cure with treatment, especially with earlier stages
- Overall good prognosis with treatment
- The prognosis of uncomplicated syphilitic aortitis is similar to that for the general population.
- Symptomatic aneurysms are associated with a poor prognosis in the absence of surgical intervention.

COMPLICATIONS
- Heart failure as a result of aortic regurgitation
- Aneurysm rupture and sudden death

PATIENT MONITORING
- With early or congenital syphilis, repeat nontreponemal tests at 3, 6, and 12 months.
- With secondary syphilis or syphilis of duration more than 1 year, repeat nontreponemal testing 24 months after treatment.
- Consider retreatment when clinical symptoms progress, nontreponemal test titers are sustained or increase, or polymerase chain reaction test result is positive.
- Echocardiogram every 6–12 months for medically managed aortic regurgitation that is severe, every 2–3 years for mild disease
- CT or MRA to evaluate progression of aortic dilation 6 months after initial examination; subsequent yearly exams if size of aneurysm is stable, every 3–6 months for enlarging aneurysms

REFERENCES
1. Halperin JL, Olin JW. Diseases of the aorta. In: Fuster V, Alexander RW, O'Rourke RA, eds. *Hurst's the Heart,* 11th ed. New York: McGraw-Hill, 2004:2301–2322.
2. Jackman JD, Radolf JD. Cardiovascular syphilis. *Am J Med.* 1989;87:425–433.
3. Kinghorn GR. Syphilis. In: Cohen J, Powderly WG, Berkley SΓ, et al, eds. *Infectious Diseases,* 2nd ed. New York: Elsevier-Mosby, 2004:807–816.
4. Lukehart SA. Syphilis. In: Kasper DL, Braunwald E, Fauci AS, et al. eds. *Harrison's Principles of Internal Medicine,* 16th ed. New York: McGraw-Hill, 2005:977–985.
5. Roberts WC, O'Rourke RA, Roldan JF. The connective tissue diseases and the cardiovascular system. In: Fuster V, Alexander RW, O'Rourke RA, eds. *Hurst's the Heart,* 11th ed. New York: McGraw-Hill, 2004:2063–2080.
6. Schoen FJ. Blood Vessels. In: Kumar V, Abbas AK, Fausto N, eds. *Robbins and Cotran Pathologic Basis of Disease,* 7th ed. Philadelphia: Elsevier-Saunders, 2005:511–554.
7. Tramont EC. Trepanoma pallidum (syphilis). In: Mandell GL, Bennett JE, Dolin R, eds. *Mandell, Douglas, and Bennett's Principles and Practice of Infectious Diseases,* 6th ed. Philadelphia: Elsevier-Churchill Livingstone, 2005:2768–2783.

CODES
ICD9-CM
093 Cardiovascular syphilis

PATIENT TEACHING
- Safe sexual practices
- Preventive or epidemiologic treatment to anyone exposed to infectious syphilis in preceding 3 months

TETRALOGY OF FALLOT

Jacqueline M. Lamour
Welton M. Gersony

BASICS

DESCRIPTION
- The tetrad of tetralogy of Fallot (TOF) includes
  - Ventricular septal defect (VSD)
  - Overriding aorta
  - Infundibular pulmonary stenosis
  - Right ventricular hypertrophy
- The severity of infundibular obstruction ranges from mild stenosis to pulmonary atresia (PA).

EPIDEMIOLOGY
TOF occurs in about 5–10% of infants born with congenital heart disease The defect occurs sporadically.
- Found in higher frequency of siblings than would be expected in the general population
- No bias to age, race, or sex

Prevalence
Found in about 1 per 3,000 live births

Genetics
Occasionally associated with chromosome 22q deletion (DiGeorge syndrome)

PATHOPHYSIOLOGY
- Systemic venous return to the right atrium and right ventricle is normal.
- Pressures in the right and left ventricle are equal.
- A right to left (R-L) shunt access across the VSD.
- Pulmonary artery pressure is lower than normal.
- When the pulmonary stenosis is moderate, a balanced shunt occurs across the VSD and the patient may not be visibly cyanotic.
- When the right ventricle contracts in the face of marked pulmonary stenosis, blood is shunted through the VSD into the aorta, resulting in cyanosis.
- When severe pulmonary stenosis is present, bronchial collaterals or a patent PDA may be present.

ASSOCIATED CONDITIONS
- Although not part of specific hereditary syndromes or chromosomal anomalies, it is commonly found in cardiofacial, VACTERL, and CHARGE syndrome.
- TOF can be associated with other cardiac malformations, including atrioventricular canal defect (4%) and absent pulmonary valve (2%).

DIAGNOSIS

SIGNS AND SYMPTOMS
- Depends on the degree of right ventricular outflow tract (RVOT) obstruction
- Acyanotic TOF (left-to-right shunt) is usually asymptomatic; these children almost always evolve to cyanotic TOF, usually later in infancy or childhood.
- Shunts may remain balanced, with the patient showing only minimal cyanosis for decades.
- Cyanotic TOF [right-to-left (R-L) shunt] may exhibit clubbing, dyspnea on exertion and squatting.
- Hypoxemic spells are episodes of transient, usually brief, hyperpnea unconsciousness. They are caused by a decrease in systemic vascular resistance or an increase in infundibular obstruction, which results in increased R-L shunt with an increase in cyanosis

and a decrease in intensity of the RV outflow murmur. This in turn leads to lower pO_2 and elevated pCO_2, causing hyperpnea.
  - Usually in acyanotic or minimally cyanotic TOF
  - Frequently in the morning
  - Usually self-limited and responsive to treatment; however, rarely a severe spell may result in syncope, seizures, or death.
  - Historically, spells disappear after 2 or 3 years of age.
- Absent PV syndrome
  - Respiratory distress due to bronchial compression from enlarged aneurysmal pulmonary arteries may be a major problem in neonates and infants.

History
- Cyanosis
- Decreased exercise tolerance
- May be asymptomatic

Physical Exam
- Depends on the degree of RVOT obstruction
- Acyanotic TOF: A long, intense systolic murmur along the left sternal border (LSB)
- Cyanotic TOF (R->L shunt) may have clubbing, and a loud and single S2 with a systolic ejection murmur at the upper LSB.
  - TOF/pulmonary atresia: Continuous murmurs over both lungs may represent major aorta pulmonary collateral arteries (MAPCA) flow.
  - TOF/absent pulmonary valve: To-and-fro murmur along left sternal border

TESTS
ECG
- Right axis deviation
- Right ventricular hypertrophy
- Electrophysiology
- Evaluate postoperative patients with syncope or suspected arrhythmia

Lab
- In cyanotic patients, a complete blood count identifies polycythemia. In cyanotic patients, iron deficiency anemia may mask degree of desaturation.
- Resting arterial oxygen saturation in asymptomatic patients may be 70–90%.

Imaging
- Chest radiograph
  - Cyanotic TOF: Boot-shaped heart caused by an enlarged right ventricle with absence of an apparent radiographic main pulmonary artery segment
  - Decreased pulmonary vascular markings (PVMs)
  - Acyanotic TOF and TOF/pulmonary atresia with MAPCAs; normal to increased PVMs
  - Absent PV, mildly enlarged cardiac silhouette, markedly dilated PAs, hyperinflated lungs
- Echocardiography
  - Aortic override of the ventricular septum; aortic root appears large with fibrous continuity between the mitral and aortic valve
  - Degree of infundibular, main PA and PV stenosis
  - Demonstrate PA continuity; PAs may be discontinuous and connected to the aorta by a patent ductus arteriosus (PDA) or MAPCAs

- Exclude multiple VSDs
- Determine arch sidedness, right-sided in 25%
- Absent PV, enlarged right ventricle and main PA with pulmonary insufficiency; absence of PDA common
- Postoperative serial studies, presence of pulmonary and/or tricuspid insufficiency, residual or progressive RVOT obstruction; RV dysfunction and residual VSDs
- Magnetic resonance imaging
  - Can be used serially postoperatively to assess RV dilatation and ejection fraction, pulmonary artery regurgitate fraction, pulmonary artery anatomy, residual or progressive RVOT obstruction

Diagnostic Procedures/Surgery
- Cardiac catheterization
  - RV pressure equals left ventricular pressure
  - Measure PA pressure in previously shunted patients at risk for pulmonary hypertension.
  - Angiography defines various levels of RVOT obstruction, anatomy of PAs, presence of multiple VSDs and coronary anomalies
  - TOF/pulmonary atresia: Collaterals originate commonly in the descending thoracic aorta; selective injections are necessary to demonstrate size, distribution, and areas of stenosis in each vessel.
  - Pulmonary wedge angiography is sometimes necessary to demonstrate true PAs.
- Interventional catheterization
  - Preoperative balloon dilatation of a stenotic PV may allow for growth of PAs, delaying need for surgical intervention.
  - Postoperative use of balloons and stents to relieve native distal areas of pulmonary obstruction or those created at distal anastomotic sites or within conduits
  - Coil embolization of MAPCAs

DIFFERENTIAL DIAGNOSIS
The differential diagnosis of TOF depends on the degree of RVOT obstruction, but includes small VSD, isolated pulmonic stenosis or pulmonary artery (PA) defect, or VSD with MAPCAs.

TREATMENT

GENERAL MEASURES
- Medical management involves the effects of hypoxia in individuals with significant RVOT obstruction or hypoxemic spells.
- For adequate oxygen saturations, hemoglobin level 15–17 g/dL, hematocrit 45–50%
- When hematocrit reaches 65%:
  - Changes in clotting status
  - Increased viscosity of blood and R-L shunt increases risk of neurologic events (headaches, seizures, and cerebrovascular accidents).
  - Rarely, phlebotomy and exchange transfusion with a plasma substitute may be needed.
  - Cyanotic patients are prone to infectious endocarditis and brain abscesses.
  - Headaches in an afebrile patient may represent a brain abscess.

MEDICATION (DRUGS)

First Line

- Patients with relative anemia (<15 g/dL) are at risk for neurologic events and should receive supplemental iron.
- Treatment of hypoxemic spells include:
  - Place patient in a knee-chest position
  - Oxygen
  - Other measures that may be used:
    - Morphine sulfate 0.1 mg/kg intramuscular (IV or SC)
    - $NaHCO_3$ 1 mEq/kg
    - Volume, normal saline or albumin 10 mL/kg
    - Propranolol
    - Phenylephrine
  - Bacterial endocarditis prophylaxis is needed as recommended by the American Heart Association.

SURGERY

- The ultimate goal for patients with TOF and TOF/pulmonary atresia is complete repair.
- TOF
  - Open heart repair in the latter 1/2 of the 1st year after birth
  - Patients with significant resting hypoxia and hypoxemic spells are treated surgically on an urgent basis.
  - Single-stage repair is optimal, but factors may prohibit this: Size of patient, small PAs, and coronary anomalies.
  - Palliative surgery increases PBF by placing an aorta to pulmonary connections, usually a Blalock shunt. Reserved for infants with small PAs, multiple VSDs, or other contraindications for early repair.
  - Increased PBF may encourage PA growth.
  - Complete repair involves patch-closing the VSD and relieving RVOT obstruction.
- TOF/pulmonary atresia
  - If true PAs are confluent and of sufficient size and distribution to permit complete repair, establishing continuity between the RV and PA with a conduit or direct anastomosis and closing the VSD is the procedure of choice.
  - If the PAs are adequate and dual pulmonary blood supply is present, collateral vessels can be ligated at surgery or embolized at cardiac catheterization.
- In the presence of MAPCAs with small PAs, unifocalization procedures incorporating as many collateral vessels to the true pulmonary arteries are used.
- Lungs totally supplied by unobstructed MAPCAs are at risk for developing pulmonary vascular disease.
- Use early complete repair when possible to allow optimal PA growth, rather than staged approach.
- If true PAs are hypoplastic or maldistributed, staged surgery may be necessary, connecting RV to PAs while leaving the VSD open to increase PBF and increase PA size.
- Care should be taken to assess PA continuity and intervene appropriately, especially in infants, in whom the PDA provides flow to the left PA. If the PDA closes, the left pulmonary artery stenosis may be lost.

- Success of surgical repair is directly related to the PA size and distribution.
- TOF with absent PV
  - Patch closing the VSD with a transannular patch
  - PA angioplasty to reduce size of PAs and relieve bronchial obstruction
  - Some clinicians advocate a valved conduit in the pulmonary position to decrease degree of pulmonary insufficiency, but this is not usual until later in childhood or adult life.

 FOLLOW-UP

DISPOSITION

- Patients need admission to a hospital for treatment of medical complications such as polycythemia, neurologic events, bacterial endocarditis, or arrhythmia.
- Surgical complications also may warrant hospital admission.

Discharge Criteria

Discharge is determined by treatment course.

PROGNOSIS

- Unoperated patients are unlikely to survive into their third decade.
- A small group survives to adulthood, unoperated or with only a palliative procedure.
- Survival through adult life is anticipated following excellent repair.
- Patients at risk for poor prognosis include:
  - Small PAs, so that shunts and relief of outflow obstruction do not improve cyanosis
  - Development of PVD after a prolonged course with large systemic–pulmonary shunt
  - TOF/pulmonary atresia with no primary PAs
  - Poor RV function
  - Ventricular arrhythmias
- Early postoperative mortality is low.
- Postoperative complications:
  - Residual RVOT obstruction, VSD, or both
  - Atrioventricular conduction abnormalities
  - Right bundle branch block
  - Ventricular arrhythmia
  - Pulmonary regurgitation; well tolerated in most patients, but associated with tricuspid regurgitation, RV failure, and arrhythmias in some. PV replacement in adult life is common.
  - Risk of sudden death following complete repair is small; when occurring, probably due to sudden arrhythmia.
- Routine stress testing and Holter monitoring performed serially following repair
- Absent PV syndrome, prognosis depends on respiratory status in newborns.

PATIENT MONITORING

- Close regular visits for assessment of progressive cyanosis
- Elective surgery in the latter part of first year
- In TOF/pulmonary atresia with MAPCAs, early cardiac catheterization to define anatomy
- Watch for signs of early CHF (increased PBF via MAPCAs) or increasing cyanosis (decreased PBF) to determine optimal timing of surgery.
- Postoperative, regular follow-up to assess right ventricular function and occurrence of arrhythmia

Pregnancy Considerations

- Women with good surgical results following complete repair should do well with pregnancy.
- Those palliated and remaining cyanotic are at increased risk for maternal and fetal mortality, as well as increased morbidity associated with bacterial endocarditis and cardiovascular deterioration.

REFERENCES

1. Garson A Jr., et al. *The science and practice of pediatric cardiology,* 2nd ed. Baltimore: Lippincott Williams & Wilkins, 1998.
2. Meijer JM, Pieper PG, Drenthen W, et al. Pregnancy, fertility, and recurrent risk in corrected tetralogy of Fallot. *Heart.* 2005:91; 801–805.
3. Snider AR, et al. *Echocardiography in pediatric heart disease.* St. Louis: Mosby Year Book, 1997.
4. Warner KG, O'Brien PK, Rhodes J, et al. Expanding the indications for pulmonary valve replacement after repair of tetralogy of Fallot. *Ann Thorac Surg.* 2003;76:1066–1072.

 MISCELLANEOUS

CODES
ICD9-CM
745.2 TOF

PATIENT TEACHING

- Educate parents about the symptoms of hypoxemic spells and what to do if they occur in affected infants.
- An estimated 2,140 sites are available on the Internet concerning TOF.

Activity

Adequate rest and reasonable physical activity

THROMBOPHLEBITIS

Rajesh Dash

 BASICS

DESCRIPTION

Thrombophlebitis is the presence of thrombus within a superficial or deep vein and the associated vessel wall inflammatory response.

- Deep venous thrombosis (DVT) is diagnosed in only 50% of the clinical cases.
- Approximately 45% of femoral and iliac deep venous thromboses embolize to the lungs (pulmonary embolism; PE).
- Superficial vein thrombosis does not confer increased risk of pulmonary embolism
- System(s) affected: Venous, pulmonary

EPIDEMIOLOGY

- Predominant age: Incidence increases with age.
- Predominant sex: None
- Approximately 260,000 patients are diagnosed and treated for DVT and PE in the United States each year.

Pediatric Considerations
Rare

Geriatric Considerations
Increased incidence and complications

RISK FACTORS

As described by Virchow, risk factors include stasis, vascular injury, and a hypercoagulable state.

- Clinical factors
  - Age >40 years
  - Prior history of thrombosis
  - Prior major surgery or trauma
  - Immobilization or paralysis
  - Venous stasis
  - Varicose veins
  - Congestive heart failure
  - Myocardial infarction
  - Obesity
  - Oral contraceptive therapy
  - Cerebrovascular accident
  - Cancer
  - Paroxysmal nocturnal hemoglobinemia
  - Antiphospholipid antibody syndrome
  - Inflammatory diseases (e.g., Crohn disease, systemic lupus erythematosus, thromboangiitis obliterans)
  - Intravascular catheters
  - Disseminated intravascular coagulation
  - Pregnancy (especially the 3rd trimester)
- Heritable factors
  - Antithrombin III (ATIII) deficiency
  - Factor V Leiden mutation
  - Protein S deficiency
  - Protein C deficiency
  - Dysfibrinogenemia
  - Plasminogen disorders
  - Elevation of concentration of factor VIII

Genetics
Hypercoagulable state may be inherited.

ETIOLOGY

- Venous stasis
- Vascular injury
- Hypercoagulable state
- Antithrombin deficiency is an autosomaldominant trait.
- Protein C deficiency is an autosomal-dominant trait.
- Protein S deficiency is an autosomal-dominant trait.
- Factor V Leiden mutation is a genetic polymorphism present in approximately 4–6% of the population.

Pregnancy Considerations

Venous thrombosis is increased in pregnancy

- Increased clotting factor
- Increased platelet aggregation
- Decreased fibrinolysis

 DIAGNOSIS

SIGNS AND SYMPTOMS

History
- Unilateral leg swelling
- Warmth
- Erythema
- Pain
- Sudden chest pain or dyspnea if presenting with PE

Physical Exam
- Leg tenderness
- Erythema
- Palpable cord
- Increased skin turgor
- Distention of superficial veins
- Pedal edema
- Homan sign (increased pain or resistance with dorsiflexion of foot) is insensitive
- Chronic stasis dermatitis

TESTS

- Patients presenting with PE may require additional tests.
- Wells pretest probability score helps identify those who are at low risk of DVT.

Lab
- D-Dimer (low sensitivity and specificity in detecting thrombosis); better test for ruling out DVT
- Specific factor levels in heritable causes (e.g., factor V Leiden, proteins C and S, ATIII)
- Antiphospholipid antibodies
- Lupus anticoagulant

Imaging
- Contrast venography (>90% positive predictive accuracy for deep veins
- Venous plethysmography (83% positive predictive accuracy for deep veins)
- Doppler ultrasonography and B-mode ultrasonography (95% positive predictive accuracy for deep veins)
- ^{125}I-fibrinogen scanning (rarely used but better at detecting calf vein thrombosis)
- Impedance plethysmography and duplex ultrasonography are the most commonly used.

Pathologic Findings
Venous thrombosis and inflammation

DIFFERENTIAL DIAGNOSIS

- Muscle trauma
- Bacterial cellulites
- Venous valvular insufficiency
- Ruptured popliteal (Baker) cyst
- Lymphedema
- Arterial occlusive disorders

 TREATMENT

GENERAL MEASURES

- Superficial thrombophlebitis or lower extremity DVT can be managed as an outpatient.
- Patients with more proximal DVT or suspected PE should be hospitalized initially.
- Minor symptoms attributable to varicose veins, superficial thrombosis, or calf deep vein thrombosis can be controlled medically as an outpatient with heat, elevation, and nonsteroidal anti-inflammatory medications because patients are at no increased risk of PE.
- Documented or suspected DVT requires aggressive management with anticoagulation because there is significant risk of PE (inpatient and outpatient regimens are shown in subsequent sections).
- Documented or suspected PE requires prompt hospitalization and monitoring for possible hemodynamic and respiratory compromise.

MEDICATION (DRUGS)

First Line
- Inpatient
  - Unfractionated heparin bolus of 80 U/kg followed by infusion of 18 U/kg adjusted to activated partial thromboplastin time (APTT) of 1.5–2 times control for at least 5 days or low molecular weight heparin
  - Low-molecular-weight heparin (LMWH): Dose depends on product and is adjusted for renal insufficiency for at least 5 days
  - Simultaneous administration of warfarin dosed daily at 5 or 10 mg PO to achieve prothrombin time (PT) to 1.3–1.5 times control or international normalized ratio (INR) of 2–3 for 6 months
  - Overlap of heparin and warfarin for 3–4 days: 5,000–10,000 U of heparin given subcutaneously can be given to those where warfarin in contraindicated (adjusted to PTT 1.5–2 times control)
- Outpatient
  - Simultaneous administration of warfarin dosed to achieve PT to 1.3–1.5 times control or INR of 2–3 for 6 months
  - Overlap of heparin and warfarin for 3–4 days
  - Warfarin therapy for 3–6 months
  - Treatment of massive DVT
  - Thrombolytic agents can be considered.
  - Streptokinase 250,000 U intravenous (IV) loading over 30 minutes followed by 100,00 U per hour infusion for 24 hours
  - Urokinase 4,400 U bolus IV with 4,400 U per hour infusion for 12–24 hours
  - Tissue plasminogen activator IV infusion 100 mg over 2 hours
  - Recurrent DVT or PE
  - Occurs in 9.5% of patients after 6 months of therapy
  - May require life-long anticoagulation
  - Contraindications
    - Active bleeding, recent major surgery, and recent stroke are contraindications for anticoagulation.
    - Precautions
    - Bleeding with anticoagulation (especially thrombolytics)
    - Heparin-induced thrombocytopenia (HIT) with platelet count less than 150,000/mm³ occurs in 5–10% of patients given unfractionated heparin secondary to heparin-dependent antibodies.
  - Significant possible interactions
    - Warfarin can interact with many drugs. (See manufacturer's literature.)

Second Line
Low-molecular-weight heparin can be given if warfarin contraindicated and may have a lower incidence of HIT than unfractionated heparin.

SURGERY
Inferior venal caval (IVC) filters for patients with strict contraindication to anticoagulation, or for recurrent DVT despite adequate anticoagulation

FOLLOW-UP

DISPOSITION
Admission Criteria
Once the diagnosis of DVT is made, indications for inpatient therapy include:
- Symptoms of pulmonary embolism (dyspnea, syncope, chest pain, and pleurisy)
- High comorbid risk for bleeding
- Active bleeding
- History of noncompliance
- Allergy to LMWH, heparin, or pork products
- Comorbidities that complicate outpatient therapy: Active malignancy, infection, stroke
- No clear follow-up plan

Discharge Criteria
- After at least first dose of LMWH administered
- No contraindication to outpatient therapy
- Appropriate anticoagulation and primary care follow-up arranged

Issues for Referral
- Consider IVC filter for recurrent DVT on anticoagulation.
- Consider thrombophilia testing for: 1st idiopathic DVT at age <50, recurrent DVT, or 1st- degree relative with idiopathic DVT at age <50 years.

PROGNOSIS
- Majority have resolution of symptoms and recannulization of thrombosis
- Recurrence in 9.5% after 6 months of anticoagulation
- Recurrence more likely in patients with ongoing coagulopathy

COMPLICATIONS
- Cellulitis
- Chronic stasis dermatitis

PATIENT MONITORING
- Improvement of presenting symptoms and for recurrence after therapy concluded
- High-risk patients may require repeated imaging to determine response to therapy.

CODES
ICD9-CM
- 451.9 Thrombophlebitis
- 451.19 Deep vein thrombosis
- 415.19 Pulmonary embolus
- See also: Pulmonary embolus

PATIENT TEACHING
Activity
Once pain and swelling symptoms have resolved, patient is encouraged to ambulate.

Prevention
- High-risk hospitalized patients should receive DVT/PE prophylaxis, including early postoperative ambulation, pneumatic compression of the lower extremities, or low-dose subcutaneous heparin 5,000 U q8h or q12h.
- LMWH (e.g., Enoxaparin 30 mg q12h) has been shown to be effective for DVT/PE prophylaxis in surgical patients.

FAQ
A. Is it true that the majority of patients with symptomatic proximal DVT and NO chest symptoms have PE on lung scans?
Q. True, 75% will test positive for PE.
A. Is LMWH acceptable for patients with HIT type 2?
Q. False, all forms of heparin are contraindicated for patients with HIT type 2.

TRICUSPID REGURGITATION

Stephen Kuehn
Steven C. Herrmann
Bernard R. Chaitman

 BASICS

DESCRIPTION
Tricuspid regurgitation is incompetence of the tricuspid valve resulting in retrograde flow from the right ventricle (RV) into the right atrium (RA) during systole.

Pregnancy Considerations
Tricuspid regurgitation generally is well tolerated during pregnancy.

EPIDEMIOLOGY
Age: Childhood cases are generally associated with congenital heart disease or pulmonary vascular disease. Most cases are diagnosed in adulthood.

Prevalence
Common

RISK FACTORS
Intravenous drug abusers susceptible to *Staphylococcus* endocarditis with resultant tricuspid regurgitation

ETIOLOGY
- Secondary tricuspid regurgitation generally results from dilation of the RV and subsequent annular enlargement.
- Common causes of annular dilation with an anatomically normal tricuspid valve include RV failure, left ventricular failure, pulmonic stenosis, primary pulmonary hypertension, RV infarction, Eisenmenger's syndrome, cor pulmonale, and mitral stenosis (MS).
- Primary tricuspid regurgitation with abnormal valvular apparatus is seen in rheumatic disease, infective endocarditis, Ebstein's anomaly, Marfan's syndrome, carcinoid syndrome, and tricuspid valve prolapse.
- Rare causes include cardiac tumors, methysergide treatment, systemic lupus erythematosus, atrioventricular canal, isolated congenital lesion, and endomyocardial fibrosis.

 DIAGNOSIS

SIGNS AND SYMPTOMS
- Tricuspid regurgitation is well tolerated unless pulmonary hypertension develops, at which time cardiac output begins to decline.
- Right-sided heart failure symptoms result from decreased cardiac output and congestion, which include dyspnea on exertion, edema, ascites, hepatomegaly, splenomegaly, and venous distention.
- Occasionally, throbbing pulsations in the neck and eyes are described. Weight loss, cachexia, cyanosis, jaundice are common. Dyspnea on exertion is frequent, but paroxysmal nocturnal dyspnea is often absent unless concomitant left heart disease exists.

Physical Exam
- Physical examination of the venous pulse shows both a prominent V-wave and steep Y-descent, both of which increase with inspiration.
- Occasionally, the RA is palpable along the right sternal border.
- The RV is usually hyperdynamic and may have a lift.
- An S3 gallop over the RV may be heard; this is louder with inspiration (Carvallo's sign).
- The tricuspid regurgitation murmur is holosystolic, high-pitched, and best auscultated in the fourth interspace along the parasternal border.
- The murmur is harsher and longer when tricuspid regurgitation is associated with pulmonary hypertension.
- Tricuspid regurgitation increases under conditions such as inspiration, Mueller maneuver (forced inspiration with a closed glottis), liver compression, leg raise, and amyl nitrate inhalation.

TESTS
- The ECG is not specific but may include an incomplete right bundle branch block, RA enlargement, and a Q-wave in V1.
- Atrial fibrillation is common.

Imaging
- Chest radiographs often show both RA and RV enlargement.
- The azygous vein may be dilated if RA pressure is elevated.
- Liver congestion often causes right hemidiaphragm elevation.
- Echocardiography usually demonstrates RA, RV, and annulus enlargement.
- RV diastolic overload pattern is common.
- Tricuspid valve prolapse may be noted.
- Doppler echocardiography shows retrograde flow from the ventricle into the atrium as well as systolic flow reversal in the hepatic vein.

Diagnostic Procedures/Surgery
- Cardiac catheterization shows elevated end-diastolic pressure in the RV.
- The atrial pressure wave form is ventricularized with prominent V-waves or fusion of the C- and V- waves. The X-descent is small, and the Y-descent is steep.
- High pulmonary artery pressures are generally associated with secondary tricuspid regurgitation.

Pathologic Findings
- Ebstein abnormality is associated with downward displacement of the tricuspid valve and anomalous attachment of the leaflets.
- Tricuspid valve tissue is dysplastic, and the apical portion of the RV is atrialized.
- Rheumatic disease results in a calcified valve with fusion of the commissures.
- Carcinoid disease is associated with diffuse fibrinous deposits on the valve leaflets.
- Myxomatous degeneration is common with tricuspid valve prolapse.

DIFFERENTIAL DIAGNOSIS
- Mitral regurgitation
- Pulmonic regurgitation

TREATMENT

GENERAL MEASURES

- Mild to moderate tricuspid regurgitation without pulmonary hypertension is generally well tolerated.
- Symptomatic tricuspid regurgitation with annular dilation is usually treated surgically with tricuspid annuloplasty.
- Rheumatic disease may require commissurotomy if the commissures are fused.
- Endocarditis and Ebstein abnormality usually require tricuspid valve replacement, although the risk of thrombosis is high in this position because of the low flow rate.
- A large porcine heterograft, without systemic anticoagulation, is preferred.

 MEDICATION (DRUGS)

- Loop diuretics are the drug of choice for edema formation.
- Digoxin can be used for RV failure.
- Peripheral vasodilators are helpful if the tricuspid regurgitation is secondary to left ventricle failure.
- Precautions: Endocarditis prophylaxis is required.
- Low potassium caused by loop diuretic use may potentiate digoxin toxicity.

 FOLLOW-UP

PROGNOSIS

- Generally favorable
- Results of prosthetic tricuspid valve replacement are not as good as annuloplasty, with 30-day morbidity approximately 15% with artificial valve replacement.

PATIENT MONITORING

Routine echocardiography is not recommended unless a change in symptomatology occurs.

REFERENCES

1. Alexander RW. *Hurst's the heart*. New York: McGraw-Hill, 1998.
2. Bonow RO, Carabello B, de Leon AC Jr, et al. ACC/AHA 2006 guidelines for the management of patients with valvular heart disease: A report of the American College of Cardiology/American Heart Association Task Force on Practice Guidelines (Writing Committee to Revise the 1998 Guidelines for the Management of Patients With Valvular Heart Disease). American College of Cardiology Web Site. Available at: http://content.onlinejacc.org/cgi/reprint/48/3/e1
3. Bonow RO, Cheitlin MD, Crawford MH, Douglas PS. Task Force 3: Valvular heart disease. *J Am Coll Cardiol*. 2005;45:1334–1340.
4. Braunwald E, ed. *Heart disease: A textbook of cardiovascular medicine*, 6th ed. Philadelphia: WB Saunders, 2005.
5. Topol EJ, ed. *Textbook of cardiovascular medicine*. Philadelphia: Lippincott-Raven, 1998.

 MISCELLANEOUS

See also: Ebstein's Anomaly; Rheumatic Heart Disease

CODES
ICD9-CM
424.2

PATIENT TEACHING
Diet
Low-sodium diet, especially in the face of edema

Activity
No limitations until cardiac output decreases as pulmonary pressures increases

Prevention
Endocarditis prophylaxis

TRICUSPID STENOSIS

Stephen Kuehn
Steven C. Herrmann
Bernard R. Chaitman

 BASICS

DESCRIPTION
Tricuspid stenosis (TS) results in a limitation of diastolic right ventricle (RV) filling imposed by a narrowed tricuspid valve.

Pregnancy Considerations
Anticoagulation with warfarin is contraindicated in pregnancy, and therefore should not be used in pregnant patients with mechanical prostheses.

EPIDEMIOLOGY
Incidence
- Age: In the U.S., it is most commonly diagnosed between the ages of 20–60 years.
- Sex: Female > Male

Prevalence
- Found in 15% of autopsy specimens in patients with documented rheumatic heart disease
- Clinically significant tricuspid stenosis occurs in less than 5% of those autopsied with rheumatic disease.
- More commonly seen in India (1/3 of autopsied hearts with rheumatic disease) than in U.S. or Western Europe.

PATHOPHYSIOLOGY
TS leads to increased right atrial (RA) pressure and a significant pressure gradient between the RA and RV during diastole.

ETIOLOGY
- Almost exclusively rheumatic in origin, with or without associated tricuspid regurgitation
- Very rare as the only valve affected by rheumatic disease
- Other causes include infective endocarditis, carcinoid, myxoma/thrombus, Fabry disease, Whipple disease, systemic lupus erythematosus (SLE), and previous methysergide treatment.
- Congenital tricuspid atresia is a rare cause.

DIAGNOSIS

SIGNS AND SYMPTOMS
- Low cardiac output results in fatigue and dyspnea with exertion. Cardiac output does not increase significantly with exercise due to limitation in right-sided filling.
- Patients may complain of generalized anorexia due to GI congestion.
- Orthopnea and paroxysmal nocturnal dyspnea are rare without concomitant mitral valve disease.
- Passive congestion of the liver and spleen results in abdominal pain.
- Peripheral edema may progress toward anasarca.
- Fluttering in the neck is a result of large RA A-waves.
- With co-existing severe tricuspid stenosis and mitral stenosis (MS), hemoptysis, paroxysmal nocturnal dyspnea, and pulmonary edema (associated with mitral valve stenosis) usually are absent because of decreased right-sided flow across the stenotic tricuspid valve.

Physical Exam
- In patients with normal sinus rhythm, a prominent A-wave in the venous pulsation with blunted Y-descent
- Presystolic hepatic pulsation and enlargement along with splenomegaly is common.
- The RA may be palpable along the right sternal border, with a diastolic thrill that increases with inspiration.
- An opening snap of the tricuspid valve may be appreciated, but is usually masked by the mitral valve examination in coexisting mitral valve stenosis.
- The diastolic murmur of TS is best heard along the left parasternal border in the fourth intercostal space and is crescendo-decrescendo in quality.
- Inspiration (Rivero-Carvallo sign), right lateral decubitus positioning, leg lift, amyl nitrate, and isotonic exercise increase the auscultatory findings of TS. The murmur of TS is reduced with maneuvers that reduce venous return, such as the early phase of the Valsalva maneuver and during quiet expiration.
- Pulmonic valve closure is normal.

TESTS
- EKG usually shows sinus rhythm with evidence of RA enlargement without RV hypertrophy.
- PR segment often is depressed because of abnormal P-wave repolarization.
- Biatrial enlargement is common because of coexisting mitral valve stenosis.
- QRS amplitude may be small in V1 because of the large amount of RA tissue between the electrode and ventricle.
- Transthoracic echocardiogram reveals diastolic doming of the tricuspid leaflets, with decreased mobility and thickening of the valve apparatus.
- The tricuspid valve orifice is small. Doppler echocardiography shows increased diastolic velocity with a prolonged deceleration time slope.
- M-mode echocardiography shows reduced E-F slope with increased shadowing of the valve leaflets.

Imaging
- Chest radiography shows prominence of the RA component of the right heart border. Dilation of the azygous vein and superior vena cava may be noted in patients with high RA pressure.
- Pulmonary artery size is normal.
- Pulmonary congestion usually is absent.
- Left atrial enlargement may be noted with coexisting MS.

Diagnostic Procedures/Surgery
- Cardiac catheterization reveals a diastolic gradient between the tricuspid valve and RA.
- A mean diastolic gradient of 2 mm Hg is sufficient for diagnosis.
- The transvalvular gradient increases as a function of flow during exercise, inspiration, infusion of saline, or administration of atropine.
- Significant tricuspid stenosis can mask many of the hemodynamic findings in associated severe MS secondary to decreased pulmonary venous return to the left atrium.
- Contrast angiography in the right anterior oblique projection may reveal thickening of the valve leaflets and the decreased orifice between the RA and ventricle as well as the enlarged RA.

Pathologic Findings
- RA enlargement with thickened chorda and fibrosis/contracture of the tricuspid valve leaflets and commissural fusion
- Tricuspid valve calcification is rare.
- Mitral valve and aortic valve disease is coexistent in the majority of cases.

DIFFERENTIAL DIAGNOSIS
Congenital tricuspid atresia, RA tumors, carcinoid syndrome, endomyocardial fibrosis, tricuspid valve vegetations, cor-triatriatum, extracardiac tumors

TREATMENT

GENERAL MEASURES

Primary therapy for symptomatic tricuspid valve stenosis is tricuspid valve replacement or open valvulotomy (see Surgery).

 MEDICATION (DRUGS)

First Line
Loop diuretics

Second Line
• Thiazides
• Diuretics
• Digoxin

SURGERY

• Decision for surgery versus valvotomy often is influenced by operative necessity of coexisting valve lesions.
• Candidates for surgery include symptomatic patients with a mean diastolic gradient of 5 mm Hg and/or a valve orifice of less than 2 cm^2.
• Simple finger commissurotomy may result in severe tricuspid regurgitation and is not recommended.
• Porcine prosthesis is recommended over mechanical valves because of the high incidence of thrombosis.
• Tricuspid valve balloon valvuloplasty has been used with favorable results.
• With coexisting tricuspid and MS, the tricuspid lesion should not be repaired alone, because severe pulmonary congestion may occur.

 FOLLOW-UP

PROGNOSIS

After valve replacement or repair, outcome is favorable.

COMPLICATIONS

• Valve thrombosis if mechanical valve prosthesis used
• Tricuspid regurgitation if commissurotomy or balloon angioplasty performed

PATIENT MONITORING

• Echocardiography is recommended in the presence of clinical symptoms and the presence of a diastolic murmur consistent with TS for diagnosis.
• Follow-up echocardiography examinations are based on changes in symptomatology.

REFERENCES

1. Alexander RW, ed. *Hurst's the heart.* New York: McGraw-Hill, 1998.
2. Bonow RO, Carabello B, de Leon AC Jr, et al. ACC/AHA 2006 guidelines for the management of patients with valvular heart disease: A report of the American College of Cardiology/American Heart Association Task Force on Practice Guidelines (Writing Committee to Revise the 1998 Guidelines for the Management of Patients With Valvular Heart Disease). American College of Cardiology Web Site. Available at: http://content.onlinejacc.org/cgi/reprint/48/3/e1
3. Braunwald E, ed. *Heart disease: A textbook of cardiovascular medicine,* 6th ed. Philadelphia: WB Saunders, 2005.
4. Topol EJ, ed. *Textbook of cardiovascular medicine.* Philadelphia: Lippincott-Raven, 1998.

 MISCELLANEOUS

See also: Mitral Stenosis; Rheumatic Heart Disease

CODES
ICD9-CM
424.2

PATIENT TEACHING
Diet
Low-sodium diet and diuretic therapy for congestive symptoms

Activity
Patients with severe TS have marked exercise limitations and should avoid strenuous activity.

TRUNCUS ARTERIOSUS

Zvi S. Marans
Welton M. Gersony

 BASICS

DESCRIPTION

Truncus arteriosus (TA) is a severe form of congenital heart disease in which a common arterial trunk arises as the sole outlet from both ventricles.

- The common trunk gives rise to the aorta and pulmonary arteries.
- A large ventricular septal defect (VSD) permits unrestricted blood flow from both ventricles to the common trunk.
- TA is classified by the different locations of the origin of the pulmonary arteries from the common trunk.
  - Type I: A common pulmonary artery arises from the left side of the common trunk.
  - Type II: Separate branch pulmonary arteries arise close to each other from the left posterolateral aspect of the common trunk.
  - Type III: Separate branch pulmonary arteries arise from widely separated origins from the common trunk.

EPIDEMIOLOGY

1–4% of all cardiac deformities

Incidence

Approximately 1/10,000 incidence in the general population

Genetics

1/3 of all cases of TA are associated with DiGeorge syndrome (a severe form of 22q11 deletion).

PATHOPHYSIOLOGY

- Systemic and pulmonary venous blood mix in the common ventricular chamber and enter the truncus. The degree of cyanosis is dependent on the amount of pulmonary blood flow. In most cases, cyanosis is minimal, but may be exacerbated in the presence of congestive heart failure (CHF).
- CHF develops due to decreased pulmonary vascular resistance (PVR) and increased pulmonary blood flow.
- There is increased loading of the ventricles due to increased pulmonary blood flow, and, in some cases, due to the presence of significant truncal valve insufficiency.

ETIOLOGY

- TA is an early embryonic structure that evolves into the aorta and pulmonary artery.
- There is failure of the TA to separate into the 2 great vessels.
- Truncal valve does not split into the aortic and pulmonic valves.
- Truncal valve does not migrate inferiorly to meet the left ventricular outflow.
- Crista supraventricularis does not form.
- There is a single, overriding truncus with a single truncal valve and an outlet VSD.

ASSOCIATED CONDITIONS

Associated cardiac defects:

- Absent patent ductus arteriosus (50%)
- Right aortic arch (21–36%)
- Interrupted aortic arch (11–19%)
- Aortic arch hypoplasia ± coarctation (3%)

 DIAGNOSIS

SIGNS AND SYMPTOMS

- In the early newborn period, babies are usually asymptomatic (due to restricted pulmonary flow secondary to high PVR).
- Babies may present in the newborn nursery with cyanosis or, less likely, with a significant murmur.
- Cyanosis is usually minimal due to complete mixing of saturated and unsaturated blood in the setting of increased pulmonary blood flow.
- If not diagnosed in the newborn nursery, babies usually present in the first few days or weeks after birth with signs and symptoms of pulmonary overcirculation and CHF, and occasionally with truncal valve insufficiency.
- Some unoperated survivors will develop signs and symptoms of Eisenmenger disease.

History

- Increased respiratory rate and effort
- Poor feeding with tiring and sweating
- Poor weight gain

Physical Exam

- Respiratory distress
- Mild cyanosis
- Hyperdynamic precordium
- Systolic murmur and occasional diastolic murmur (pulmonary flow and/or truncal insufficiency)
- Hepatomegaly
- Bounding pulses

TESTS

Lab

- Hemoglobin often mildly increased
- Fluorescent *in situ* hybridization for 22q11 deletion
- ECG
  - Usually normal in the first few days after birth
  - Biventricular enlargement, as pulmonary vascular resistance decreases and pulmonary overcirculation progresses

Imaging

- Chest x-ray
  - May be normal in the first few days after birth
  - Findings of CHF as PVR decreases; cardiomegaly and increased pulmonary vascular markings
- Echocardiogram; definitive diagnostic study
  - Determines the location of the origins of the pulmonary arteries
  - Pulmonary arteries rarely may be stenotic at their origins
  - Assesses the status of the truncal valve, especially for truncal valve insufficiency
  - Right aortic arch is common.
  - Large, unrestrictive VSD is always present.
- Cardiac catheterization
  - Usually unnecessary unless the diagnosis is in question or the pulmonary artery anatomy is not well defined by echocardiography

DIFFERENTIAL DIAGNOSIS

- Isolated large VSD
- Pulmonary atresia with VSD (extreme tetralogy of Fallot), with secondary source of pulmonary blood flow, such as a patent ductus arteriosus (PDA) or major collateral vessel. In the past, some patients labeled as type IV truncus, a term not appropriate for this diagnosis
- Large PDA
- Aorticopulmonary window

TREATMENT

GENERAL MEASURES

- If infant presents in the newborn period, surgical intervention is planned within the first few weeks after birth.
- When signs and symptoms of CHF develop, treatment with digoxin and furosemide is indicated and usually beneficial.

MEDICATION (DRUGS)

- Digoxin and furosemide, for treatment of signs and symptoms of CHF
- Angiotensin-converting enzyme inhibitors may be useful.

SURGERY

- Open heart repair is performed in early infancy, usually in neonatal period
- Surgery consists of:
  - VSD closure
  - Detaching pulmonary arteries from the arterial trunk
  - Placement of right ventricle (RV) to pulmonary artery (PA) extracardiac conduit (homograft or xenograft) or establishing a direct, nonconduit anastomosis between RV and PA
  - Attaching pulmonary arteries to distal end of the RV-PA connection
  - Aortic (truncal) valvuloplasty or replacement may be required in some cases
- When severe truncal valve insufficiency is not repairable, and aortic valve replacement is not possible, cardiac transplantation is the only surgical option.

PROGNOSIS

- Surgical mortality of complete repair in infancy is approximately 5%.
- If patient does well clinically and ventricular function is excellent in the early postoperative period, long-term prognosis is good.
- Reoperations will be required, usually within 10 years, to revise RV-PA conduit or the direct RV-PA anastomosis.
- Significant truncal valve insufficiency may require aortic valve replacement.
- Unoperated survivors will eventually develop pulmonary vascular disease.

COMPLICATIONS

- Ventricular dysfunction secondary to aortic and/or pulmonary insufficiency
- Increased PVR (Eisenmenger syndrome).

PATIENT MONITORING

- Prior to surgery, monitoring patient for signs and symptoms of CHF, and scheduling surgery prior to deterioration
- In early postoperative period, close follow-up is maintained, including serial physical examinations and appropriate noninvasive laboratory studies.
- In the absence of significant problems, yearly follow-up visits are important, with specific observations for:
  - Progressive abnormalities with the RV-PA connection, such as pulmonary stenosis or insufficiency
  - Truncal valve insufficiency
  - Decreased left and/or right ventricular function
  - Increased PVR
- Surveillance testing usually includes surface ECG, ambulatory ECG, echocardiography, and treadmill exercise testing. Cardiac catheterization is indicated only if hemodynamic data are required for decision making.

REFERENCES

1. Anderson RH, et al., eds. *Paediatric Cardiology*, 2nd ed. New York: Churchill Livingstone, 2000.
2. Allen HD, et al. eds. *Moss and Adams' Heart Disease in Infants,* Children and Adolescents, 6th ed. Baltimore: Lippincott Williams & Wilkins, 2001.
3. Goldmuntz E, et al. Frequency of 22q11 deletions in patients with conotruncal defects. *J Am Coll Cardiol.* 1998;32:492–498.
4. McElhinney DB, et al. Trends in the management of truncal insufficiency. *Ann Thorac Surg.* 1998:65:517–524.
5. Williams JM, et al. Factors associated with outcomes of persistent truncus arteriosus. *J Am Coll Cardiol.* 1999;34:545–553.

CODES

ICD9-CM
745.0

PATIENT TEACHING

- Subacute bacterial endocarditis prophylaxis
- Significant symptoms, such as syncope or chest pain, require immediate medical attention.

Activity

- Routine recreational exercise is usually permitted and encouraged in patients who have had good surgical results.
- Avoid sedentary lifestyle, significant weight gain.

TURNER'S SYNDROME

Eric D. Fethke
Welton M. Gersony

 BASICS

DESCRIPTION
- Turner syndrome (TS) is the most common chromosomal abnormality in females and is caused by an aneuploidy disorder with only one fully functioning X chromosome. It presents in its classic form with a characteristic phenotype.
- It was first described in 1938 by Dr. Henry Turner.
- System(s) affected: Cardiovascular; Lymphatic; Endocrine; Renal; Gastrointestinal; Otologic; Hematologic; Neuropsychological
- Synonym(s): XO gonadal dysgenesis; Gonadal dysplasia; Ovarian agenesis

GENERAL PREVENTION
Prenatal counseling

EPIDEMIOLOGY
- Age at presentation:
  - 10% spontaneous miscarriages
  - Fetal to adult
- Sex: Female only

Incidence
The overall incidence is 1/2,000 phenotypic females.

RISK FACTORS
Abnormal maternal serum triple-quadruple screen

Genetics
Complete absence or partial deletion of X chromosome; chromosome constitution consisting of monosomy X (45,X) karyotype (40–60% liveborn) or isochromosome (12–20%) translocation; full penetrance (45,X) or mosaicism (45,X/46,XX or 45,X/46,XY)

PATHOPHYSIOLOGY
- Prenatal: Placental dysfunction
- Postnatal: Gonadal/hormone deficiency

ETIOLOGY
Genetics:
- Absence of Y-chromosome
- Development of embryonic ovary

ASSOCIATED CONDITIONS
- Cardiovascular (22–35%):
  - Coarctation of the aorta: 5–15%
  - Aortic valve disease, stenosis or incompetence: 3–5%
  - Bicuspid aortic valve: 15–35%
  - Aortic root dilatation with possible dissection or ruptures: 6%
  - Partial anomalous pulmonary venous return: 3%
  - Hypoplastic left heart
  - Idiopathic systemic hypertension
  - Coronary artery disease: Secondary to increased incidence of obesity, systemic hypertension, and gonadal/estrogen deficiency

- Endocrine/reproductive
  - Gonadal dysfunction, ranging from abnormal menstruation to infertility
  - Short stature
  - Osteoporosis
  - Autoimmune thyroiditis
  - Carbohydrate intolerance with insulin resistance
- Gastrointestinal
  - Inflammatory bowel disease
- Renal (50%)
  - Horseshoe kidney most common
- Otologic
  - Conductive and sensorineural hearing deficits
- Neuropsychological
  - Mental retardation (rare)
  - Developmental problems: Speech delay, autism, neuromotor deficits, and learning disabilities

 DIAGNOSIS

SIGNS AND SYMPTOMS
- The phenotype varies with age at presentation.
- Fetal
  - Possible hydrops
  - Pleural effusion
  - Polyhydramnios/oligohydramnios
  - Cystic hygroma
  - Typical karyotype on amniocentesis
  - Brachycephaly or growth retardation
  - Cardiac and renal abnormalities
  - Spontaneous abortion
- Infant
  - Edema of hands and feet
  - Neck webbing
  - Wide-spaced nipples
  - Typical facies: Large low-set ears, hypertelorism, epicanthal folds, down-slanting palpebral fissures
  - Cardiovascular malformations: Predominantly coarctation of the aorta or hypoplastic left heart
- Childhood
  - Short stature
  - Otherwise few dysmorphic features
  - Developmental problems
- Adolescence
  - Delay or absence of puberty: Primary or secondary amenorrhea, lack of secondary sexual characteristics
- Adult
  - Short stature
  - Obesity
  - Gonadal dysgenesis resulting in amenorrhea, infertility, osteoporosis, and premature menopause
  - Hypertension
  - Autoimmune thyroiditis
  - Atherosclerotic coronary artery disease

History
- Prenatal
  - Amniocentesis or ultrasound
- Postnatal
  - Typical dysmorphic features
  - Cardiac murmurs

Physical Exam
Varies with age
- Typical dysmorphic features
- Abnormal cardiac auscultation

TESTS
- ECG
  - Left ventricular hypertrophy or dilatation (manifested by increased R-wave voltage in left precordial leads and increased S-wave voltage in right precordial leads) in left heart lesions, causing either increased afterload or volume load on the left ventricle
  - Diminutive left ventricular forces in association with hypoplastic left-heart syndrome
  - May be normal if neither of the above hemodynamics is present
- Audiometry
  - Sensorineural or conductive hearing losses
- Developmental/psychosocial testing
  - May reveal varying degrees of cognitive, behavioral, and psychosocial deficits

Lab
- Chromosome studies of peripheral blood cells (lymphocytes) or other body tissues, including skin, fetal chorion villus, or amniocentesis sample revealing either the 45X0 karyotype (40–60% of liveborn TS patients) or a mosaic karyotype (30–40%)
- Abnormal triple-quadruple maternal serum screening
- Endocrine studies, such as thyroid function tests, growth hormone, and estrogen levels
- Renal function tests
  - Urine specific gravity and electrolytes
  - Blood urea nitrogen (BUN), creatinine, and electrolyte concentrations

Imaging
- Fetal ultrasonography
  - Subcutaneous edema of nuchal skin folds
  - Generalized fetal edema
  - Poly- or oligohydramnios
  - Brachycephaly
  - Renal abnormalities
  - Growth retardation
  - Cardiac abnormalities
- Transthoracic or fetal echocardiography
  - Aortic coarctation, aortic valve stenosis or insufficiency, bicuspid aortic valve, or hypoplastic left heart
  - Anomalous pulmonary venous return
  - Left ventricular hypertrophy secondary to chronic systemic hypertension
  - Aortic root dilatation or dissection

- Renal ultrasonography and voiding cystourethrography
  - Structural renal abnormalities
- Roentgenograms
  - Chest: Enlarged cardiac silhouette secondary to left ventricular hypertrophy or dilatation
  - Extremity: Bone age studies in association with growth hormone therapy for growth retardation

Diagnostic Procedures/Surgery
Cardiac catheterization usually is not required for cardiovascular diagnosis.

DIFFERENTIAL DIAGNOSIS
- Other forms of gonadal dysgenesis syndromes, such as XY or mixed gonadal dysgenesis, male pseudohermaphrodism, and male TS
- Noonan syndrome
- The specific diagnosis can be established via both phenotypic differences, such as characteristic associated congenital heart defects, and appropriate chromosomal studies.
- Criteria
  - An abnormal karyotype in at least 1 tissue characterized by partial or complete absence of the 2nd sex chromosome, usually in association with characteristic phenotypic features

 TREATMENT

GENERAL MEASURES
Treatment depends on age of diagnosis and/or presentation to medical attention

- Prenatal: Parental counseling is advised regarding potentially affected systems, especially cardiac and renal. Timing and mode of delivery should be organized through the efforts of a high-risk perinatal team.
- Newborn: Patients with fetal hydrops should receive supportive, nutritional, and respiratory care in an experienced center where neonatal, renal, and cardiac care can be provided.
- Infancy and childhood: Early recognition of and intervention for cognitive or developmental delays; identification and management of hearing deficits
- Adolescence and adulthood
  - Early evaluation and recognition of growth delay
  - Appropriate referral for management of failure to initiate puberty, amenorrhea, absence of secondary sexual characteristics, infertility, or osteoporosis
  - Identification and aggressive management of progressive systemic hypertension
  - All individuals with heart lesions associated with an increased risk for endocarditis should receive appropriate prophylaxis prior to dental or invasive procedures.

 MEDICATION (DRUGS)

- Diuretics, digoxin, and/or afterload-reducing medications for appropriate left-heart lesions
- Growth hormone therapy beginning as early as 8 years of age for children with growth retardation/short stature
- Hormone/estrogen replacement therapy for delayed puberty, amenorrhea, absence of secondary sexual characteristics, or osteoporosis
- Estrogen replacement therapy for infertility
- Antihypertensive medications for systemic hypertension

SURGERY
- Cardiac
  - Repair of left-sided heart lesion
  - End-to-end anastomosis of discrete coarctation of the aorta
  - Norwood, Glenn, and Fontan procedures for hypoplastic left-heart syndrome
  - Balloon or surgical valvuloplasty for aortic valve stenosis
  - Aortic valve replacement or Ross procedure for severe aortic valvar stenosis or insufficiency
  - Aortoplasty for severe or progressive aortic dilatation or disruption.
- Orthopedic
  - Leg-lengthening procedures for short stature
- Otologic
  - Placement of hearing-aid devices for sensorineural deficits or myringotomy tubes for conductive hearing loss
- Reproductive
  - Assisted reproduction therapy, such as ovum donation and hormone replacement

 FOLLOW-UP

PROGNOSIS
- Overall, the prognosis and outcomes have improved significantly due to early recognition and treatment of associated cardiac malformations, short stature, infertility, systemic hypertension, and osteoporosis.
- Aortic dissection and rupture is a potentially lethal abnormality, but is not necessarily associated with a cardiovascular malformation such as bicuspid aortic valve, aortic coarctation, or systemic hypertension.
- Genetic guidance is indicated in pregnant women suspected of carrying a fetus with TS or a woman with TS planning to conceive.

Pregnancy Considerations
- Full term pregnancy rare
- A large incidence of miscarriages or infants born with malformations (e.g., TS, trisomy 21)
- 38% of pregnancies result in healthy newborns.

PATIENT MONITORING
Routine life-long outpatient visits are recommended, with attention to systems discussed, especially cardiovascular, renal, endocrine, and otologic. A well-coordinated multidisciplinary approach is required.

REFERENCES
1. Albertson-Wikland K, Ranke MB, Turner syndrome in a life span perspective: Research and clinical aspects. Proceedings of the 4th International Symposium on Turner Syndrome, Gothenburg, Sweden, May 18–21, 1995. Amsterdam: Elsevier.
2. Lin AE, Lippe B, Rosenfeld RG, et al. Further delineation of aortic dilation, dissection, and rupture in patients with Turner syndrome. Pediatrics. 1998;102(1):e12.
3. Stenberg AE, et al. Otological problems in children with Turner's syndrome. Hearing Res. 1998;124: 85–90.
4. Tarani L, et al. Pregnancy in patients with Turner's syndrome: Six new cases and review of literature. Gynecol Endocrinol. 1998;12:83–87.
5. Telvi L, et al. 45,X/46,XY mosaicism: Report of 27 cases. Pediatrics. 1999;104(part 1):304–308.

PATIENT TEACHING
Diet
No dietary restrictions

Activity
No restrictions in absence of cardiac disease

Prevention
- If cardiac defects present, administer bacterial endocarditis prophylaxis for dental and invasive procedures according to American Heart Association guidelines.
- Aortic disruption or dissection: Treat hypertension in cases of dilation of the aorta; monitor closely.
- Short stature: Treat early with growth hormone in collaboration with a pediatric endocrinologist.
- Amenorrhea, infertility, and osteoporosis: Treat with estrogen replacement under obstetric or endocrinologic guidance; artificial fertilization possible.
- Pregnancy: Birth control measures are indicated in TS because, although rare, pregnancy is possible.

VALVULAR CARDIAC SURGERY

Jennifer Lash
Steven Herrmann
Bernard R. Chaitman

 BASICS

Aortic stenosis (AS)

Description
- Severity of aortic stenosis is related to aortic valve area:
  - Normal aortic valve area ~3.0–4.0 cm^2
  - Mild AS: >1.5 cm^2
  - Moderate AS: 1.0–1.5 cm^2
  - Severe AS: <1.0 cm^2
- In patients with a larger body habitus, the same valve area may result in a more significant limitation to ventricular outflow than that seen in a smaller individual. Some experts recommend normalizing aortic valve area per meter squared of body surface area.
- The timing of surgery is based on symptoms of angina, syncope, heart failure, or degree of critical narrowing of the valve.

AORTIC REGURGITATION (AR)
Description
Qualitative assessment of severity by cardiac catheterization depends on regurgitation of contrast from aorta to left ventricle (LV) and can be classified as follows:
- Mild (1+): Small amount of contrast enters the left ventricle in diastole, is essentially cleared with one beat, and never fully opacifies the LV.
- Moderate (2+): More contrast enters the LV with each diastole, and faint opacification of entire chamber occurs.
- Moderately severe (3+): Left ventricle chamber is well opacified and is equal in density with the ascending aorta.
- Severe (4+): Complete dense opacification of LV chamber with the first beat and appearance that the left ventricle is more densely opacified than ascending aorta.
  Echocardiography is useful to assess the severity of the regurgitation, the valve morphology, the LV size and function, and the aortic root.

MITRAL STENOSIS
Description
- Severity of mitral stenosis is based on the calculated mitral valve area by echocardiography or cardiac catheterization.
  - Mild MS: >1.5 cm^2
  - Moderate MS: 1.1–1.5 cm^2
  - Severe MS: <1.0 cm^2

MITRAL REGURGITATION (MR)
Description
Echocardiography with Doppler interrogation of the mitral valve gives a qualitative and quantitative assessment of regurgitant volume and fraction. It is also useful in determining the left ventricular size and function as well as the left atrial size.

Qualitative assessment of severity by cardiac catheterization depends on opacification of left atrium (LA) and can be classified as:
- Mild (1+): Never opacifies entire LA and clears with each beat
- Moderate (2+): Opacifies LA after several beats, but opacification is less than that in LV and does not clear with one beat
- Moderately Severe (3+): LA is completely opacified and is equal to opacification of LV.
- Severe (4+): Opacification of entire LA with one beat, progressively more dense with each beat, and contrast can be seen refluxing into pulmonary vein

Pregnancy Considerations
Refer to chapter on Aortic Stenosis, Adult.

ETIOLOGY
Refer to chapters on Aortic Stenosis.

 TREATMENT

GENERAL MEASURES
- Aortic stenosis
  - See chapter on Prosthetic Valves.
- Aortic regurgitation
  - See chapter on Prosthetic Valves.

SURGERY
Aortic Stenosis
- Aortic valve replacement (AVR)
  - AVR is definitely indicated in:
    - Symptomatic patients with severe AS
    - Patients with severe AS and undergoing coronary artery bypass surgery
    - Patients with severe AS and undergoing surgery on the aorta or other heart valves
  - AVR also may be indicated in patients with moderate AS and undergoing coronary artery bypass surgery or undergoing surgery on the aorta or other heart valves.
  - AVR may be indicated in asymptomatic patients with severe AS and
    - LV systolic dysfunction
    - Abnormal response to exercise (e.g., hypotension).
    - Significant arrhythmias (e.g., ventricular tachycardia)
    - Marked or excessive LV hypertrophy (>15 mm)
    - Valve area <0.6 cm^2

- Aortic balloon valvuloplasty
  - Infrequently used in adults because of a significant complication rate
  - American College of Cardiology indications in adults
    - A bridge to surgery in hemodynamically unstable patients who are at high risk for AVR (cardiogenic shock or moderate/severe heart failure)
    - Palliation in patients with serious comorbid conditions
    - Patients who require urgent noncardiac surgery
- Aortic valve replacement
  - According to the American College of Cardiology, AVR is definitely indicated in:
    - Patients with NYHA functional class III or IV symptoms and preserved LV systolic function, defined as normal ejection fraction (EF) at rest (EF >50%)
    - Patients with NYHA functional class II symptoms and preserved LV systolic function (EF >50% at rest) but with progressive LV dilatation, declining EF at rest on serial studies, or declining effort tolerance on exercise testing
    - Patients with Canadian Heart Association functional class II or greater angina with or without coronary artery disease
    - Asymptomatic or symptomatic patients with mild to moderate LV systolic dysfunction at rest (EF 25–49%).
    - Patients undergoing coronary artery bypass surgery or surgery on the aorta or other heart valves
  - According to the American College of Cardiology, AVR also may be indicated in:
    - Patients with NYHA functional class II symptoms and preserved LV systolic function (EF >50% at rest) with stable LV size and systolic function on serial studies and stable exercise tolerance.
    - Asymptomatic patients with normal LV systolic function (EF >50%) but with severe LV dilatation (end-diastolic dimension >75 mm or end-systolic dimension >55 mm) or high left ventricular end-diastolic volume index ($\geq$150 mL/m^2) + PA wedge pressure $\geq$20 mm Hg, or declining EF on stress testing

Mitral Stenosis
- Percutaneous mitral valvotomy
  - American College of Cardiology indications include:
    - Patients with mitral stenosis (mitral valve area <1.5 cm^2) and NYHA class II or more symptoms and valve morphology suitable for balloon valvotomy in the absence of atrial thrombus and moderate to severe
    - Patients with mitral stenosis (mitral valve area <1.5 cm^2) and pulmonary hypertension (pulmonary artery systolic pressure >50 mm Hg at rest and 60 mm Hg during exertion) and valve morphology suitable for balloon valvotomy in the absence of atrial thrombus and moderate to severe mitral regurgitation
    - Patients with mitral stenosis (mitral valve area <1.5 cm^2) and NYHA class III or more symptoms and a nonpliable calcified valve who are at high risk for surgery in the absence of atrial thrombus and moderate to severe mitral regurgitation
    - Asymptomatic patients with mitral stenosis (mitral valve area <1.5 cm^2) and valve morphology suitable for balloon valvotomy who have new-onset atrial fibrillation in the absence of atrial thrombus and moderate to severe mitral regurgitation
- Mitral valve repair
  - American College of Cardiology indications include:
    - Patients with NYHA functional class III–IV symptoms, moderate or severe mitral stenosis (mitral valve area ≤1.5 cm^2), and valve morphology favorable for repair of percutaneous mitral balloon valvotomy is not available.
    - Patients with NYHA functional class III–IV symptoms, moderate or severe mitral stenosis (mitral valve area ≤1.5 cm^2), and valve morphology favorable for repair if left atrial thrombus is present despite anticoagulation.
    - Patients with NYHA functional class III–IV symptoms, moderate or severe mitral stenosis (mitral valve area ≤1.5 cm^2), and a nonpliable or calcified valve with the decision to proceed with repair or replacement made at the time of the operation.
- Mitral valve replacement
  - American College of Cardiology indications include:
    - Patients with moderate or severe mitral stenosis (mitral valve area ≤1.5 cm^2) and NYHA functional class III-IV symptoms who are not considered candidates for percutaneous balloon valvotomy or mitral valve repair
    - Patients with severe mitral stenosis (mitral valve area ≤1 cm^2) and severe pulmonary hypertension (pulmonary artery systolic pressure >60–80 mm Hg) with NYHA functional class I–II symptoms who are not considered candidates for percutaneous balloon valvotomy or mitral valve repair

Mitral Regurgitation
- 3 different mitral valve operations are currently being used for correction of MR:
  - Mitral valve repair
  - Mitral valve replacement (MVR) with preservation of all or part of the mitral apparatus
  - MVR with removal of mitral apparatus

Acute Severe MR
- The patients with acute severe MR are almost always symptomatic.
- These patients need to be assessed by transthoracic or transesophageal echocardiogram for valve morphology.
- If ischemia is not the cause of MR, the patient can have mitral valve repair without the need for cardiac catheterization.

Chronic Severe MR (Nonischemic)
- Surgery is definitely indicated in following patients:
  - Acute symptomatic MR in which repair is likely
  - Patients with NYHA functional class II, III, or IV symptoms with normal LV systolic function defined as EF >60% and end-systolic dimension <45 mm.
  - Symptomatic or asymptomatic patients with mild LV systolic dysfunction, EF 50–60%, and end-systolic dimension 45–50 mm
  - Symptomatic or asymptomatic patients with moderate LV systolic dysfunction, EF 30–50%, and/or end-systolic dimension 50–55 mm
- Surgery also may be indicated in the following patients:
  - Asymptomatic patients with preserved LV systolic function and atrial fibrillation
  - Asymptomatic patients with preserved LV systolic function and pulmonary hypertension (pulmonary artery systolic pressure >50 mm Hg at rest or >60 mm Hg with exercise).
  - Asymptomatic patients with EF 50–60% and end-systolic dimension <45 mm and asymptomatic patients with EF >60% and end-systolic dimension 45–55 mm
  - Patients with severe LV systolic dysfunction (EF <30% and/or end-systolic dimension >55 mm) in whom chordal preservation is highly likely

Tricuspid Regurgitation
- Surgical options available for tricuspid regurgitation are:
  - Tricuspid valve and chordal reconstruction
  - Tricuspid valve annuloplasty
  - Tricuspid valve replacement
- Indications
  - Annuloplasty for severe longstanding TR and pulmonary hypertension in patients with mitral valve disease requiring mitral valve surgery
  - Valve replacement for severe TR secondary to diseased/abnormal tricuspid valve leaflets not amenable to annuloplasty or repair
  - Valve replacement or annuloplasty for severe TR with mean pulmonary artery pressure <60 mm Hg when symptomatic; bioprosthesis is preferred over mechanical prosthesis
  - In drug addicts with tricuspid valve regurgitation due to endocarditis, total excision of the tricuspid valve is usually well tolerated in the absence of pulmonary hypertension.

Tricuspid Stenosis
- Surgical options available for tricuspid stenosis are:
  - Tricuspid commissurotomy (closed or open)
  - Tricuspid valve replacement

Pulmonary Regurgitation
- Surgical treatment of pulmonary regurgitation is rarely if ever required for intractable right heart failure, and is usually for patients after multiple surgeries for congenital heart disease.
- Bioprosthesis is preferable because of mechanical valve thrombosis in this position.

Pulmonary Stenosis
- Surgical options available for pulmonic stenosis are either balloon valvuloplasty or valve replacement with or without surgical correction of other abnormalities.
- Balloon valvuloplasty is the treatment of choice for congenital pulmonic stenosis in symptomatic patients with a peak-to-peak gradient of 50 mm Hg.
- Surgery is indicated in patients with exertional dyspnea, angina, syncope, or presyncope.
- Valve replacement is required in patients with dysplastic valve with or without correction of other abnormalities like in patients with Noonan syndrome.

Aortic Stenosis
- Complications of AVR
  - Significant complications occur at a rate of 2–3% per year, whereas death due directly to prosthesis occurs at a rate of ~1% per year.
  - Risk and complications of anticoagulation for prosthetic metallic heart valve

REFERENCES

1. Bonow RO, Carabello B, de Leon AC Jr, et al. ACC/AHA 2006 guidelines for the management of patients with valvular heart disease: A report of the American College of Cardiology/American Heart Association Task Force on Practice Guidelines (Writing Committee to Revise the 1998 Guidelines for the Management of Patients With Valvular Heart Disease). American College of Cardiology Web Site. Available at: http://content.onlinejacc.org/cgi/reprint/48/3/e1
2. Feigenbaum H, et al. *Feigenbaum's Echocardiography*, 6th ed. Philadelphia: Lippincott Williams & Wilkins, 2005.
3. Enriquez-Sarano M, Avierinos JF, Messika-Zeitoun D, et al. Quantitative determinants of outcome of asymptomatic mitral regurgitation. *N Engl J Med*. 2005;352:875–883.
4. Enriquez-Sarano M, Tajik AJ. Aortic regurgitation. *N Engl J Med*. 2004;351:1539–1546.
5. Zoghbi WA, Enriquez-Sarano M, Foster E, et al. Recommendations for evaluation of the severity of native valvular regurgitation with two-dimensional and Doppler echocardiography. *J Am Soc Echocardiogr*. 2003;16:777–802.

CODES
ICD9-CM
- 424.1
- 424.0
- 396.3
- 394.0
- 396.8

VENTRICULAR SEPTAL DEFECT

Donald Leichter
Welton M. Gersony

 BASICS

DESCRIPTION

A ventricular septal defect (VSD) is an anatomic defect that allows intracardiac shunting of blood. VSDs may occur at various positions in the ventricular septum:

- Posterior: Inlet distal to the tricuspid valve (endocardial cushion type), may exist as an isolated anomaly or as part of an atrioventricular canal.
- Subaortic (membranous)
- Subpulmonary (supracristal): Associated with aortic valve prolapse
- Muscular: Mid or apical; may be multiple

Pediatric Considerations
Careful evaluation for possible pulmonary hypertension prior to 2 years of age

EPIDEMIOLOGY
- VSD is the most common congenital heart defect, excluding bicuspid aortic valve without obstruction.
- Predominant sex: Female > Male (56%)

Incidence
Incidence is 1.5–3.5/1,000 term births

Prevalence
- Overall prevalence in children is 1.4/1,000 live births.
- The smaller prevalence in children largely represents spontaneous closure, occurring commonly in the 1st year of age, but also as late as adult life.

RISK FACTORS
- Family history of congenital heart disease
- Associated with chromosomal anomalies
- Exposure to teratogens during gestation

Pregnancy Considerations
- Pulmonary hypertension poorly tolerated
- 2–3% risk of congenital heart disease in offspring

Genetics
- 90% of VSDs are "multifactorial" in etiology and not associated with specific chromosomal anomalies.
- 8% have chromosomal anomalies (trisomy 13,18, 21, etc.).
- 2% may be attributable to environmental causes.

PATHOPHYSIOLOGY
Left to right shunt
- Congestive heart failure
- Alterations in pulmonary vascular resistance (PVR)
- Volume overload
- Pulmonary congestion
- Altered pulmonary compliance
- Hyperkinetic pulmonary hypertension
- Pulmonary vascular obstructive disease
- Late right heart dilation and hypertrophy
- Aortic regurgitation in 5% of patients (40% in Asians)
- Infundibular stenosis in up to 7% (evolving tetralogy physiology)

ETIOLOGY
- Congenital (most common)
- Traumatic
- Ischemic

ASSOCIATED CONDITIONS
- Failure to thrive
- Congestive heart failure (CHF)
- Pulmonary hypertension
- Pulmonary vascular obstructive disease

 DIAGNOSIS

SIGNS AND SYMPTOMS
- Small restrictive VSD
  - Asymptomatic
- Large unrestrictive VSD with significant shunting (>2:1 Qp/Qs) and hyperkinetic pulmonary hypertension
  - CHF beginning about 4–8 weeks of age with:
    - Tachypnea
    - Tachycardia
    - Fatigue with feeding
    - Poor weight gain
    - Diaphoresis

History
- Murmur
- CHF during infancy (large defects)
- CHF may diminish
  - With decreasing VSD size
  - With increasing pulmonary vascular resistance (PVR)
  - With development of right ventricular (RV) outflow obstruction
- Spontaneous closure may occur, usually in small (but occasionally in large) VSDs. Closure occurs by:
  - Membranous aneurysm formation
  - Fibrous proliferation
  - Muscle bundle hypertrophy with formation of a double-chambered right ventricle
  - Prolapse of aortic valve leaflet into defect
- Pulmonary vascular obstruction may evolve in unrepaired patients as early as 2 years of age

ALERT
- In high altitude or with trisomy 21, elevated pulmonary vascular resistance (PVR) may develop in infancy.
- A recognizable period of congestive failure may not occur.

Physical Exam
- Small restrictive VSD
  - Pansystolic murmur along left lower sternal border
  - Systolic thrill (occasionally)
- Large unrestrictive VSD with significant shunting (>2:1 Qp/Qs) and hyperkinetic pulmonary hypertension
  - Loud pansystolic murmur along the left sternal border
  - Systolic thrill (often)
  - Diastolic rumble at apex (increased diastolic blood flow across mitral valve)
  - CHF beginning about 4–8 weeks of age with:
    - Tachypnea
    - Tachycardia
    - Hepatomegaly
    - Rales
    - Diaphoresis
- Large unrestrictive VSD with elevated pulmonary vascular resistance and shunting <2:1 Qp/Qs
  - Loud second heart sound (S_2)
  - Little or no holosystolic murmur from VSD
  - Failure to thrive
- Large unrestrictive VSD with pulmonary vascular disease and reversal of shunt
  - Loud P2
  - Cardiac murmur less prominent as L-R shunt decreases
  - Cyanosis as shunt reverses (see chapter on Eisenmenger's Syndrome).

TESTS
- Electrocardiogram (ECG)
  - Small shunts: ECG usually normal
  - Large shunts: Left atrial enlargement and left ventricular hypertrophy evident; prominent Q waves in the inferior and left lateral leads. In infants, mid-precordial leads may show biventricular enlargement (Katz-Wachtel sign).
  - Pulmonary vascular disease: Right ventricular hypertrophy (RVH) will dominate.

Lab
- Hyponatremia is seen in CHF due to water retention.
- A peptide, NT-proBNP is elevated in the presence of congestive heart failure.
- In severe failure, hyperkalemia and lactic acidosis may occur.
- Loop diuretics may result in hypochloremia and elevations in bicarbonate.

Imaging
Chest x-ray
- Isolated small VSD: Normal heart size and vascularity
- Moderate defects with normal pulmonary arterial pressures but high flow: Increased vascular markings and varying degrees of cardiomegaly
- Large defects with significant left-to-right shunting: Increased pulmonary vascular markings, cardiomegaly, prominent pulmonary artery segments, splaying of the right and left bronchi, and left atrial enlargement
- Large defects with pulmonary vascular disease: RVH with upturned apex and prominent proximal pulmonary artery segments in the absence of increased vascular markings in the periphery. Heart size often appears to be normal.

Echocardiography
- Sector scan
  - Number, location of VSDs
  - Chamber enlargement or hypertrophy
  - Associated lesions
- Doppler
  - Pulse wave blood flow evaluation
    - VSD demonstrated
    - Valves evaluated
    - Aorta and pulmonary artery anatomy demonstrated
  - Continuous wave Doppler evaluation
    - Trans-septal gradient determines whether VSD is restrictive.
    - Tricuspid regurgitant gradient estimates RV pressure.
  - Color flow Doppler
    - Shunt location documented
    - Qualitative estimate of shunt
- Real-time 3D echocardiography
  - Further defines size, shape, and relationship of VSD to other cardiac structures

Cardiac catheterization
- Not routinely indicated in uncomplicated VSD.
- Useful if the VSD is not clearly "restrictive" or has complex associated lesions
- Important data measured or calculated include:
  - Shunt quantitation
  - Pulmonary artery pressure
  - Pulmonary wedge pressure
  - Left ventricular end-diastolic pressure
  - Pulmonary and systemic resistances

- Angiography
  - Documents locations of septal defect(s)
  - Qualitative evaluation of shunt
  - Determination of left and right ventricular function
  - Identification of associated defects
- Interventional device closure of muscular
- VSDs may be appropriate in special circumstances

Pathologic Findings
- Anatomic locations
  - Subaortic, perimembranous
  - Subpulmonic, outlet
  - Endocardial cushion, inlet
  - Muscular (midseptal, apical, multiple)
- Physiologic findings

DIFFERENTIAL DIAGNOSIS
The differential diagnosis of a pansystolic murmur along the left lower sternal border includes atrioventricular valve insufficiency and subaortic stenosis, as well as VSD.

- The infant with CHF and a large left-to-right shunt may have communications between the left and right heart/great arteries other than VSD (atrioventricular canal defect, double-outlet right ventricle, patent ductus arteriosus, single ventricle anatomy without pulmonary stenosis, aortopulmonary window, truncus arteriosus).
- CHF due to severe mitral insufficiency also can be confused with VSD. In addition, other cardiac lesions frequently coexist with VSD.

TREATMENT

GENERAL MEASURES
- Outpatient other than for surgery or management of complications
- Antibiotic prophylaxis
- Small VSDs: Spontaneous closure may occur, no risk for CHF or pulmonary hypertension. Reassurance should be provided. Although occasional re-evaluation may be indicated, in general these patients should not require close follow-up.
- Large VSDs: Close follow-up of infants with large defects is necessary. The clinical course may diverge widely.
- Development of progressive CHF, which responds to medical therapy, allowing time for spontaneous closure or subsequent surgical closure prior to 18–24 months of life
  - Development of progressive CHF, which does not respond to medical therapy; early surgical closure is required
  - Defects close or become hemodynamically insignificant.
  - Unoperated patients with unrestrictive VSDs may develop increased PVR and decreased shunting.
  - RV infundibular hypertrophy may develop, decreasing left-to-right shunting with eventual development of tetralogy physiology.
  - RV muscle bundles may hypertrophy and partially or fully close the VSD, creating a high-pressure subchamber (double-chamber right ventricle).

MEDICATION (DRUGS)

First Line
- Digoxin as an oral cardiotonic agent
- Lasix combined with Aldactone for diuretic management of CHF
- Angiotensin-converting enzyme inhibitors may be used for afterload reduction.
- Antibiotic prophylaxis

SURGERY
- Surgical closure is indicated in infants with CHF refractory to medical therapy.
- Older infants with large defects and significant shunts, stable on medical management, still require surgical closure if their defect does not become restrictive. Such patients not repaired by 2 years of age are at significant risk for developing pulmonary vascular disease.
- Timing of surgical closure prior to the end of the 2nd year of age is strongly recommended.
- In contrast, an asymptomatic patient with normal pulmonary arterial pressures rarely will require surgical closure.
- Patients with significant shunts, but normal pulmonary arterial pressures may require closure if failure to thrive, recurrent pulmonary infections, or bronchial compression due to atrial or pulmonary artery dilation become an issue.
- Subaortic VSDs with aortic valve prolapse and progressive aortic regurgitation (AR) require repair.

PROGNOSIS
- Small defects have a benign prognosis. Some will close spontaneously.
- Large defects diagnosed in the 1st year of age and requiring surgical closure will be repaired prior to 2 years of age. The expected operative mortality should be less than 3%. Long-term prognosis for a "normal life" is excellent.
- Large defects unrepaired or repaired late with pulmonary vascular disease will have a guarded prognosis.

COMPLICATIONS
- CHF and pulmonary edema
- Pulmonary hypertension and pulmonary vascular disease
- Endocarditis

PATIENT MONITORING
- Small defects: Close follow-up unnecessary; no restriction of activities
- Large defects: Close follow-up for assessment of developing CHF and/or pulmonary hypertension over the 1st year of age; follow-up after closure; regular activity
- Pulmonary vascular disease: See chapter on Eisenmenger's Syndrome.

REFERENCES
1. Dajani A, et al. AHA medical/scientific statement: Prevention of bacterial endocarditis. *Circulation.* 1997;96:358–366.
2. Elliot LP. *Cardiac Imaging in Infants, Children and Adults.* Philadelphia: JB Lippincott, 1991.
3. Emmanouilides G, et al., eds. *Heart Disease in Infants, Children and Adolescents,* 5th ed. Baltimore: Williams & Wilkins, 1995.
4. Silverman NH. *Pediatric Echocardiography.* Baltimore: Williams & Wilkins, 1992.
5. Task Force 6. Arrhythmias. *J Am Coll Cardiol* 1994;24:845–899.
6. Weidman WH, et al. Second natural history study of congenital heart defects. *Circulation.* 1993;87(suppl I):1–120.

ADDITIONAL READING
Van den Bosch AE, Ten Harkel DJ, McGhie JS, et al. Feasibility and accuracy of real-time 3-dimensional echocardiographic assessment of ventricular septal defects. *J Am Soc Echocardiogr.* 2006;19:7–13.

CODES
ICD9-CM
745.4 Ventricular septal defect

PATIENT TEACHING
- Subacute bacterial endocarditis prophylaxis
- Reassurance with small VSDs
- Emphasize close follow-up of large defects in infancy.
- Anticipate surgical repair of large defects.

Diet
Adequate calories (139–150 calories/kg/day) should be provided.

Activity
- Small VSD: Unrestricted activity
- Large repaired VSD, no pulmonary vascular disease: If without significant residua (shunt, pulmonary hypertension, myocardial dysfunction), may participate in all activities within 6 months of repair
- Large VSD, repaired, significant arrhythmias: Follow recommendations for specific arrhythmia.

Prevention
- Antibiotic prophylaxis (see preceding text)
- Avoid known teratogens during pregnancy.
- Fetal echocardiography for patients with fetus at increased risk for CHD

FAQ
Q. Why aren't all VSDs evident on auscultation at birth?

A. In the presence of elevated PVR a significant L-R shunt and turbulent flow at the VSD may not be obvious. With time, PVR drops and the shunt becomes apparent.

Q. An asymptomatic and well appearing 2 year old is noted to have a prominent cardiac silhouette on chest x-ray, left ventricular enlargement (LVE) on ECG and a perimembranous VSD on ultrasound with a gradient across the VSD estimated at 75 mmHg. How urgent is surgical closure?

A. This patient has evidence of increased left heart volume but no suggestion of elevated pulmonary artery (PA) pressures. In the absence of pulmonary hypertension or symptomatic CHF, there is no urgency to surgical closure. Some of these patients will go on to have progressive diminution of the VSD shunt over time.

Q. A 4 month old with trisomy 21 has a diagnosis of a large VSD made at birth. No evidence of CHF has been noted and a VSD murmur is not easily appreciated. Does this patient require further cardiac evaluation?

A. Infants with trisomy 21 frequently exhibit early elevation of pulmonary vascular resistance and may not demonstrate significant VSD shunting or CHF. They are at high risk to develop permanent pulmonary vascular changes and early Eisenmenger syndrome if not repaired in the first 6 months after birth.

Activity Recommendations in Patients with Congenital Aortic Stenosis

Mild (gradient ≤20 mmHg) No LVH, no symptoms **Moderate** Mild LVH, no symptoms	Low static/moderate dynamic sports (baseball, tennis, or volleyball), low dynamic/moderate static activities (diving or equestrian activities)
Severe Severe LVH, symptoms Full participation in recreational and competitive sports	No competitive, limited recreational sports

LVH, left ventricular hypertrophy.

Classification of Severity of Pulmonary Stenosis

RV-PA GRADIENT	SEVERITY
<50 mm	Mild
50–79 mm	Moderate
80+ mm	Severe

RV-PA, right ventrical-pulmonary artery.

Drugs That Can Prolong the QT Interval

Antiarrhythmic drugs
  Quinidine (Quinidex extentabs, Quinaglute, Cardioquin, Duraquin)
  Procainamide (Pronestyl, Procan, Procan SR, Procanbid)
  Disopyramide (Norpace)
  Sotalol (Betapace)
  Amiodarone (Cordarone)
  Ibutilide (Corvert)
  Dofetilide
  Flecainide (Tambocor)[a]
  Mexiletine (Mexitil)[a]
  Tocainide (Tonocard)[a]
Calcium blockers for angina
  Bepridil (Vascor)
  Mibefradil (Posicor: Withdrawn from market)
Psychiatric drugs
  Phenothiazines [prochlorperazine (Compazine), thioridazine (Mellaril), chlorpromazine (Thorazine), fluphenazine (Prolixin), trifluoperazine (Stelazine), perphenazine (Etrafon, Trilafon), etc.]
  Tricyclics [amitriptyline (Elavil), imipramine (Tofranil), maprotiline (Ludiomil), nortriptyline (Pamelor), protriptyline (Vivactil), amoxapine (Asendin),[a] clomipramine (Anafranil),[a] doxepin (Sinequan),[a] etc.]
  Haloperidol (Haldol)
  Pimozide (ORAP)
  Risperidone (Risperdal)
  Thiothixene (Navane)
Antibiotics
  Azithromycin (Zithromax)
  Chloraquine (Aralen)
  Erythromycin (Akne-Mycin, E-Mycin, Ery-Tab, EryPeds, PCE Dispertab, and others)
  Fluconazole (Diflucan)
  Halofantrine (Halfan)
  Itraconazole (Sporanox)
  Ketoconazole (Nizoral)
  Pentamadine (Pentacarinat, Pentam, NebuPent)
  Trimethoprim-sulfa (Septra, Bactrim)
Antihistamines (especially with antifungals, such as ketoconazole)
  Terfenadine (Seldane)
  Astemizole (Hismanal)
  Clemastine (Tavist)[a]
  Diphenylhydramine (Benadryl)[a]
Antihyperlipidemics
  Probucol (Lorelco)
Toxins
  Arsenic
  Organophosphate insecticides
  Liquid protein diets
Anesthetics/antiasthmatics
  Adrenaline/epinephrine
Miscellaneous (and potentially risky)
  Amantadine (Symmetrel)
  Diuretics without potassium, and sometimes magnesium, supplementation, especially indapamide (Lozol)
  Chloral hydrate
  Cisapride (Propulsid) with ketoconazole, fluconazole, itraconazole, miconazole, erythromycin, troleandomycin, clarithromycin
  Cocaine
  Fludrocortisone (Florinef)
  Ipecac
  Tamoxifen (Nolvadex)
  Terodiline (Mictrol, Micturin)

[a] Unconfirmed or rarely reported cases of torsades de pointes ventricular tachycardia.

Interpretation of Hemodynamic Patterns in Cardiac Patients

ETIOLOGY	DECREASED PRELOAD		CARDIOGENIC				
	HYPOVOLEMIA	VASODILATION	BRADYCARDIA	LV DYSFUNCTION	RV DYSFUNCTION	TAMPONADE	SEPSIS
Hemodynamics							
RA	<8	<8	≤10	≥10	≥10	>15	<10
PCW	<15	<15	>15	>20	≤15	>15	<15
CI	<2.0	<2.0	<2.0	<2.0	<2.0	>2.0	≥2.0
SVR	>1,200	<1,000	>1,200	>1,000	>1,000	>1,000	<600
Other			HR <60		PCW >15 if LV	RA = PCW = PAd	Narrow AVO$_2$ difference
Management	Fluids; transfuse if Hgb <10; intropic drugs	Vasopressors	Cardiac pacing	Inotropic drugs; vasopressors; vasodilators; mechanical assistance	Supplemental O$_2$; pulmonary vasodilators; inotropic drugs; mechanical assistance	Reexploration; inotropic drugs; fluids	Fluids; antibiotics; vasopressors; inotropic drugs

LV, left ventricular; RV, right ventricular; Ra, right atrial; PCW, pulmonary capillary wedge; CI, cardiac index; SVR, systemic vascular resistance; PAd, pulmonary artery diastolic pressure; AVO$_2$, arteriovenous oxygen; Hgb, hemoglobin.

Adapted from Antman E. Medical management of the patient undergoing cardiac surgery. In: Braunwald, E, ed. Heart disease: A textbook of cardiovascular medicine, 6th ed. Philadelphia: WB Saunders, 2005:1726; with permission.

Intravenous Positive Inotropic Agents

MEDICATION	DOSAGE	COMMENTS
Dopamine	2–20 μg/kg/min	Low dose: dopaminergic effect Moderate dose: inotropic effect High dose: vasopressor effect
Dobutamine	2–20 μg/kg/min	Inotropic drug
Epinephrine	1–4 μg/min	Inotropic drug
Amrinone	10–15 μg/min	Inotropic drug
Milrinone	12.5–75 μg/kg/min	Inotropic drug
Isoproterenol	0.5–10 μg/min	Inotropic and chronotropic drug
Norepinephrine	2–12 μg/min	Vasopressor and inotropic drug
Phenylephrine	10–500 μg/min	Vasopressor

Adapted from Morris DC, St. Claire D. Jr: Management of patients after cardiac surgery. *Curr Probl Cardiol*. 1999;24: 161–228; with permission.

Diagnosis of Myocardial Infarction in Patients Undergoing Coronary Bypass Surgery

NEW Q-WAVES ON ECG	CK-MB >30 IU/L	NEW RWMA ON ECHO	DIAGNOSIS OF MI	COMMENTS
Yes	Yes	Yes	Definite	
Yes	No	Yes	Definite	CK-MB missed with infrequent sampling
Yes	Yes	No	Probable	New zone of necrosis may not be evident on echo
No	Yes	Yes	Probable	NQMI
Yes	No	No	Possible	New Q's may be false positive
No	Yes	No	Unlikely	Small NQMI cannot be entirely excluded
No	No	Yes	Unlikely	Removal of pericardium may result in new RWMA, especially high anterior septum
No	No	No	No MI	

CK-MB, creatinine kinase-MB fraction: RWMA, regional wall motion abnormality; NQMI, non-Q-wave myocardial infarction; MI, myocardial infarction.

Adapted from Antman E. Medical management of the patient undergoing cardiac surgery. In: Braunwald E, ed. *Heart disease: A textbook of cardiovascular medicine*, 7th ed. Philadelphia: WB Saunders, 2005:1724; with permission.

Risk Stratification in Hypertensive Patients

BLOOD PRESSURE STAGE (mmHg)	RISK GROUP A (NO RF; NOT TOD AND/OR CCD)	RISK GROUP B (AT LEAST 1 RF, NOT DIABETES, NO TOD OR CCD)	RISK GROUP C (TOD/CCD AND/OR DIABETES)
High-normal 130–139/85–89	Life -style modification	Life-style modification	Drug therapy[a]
Stage 1 140–159/ 90–99	Life-style modification (up to 12 mo)	Life-style modification (up to 6 mo)	Drug therapy
Stage 2–3 >169/>100	Drug therapy	Drug therapy	Drug therapy

[a] In those with heart failure, renal insufficiency, or diabetes.

TOD, target organ damage; RF, risk factor.

Adapted from The Seventh Report of the Joint National Committee on Prevention, Detection, Evaluation, and Treatment of High Blood Pressure: The JNC 7 Report. Aram V. Chobanian; George L. Bakris; Henry R. Black; William C. Cushman; Lee A. Green; Joseph L. Izzo Jr; Daniel W. Jones; Barry J. Materson; Suzanne Oparil; Jackson T. Wright Jr; Edward J. Roccella. *JAMA*. 2003;289:2560–2571.

Scientific Statements and Practice Guidelines

ACC/AHA Joint Guidelines	Acute myocardial infarction	AEDs
Aging	AHA Guidelines	Alcohol
Aneurysm	Angina	Angiography
Angioplasty	Anticoagulents	Antioxidants
Arrhythmias	Arteries	Arteriovenous malformation
Aspirin	Atherosclerosis	Athletes
Atrial fibrillation	Automated external defibrillators	Bacterial endocarditis
Behavior	Blood pressure	CPR
Carotid endarterectomy	Children	Cholesterol
Congenital Heart Defects	Coronary Artery Bypass Surgery	Coronary Artery Calcification
Critical Pathways	Defibrillation	Diabetes mellitus
Diet/Nutrition	Echocardiography	Electrocardiography
Electron Beam CT	Electrophysiology	Emergency Cardiovascular Care
Endocarditis	Exercise	Exercise testing
Fatty acids	Fibrillation	Functional capacity
Genetic testing	Heart attack	Heart failure
Heart transplant	Heparin	Homocysteine
Hypertension	Hypocholesterolemia	Imaging
Kawasaki disease	Lipids	Metabolic syndrome
Mitral valve	Myocardial infarction	Nutrition
Obesity	Oral anticoagulants	Pacemakers
Peripheral vascular disease	Physical activity	Phytochemicals
PPTA	Prevention	Protocols
PTCA/Angioplasty	Public access defibrillation	Psychotropic drugs
Regurgitation (valvular)	Resuscitation	Rehabilitation
Rheumatic fever	Risk factors	Secondary prevention
Sildenafil	Smoking	Sphygmomanometry
Stable angina	Stroke	Surgery
Thrombosis	Tomography, electron beam	Trans fatty acids
Transient ischemic attack (TIA)	'Ulstein style' reporting guidelines	Valvular heart disease
Vascular medicine	Weight management	Women

Adapted from the American Heart Association web site: www.americanheart.org

INDEX